Stress, the Aging Brain, and the Mechanisms of Neuron Death

Robert M. Sapolsky

A Bradford Book
The MIT Press
Cambridge, Massachusetts
London, England

This book was set in Palatino by Asco Trade Typesetting Ltd., Hong Kong, and was printed and bound in the United States of America.

Library of Congress Cataloging-in-Publication Data

Sapolsky, Robert M.
   Stress, the aging brain, and the mechanisms of neuron death / Robert M. Sapolsky.
      p.   cm.
   "A Bradford book."
   Includes bibliographical references and index.
   ISBN 0-262-19320-5
    1. Neuroendocrinology. 2. Brain—Aging.   3. Cell death. 4. Neurons.
   5. Glucocorticoids—Physiological effect. 6. Stress (Psychology) I. Title.
   [DNLM: 1. Aging—physiology. 2. Cell Survival. 3. Glucocorticoids. 4. Models,
   Biological. 5. Stress-physiopathology.   WK 755 S241s]
   QP356.4.S37   1992
   612.8'2—dc20
   DNLM/DLC
   for Library of Congress   91-46530
                                                                              CIP

For my father and the pain of his old age.
For the rats and the pain of these experiments.
May these pages justify the hopes of the former,
and the forced involvement of the latter.

Contents

Preface and Acknowledgments

The basic tenets of neuroendocrinology are now established beyond question. The brain can regulate the release of hormones throughout the body and hormones, in turn, can influence neural events. Naturally, the details regarding these two simple facts are turning out to be more complex and fascinating than anyone could ever have guessed—multiple hypothalamic releasing factors synergizing with each other, steroid receptor superfamilies, neural/endocrine/immune interactions, ultrashort feedback loops, and so on. This is both a pleasing and challenging time to be involved in this discipline.

This accumulation of knowledge has given us some degree of confidence as to the normal workings of neuroendocrine axes, which allows us to begin to understand neuroendocrine dysfunction. This book is about such dysfunction. It focuses on the regulation of glucocorticoids, the adrenal hormones secreted during stress. In many ways, glucocorticoids typify the contradictory lessons of stress physiology—while it is vital to mobilize glucocorticoid secretion during a physical stressor, an excess of these hormones can have profoundly damaging effects throughout the body. This book examines ways in which glucocorticoid secretion is disrupted during aging, sustained stress, and a number of neuropsychiatric disorders. Furthermore, it focuses on the emerging information regarding a new pathogenic consequence of glucocorticoid excess—damage to certain neurons in the brain.

Part I focuses on the ways in which the secretion of glucocorticoids are altered during aging in the rat, with the defect being in the direction of hypersecretion of these potent hormones. It also focuses on the causes and consequences of such secretion; the central hypothesis is that these are connected—that senescent glucocorticoid hypersecretion arises at least in part because of age-related damage to the hippocampus, and that a consequence of glucocorticoid excess includes further damage to the hippocampus. These two features—the effect of the hippocampus on glucocorticoid secretion and the effect of glucocorticoids on the hippocampus—are viewed as combining into a feedforward cascade of dysregulation that is of relevance to normal rodent aging.

Part II of the book focuses on what, to me, is the most interesting question to arise from this dysregulatory cascade, namely "How do glucocorticoids damage the hippocampus?" A considerable amount of evidence suggests that glucocorticoids need not be directly toxic to the hippocampus but may instead endanger the structure such that hippocampal neurons are less likely to survive coincident metabolic insults. Of perhaps greatest importance, these findings suggest that glucocorticoids can exacerbate the toxicity of rodent models of some of the most common neurological insults to the hippocampus. Part II finishes with the presentation of a model in which glucocorticoids compromise the ability of hippocampal neurons to survive the degenerative cascade involving excitatory amino acid neurotransmitters (such as glutamate and aspartate) and excessive mobilization of free cytosolic calcium.

Part III of the book examines the implication of these ideas. Chapter 12 reviews the sources of individual variation in patterns of glucocorticoid secretion in various organisms (as a function of genetics, diet, early experience, social rank, and so on), asking whether these sources of variability might be exploited as a means of reducing the pathologic impact of glucocorticoids during aging. Chapter 13 focuses on possible interventions to reduce the endangering impact of glucocorticoids in the aftermath of various neurological insults. Finally, chapter 14 examines the relevance of these findings to the human.

These ideas are at an intersection of a number of different disciplines, with part I being most relevant to endocrinologists and gerontologists, part II to neurologists and neurobiologists, and part III to anyone still awake at that point. Thus, I have tried to facilitate the reading of the entire book by individuals from each of these disciplines. I have done this by noting the onset of sections that will be stultifying to all but the most ardent specialist and by beginning each chapter with a summary of the book up to that point. While that device is meant to make it possible for a reader to begin the book at any chapter, such summaries omit many of the nuances, caveats, and uncertainties voiced within the main text. These are particularly important with respect to the caveats at the ends of chapter 6 (regarding the model of feedforward senescent degeneration involving the hippocampus and the adrenocortical axis) and chapter 11 (regarding the model of glucocorticoid-induced metabolic endangerment of hippocampal neurons).

I also emphasize that this is not a textbook reviewing the long-standing and well-established facts about a subject. Rather it is a monograph about a very recent body of scientific data that are still emerging, often in a rather contentious manner. I have tried to present the data as they are presently understood as accurately as possible, although in the face of any neurobiological errors, perhaps I should state "Don't be too hard on me, I'm only an endocrinologist" and, in the face of any endocrinological errors, "Come on, I'm only a neurobiologist." Moreover, parts I and II each finish with a highly speculative model synthesizing the facts presented, and while I am rather attached to these models, they may prove to be far from correct. Probably the safest thing to say regarding these speculative syntheses is that they will have served their purpose if they spur the research that will clarify how these things really work.

Many people are responsible for getting me to the point of writing this book, even if their help was, in some cases, many years removed from my being chained to this computer. First are Harry Stanton, my publisher, who approached me about this book an embarrassingly large number of years ago, and Fiona Stevens, my editor, whose peptalks and advice brought to fruition this foolish promise to Harry. It has been a pleasure working with both of you, and I am grateful for your sticking by me throughout the process. I would also like to thank the people who trained me to do science and inspired me to enjoy doing science: Howard Klar, Howard Eichenbaum, Mel Konner, Bruce McEwen, Lewis Krey, Paul Plotsky, and Wylie Vale. Thank you also to Dennis Choi, Mary Dallman, Ron de Kloet, Tuck Finch, and Peter Lipton, good friends and colleagues whose thoughtful and exhaustive critiquing of the manuscript did much to hammer it into its current shape—in some cases, the very literate wordings of ideas are their own. I also thank the anonymous reviewers of this manuscript for their assistance. I would like to emphatically thank the wonderful members of my lab, who read the manuscript, directed me to papers I had missed, put up with my negligant distractedness during its writing and, most importantly, did so much of the excellent research for which I will try to take credit in these pages: Kristin Adams, Mark Armanini, Sheila Brooke, Ingrid Chang, Elicia Elliott, Taryn Ha, Kelly Harrity, Dora Ho, Heidi Horner, Chris Hutchins, Lauren Jacobson, Ted Liu, Desta Packan, Raymond Pan, Kate Raley-Susman, Justina Ray, Debby Redish, Michael Romero, Becky Stein-Behrens, Geoff Tombaugh, Larry Tsai, CJ Virgin, Susan Yang, and Michael Yeh. Finally, and above all else, I would like to thank my wife—Lisa, you have taught me something I never could have conceived of: Life consists of more than just glucocorticoids and the hippocampus.

The work described was supported by the National Institute on Aging, the National Science Foundation, the National Institute of Mental Health, the Harry Frank Guggenheim Foundation, the Klingenstein Fund, the Alzheimer's Disease and Related Disorders Association, the Sloan Foundation, the Explorers Club, the Mathers Foundation, the Adler Foundation, and by a MacArthur Prize fellowship from the John D. and Catherine T. MacArthur Foundation. I thank them all for their generosity and faith.

Four years into writing this book and nearly four years into wishing it were done and out of my hair, I find myself in the neurotic state apparently common to many authors—I am having trouble finishing this and letting go, for fear that next week's *Current Contents* will trumpet some paper that confirms every crackpot idea in here or, worse, negate the whole thing. Nevertheless, it is time to finish this. I wish the reader fortitude; this book now contains everything I know as of January 10, 1992.

I The Glucocorticoid Cascade Hypothesis

1   The Stress-Response and the Emergence of Stress-Related Disease

Ours is not a perfect world. If it were, nations would beat their swords into plowshares, we would always find a parking spot, and the supermarket line we picked would always move the fastest. And our kidneys would filter our blood at just the right speed. But it is not a perfect world, and our bodies are forever buffeted by this imperfection. We can be seriously injured or become ill. The rains may fail, locust may swarm, and we must spend a season hungry and walking miles daily to forage. We may be menaced by predators or by the aggressiveness of our own kind. Our hearts may be broken by loss. And we are smart enough to often anticipate these perturbations, or neurotic enough to decide irrationally that they are impending.

Stress physiology is the study of the imperfections in our world and the attempts of our bodies to muddle through them. A *stressor* can be defined in a narrow, physiological sense as any perturbation in the outside world that disrupts homeostasis, and the *stress-response* is the set of neural and endocrine adaptations that help reestablish homeostasis. The original definition of a stressor must be expanded to include the psychological realm of the *anticipation* (rational or otherwise) of physical and emotional stressors. In our lives, where we spend far more time worrying about being mugged than actually experiencing such an unpleasantry, the potency and pathogenicity of psychological stress is of great importance. This will be discussed in chapter 12.

The physiology of the stress-response has, in many ways, often frustrated systems physiologists. Mainstream physiology, as usually taught and far too often conceptualized, focuses on specific organs or narrowly related systems and specific physiological problems—filtering of blood, exchanging of oxygen, forming a clot, and so on. The stress-response, in contrast, is a disparate, bodywide set of adaptations. It does not so much respond to a specific problem as to the magnitude of a problem (i.e., a system that can be equally activated by being very cold or very hot), and does not so much regulate a single organ system as set and reset priorities for organs throughout the body during an emergency.

This disparateness might suggest that this is not a physiological system of great importance, but that would be incorrect. Its importance is encompassed in its two-edged quality: If an organism is faced with an acute physical stressor and cannot appropriately turn on the stress-response, the consequences are typically fatal. In contrast, if the stress-response is activated chronically, it can be the cause of a variety of diseases.

It was Claude Bernard (1813–1878) who oriented physiologists toward these issues. Bernard, in coining the term *internal milieu*, emphasized that organisms have evolved to become more independent of the outside environment, and that a goal of physiological systems is to buffer the internal environment or milieu from environmental perturbations. Walter Cannon (1871–1945) extended these ideas and focused attention on the adaptive nature of the stress-response in coping with such challenges to the internal milieu, or *homeostasis*, as he called it. The "flight or fight" response, as he termed the stress-response, was logical and effective, and Cannon's writing was suffused with a physiological optimism that was reflected in the titles of his popular works, such as *The Wisdom of the Body*. The adaptiveness could be appreciated in considering the physiological responses of mammals undergoing acute physical stressors. Consider a scenario: A zebra is mauled by a lion, badly injured, yet manages to escape. For the next hour it must evade the still-stalking lion. The lion, half-starved, must find the strength to chase down a meal or not survive the night. In both cases, there is likely to be a fairly convergent set of physiological responses occurring, and they are relatively logical. There is secretion of sympathetic catecholamines such as epinephrine and norepinephrine at such times (a subject pioneered by Cannon). In addition, glucocorticoids are secreted by the adrenal cortex. Typically, there will also be secretion of β-endorphin, prolactin, and vasopressin by the pituitary, and glucagon by the pancreas (to list only the most prominent of the stress-responsive hormones). Conversely, activity of the parasympathetic nervous system will be suppressed, as will be sex hormone secretion and (with prolonged stress and in most species) growth hormone. (For a review of the endocrine responses to stress, as well as to the emerging view that all stressors are not equivalent in activating the identical profile of hormonal changes, see Frankenhaeuser 1980; Rose 1985; Sapolsky 1992a.)

Collectively, these endocrine changes aid adaptation to this acute physical stressor. *Energy is mobilized* from storage tissues and further energy storage is halted. This is part of the obvious strategy to divert nutrients from storage sites and to shunt them, instead, to exercising muscle. Thus, uptake of glucose, amino acids, free fatty acids, and glycerol is inhibited in fat and liver; triglyceride, glycogen, and protein synthesis is suppressed; preexisting stores of those compounds are lysed and their constituents released into the circulation, and gluconeogenesis is stimulated in the liver (Goodman 1980). *Cardiovascular and pulmonary tone are increased*, to facilitate the delivery of oxygen and glucose to whichever muscles are exercising. *Anabolism is suppressed* until the acute emergency is survived—in effect, during a crisis like this, the body has better things to do with its energy than to extend long bones or reach puberty. Thus, digestion, growth, reproduction, and immunity are suppressed (as will be discussed in later chapters, this conceptualization of the logic of stress-induced immunosuppression is too simplistic) (Munck et al. 1984; Sapolsky 1987; Reid 1989). *Inflammatory responses* are suppressed as well. As a further feature of the stress-response, pain perception can be blunted, and the neuro-chemistry of *stress-induced analgesia* is well understood (Brush and Nagase Shain 1989). Finally, there is *altered cognition*, with a tendency toward sharp-ened sensory thresholds—again, a logical adaptation for coping with an emergency.

These responses are logical for responding to an acute physical stressor: Energy is mobilized and delivered to where it is needed, unessential anabolism is curtailed, pain is blunted, and cognition is sharpened. These same responses, however, are highly deleterious when activated chronically, especially in the face of psychological rather than physical stressors.

Attention was focused on these pathogenic features of the stress-response by Hans Selye (1907–1982). Selye, whose work concentrated more on the adrenocortical component of the stress-response (i.e., the secretion of gluco-corticoids) than on the sympathetic catecholaminergic response, was among the first to note that chronic stress caused disease. In his classic initial studies (Selye 1936), he observed that a variety of chronic stressors would cause peptic ulcers, adrenal hypertrophy, and immune collapse. Selye's discovery of stress-related disease was of extraordinary importance, and a half-century later, we now recognize the tremendous number of diseases that can be exacerbated by chronic stress. A notable failure of Selye's, however, was his concept of *why* stress-related disease occurred.

Selye conceptualized the stress-response as potentially having three compo-nents (cf. Selye 1976). In the initial *alarm* stage, the stressor is noted. The second stage, *resistance*, consisted of successfuly dealing with the short-term physical insult. The third stage was where disease started, when the stressor became chronic. Selye termed this stage *exhaustion*. In his speculative view, disease emerges because the capacity to mount a stress-response had been depleted. In specific endocrinological terms, there are no longer sufficient catecholamines, glucocorticoids, and the like, to combat the stressor, which can now damage the body unhindered. In his view, then, stress-related disease was due to the stressor itself attacking the undefended body.

In actuality, there is little evidence of such a global Selyian exhaustion of the hormones of the stress-response. Chronic stress is not pathogenic because the body's defenses fail but because, with chronic enough stress, those de-fenses themselves become damaging. Basically, most of the features of the stress-response are catabolic and inefficient. During a short-term stressor, their costs can be contained, but with chronic activation, they eventually exact a toll.

This can be seen if the logical, hour-long responses of the zebra or lion, discussed above, are instead activated for months during a chronic psychologi-cal stressor. The short-term adaptation of mobilizing energy will, when carried out over time, impair energy storage; an economy built on extreme catabolism cannot be afforded for long. Thus, myopathy, fatigue, and increased risk of adult-onset diabetes ensue (Goodman 1980; Krieger 1982; Munck et al. 1984). Shifting to the cardiovascular component of the stress-response, the short-term logic of being hypertensive when sprinting across the savannah will obviously become deleterious when activated chronically. Continuing in this vein, if anabolism is constantly curtailed for more auspicious times, nothing is built or repaired. Peptic ulceration and colitis become more common; growth can be disrupted in children to the point of psychogenic dwarfism, while in adults, the equivalent is suppression of recalcification of bones, eventually producing osteoporosis (Rose 1985; Reid 1989). With sufficiently chronic stress, reproductive behavior and physiology will be curtailed, producing irregular or absent cycles in females and impotency, premature ejaculation, and suppressed sperm count in males (Warren 1983; Sapolsky 1987). Finally, profound and chronic immunosuppression carries with it impaired resistance to disease (for example, as seen in AIDS), and the current fevered interest in psychoimmunology arises, in part, from the possibility that psychologic modulation of the stress-response, and thus the immune system, can have a significant impact on disease processes (Dunn 1989).

To reiterate what strike me as the two most important facts about stress physiology, (1) if an organism cannot appropriately initiate a stress-response during an acute physical stressor, the consequences can be extremely deleterious; (2) if an organism cannot appropriately terminate a stress-response at the end of stress, or if it activates the system too much because of repeated or chronic stressors, numerous stress-related diseases can emerge. The stress-response is a vital set of responses on the part of the body, but a dangerous one (table 1.1).

It is this two-edged quality of the stress-response that has attracted the attention of gerontologists for decades, and gerontological theorizing about stress has generally taken two forms.

1. Aging can be thought of as a time of decreased capacity to respond appropriately to stressors. This can take various forms. First, the aged organism might require less of an exogenous insult for homeostasis to be disrupted. Such a case occurs with performance on mental tests at different ages. In all age groups, performance quality declines as tasks are done under increasing time pressure. Although initial quality may not differ by age, as the speed of required performance increases, the decline is typically more dramatic in aged populations (Birren and Schaie 1985). As a more physiological example, while concentrations of lactate, phosphocreatine, ATP, and total energy charge do not differ by age in the rat brain or synaptosomal preparation, these measures

Table 1.1. The stress-response and its consequences

Stress-response	Stress-related disorder
Mobilization of energy	Myopathy, fatigue, steroid diabetes
Increased cardiovascular tone	Stress-induced hypertension
Suppression of digestion	Ulceration
Suppression of growth	Psychogenic dwarfism
Suppression of reproduction	Amenorrhea, impotency, loss of libido
Suppression of immune system	Increased disease risk
Sharpening of cognition	Neuron death

are far more disrupted by hypoxia in tissue from aged rats than from young ones (Hoffman et al. 1985; Benzi et al. 1987). Thus, basal function may not differ by age, but the vulnerability to disruption of homeostasis may increase in senescent organisms. As a second way in which there can be an inappropriate stress-response in aged organisms, it may take them longer to reestablish homeostasis, once the stressor has occurred. As an example of this, while young and aged humans have similar basal body temperatures, the time needed to reattain that temperature after a cold or heat challenge increases with age (Shock 1977). Finally, once homeostatic balance is reattained, it may take aged organisms longer to terminate the endocrine stress-response. An example of this is seen with the sympathetic nervous system and catecholamine secretion after the end of a stressor (McCarty 1986). Thus, there is evidence that aged organisms respond to stress less adaptively than do young organisms.

2. Chronic stress may accelerate some of the degenerative aspects of aging. "Rate of living" hypotheses of aging—in effect, if you live fast, you die young—arose around the time of Weismann (1889) and was later given experimental support by the classic studies of Rubner (1908); he showed an inverse correlation between the life span of various species and their metabolic rate (when expressed per unit body weight). This interspecies correlation (which, it should be noted, is at best a rough one) was soon posited as applying within species. Rate of living hypotheses were quickly intertwined with various "wear and tear" hypotheses of aging (Pearl 1929), and the later theories of Selye and colleagues (cf. Selye and Tuchweber 1976). Collectively, these investigators posited that the rate of senescent degeneration could be paced by one's rate of living (a term that was defined more precisely in far too few cases) or by the rate of exogenous insults encountered during the lifetime.

This book reposes these two questions—Do aged organisms respond to stress adaptively? Can stress accelerate aging?—in light of some very recent and exciting data. These findings focus on glucocorticoids, the steroid hormones which, along with the sympathetic catecholamines, dominate both the adaptive and pathogenic nature of the stress-response. Glucocorticoids (in the human, the principal one being cortisol [also known as hydrocortisone], in the rat, corticosterone) are secreted by the adrenal gland in response to a wide variety of stressors. Such secretion is the final step in a classic neuroendocrine cascade beginning in the brain, proceeding to the pituitary and then to the adrenal (see chapter 2). These steroids are absolutely central to the metabolic stress-response (with their name reflecting the capacity of *gluco*corticoids to mobilize glucose during stressors). They accomplish this by inhibiting transport of nutrients into target tissues, by promoting catabolism of proteins, glycogen, and triglycerides, and mostly by stimulating gluconeogenesis (Goodman 1980; Krieger 1982). They augment the cardiovascular effects of catecholamines, both at target tissues and by enhancing epinephrine synthesis (Wurtman and Axelrod 1966). Finally, they suppress growth, digestion, inflammation, and immunity through an astonishing array of mechanisms (Krieger 1982; Warren 1983; Munck et al. 1984; Rose 1985; Sapolsky 1987;

Dunn 1989). In summary, while a variety of physical stressors are typically fatal to organisms lacking glucocorticoids and low basal concentrations of the hormones exert many anabolic effects (Devenport et al. 1989), excessive exposure to glucocorticoids is extremely damaging.

This book is about how regulation of glucocorticoid secretion fails during aging, producing excessive secretion of these hormones, and how an only recently recognized consequence of that glucocorticoid excess is damage to the brain. These two features combine to form a complex cascade of degeneration during aging, the focus of part I of the book. Moreover, the potential for glucocorticoid neurotoxicity appears to have considerable implications for neurology, the focus of part II.

In order to begin to appreciate this literature, it is necessary to review the basic features of the adrenocortical axis and the regulation of glucocorticoid secretion. This is the subject of the next chapter.

CHAPTER SUMMARY

Stressors are physiological or psychological perturbations that throw us out of homeostatic balance, and the stress-response is the set of neural and endocrine adaptations that help us reestablish homeostasis. This stress-response is surprisingly convergent, in that stressors as varied as being injured, starving, too hot, too cold, or anxious will provoke a somewhat similar stress-response. This convergence is logical; in the face of most stressors, energy must be mobilized from storage sites, such energy substrates need to be delivered to the appropriate target tissues more rapidly, and long-term anabolic processes should be deferred until after the costly immediate crisis is finished. By mediating these adaptations, the stress-response is ideal for responding to acute physical stressors.

With prolonged stress, however, the stress-response can become as damaging as the stressor itself. This reflects the essentially catabolic nature of these responses. Thus, with chronic overactivation of the stress-response, there is emergence of stress-related diseases such as myopathy, steroid diabetes, hypertension, peptic ulcers, reproductive impairment, psychogenic dwarfism, or immunosuppression.

These findings generate two important conclusions. First, it can be disastrous to be faced with an acute physical stressor and to be unable to appropriately initiate a stress-response. Second, overactivation of the stress-response, whether due to exposure to too much stress or due to an inability to appropriately terminate secretion at the end of stress, can ultimately be quite disastrous as well.

This two-edged quality to stress physiology has provoked speculation about its interaction with aging. Principally, such speculation has taken two forms. (1) Aging can be defined as a time of impaired capacity to respond to stress. (2) Stress, especially prolonged stress, can accelerate some of the degenerative aspects of aging. This book will examine the validity and interactions of these two ideas, especially with regard to senescent degeneration of the brain, as well as the general mechanisms of neuronal death during neurological insults. This recent synthesis has centered on glucocorticoids, the adrenal steroids that, along with sympathetic catecholamines, dominate the stress-response. The next chapter reviews the general features of glucocorticoid regulation and actions as a prelude to examining glucocorticoids and aging.

2 An Introduction to the Adrenocortical Axis

A BRIEF OVERVIEW

As is the case with many peripheral glands that secrete hormones, adrenal secretion of glucocorticoids is not autonomous. Instead, the adrenal is ultimately under the control of the brain.

With the onset of stress, corticotropin releasing factor (CRF) is secreted from the hypothalamus into the hypophysial-pituitary portal circulation. For most stressors, an afferent pathway must be stimulated. That is to say that, for example, the stressful news about a painful injury to the foot must be carried to the hypothalamus via relevant neural circuits. Some stressors, however, can be detected directly in the hypothalamus; hypoglycemia is an example of this (Widmaier et al. 1988). CRF secretion occurs within seconds and triggers pituitary release of adrenocorticotropic hormone (ACTH) within about 15 seconds. CRF was the first of the hypothalamic releasing hormones whose existence was inferred physiologically (in 1955). Its isolation and characterization, however, took until 1981, in part because of its large size (41 amino acids) (Vale et al. 1981). Its isolation triggered a vast number of studies of its mechanism of action, and they confirmed a sense that had been emerging in the field for years—CRF is but one of a number of hormones that cause ACTH release. It is now known that a variety of such "secretagogs" (releasers of ACTH) exist, with CRF merely being the most important one (in most, but not all species). In descending order of importance, the other main secretagogs include vasopressin, oxytocin, and catecholamines (epinephrine and norepinephrine).

Once ACTH is released, it rapidly triggers adrenocortical synthesis and release of glucocorticoids. With the onset of stress, circulating glucocorticoid concentrations rise within a few minutes. Glucocorticoids then exert their effects on target tissues throughout the body. Principally, this is accomplished by interacting with cytosolic receptors which, upon binding the hormone, translocate to the nucleus and regulate genomic events. Therefore, glucocorticoids can increase or decrease transcription of particular genes. As discussed, glucocorticoid actions are central to the stress-response. They block energy storage and help mobilize energy from storage sites, increase cardiovascular tone, and inhibit anabolic processes such as growth, reproduction, inflammation, and immunity.

The adrenocortical axis is under end-product control, in that glucocorticoid concentrations in the bloodstream influence subsequent adrenocortical activity. This makes sense: The brain, in initiating an adrenocortical stress-response, is many steps removed from the bottom line—how much glucocorticoid winds up in the circulation. Therefore, the brain (and, to a lesser extent, the pituitary) must be able to measure the concentrations of circulating glucocorticoids to insure that the desired levels are reached. If circulating concentrations are not yet at a level appropriate to the circumstance, secretagogs and ACTH are still released. In contrast, once that "feedback threshold" is reached, subsequent secretion is inhibited. In this general way, such feedback regulation is identical to that seen in most endocrine systems and in the end-product inhibition of most biochemical pathways (and, in fact, in the way that thermostats regulate temperature and even how toilet bowls fill up but do not overflow). Intrinsic to different concentrations of glucocorticoids being achieved at different times (circadian trough, circadian peak, at the height of a stressor, in the recovery period after a stressor) is that the threshold for feedback can shift.

SOME MINOR COMPLICATIONS

This review is about as simplistic as one can be about the adrenocortical axis, and the individual steps in the axis are far more complex than described above. Rather than try to explore all of these complexities in exhaustive detail, I will touch on those that are most relevant to this book and direct the reader to more detailed reviews.

Linearity Versus All-or-None Effects in the Adrenocortical Axis

Various stressors cause secretion of the secretagogs, ACTH, and glucocorticoids. Is this a linear or a threshold phenomenon? For example, do roughly equal (and large) amounts of secretion occur once the degree of hypotension passes a certain threshold, or does an incremental increase in the severity of the hypotension increase the magnitude of the adrenocortical response? The latter appears to be the case, with ACTH or glucocorticoid secretion being impressively linear in response to the severity of hypoglycemia, hypoxia, hypotension, or environmental novelty (figure 2.1; Dallman et al. 1987; also see Levine et al. 1989, for a discussion of responses to psychologic stressors). (*Linearity* here is used rather loosely, in that the data might actually be sigmoidal, curvilinear, and so on, and require transformation to be linearized. More correct is to say that there is a *dose-response* relationship between the severity of the stressor and the magnitude of the adrenocortical response.)

The dose-responsiveness suggests that the adrenocortical axis can differentiate between stressors of different sizes. Logically, this sensitivity should be translated into target tissue effects—it would be illogical if subtle differences

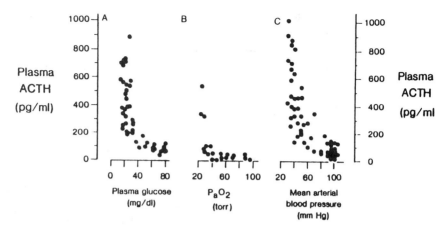

Figure 2.1. ACTH responses are proportional to stimulus intensity. (*A*) ACTH response to insulin-induced hypoglycemia in conscious dogs. (*B*) ACTH responses to hypoxemia in pentobarbital-anesthetized, paralyzed, and ventilated dogs. (*C*) ACTH responses to hemorrhage-induced hypovolemia and hypotension in conscious rats. (From Dallman et al., 1987, Recent Prog Horm Res 43, 113. Reprinted courtesy of Academic Press.)

in the severity of, for example, hypoglycemia produced subtle differences in the amount of circulating glucocorticoids, yet all sorts of different high circulating levels caused the same degree of glucose mobilization. Despite this, glucocorticoids were long thought to be rather "permissive" and all-or-none in their effects, rather than having linear, dose-response effects on target tissues. Recently, more sensitive assay techniques have shown glucocorticoids to exert numerous dose-response effects on the body, as measured by such disparate endpoints as body weight, circulating glucose concentrations, pancreatic amylase concentrations, vertebral bone calcium content, plasma angiotensinogen, renin, angiotensin II concentrations, thymus weight, extent of skeletal muscle myopathy, glucose transport, glycogen content, and liver enzyme activity (Munck 1971; Munck et al. 1984; Dallman et al. 1987).

In summary, the adrenocortical axis can differentiate between stressors of different sizes, and can communicate those differences throughout the body. Another way of stating this is that moderate differences in circulating glucocorticoid concentrations have consequences for target tissues, and regulation of such circulating concentrations must be extremely precise. This will be shown to be the case with a vengeance.

The Multiplicity of ACTH Secretagogs

The recognition that CRF, vasopressin, oxytocin, and catecholamines can all release ACTH spurred an enormous amount of research. An immediate question was whether there are other secretagogs. Three types of evidence would make a particular factor a likely candidate. First, it must release ACTH from the pituitary. Second, its concentrations in the hypothalamic portal circulation must rise following some type of stressor. Finally, the elimination of that factor during a stressor (by lesioning, blocking its receptor in the pituitary, or immunoneutralization) must attenuate the normal secretion of ACTH to that stressor. This final requirement of attentuation is the most stringent, in that it focuses not only on whether a factor *could* release ACTH, but whether it does so under physiologic circumstances. While a number of factors meet at least one of these criteria (e.g., angiotensin II, cholecystokinin, vasoactive intestinal polypeptide), CRF, vasopressin, oxytocin, and the catecholamines are the most convincing physiologic secretagogs (Antoni 1986; Plotsky et al. 1989).

The localization of the various secretagogs within the brain casts light on their regulation. While CRF is secreted from axon terminals in the median eminence, the cell bodies of these neurons are located in the paraventricular nucleus (PVN) of the hypothalamus (figure 2.2; Sawchenko 1991). Vaso-pressin-secreting neurons occur in both the PVN and the supraoptic nucleus. The latter is mostly the source of vasopressin destined for the posterior pituitary (i.e., the classic endocrine role for this hormone). Vasopressin des-tined for an ACTH-secretagog role in the portal circulation has been thought to be almost exclusively derived from the PVN, although some recent work implicates peptide from the supraoptic nucleus as well (Antoni et al. 1990). Oxytocin appears to have a similar distribution as vasopressin. Within the PVN, about half the CRF neurons also synthesize vasopressin, and the two hormones are often colocalized in secretory granules in the median eminence (Whitnall et al. 1987, Whitnall 1988, 1990). This partial coexpression sug-

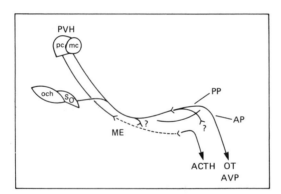

Figure 2.2. Schematic sagittal view of the basal diencephalon and pituitary shows the organiza-tion of magnocellular (mc) and parvocellular (pc) neurosecretory components of the paraventri-cular nucleus of the hypothalamus (PVH), and potential sites at which secretions of magno-cellular neurons may interact with the parvocellular system. CRF contained in axonal projections from the parvocellular division of the PVH to the external zone of the median eminence (ME) is transported to the anterior pituitary (AP) via the portal vasculature (dashed line). Projections of magnocellular neurosecretory neurons from the PVH and the supraoptic nucleus (SO) pass through the internal lamina of the median eminence en route to the posterior lobe (PP), where oxytocin (OT) and vasopressin (AVP) are released into the systemic circulation. Magnocellular secretions may gain access to the portal vasculature via exocytotic release at the level of the median eminence or via vacular links between the posterior and anterior lobes (question marks). (From Sawchenko, 1991, in M Brown, et al. (eds), Stress: Neurobiology and Neuroendocrinology. Marcel Dekker, New York.)

gests that the brain can regulate whether CRF is secreted with or without vasopressin. The expression of vasopressin in CRF cells becomes more pronounced after adrenalectomy (Tramu et al. 1983; Kiss et al. 1984; Sawchencko et al. 1984), with neurons previously expressing only CRF now expressing both hormones. (This shows that glucocorticoid feedback regulation inhibits vasopressin expression more vigorously than it does CRF expression; the implications of this are explored in subsequent chapters, as it generates some predictions as to which secretagogs might be hypersecreted when feedback fails.) In contrast to the hypothalamic origin of the other secretagogs, the epinephrine and norepinephrine that serve as secretagogs arise from the brain stem and sympathetic ganglia (reviewed in Plotsky et al. 1989; Pesce et al. 1990).

All of this complexity raises the most obvious question—Why have multiple secretagogs? Why isn't CRF sufficient? An important answer to this came with the recognition that different stressors trigger different *combinations* of secretagog release. For example, hemorrhage stimulates the secretion of CRF, vasopressin, oxytocin, and catecholamines (Plotsky et al. 1985a). In contrast, hypotension stimulates only CRF (Plotsky et al. 1986), while insulin-induced hypoglycemia only stimulates the secretion of vasopressin (Plotsky et al. 1985b).

Stressor-specific patterns of secretion have been examined with hypophysial-pituitary portal cannulation, a surgical technique in which the small private vascular system connecting the hypothalamus with the pituitary is exposed and vessels are cannulated. This is a highly invasive procedure and precludes ever measuring portal concentrations of secretagogs secreted in response to anything other than the major physical stressors just discussed. Therefore, it is not known how the brain "orchestrates" secretagog release in response to psychologic stressors such as novelty, social subordinance, or anxiety (nor, for that matter, whether the patterns of secretion for the somatic stressors discussed in the previous paragraph were altered by the trauma of the surgical procedure).

There are some possible reasons to have the orchestration of multiple secretagogs, rather than just CRF alone. The multiplicity provides a safety net for maintaining adrenocortical function in case of damage to secretagog-synthesizing neurons; for example, following lesion of the paraventricular nucleus, there appears to be a transient increase in the secretion of other secretagogs (most probably catecholamines), maintaining ACTH concentrations (Makara et al. 1986). However, it is not clear how often this situation arises. In some ways, the multiplicity of secretagogs is an arbitrary solution to a problem that could have been solved in other ways. Two different stressors (for example, hypoglycemia and hemorrhage) stimulate afferent pathways that reach and travel through the brain through separate routes. Both stimulate the same endpoint of ACTH secretion by the pituitary. Therefore, it could have evolved that the two separate pathways converge at the level of the hypothalamus, both triggering the release of a single CRF-like hormone. Alternatively, the two separate pathways could still be differentiated at the hypothalamic level, and release different secretagogs or different combinations of secretagogs; in the latter case, the convergence occurs at the pituitary level, with the various secretagogs collectively releasing ACTH. Evolution seems to have favored the latter pattern.

In addition, the multiplicity of secretagogs may not just be an arbitrary solution to a problem. While it may be logical for hypoglycemia and hypotension (for example) to both provoke ACTH secretion, in some ways, the physiologic responses to these two very different stressors must differ. Conceivably, the various secretagogs may all release ACTH, but may do additional and differing things at the anterior pituitary, designed to meet the specific as well as the general demands of different stressors. I do not know of any data supporting this idea, however.

Thus, the synthesis, storage, and patterns of release of the various secretagogs remains an ongoing topic of intensive research (for example, there is emerging evidence for the existence of *CIF*, a hypothalamic corticotropin *inhibiting* factor [Grossman and Tsagarakis, 1989], which would add a further complexity to this story [see Graf et al. 1985; Okajima and Hertting, 1986 for the CIF-like role for delta-sleep—inducing peptide; Grossman et al. 1986 for a CIF-like role for metenkephalin; Kovacs and Antoni 1990 for evidence concerning atriopeptin]). These various relations are summarized in figure 2.3 (Plotsky 1988), including information regarding the likely neurotransmitters mediating the release of these secretagogs. All of this is relevant, as this book will focus on a number of disorders of glucocorticoid hypersecretion that are driven at the level of the brain. To understand better what neural defects lead to these cases of hypersecretion, one must know which secretagogs mediate the hypersecretion.

Interactions Among Secretagogs in the Release of ACTH

The recent research regarding the multifactorial control of ACTH secretion has confirmed a fascinating observation that predates the characterization of CRF: While vasopressin, oxytocin, and catecholamines individually have some intrinsic capacity to release ACTH, what they are best at is potentiating the effect of CRF. The ability of these secretagogs to increase the potency of CRF manyfold has been demonstrated in vivo and in vitro, in both rats and humans (Yates et al. 1971; Gillies et al. 1982; Rivier and Vale 1983a; Mezey et al. 1983; Antoni et al. 1983a; Giguere and Labrie 1983; Vale et al. 1983; Gibbs et al. 1984; Abou-Samra et al. 1986a; Gibbs, 1986; Bilezikjian and Vale, 1987; Labrie et al. 1987; Watabe et al. 1988). It is certainly a major challenge to understand the physiological implications of these synergies. Of at least equal interest is how these synergies work within the corticotrope (the pituitary cell type that secretes ACTH). While some corticotropes have receptors for only a single secretagog (Schwartz et al. 1989) and secrete ACTH in response to single secretagogs (Jia et al. 1991), most corticotropes contain receptors for more than one secretagog (Childs et al. 1987) and respond synergistically to combinations of secretagogs (Jia et al. 1991).

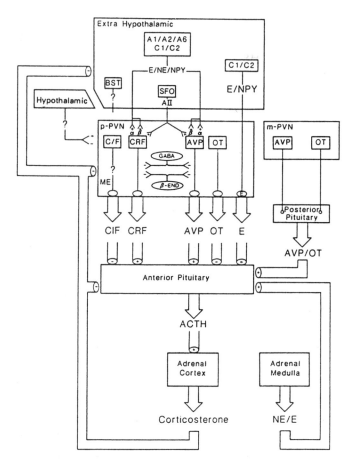

Figure 2.3. Schematic diagram of the hypothalamic-pituitary-adrenal axis based on currently available literature (as reviewed in the text). A1, ventrolateral medullary noradrenergic cell group; A2, noradrenergic cell group of the nucleus tractus solitarious; A6, noradrenergic group of the locus coeruleus; BST, bed nucleus of the striae terminalis; C1, ventrolateral medullary adrenergic cell group; C2, adrenergic cell group of the nucleus tractus solitarius; E, epinephrine; NE, norepinephrine; NPY, neuropeptide Y; CIF, proposed corticotropin inhibiting factor; ME, median eminence; m-PVN, magnocellular region of the paraventricular nucleus; p-PVN, parvocellular division of the paraventricular nucleus. (From Plotsky, 1988, in G Chrousos, et al. (eds), Mechanisms of Physical and Emotional Stress, Plenum Press, New York. Reprinted with permission of Plenum Publishing Corp.)

How these synergies work remains an open question, but some of the critical second messengers in the synergies have been identified. CRF, for example, exerts its actions through the cAMP/protein kinase-A pathway. The peptide causes cAMP accumulation in corticotropes (Labrie et al. 1982; Giguere et al. 1982; Bilezikjian and Vale, 1983; Aguilera et al. 1983), and exogenous cAMP stimulates ACTH synthesis and release (Vale et al. 1983; Aguilera et al. 1983; Loeffler et al. 1986; Dave et al. 1987; Wand and Eipper 1987; Gagner and Drouin 1987; Eberwine et al. 1987; Wand et al. 1988; Suda et al. 1980). In contrast, vasopressin releases ACTH through the phosphotidylinositol/protein kinase-C pathway (Raymond et al. 1985; Bilezikjian et al. 1987). Therefore, at least two independent intracellular second messenger cascades can trigger ACTH release. As an intracellular version of these synergies, neither vasopressin nor the catecholamines cause cAMP accumulation, but both augment CRF-induced cAMP accumulation (Giguere and Labrie 1982; Aguilera et al. 1983; Abou-Samra et al. 1987; Bilezikjian et al. 1987), and this synergistic effect on CRF's actions can be mimicked with protein kinase-C (Raymond et al. 1985; Abou-Samra et al. 1986a; Bilezikjian et al. 1987b; Labrie et al. 1987).

To complicate the picture further, there also appear to be autocrine factors released by the pituitary itself that will modulate corticotrope responsiveness to secretagogs. For example, chromogranin A, a pituitary glycoprotein, appears to inhibit responsiveness to CRF (Wand et al. 1991). The cellular basis of this effect is not known, nor is its physiological relevance, although of interest for the latter, chromogranin A secretion is stimulated by glucocorticoids (Wand et al. 1991), suggesting that it might mediate glucocorticoid feedback inhibition at the pituitary (see chapter 3). As a final complication, there appears to be paracrine communication among corticotropes, in that one cell appears capable of regulating the sensitivity of another to secretagogs (Jia et al. 1992).

ACTH Release of Glucocorticoids: The Adrenal as an Integrator of the ACTH Signal

A puzzling feature of ACTH action is that relatively low concentrations of ACTH stimulate maximal glucocorticoid secretion. Therefore, while raising ACTH concentrations from 10^{-12} to 10^{-8} M causes a linear increase in cAMP accumulation in the adrenal. the glucocorticoid secretory response is already saturated by 10^{-11} M ACTH (Buckley and Ramachandran 1981). This seems rather illogical. This mystery was solved recently. Once saturation occurs, a further increase in ACTH concentrations does not lead to a *larger* glucocorticoid secretory response, but rather to a *longer* one (Keller-Wood et al. 1983a; Keith et al. 1986). Thus, the adrenal gland can integrate the ACTH signal. This becomes relevant in the next chapter with the demonstration that the aged rat hypersecretes ACTH. In agreement with the data just discussed, this produces a prolonged, rather than a larger glucocorticoid stress-response, larger rise during the circadian trough (Yasuda et al. 1976; Engeland et al. 1977; Kant et al. 1986; Bradbury et al. 1991).

This also raises the issue of whether sensitivity to negative feedback inhibition shifts over the circadian cycle. This is the case, and will be reviewed in chapter 3.

Negative Feedback Regulation of the Adrenocortical Axis

As described earlier, the adrenocortical axis is a closed-loop endocrine system, in that elevated circulating concentrations of glucocorticoids will decrease the likelihood of subsequent secretion within the axis. This turns out to be such an appallingly complex subject that it will be considered separately in chapter 3; this subject has great relevance to what goes wrong in the aged adrenocortical axis.

Repeated Stressors: Interactions Between Feedback and Feedforward Elements of the Axis

Amid the intricacies of negative feedback regulation that will be covered in the next chapter, a basic feature holds—if you infuse a rat with glucocorticoids, you will generally inhibit the responsiveness of the axis to a subsequent stressor. This, then, predicts that if circulating glucocorticoid concentrations are raised through more physiologic means (i.e., during stress), the same should hold—one stressor should inhibit the magnitude of the response to a subsequent stressor. However, this is usually not the case. Instead, a stressor often provokes the same magnitude of response, regardless of whether it is the first or the umpteenth stressor in a series (Knigge et al. 1959; Jones and Stockham 1966; Zimmermann and Critchlow 1969; Fortier et al. 1970; Dallman and Jones 1973a,b; Raff et al. 1982). Dallman and Jones (1973a), in viewing these data, proposed that *facilitation* occurs. In this scenario, the tendency for the elevated glucocorticoid concentrations provoked by previous stressors to inhibit the axis is offset by an approximately counterbalancing facilitation. If facilitation occurs, then an adrenalectomized rat exposed to repeated stressors (i.e., one in which this is occurring in the absence of glucocorticoid feedback inhibition) should show larger ACTH responses with repetition of a stressor. This has been observed (Dallman and Jones 1973a; de Souza and van Loon, 1989).

The mechanisms for the facilitation are probably numerous. Some occur at the hypothalamus. While it has yet to be demonstrated, most investigators assume that with repeated stressors (in the absence of confounding glucocorticoid feedback inhibition) there is enhanced secretion of some secretagog. As an indirect measure of this, with repeated stressors, the number of vasopressin-positive median eminence neurons increases, as does the amount of vasopressin stores (while equivalent changes in CRF were not observed) (de Goeij et al. 1991).

contributing to the fact that aged rats are impaired in terminating their stress-response at the end of stress.

As additional adrenal complexities, there is increasing evidence that ACTH is not the sole regulator glucocorticoid secretion. Peptides, termed *corticostatins*, secreted from leukocytes, inhibit adrenal glucocorticoid release (cf. Tominaga et al. 1990), while the sympathetic nervous system inputs into the adrenal can modulate adrenal sensitivity to ACTH (Charlton 1990). There have also been reports of direct release of glucocorticoids or augmentation of ACTH action by angiotensin II (Keller-Wood et al. 1986), interleukin-1-β (Andreis et al. 1991), and even CRF itself (Jones and Edwards 1990). The physiological relevance of any of these adrenal effects is not clear, with the exception of CRF, which does appear to directly contribute to glucocorticoid release under physiological circumstances (van Oers et al. 1992).

Glucocorticoid Transport in the Bloodstream

Steroid hormones such as glucocorticoids are far more hydrophobic and lipophilic than are peptide hormones. This has the important implication that steroids permeate through the cell membrane quite readily. Therefore, steroid hormones can interact with intracellular receptors, in contrast to peptide hormones, which typically interact with membrane-bound receptors.

The same features of steroid hormones make them unable to travel freely in the bloodstream. Instead, they are typically bound to carrier proteins. Most circulating glucocorticoids are noncovalently bound to corticosteroid binding globulin (CBG, also known as *transcortin*) and are not biologically active at that time. Only when released near the target cell can they permeate the membrane and exert their actions. It is not clear whether CBG must be cleaved to release glucocorticoids, or whether it interacts with a membrane-bound CBG receptor (Hammond 1990; Rosner 1990). As an added complexity, there is the suggestion that CBG is not always "merely" a carrier, but can serve as, in effect, a sponge within the circulatory system—by binding large quantities of (now inactive) glucocorticoids, CBG can be a reservoir, able to release them rapidly during stress (Rosner 1990). In some cases, CBG can also be internalized and bind glucocorticoids intracellularly. Because such binding does not lead to the classic events arising from glucocorticoid interaction with the typical receptor, the intracellular CBG can serve as a buffer against glucocorticoid action. This situation is best documented in the pituitary, where postnatal shifts in the levels of such "CBG-like" receptors have considerable consequences for pituitary responsiveness to glucocorticoids (Sapolsky and Meaney 1986).

Of greatest interest are the quantitative dynamics of glucocorticoid/CBG interactions. Under normal basal conditions, approximately 95% of glucocorticoids in the circulation are bound to CBG, and approximately 5% of glucocorticoids form the biologically active pool. An important implication of this is that if CBG levels are held constant and total glucocorticoid concentrations increase a mere 5% higher, the free fraction will have doubled (Westphal

1971). This is ideal for a system designed for very rapid responses to emergencies—the first minute increase in glucocorticoid secretion is "heard" throughout the body. An additional piece of regulation exaggerates this pattern even further: Glucocorticoids decrease the levels of CBG in the circulation (by altering both their rate of production and breakdown) (Schlechte and Hamilton 1987; Frairia et al. 1988). Therefore, when glucocorticoids rise during stress, there is a vast increase in the amount of free steroid reaching target tissues. For example, doubling circulating glucocorticoid concentrations from 5 to 10 μg/dl in the rat (a change from moderate basal to very low stress levels) causes an almost *hundredfold* increase in the calculated free glucocorticoid fraction (Dallman et al. 1987).

The most striking implication of these dynamics is that even small increases in glucocorticoid concentrations matter. This becomes critical; one of the themes that will emerge in subsequent chapters is that aging rats have moderately increased basal glucocorticoid concentrations.

The Cellular Mechanisms of Glucocorticoid Action

While most steroid hormone action is thought to be mediated by interaction with cytosolic receptors and subsequent regulation of genomic events, there are proving to be exceptions. As will be reviewed in chapter 4, these include interactions with membrane-bound steroid receptors (which probably exert their effects through second messengers), with receptors for neurotransmitters, and through nonspecific fluidization of membranes. This will become relevant in considering how to counter or mimic various glucocorticoid actions—only some are likely to be prevented by antagonizing the classic cytosolic receptors.

Currently, even the well-established genomic picture of glucocorticoid action is increasing in complexity. In the basic model, a "glucocorticoid responsive element" in the DNA binds the hormone/receptor complex, leading to enhanced or decreased transcription of a gene closely downstream. As will be discussed in a subsequent chapter, this is a simplification, and for a logical reason.

Circadian Rhythmicity to Glucocorticoid Release

Like most endocrine systems, the adrenocortical axis exhibits circadian rhythmicity, with glucocorticoid concentrations at their trough around the onset of sleep and at their peak shortly after waking. This is seen in both diurnal and nocturnal species, and probably reflects the need to mobilize energy stores when beginning the day's activity (i.e., even on an unstressful day, it is somewhat stressful to merely start functioning). The glucocorticoid rhythmicity is fairly striking: Circadian trough levels in the rat are typically less than 1 μg/dl, while peak levels are typically 15 to 20 μg/dl (Dallman et al. 1987).

The generation of the glucocorticoid rhythm is quite complex. Part of the rhythmicity arises from the adrenal. Adrenal sensitivity to ACTH shifts throughout the circadian cycle; at the peak, the adrenal is 2.5 times [more] sensitive to the peptide than at the trough (Dallman et al. 1978; Kaneko [et al.] 1980, 1981). The basis for this shift is not yet understood, although it [does] not involve ACTH itself or autonomic innervation of the adrenal (Dallman [et] al. 1978; Wilkinson et al. 1981).

At the pituitary level, there is disagreement as to whether there is a [shift] over the circadian cycle in pituitary sensitivity to CRF, to the other [se]cretagogs, or to stress (Akana et al. 1986). Importantly, the pituitary [can] secrete ACTH autonomously, independent of hypothlamic stimulation. [This] appears to be the case during the circadian trough. Thus, following lesion[s of] the mediobasal hypothalamus (destroying the source of secretagogs), [the] circadian peak of ACTH secretion is destroyed, but ACTH concentration[s at] the circadian trough are normal (Kaneko et al. 1980; Dallman et al. 1987). [This] generates the prediction that during the circadian trough, there should b[e no] secretagogs in the portal circulation. This is not testable, since it is not pos[sible] to do the surgery neccesary to cannulate the circulation without stressing [the] animal. However, a circadian rhythm in median eminence content of CRF [has] been demonstrated (Hiroshige and Sato 1970).

Within the brain, the source of the circadian rhythmicity is most l[ikely] the suprachiasmatic nucleus (SCN) of the hypothalamus, which is the [best] documented of neural circadian rhythm generators. Lesions of the SCN ab[olish] circadian rhythms throughout the adrenocortical axis (Moore and Ei[chler] 1972; Stephen and Zucker 1972; Krieger et al. 1977; Abe et al. 1979, C[ascio] et al. 1987). It is not known by what neuroanatomical route the SCN influe[nces] secretagog release. Moreover, in my reading of the literature, it is not [clear] whether the SCN solely inhibits secretagog release during the circa[dian] trough, stimulates during the peak, or both. Finally, some of the adrenoco[rtical] rhythmicity generated by the SCN might be mediated by rhythmic flu[ctua]tions in food consumption, as such rhythms can entrain the adrenocortical [axis] (reviewed in Dallman et al. 1987).

Does the size of the stress-response vary over the circadian cycle? Po[ten]tially, the purpose of a stress-response could be to achieve circulating gl[uco]corticoids concentrations of, say, 25 μg/dl in response to a certain degre[e of] hemorrhage. In that scenario, there would be a vast increase in glucocorti[coid] secretion in response to that hemorrhage during the circadian trough, b[ut a] much smaller response at the peak. Alternatively, the purpose of the st[ress] response might be to, for instance, elevate glucocorticoid concentration[s x] μg/dl in response to this stressor, regardless of the initial circulating concen[tra]tions. This issue appears somewhat unsettled at this point. One study indic[ates] that there is no difference in the magnitude of the ACTH stress-response [as a] function of time of day (Wilson et al. 1983), whereas quite a few stu[dies] indicate that the size of the stress-response (as measured either by ACT[H or] corticosterone concentrations) does indeed differ. The confusion, howeve[r, is] that some of them indicate that the response is greater during the circa[dian] peak (Zimmermann and Critchlow 1967; Gibbs 1970), while others sho[w]

At the pituitary level, a single exposure to a stressor (Rivier and Vale 1983b) and repeated stressors (Hauger et al. 1990) blunt pituitary responsiveness to CRF a few hours later. In an in vitro equivalent of this observation, pituitary explants or cultures become less sensitive to CRF following a prior CRF challenge (Reisine and Hoffman 1983; Holmes et al. 1984). Thus, any facilitation at such times could not be driven by enhanced sensitivity to CRF, and recent work suggests that such facilitation involves enhanced sensitivity to vasopressin (Scaccianoce et al. 1991).

In contrast, facilitation following *multiple or prolonged* stressors may indeed be at least partially driven by enhanced sensitivity to CRF, since repeated or prolonged exposure to CRF increases corticotrope number (Siperstein and Miller 1970; Kracier et al. 1973; Gertz et al. 1987; Sasaki et al. 1990), and enhances their responsiveness to CRF (Wynn et al. 1985). Facilitation at the level of the pituitary might also arise from a blunting of pituitary sensitivity to the inhibitory effects of glucocorticoid feedback. In support of this view, CRF down-regulates glucocorticoid receptor expression in corticotropes (Sheppard et al. 1991).

At the level of the adrenal. facilitation can occur as well, in that prolonged ACTH exposure causes adrenal hypertrophy and hyperplasia (Dallman et al. 1981) and enhanced responsiveness to ACTH (Raff et al. 1982; Engeland et al. 1981).

In summary, various "feedforward" elements might contribute to the facilitation that counterbalances the glucocorticoid feedback inhibition. However, the feedforward components are not purely facilitatory; some will work with the glucocorticoids to inhibit the system. For example, each secretagog (e.g., CRF or vasopressin) will down-regulate the number of its own receptors in the pituitary (Wynn et al. 1985; Koch and Lutz-Bucher 1985; Antoni et al. 1985). Moreover, different secretagogs will inhibit the release of other secretagogs, via "ultrashort" feedback loops (reviewed in Taylor and Fishman 1988). At the adrenal, at the same time that chronic ACTH exposure is causing hypertrophy and hyperplasia, there is also down-regulation of ACTH receptor number (Dallman 1985).

This is obviously complex, and it is not possible to predict, a priori, how the various inhibitory and facilitory pieces will add up for particular instances of repeated stressors. Therefore, sometimes facilitation occurs—a stressor will cause a larger adrenocortical response than usual if it comes in the aftermath of other, previous stressors (Dallman and Jones 1973b; Sakellaris and Vernikos-Danellis 1975; Gann et al. 1977; Kartoszi et al. 1982; Bereiter et al. 1982; Raff et al. 1982, 1986; de Souza and van Loon 1982). Sometimes, the inhibitory and facilitory components balance out, and the size of the stress-response is not sensitive to prior stressors (Dallman and Jones 1973a,b; Jones and Stockham 1966; Knigge et al. 1959; Zimmermann and Critchlow, 1969; Fortier et al. 1970; Raff et al. 1982). In some cases, the inhibition seems to be stronger (Gann et al. 1977; Keller-Wood et al. 1983b). The balancing reflects the timing of the repeated stressors, and the type of stressor involved (Keller-Wood and Dallman 1984).

Do Glucocorticoids Mediate the Stress-Response or the Recovery from the Stress-Response?

In chapter 1, when introducing the logic of the stress-response and of glucocorticoid actions during stressors, I presented a view that was fairly derivative of the ideas of Selye from half a century ago. Glucocorticoids, by helping to mobilize energy, increase cardiovascular tone, and suppress unessential anabolism, constitute the stress-response—the means by which the organism survives a physical stressor.

This is the general textbook dogma regarding the teleology of glucocorticoid physiology. In recent decades, there has not been a rejection of this teleologic framework, as much as a loss of interest in it. Instead, the focus now is often on the biochemistry, cell biology, or molecular biology of glucocorticoid action—the structure of the glucocorticoid receptor and the receptor superfamily to which it belongs; the mechanisms of glucocorticoid-induced lymphocytolysis as a convenient model for studying programmed cell death; the use of glucocorticoids as a tool for studying the role of the receptor as a ligand-activated transcriptional factor, and so on.

There are a number of explanations for this loss of interest. Reductionist biology is extremely in vogue. Few scientists are interested in integrating pieces into large physiological wholes. Furthermore, as more disparate glucocorticoid actions in a plethora of tissues have been uncovered, it becomes daunting to attempt such a synthesis (and as a result, many physiologists have relegated these nonintuitive, obscure glucocorticoid actions to pharmacology and thus washed their hands of the inconvenience). Finally, Selye, as the most voluble of early glucocorticoid endocrinologists, made some highly visible mistakes in his formulations, which tended unfortunately to discredit all of his work.

This historical trend and its underlying reasons were reviewed in a landmark paper by Allan Munck and colleagues (1984). Munck, one of the most respected and productive of endocrinologists, wrote not merely to lament the subordinance of physiological thinking about glucocorticoids, but to propose a paradigm shift that would integrate the various pieces of glucocorticoid action into a new, coherent physiological whole.

Specifically, the authors rejected the idea that glucocorticoids help *mediate* the stress-response. Instead, they proposed that glucocorticoids cause the *recovery* from the stress-response. To quote:

We propose that: (1) the physiological function of stress-induced increases in glucocorticoid levels is to protect not against the source of stress itself, but against the normal defense reactions that are activated by stress; and (2) the glucocorticoids accomplish this function by turning off those defense reactions, thus preventing them from overshooting and themselves threatening homeostasis.

This influential paper has gathered many adherents. While it has made the important contribution of focusing attention on the possibility of these hor-

Table 2.1. Some physiological and biochemical processes inhibited by glucocorticoids

Immune interferon
Natural killer cell activity
Interleukin-1
Prostaglandin synthesis
Leukotriene synthesis
Insulin secretion
β-Endorphin secretion
Vasopressin secretion
Growth hormone secretion
Glucose transport and glycogen synthesis
Calcium transport into bone
Macrophage activating factor
Lymphocyte activating factor
T cell growth factor
Thromboxane synthesis
Bradykinin synthesis
CRF secretion
ACTH secretion
Gonadal responsiveness to LH
Insulinlike growth factor secretion
Amino acid transport and protein synthesis
Triglyceride synthesis

Data from Krieger (1982), Munck et al. (1984), and Sapolsky (1986).

mones mediating recovery, I still believe that the bulk of glucocorticoid actions constitute the stress-response itself.

How does one determine this? A number of criteria come to mind:

1. Glucocorticoids inhibit numerous physiological and biochemical processes in the body (see table 2.1 for a sampling of these). If glucocorticoids form the recovery from the stress-response, then these physiological and biochemical processes must constitute the stress-response. In other words, during the time lag between the onset of a stressor and the onset of the glucocorticoid action, is there a dramatic activation of these processes? It should be noted that this criterion requires that those processes be turned on in response to a majority of the various psychological and somatic stressors that exist.

2. When there are pathologic shortages of glucocorticoids (such as in Addison's disease, due to adrenal failure), do the physiological and biochemical processes in table 2.1 wildly overshoot their normal bounds and damage the body?

3. Some of the most critical hormones of the stress-response (e.g., CRF, ACTH, and catecholamines) are secreted and have their actions within seconds. In contrast, it takes minutes for glucocorticoids to be secreted and, in some cases, hours for their peak actions to occur. This lag time seems a strong reason to suspect that glucocorticoids are not the stress-response as much as

the recovery. In that regard, one must compare glucocorticoid actions with those of the faster hormones. Are glucocorticoid actions similar to, opposite of, or merely different from those of the fastest of the stress-responsive hormones (CRF, ACTH, catecholamines)? If they are the same, then glucocorticoids must be mediating the stress-response just as surely as these other hormones do—glucocorticoids merely form a slower second wave of defense. If glucocorticoids do exactly the opposite of those hormones, the steroids are indeed probably mediating the recovery from the stress-response. If glucocorticoids do something *different* (but not opposite), they may still be mediating the stress-response; to use a military metaphor, catecholamines may mobilize defenses to an invasion over seconds by handing out rifles, while glucocorticoids may mobilize defenses to an invasion over hours by stimulating the lengthy construction of forts and trenches. The latter, while slower, is still most certainly a "stress-response," rather than a recovery from it.

By these criteria, in some cases, glucocorticoids probably do indeed mediate the recovery from the stress-response. A classic example is in glucocorticoid inhibition of inflammation after, for example, our proverbial zebra's knee is injured. In the absence of glucocorticoids, inflammation would occur to the point of making the knee stiff and unusable. If physical activity (e.g., escape) is still required, this is maladaptive. Therefore, this seems a convincing case where glucocorticoids prevent the inflammatory response to an injurious stressor from overshooting and becoming endangering itself.

A second example where glucocorticoids probably mediate recovery from the stress-response is during hemorrhage. In the absence of glucocorticoids, there is intense vasopressin secretion during hemorrhage. This causes excessive hepatic vasoconstriction, hepatic ischemia, and death (Darlington et al. 1990a,b). Thus, by inhibiting vasopressin secretion, glucocorticoids prevent this stress-response from overshooting to a fatal degree.

However, in most cases, I think glucocorticoids do not mediate recovery from the stress-response. This is most striking in three areas (of a larger number that could have been chosen).

Reproductive Physiology   Glucocorticoids inhibit reproduction in a variety of ways, reducing concentrations of estrogen, progesterone, testosterone, and so on. Does secretion of estrogen and testosterone constitute a logical stress-response that must be reined in by glucocorticoids? There is little evidence that these reproductive hormones are hypersecreted during the first few minutes of a stressor. Furthermore, Addisonian patients do not hypersecrete these sexual hormones. Finally, the most rapid hormones of the stress-response also inhibit reproduction (reviewed in Sapolsky 1987, 1991). Therefore, glucocorticoid inhibition of reproduction seems to constitute a stress-response, and this makes sense—costly and anabolic reproduction cannot be afforded during a stressful emergency.

Immunity   As noted, glucocorticoids inhibit immunity in a vast number of ways (reviewed in Munck et al. 1984). This inhibition is, in some ways, the centerpiece of the theory by Munck and colleagues. Most explicitly, they hypothesized that stressors stimulate the immune system, and that gluco-corticoids inhibit the immune system to prevent it from overshooting into uncontrolled autoimmunity at such times. To my knowledge, however, there is little evidence that immediately after the onset of any of a broad array of stressors, there is dramatic immune activation. Furthermore, in the aftermath of their adrenal insufficiency, Addisonian patients do not develope auto-immune disorders (a critical prediction generated by the Munck hypothesis).

Metabolism   Glucocorticoids block glucose transport, block energy storage (by blocking synthesis of triglycerides, glycogen, proteins), and promote energy mobilization (by promoting the breakdown of preexisting trigly-cerides, glycogen, and proteins, and the hepatic regeneration of glucose) (reviewed in Goodman, 1980). There is no evidence that immediately after the onset of a stressful emergency (before glucocorticoids begin to work), the body begins to store energy. Furthermore, Addisonian patients do not do this to a pathologic extent (in fact, they become pathologically lean). Finally, the fastest hormones of the stress-response (the catecholamines) mobilize energy from storage sites just as glucocorticoids do. Teleologically, glucocorticoid actions on metabolism make perfect sense as helping to mediate the response to an immediate stressful emergency—mobilize energy from storage sites so that it can be utilized immediately.

Thus, at this point, I would advocate the not very radical view that both the classic Selyian view and this more recent revisionism have some validity. In general. glucocorticoids appear to help the recovery from the response to very *specific* stressors—hemorrhage, a joint injury, perhaps an infectious stressor. However, they appear to help mediate the primary stress-response to a far broader array of stressors, in that they mobilize energy and block costly anabolism. It is also possible that glucocorticoids, because of their relatively slow time course, may mostly prepare the body for responding to *subsequent* stressors (an idea of M. Romero, a member of my laboratory); this idea has not been explored.

3 Glucocorticoid Concentrations in the Aged Rat: A Problem of Hypersecretion

SUMMARY OF THE BOOK SO FAR

The stress-response is the set of neural and endocrine adaptations by which the body maintains homeostatic balance during stress. While the stress-response is ideal for adapting to acute physical stressors, overactivation of this stress-response can be extremely damaging, and a large percentage of what we think of as "stress-related" diseases are disorders of an overabundance of the stress-response. This emphasizes the need for the exquisitely tight regulation of the magnitude and duration of the stress-response.

Given the difficulty of regulating the stress-response, and the adverse consequences when it is not adequately regulated, gerontologists have focused on two types of interactions between the stress-response and the biology of aging. The first is the notion that aging is associated with an impaired capacity to deal with stress optimally. The second is that prolonged stress can accelerate some of the degenerative features of aging. This book focuses on the considerable evidence for these two ideas and their interactions in mediating neural degeneration during aging.

Rather than focusing on the generic "stress-response," the focus will be on the class of hormones that are central to both the adaptive and pathogenic properties of the response. These hormones, glucocorticoids, are secreted by the adrenal gland. This is the final step in a neuroendocrine cascade that begins in the brain. As the first step in this "adrenocortical axis," stressors are perceived in the brain and, within seconds, stimulate the secretion of CRF, vasopressin, and other secretagogs into the hypothalamic-pituitary portal circulation. This triggers pituitary release of ACTH within perhaps 15 seconds which, in turn, triggers adrenal secretion of glucocorticoids.

This, naturally, represents a vast simplification of this axis. Some of the complexities of relevance to the remainder of this book include the following: (1) The impressive degree of colinearity among the magnitude of a stressor, the magnitude of the adrenocortical stress-response, and the magnitude of target tissue responses to these hormones; (2) The multiplicity of hypothalamic secretagogs and their synergies in releasing ACTH; (3) The dynamics of glucocorticoid transport in the circulation, which cause small increases in hormone concentrations to have an enormous effect on target tissues. (4) Negative-feedback regulation of the adrenocortical axis by glucocorticoids, and the interaction between this feedback inhibition and feedforward stimulation. (5) The complex teleologic issue of whether glucocorticoids primarily constitute the stress-response or the brake on the stress-response.

With this outline of glucocorticoid secretion and actions, it is possible to ask the initial question, Can aged rats appropriately initiate and terminate glucocorticoid secretion in response to stress?

GLUCOCORTICOID CONCENTRATIONS IN THE AGED RAT

(Note: Throughout the book, all published studies referred to were carried out on rats, unless stated otherwise. Throughout, "young" refers to rats 3 to 6 months of age, "mid-aged," those 10 to 15 months of age, and "aged" or "senescent" to those 20 or more months of age. See the brief appendix at the end of this chapter.)

Given the absolutely critical role that glucocorticoids play in mediating survival from physical stressors, it is fair to ask whether aged rats can appropriately initiate glucocorticoid secretion during stress. This appears to be the case. Circulating concentrations of corticosterone (the principal glucocorticoid of rats) are similar in young and aged male rats being stressed with immobilization or cage transfer (which are predominately psychological stressors), or more somatic stressors such as laparotomy, shock, immobilization, cold, or ether exposure (Rapaport et al. 1964; Hess and Riegle, 1972; Riegle and Hess 1972; Riegle 1973; Sencar-Cupovic and Milkovic 1976; Tang and Phillips 1978; Sapolsky et al. 1983a; Brodish and Odio 1989; Sabatino et al. 1991; however, see Lorens et al. 1990 for a demonstration of an enhanced glucocorticoid response to a conditioned emotional stressor in aged rats). The speed of the response has not been studied in a great deal of detail, but appears to be normal (Sapolsky et al. 1983a; Brodish and Odio 1989; Sabatino et al. 1991). Moreover, reserve capacity of the adrenocortical axis appears intact (i.e., aged rats still respond to a novel stressor after previous chronic stress) (Sapolsky et al. 1983a), and there is still a circadian rhythm in corticosterone concentrations (Sapolsky et al. 1983a; Oxenkrug et al. 1984b; Issa et al. 1990; Sabatino et al. 1991).

A roughly similar story holds for aging female rats. Superficially, there appears to be a major decline in stress-induced corticosterone concentrations with age in the female rat, which has been interpreted as a diminished adaptive capacity during aging (Hess and Riegle, 1970, 1972; Wilson 1985; Brett et al. 1983; no decline in the magnitude of stress-response: Sencar-Cupovic and Milkovic 1976; Erisman et al. 1990). This is probably not the case, however. As discussed, glucocorticoids are transported in the circulation bound to CBG. Estrogen is a powerful inducer of CBG production (Sandberg and Slaunwhite 1959). With the declining concentrations of estrogen in the aged female rat, both CBG-bound and total glucocorticoid concentrations decline. However, if the size of the free, active compartment does not change, the strength of the glucocorticoid signal should not decline. This idea has yet to be tested explicitly, however.

Thus, aged rats elevate corticosterone concentrations normally during stress. When I began work in this field, I found this to be disappointing, since an inability to turn on a stress-response would be a dramatic age-related impairment. However, it would not be particularly commensurate with the picture of aging—the consequences of a failure to initiate glucocorticoid secretion during a major physical stressor are usually immediate and catastrophic. In contrast, the normative picture of aging is one of slow decrement and gradual accumulation of damage. The defect in the aged adrenocortical axis turns out to be one of *excessive* glucocorticoids, and this fits the picture of aging far better than would a failure of the stress-response.

As a first defect, aged rats have elevated *basal* corticosterone concentrations. This has been observed frequently, although often without reaching statistical significance. This has led to some disagreement as to whether there is an increase. Rather than listing those studies either showing or failing to show a significant increase, I summarize the magnitude of age-related increases from these varied reports in table 3.1. Collectively, they consistently report increased basal corticosterone concentrations in aged rats. As just discussed, the declining CBG concentrations in the aged female would tend to lead to a decrease in total glucocorticoid concentrations; thus, the small but consistent increases in concentrations in the aged female are actually quite impressive.

Why has the increase in circulating corticosterone concentrations with age, which appears so consistent when gathered in table 3.1, so often failed to reach significance in individual studies? Part of this arises from the massive variability intrinsic to aging studies. This has been noted and bemoaned by gerontologists for decades; only recently has it been viewed as an indicator of interesting heterogeneity within aged populations (see chapter 12). In reviewing these many studies, I have found that sex, time of day, and strain cannot explain the varying results regarding the effects of age on basal corticosterone. However, I have noted one additional factor that is likely to give rise to the variability.

Table 3.1 lists the studies (when grouped by sex and time of day) progressing from those reporting the lowest basal corticosterone concentrations in young rats to those reporting the highest. The variability is considerable; for example, among males studied during the circadian trough, there is a 40-fold range of values reported, and the ones in the upper range are clearly above nonstressed, basal values (Dallman et al. 1987). This might reflect the method by which blood was obtained, some stressful feature of the social housing of the animals, a recent disturbance in the animal room prior to sampling, and so on. When studies are divided as to whether reported corticosterone values for young animals are truly in the basal range (very liberally defined as < 10 and < 15 μg/dl during the circadian trough and peak, respectively), a striking pattern emerges (figure 3.1): When corticosterone is measured under (apparently) truly nonstressed conditions, the circulating concentrations rise markedly with age (and the few studies that have studied a variety of ages suggest that this rise is fairly progressive throughout the lifetime). Under conditions where basal values are already in the moderate stress range, there is no age difference. This latter observation is not surprising, given the literature (just discussed) showing that young and aged rats achieve

Table 3.1. Changes in basal corticosterone concentrations in aged rats

| Study | Basal corticosterone concentrations | | | |
	Young	Old	Change with age	Strain
Studies of Female Rats				
A. *Studies conducted during circadian trough*				
Sencar-Cupovic and Milkovic, 1976	4.8	8.5	+3.7	F
Riegle, 1973	9.6	23.0	+13.4	F
Brett et al., 1983	15.0	22.0	+7.0	F
Brett et al., 1986	25.0	25.0	0	F
B. *Studies conducted during circadian peak*				
Meaney et al., 1991	8.8	17.8	+9.0	LE
C. *Studies conducted at indeterminate time*				
Hess and Riegle, 1970	9.6	11.5	+1.9	F
Studies of Male Rats				
A. *Studies conducted during circadian trough*				
Oxenkrug et al., 1984b	0.5	6.0	+5.5	SD
Scaccianoce et al., 1990	1.5	7.0	+5.5	SD
Tang and Phillips, 1978	1.8	3.9	+2.1	SD
DeKosky et al., 1984	2.0	4.0	+2.0	SD
Sencar-Cupovic and Milkovic, 1976	3.5	9.5	+6.0	F
Landfield et al., 1978	4.2	8.0	+3.8	F
Meaney et al., 1988	6.0	13.0	+7.0	LE
Sapolsky et al., 1983	6.0	11.5	+5.5	F
Riegle, 1973	6.4	13.8	+7.4	LE
Britton et al., 1975	8.0	10.3	+2.3	SD
Sonntag et al., 1987	10.0	11.0	+1.0	F
Brett et al., 1983	15.0	16.0	+1.0	F
Lorens et al., 1990	17.0	22.0	+5.0	F
Brett et al., 1986	20.0	21.0	+1.0	F
B. *Studies conducted during circadian peak*				
DeKosky et al., 1984	10.0	20.0	+10.0	SD
Oxenkrug et al., 1984	12.0	24.0	+12.0	SD
Sapolsky et al., 1983	13.0	21.0	+8.0	F
Sonntag et al., 1987	17.0	17.0	0	F
C. *Studies conducted at indeterminate time*				
Hess and Riegle, 1970	4.9	5.6	+0.7	LE
Chiueh et al., 1980	19.0	26.0	+7.0	F

Corticosterone concentrations and change with age both expressed as μg/dl. Abbreviations: SD, Sprague-Dawley; F, Fischer-344; LE, Long Evans. "Circadian trough" indicates studies conducted during the first 8 hours of the light cycle; "circadian peak" indicates studies conducted during the first 8 hours of the dark cycle.

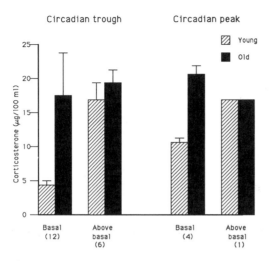

Figure 3.1. Comparison of age effects in studies in which basal corticosterone concentrations of young subjects were truly in the basal range (less than 10 μg/dl in the circadian trough; less than 15 μg/dl in the circadian peak) versus those in which values were above basal range. (From Sapolsky, Do glucocorticoid concentrations rise with age in the rat? Neurobiol Aging, 1991, vol. 13, p. 171. Copyright 1991, Pergamon Press plc.)

roughly equal corticosterone concentrations during stress. Therefore, I feel that some of the confusion in the literature has arisen from animals being studied under nonbasal conditions, and that there is, in fact, a robust increase in basal corticosterone concentrations with age. (An additional recent study of male Wistar rats supports these conclusions but was not included in the analysis in figure 3.1 because the youngest age included was 12 months of age [Dellwo and Beauchene 1990], as does another study of male Fischer rats, which arrived after the analysis in figure 3.1 was completed [Sabatino et al. 1991] However, another such recent study with male brown Norway rats does not support these conclusions [van Eekelen et al. 1991]).

The analysis in figure 3.1, as noted, compares only two ages of rats. Is the increase in basal corticosterone concentrations with age progressive, in that each succeeding age group shows more pronounced hypersecretion? Few studies have examined multiple ages, in particular those in the 15 to 30 month age range. Of the two that have, one showed that the senescent corticosterone hypersecretion had already plateaued by 18 to 19 months of age (Sabatino et al. 1991), while another showed a mild worsening of the hypersecretion problem from 16 to 24 months of age (Meaney et al. 1988a). The implications of this will be considered in chapter 6.

This age-related increase in circulating corticosterone concentrations is likely to be even more pronounced when one considers the free fraction, rather than the total pool. Circulating CBG concentrations have been reported to show either a substantial (van Eekelen, 1990) or mild (Sabatino et al. 1991) decrease. Thus, the free fraction should increase considerably with age, as has been reported (Sabatino et al. 1991).

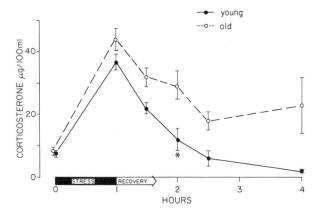

Figure 3.2. Corticosterone concentrations in young and aged rats during 60 minutes of immobilization stress, followed by 3 hours of recovery. Subjects were immobilized one hour into the light cycle. * indicates point at which concentrations in young subjects had returned to basal values; aged subjects did not recover to basal values. (From Sapolsky et al., 1984, Proc Natl Acad Sci USA 81, 6174.)

A second instance of corticosterone hypersecretion occurs in aged rats as well. While aged rats can generate normal glucocorticoid concentrations during stress, they have an impaired capacity to *terminate* the stress-response, and there are excessive corticosterone concentrations during this recovery period. In young rats, with the abatement of the stressor, corticosterone concentrations decline rapidly as a function of the clearance rate from the blood. Aged rats, in contrast, hypersecrete the hormone for hours after the end of the stressor (figure 3.2; Sapolsky et al. 1983; see also Chiueh et al. 1980; Ida et al. 1984; Brodish and Odio 1989 [where the recovery problem is apparent, but not noted; see figure 2]; Erisman et al. 1990; Sabatino et al. 1991 [but also see van Eekelen et al. 1991, for no change in recovery of total corticosterone concentrations post stressor with age]; a similar inability to shut off the sympathetic stress-response also occurs in aged rats: McCarty, 1986). This has been shown for both sexes; furthermore, the ACTH recovery from the stress-response is also delayed in aged rats (Erisman et al. 1990; van Eekelen et al. 1991). In their report of a substantial decline in CBG with age, van Eekelen and colleagues (1991) showed that the recovery time for the free corticosterone fraction is even more dramatically delayed in aged rats. In addition, corticosterone secretion habituates to mild stressors more slowly in aged rats (Sapolsky et al. 1983a; Odio and Brodish, 1989; also see Methods section of Kerr et al. 1991, reporting the same). As a probable consequence of this, the metabolic stress-response (e.g., changes in glucose and free fatty acid concentrations) also habituates more slowly in aged rats (Odio and Brodish 1988).

Therefore, the aged rat has elevated circulating concentrations of glucocorticoids both basally and during the recovery period after the end of stress. What point in the adrenocortical axis is malfunctioning? Evidence suggests that there is some defect at the neural level.

To begin, the elevated glucocorticoid concentrations could be due to impaired clearance of them from the circulation, and/or to enhanced secretion. Arguing against the former, the half-life of circulating corticosterone does not change with age in the rat (24-month-old rats; Sapolsky et al. 1983a). Given this, plus the fact that there is a large increase in blood volume with age in some of the strains in which hypersecretion occurs (Britton et al. 1975), the aged adrenal must be secreting greatly increased amount of the steroid. Supporting this, the adrenal cortex is hyperplastic in the old rat.

These data shift the emphasis to the level of the adrenal or higher. Potentially, the hypersecretion of glucocorticoids could be purely adrenal in origin; that is, ACTH concentrations could be normal in aged rats, but the adrenal is hyperresponsive to the peptide. Surprisingly, adrenal responsiveness to ACTH decreases with age both in vivo and in vitro (Britton et al. 1975; Hess and Riegle 1970, 1972; Malamed and Carsia 1983; Popplewell et al. 1986, 1987; Pritchett et al. 1979; Tang and Phillips 1978a; Cheng et al. 1990. No loss of sensitivity reported by Riegle 1973; Sonntag et al. 1987; increased in vivo sensitivity reported by Brodish and Odio 1989). The mechanisms underlying this loss of sensitivity are quite complex. There is no decline in the numbers of adrenal ACTH receptors, or of ACTH activation of cAMP (Popplewell et al. 1986). Instead, there is decreased activity of cholesterol esterase, which converts stored cholesterol esters to cholesterol for steroidogenesis, and of HMG-CoA reductase, which is essential for de novo synthesis of cholesterol (Popplewell and Azhar 1987; Popplewell et al. 1987). Thus, there is less delivery of cholesterol to adrenal mitochondria for conversion by cytochrome $P450_{scc}$ to pregnenolone to begin the pathway to corticosterone. To confuse things, activity of that latter enzyme, which is rate-limiting in the pathway, *increases* with age, although by a magnitude insufficient to counteract the diminished delivery of cholesterol to mitochondria (Popplewell and Azhar 1987; Popplewell et al. 1987). The net result of this is that within any given adrenocortical cell, ACTH stimulates less corticosterone synthesis and secretion.

It is important to note here that some researchers have considered this decreased adrenal sensitivity on a cellular level during aging to mean that the stress-response is decreased. That is not the case—ACTH is not a stressor, and adrenal responsiveness to ACTH is merely one step in a cascade. Conclusions about entire physiological systems require putting the various pieces together. When that is done, the decreased adrenal responsiveness is probably best viewed as an only somewhat successful compensation for hypersecretion at higher points in the axis. It is only partially successful because of the adrenal hyperplasia—despite individual adrenal cells being less responsive to ACTH, there are more such cells—and because of a greatly enhanced ACTH signal originating from the aged pituitary (Tang and Phillips 1978a; Issa et al. 1990; van Eekelen et al. 1991; Dellwo and Beauchene 1990, although it should be noted that values were extremely high in this last study). Given the fact that elevated concentrations of ACTH manifest themselves in prolonged plateaus of glucocorticoid secretion, rather than higher plateaus (see chapter 2), this fits nicely with the observation of a prolonged glucocorticoid stress-response in aged rats after the end of stress.

Moving higher in the axis, the elevated ACTH concentrations could arise from elevated concentrations of any of the hypothalamic secretagogs, and/or from enhanced pituitary sensitivity to those secretagogs. The hypersecretion is probably not due to the latter mechanism—the aged pituitary is *less* responsive to CRF (Hylka et al. 1984) and has fewer CRF receptors (Heroux et al. 1991). (One study [Scaccianoce et al. 1990] shows no change with age in pituitary responsiveness to CRF. This was probably not as informative a study as that of Hylka et al. [1984], in which CRF was administered in vivo, whereas Scaccianoce et al. stimulated pituitary explants with hypothalamic extract containing variable quantities of CRF).

This suggests that the hypersecretion of the axis is driven at the level of the brain (if there is enhanced ACTH secretion yet decreased sensitivity to CRF, there must be greatly enhanced levels of CRF stimulating the pituitary). However, this fails to recognize that there are other secretagogs involved in the story, and the pituitary could have enhanced sensitivity to them. Obviously, the most direct way to implicate the brain in the hypersecretion would be to demonstrate that there are elevated concentrations of any of these hypothalamic secretagogs in the portal circulation of the aged rat. This difficult experiment has not yet been done (mainly because of the fragile state of aged animals and the traumatic nature of such surgery). However, a recent report offers important, although slightly less direct evidence for CNS hypersecretion in the aged rat (Scaccianoce et al. 1990). Hypothalamic blocks were prepared and their secretion of CRF was monitored basally and after stimulation with acetylcholine. In both conditions, there was hypersecretion from aged hypothalami.

In summary, hypersecretion of glucocorticoids in the aged rat is probably driven neurally. The theme that will unfold in subsequent chapters is the search for the neural site(s) whose senescent degeneration contributes to this hypersecretion. Before that, however, a critical question is whether the hypersecretion is tonic in nature, or whether it represents a disinhibition of feedback regulation. As discussed, the adrenocortical axis is under classic end-product control, in that circulating glucocorticoids will inhibit subsequent adrenocortical activity. Does this instance of hypersecretion arise from a damping of such feedback inhibition? In order to appreciate the studies demonstrating that to be the case, it is neccesary to review such regulation. I warn the neophyte that, in terms of endocrine complexity, this is not a subject for the fainthearted.

NEGATIVE FEEDBACK REGULATION OF THE ADRENOCORTICAL AXIS

The most succinct demonstration that the adrenocortical axis is under negative feedback control by glucocorticoids is that activity increases throughout the axis when glucocorticoids are removed. Following adrenalectomy, there are increased concentrations of various secretagogs and of their mRNAs in the hypothalamus, as well as enhanced secretion of them into the portal circulation (Stillman et al. 1977; Robinson et al. 1983; Paull and Gibbs 1983; Sawchenko et al. 1984; Kiss et al. 1984; Wolfson et al. 1985; Westlund et al. 1985; Young et al. 1986; Plotsky and Sawchenko 1987; Fink et al. 1988; Beyer et al. 1988). In the case of storage of the peptides, there is typically an initial decline before synthesis catches up with enhanced secretion. In the pituitary, there is rapidly enhanced synthesis and secretion of ACTH, and eventually, increased numbers of corticotropin cells (Eberwine and Roberts 1984; Jingami et al. 1985). A recent study has shown that the most rapid activation of the hypothalamus and pituitary after adrenalectomy is due to the stressfulness of the surgery itself, but that the delayed (i.e., approximately 18 to 20 hours) response represents true disinhibition from glucocorticoid feedback (Jacobson et al. 1989). With glucocorticoid replacement, these changes typically are eventually normalized.

As a converse example of feedback inhibition, as glucocorticoid concentrations are raised above normal, the magnitude of a subsequent stress-response is inhibited. This can be shown most clearly with the artificial circumstance of administering exogenous glucocorticoids and then stressing the individual. An elegant example of this (figure 3.3, taken from Keller-Wood et al. 1984) focused on the fact that glucocorticoid pretreatment inhibits the ACTH secretory response to hypoglycemic stress. Critically, there is a constant proportionality to this feedback. First, the authors showed that in control animals (i.e., those without glucocorticoid feedback), increasing the magnitude of the

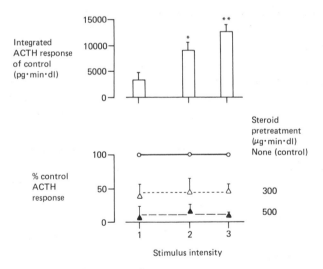

Figure 3.3. Glucocorticoid inhibition of stimulus-induced ACTH secretion is proportional to stimulus intensity. The relationship between stimulus intensity and the integrated ACTH response to insulin-induced hypoglycemia in conscious dogs is shown in the top panel. The proportionality of the feedback signal (provided by prior infusions of ACTH at three different rates) on stimulated ACTH secretion is shown in the bottom panel. (From Dallman et al., 1987, Recent Prog Horm Res 43, 113. Reprinted courtesy of Academic Press.)

hypoglycemia increased the magnitude of the ACTH response (i.e., the dose-responsiveness discussed in chapter 2). Then, by superimposing glucocorticoid feedback upon this, they showed that X amount of glucocorticoids infused caused the same percentage inhibition of ACTH response, regardless of the intensity of the hypoglycemia. This important observation suggests that glucocorticoids impair the capacity of the system to respond to this stressor, rather than cause the stressor to be sensed as "less stressful" in some absolute way.

In the more physiologic situation of a stressor occurring when circulating glucocorticoid concentrations are high due to endogenous release (i.e., in the case of repeated stressors), the feedback component is somewhat obscured by the facilitation of responsiveness that occurs with repeated stressors. This was discussed in the previous chapter.

The Differing Forms of Glucocorticoid Feedback Regulation

In summary, the adrenocortical axis is a closed-loop system of end-product inhibition; in that regard, it is just like most classic endocrine axes. Logically, the higher the circulating levels of glucocorticoids at the time of a stressor, the less likelihood there should be for a secretory response to that stressor. However, this was shown to be simplistic early on (Smelik 1963): There was not a good correlation between glucocorticoid concentrations *at the time of* the stressor and the magnitude of the subsequent stress response. In a landmark paper that was stunning in its elegance and implications, Dallman and Yates (1969) introduced the notion of a time lag in feedback control—the system is responding to what glucocorticoid concentrations were at a prior point. Moreover, they showed that there are differing types of feedback regulation, with differing time domains.

They identified a rapid form of feedback that works beginning within seconds until approximately 20 minutes after the onset of a feedback signal. Such *fast feedback* showed the novel property of being *rate-sensitive*. Specifically, it was not the absolute amount of glucocorticoids in the bloodstream that determined how much the axis was inhibited subsequently. Rather, it was the rate at which glucocorticoid concentrations increased that determined the extent of inhibition. Therefore, in a hypothetical circumstance, a shift from 10 to 12 units of glucocorticoids in the bloodstream in a unit of time would exert more of a feedback signal than a rise of from 100 to 101 units in the same amount of time (figure 3.4).

Following this is a "silent period" in which circulating glucocorticoid concentrations have no effect on secretion occurring approximately 30 minutes later. Finally, Dallman and Yates defined *delayed* feedback, which begins to work approximately 40 minutes after the onset of a feedback signal. In this more traditional type of regulation, the strength of the negative feedback signal is a function of the *level* of glucocorticoids in the bloodstream. Therefore, during that feedback domain, the more glucocorticoids in the circulation,

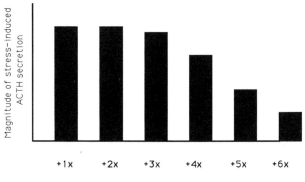

Figure 3.4. Schematic representation of rate-sensitive feedback. The magnitude of ACTH secretion in response to stress varies as a function of the rate of rise of glucocorticoid concentrations prior to the onset of the stressor.

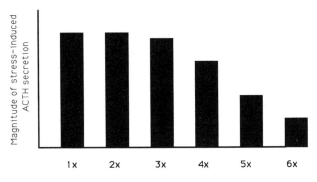

Figure 3.5. Schematic representation of level-sensitive feedback. The magnitude of ACTH secretion in response to stress varies as a function of the absolute level of glucocorticoid concentrations achieved prior to the onset of the stressor.

the stronger the feedback signal, regardless of the rate at which those levels were achieved (figure 3.5).

Subsequent work has added more complexity to this already bewildering story. During the fast feedback time domain, glucocorticoids exert their inhibitory effects only on the *secretion* of relevant hormones. Coupled with this blockade of secretion is typically a complementary increase in the tissue content of that hormone. These effects were originally thought to occur too rapidly for the classic genomic effects of glucocorticoids, and untraditional nongenomic mechanisms were posited. Currently, there is less certainty that all of fast feedback occurs too rapidly for a genomic involvement, so the issue remains unresolved. During the early parts of delayed feedback (approximately the first 2 to 10 hours), this level-sensitive feedback is inhibiting only the secretion of relevant hormones. With longer periods of feedback, there is also inhibition of the *synthesis* of the hormones and down-regulation of recep-

Glucocorticoid Concentrations in the Aged Rat

tors for hormones stimulating secretion at that tissue. In recent years, it has become fashionable to refer to the earlier level-sensitive feedback domain in which there is not yet inhibition of hormone synthesis as *intermediate* level-sensitive feedback (Dallman et al. 1987).

It should be pointed out that rate-sensitive feedback presents a fascinating problem to cellular endocrinologists—it is simply not clear how it works. It would be easy to design a cell participating in level-sensitive feedback. Above a certain level of glucocorticoids reaching the cell, a certain number of glucocorticoid/receptor complexes are generated which are sufficient to trigger a critical genomic event—for example, the inhibition of ACTH synthesis. However, it is not clear, within the recognized framework of steroid hormone action, how a cell can be sensitive to rate changes in hormone exposure— remember, in this type of regulation, the cell in effect cannot tell the difference between 10 units and 1000 units of glucocorticoids, only how much less there was some short time before that measurement. One can construct some rather complex models that would explain such regulation; it is not clear what actually occurs in target cells.

In the years following the classic Dallman and Yates paper, both forms of feedback have been demonstrated basally and during stress, at both the pituitary and CNS levels, and in various species including humans (reviewed in Keller-Wood and Dallman 1984; also see more recent examples of this in Raff et al. 1988; Won et al. 1987). Considerable information has emerged about the workings of these types of feedback. For example, structure/activity studies have shown that different parts of the glucocorticoid molecule mediate fast versus delayed feedback (Jones et al. 1974; Jones and Hillhouse, 1976; Jones and Tiptaft, 1977). Some elaborations in the parameters of the feedback have been uncovered. For example, a recent study showed that fast feedback may not just determine the height of a subsequent stress-response, but its duration as well (de Souza and van Loon 1989).

Some studies have tried to define the physiological relevance of the different forms of feedback. In the male rat, rate-sensitive feedback is triggered when the rate of change of glucocorticoids in the bloodstream becomes greater than 1.3 μg/dl/min (Jones et al. 1972), while in humans, it is triggered by cortisol at a rate of 2.7 μg/dl/min (Fehm et al. 1979). Are there any physiological circumstances in which a rise occurs this rapidly? This seems to be the case for some stressors. This then raised the questions as to the consequences and purpose of such rapid feedback. Most plausibly, it serves to limit the magnitude of the stress-response (Jones et al. 1982) or of subsequent stress-responses occurring soon afterward (as discussed in chapter 2). In contrast, the delayed feedback might serve a physiological role under the rarer circumstance of prolonged and continuous stress, or pathologic hypersecretion of glucocorticoids. As another issue, chapter 5 will discuss the evidence that the brain is more sensitive to feedback than is the pituitary, and this raises the question of how often feedback (or any type) actually occurs at the pituitary. This remains unresolved.

Feedback Regulation of Basal, Stress, and Poststress Secretion

It now becomes relevant to consider how fast and delayed feedback affect glucocorticoid secretion under different physiological conditions.

Basal Secretion   Glucocorticoids are capable of inhibiting basal secretion of the adrenocortical axis. This mostly occurs at the level of the brain. The most obvious demonstration of this would be to show glucocorticoid feedback inhibition of basal secretagog release into the portal circulation; however, because of the invasive nature of that surgery, it is never possible to obtain basal values for these hormones. However, during the circadian trough, lesion of the mediobasal hypothalamus or of the paraventricular nucleus (i.e., blocking the release of any secretagogs) has no effect on ACTH concentrations (Halasz et al. 1967; Wilson and Critchlow 1975; Kaneko et al. 1980; Dallman et al. 1985; Levin et al. 1988). This implies that normally the brain component of the adrenocortical axis is quiet during the circadian trough, and the pituitary secretes autonomously at that time. Therefore, the feedback inhibition that brings about the trough must be occurring at the level of the brain.

Among the most interesting features of glucocorticoid feedback inhibition of basal secretion is that the strength of such regulation shifts in a circadian manner. During the circadian trough, the adrenocortical axis is exquisitely sensitive to glucocorticoid feedback inhibition; this is one of the reasons that circulating ACTH concentrations are so low at that time. During the circadian trough in the rat, it takes only 0.7 nM of free corticosterone to inhibit 50% of ACTH secretion post adrenalectomy. In contrast, during the circadian peak, the axis is less sensitive to feedback inhibition, and it takes more than five times as much free corticosterone to inhibit 50% of ACTH secretion (Akana et al. 1986; figure 3.6). In subsequent chapters, I will be detailing the existence of two different classes of glucocorticoid-binding receptors in the brain. Of immediate importance, they differ markedly in their affinities; the high affinity receptor has a Kd of approximately 0.5 nM, the low affinity, approximately 5.0 nM. These are quite close to the concentrations of free corticosterone, which are 50% inhibitory of ACTH secretion in the circadian trough and peak, respectively. This led to the proposal that basal feedback inhibition during the circadian trough is mediated by the high-affinity (Type I) receptor, whereas inhibition during the peak involves both the high and low-affinity (Type II) receptor (Dallman et al. 1987). Studies using glucocorticoids with differing affinities for the two receptors and their differing capacities to exert feedback signals throughout the circadian cycle have confirmed this idea in humans and in rats (Jubiz et al. 1970; Gaillard et al. 1984; Akana et al. 1985a; Dallman et al. 1989). The roles of these two receptor types will be considered in greater detail in chapter 4.

Secretion During Stress   Glucocorticoid feedback regulation will also limit the size of the stress-response. This is shown most clearly following adrenalectomy, where the magnitude of the ACTH stress-response is greatly

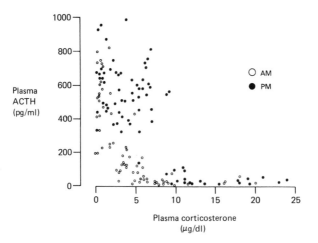

Figure 3.6. Plasma ACTH concentrations as a function of plasma corticosterone in the morning (open circles) or evening (closed circles) 5 days after adrenalectomy in rats replaced at surgery with several levels of corticosterone. There is a clear shift to the right in corticosterone feedback efficacy between morning and evening. (From Dallman et al., 1987, Recent Prog Horm Res 43, 113. Reprinted courtesy of Academic Press.)

enhanced. Feedback inhibition of basal ACTH by glucocorticoids appears to be more sensitive than inhibition of ACTH secretion during stress, as it takes less replacement glucocorticoids to normalize basal ACTH secretion than to normalize stress-induced secretion in adrenalectomized rats (Hodges and Vernikos 1960; Keller-Wood et al. 1983a; Akana et al. 1985b, 1988). This suggests a potential dissociation in the neural pathways mediating feedback upon basal versus stress-induced adrenocortical activity. As further evidence of this dissociation, the timing of the onset of the different time domains of feedback differ during basal and stressful circumstances.

As one complication already noted, in the case of repeated stressors, there are complex interactions between facilitation of subsequent stress-responses (due, in part, to an unidentified central source) and inhibition (due to the glucocorticoid feedback signal). As another complication, not all stressors are equally sensitive to glucocorticoid feedback inhibition. The bulk of stressors are sensitive to feedback regulation (i.e., the magnitude of the stress-response can be inhibited by a prior elevation of circulating glucocorticoid concentrations), and even such recent and novel stimulators of the adrenocortical axis as the immune lymphokine interleukin-1 (Sapolsky et al. 1987; Berkenbosch et al. 1987) are sensitive to feedback inhibition (Cambronero et al. 1989). However, a subset of stressors, including severe hemorrhage, endotoxins, anoxia, laparotomy, and large doses of histamine, are relatively insensitive to such feedback (Keller-Wood and Dallman 1984). Is "insensitive" a relative or an absolute term? One model is that feedback sensitive versus insensitive stressors reach the hypothalamus via separate pathways (Dallman and Yates, 1968). This would certainly make some sense for the subset of stressors detected directly at the hypothalamus, as opposed to those clearly relying on long afferent pathways carrying the stressful information. An opposing model proposes a single pathway, sensitive with a certain threshold to glucocorticoid feedback, but with feedback sensitive versus insensitive stressors stimulating it with lesser versus greater strengths, respectively (Yates et al. 1969; Yates and Maran 1974). This latter model predicts that all stressors should become feedback insensitive when strong enough. This has not proven to be the case (Gann and Cryer 1973; Keller-Wood et al. 1984) (i.e., the magnitude of the ACTH response to a stressor does not predict if that stressor will be sensitive or not to feedback).

Poststress Secretion   Glucocorticoid feedback regulation might also contribute to terminating the stress-response, in that the adrenalectomized rat has not only a larger, but a more persistent ACTH stress-response. Do adrenalectomized rats have trouble terminating the ACTH stress-response because they do not secrete glucocorticoids during the stressor, or because they do not experience fluctuations in glucocorticoid concentrations throughout the circadian cycle? In other words, is it the fact that they have not been experiencing the glucocorticoid feedback signal recently (during the stressor), or earlier in the day as part of the circadian peak, which makes it difficult to turn off the ACTH secretion post stress?

Recently, Jacobson and colleagues (1988) demonstrated that, surprisingly, it is the circadian fluctuation which is critical. In this study, three groups of adrenalectomized rats were replaced with glucocorticoids. In the *CORT-pellet* rats, corticosterone-secreting pellets were implanted subcutaneously; within a few hours after implantation, these pellets produce relatively constant levels of corticosterone in the bloodstream. Thus, these rats have neither circadian fluctuations in glucocorticoid concentrations nor stress-induced increases in glucocorticoid concentrations. In the *CORT-water* rats, corticosterone was mixed in the drinking water; because rats drink with a circadian rhythm roughly matching the normal endogenous circadian rhythm of corticosterone, these rats generated their own circadian rhythm of corticosterone. Therefore, these rats had circadian fluctuation but no glucocorticoid stress-response. In the *cyanoketone* rats, this drug was administered to intact animals at a dose that blocks stress-induced glucocorticoid secretion but is not powerful enough to blunt circadian rhythmicity. Therefore, like the "water" rats, they had a circadian fluctuation but no glucocorticoid stress-response. In pilot studies, dosages were determined such that the three groups had identical cumulative daily exposures to glucocorticoids, but simply markedly different temporal patterns. The authors observed that a constant feedback signal in the CORT-pellet rats was not sufficient to normalize the rate of recovery from stress (whereas a constant signal plus an acute rise in corticosterone concentrations at the beginning of the stressor were sufficient [Jacobson and Sapolsky 1991]). In contrast, a delayed rhythmic signal (i.e., in "water" and "cyanoketone" rats) normalized the rate of recovery from stress.

Something about a constant feedback signal is insufficient. This might be due to the fact that corticosterone levels are no longer high enough during what should be the circadian peak, and a delayed level-sensitive feedback signal is not triggered. Alternatively, levels may be too high during what should be the circadian trough, and somehow blunt the sensitivity of the axis to feedback regulation (Jacobson et al. 1988). Regardless of the mechanism, these findings show that it is not necessary to have a rise in glucocorticoid concentrations *during* a stressor in order to turn off the stress-response promptly afterward; instead, the system is sensitive to smaller rises in glucocorticoid concentrations many hours before. This is the epitome of delayed feedback.

RELATIVE INSENSITIVITY TO GLUCOCORTICOID FEEDBACK INHIBITION IN AGED RATES

This lengthy review now allows us to consider glucocorticoid feedback regulation during aging. One straightforward way of studying this would be to focus on the increased basal ACTH concentrations in aged rats. After adrenalectomy, do aged rats still have higher levels than do young rats? If both age groups then had equal (and high) ACTH concentrations after adrenalectomy, then the hypersecretion seen previously in intact aged rats (compared to intact young rats) would represent feedback resistance. In contrast, if hypersecretion persisted after adrenalectomy, it would represent increased tonic drive during aging, rather than just feedback resistance.

This study has not been possible to perform, given the extreme fragility of aged rats after adrenalectomy. Instead, feedback impairments in aged animals have been shown with a dexamethasone suppression test (Oxenkrug et al. 1984a). Rats were injected with the synthetic glucocorticoid dexamethasone, which normally exerts a feedback signal and drives down endogenous glucocorticoid secretion. The older the rat, the more resistance to the inhibitory feedback effect of dexamethasone (table 3.2; the reader should note, however, that the "aged" rats in this study were not particularly aged).

This certainly suggests a failure of feedback sensitivity in aged rats. However, a number of possible confounds emerge (which will be considered again in chapter 14 when considering dexamethasone suppression tests in human

Table 3.2. Dexamethasone suppression test in rats of 2 to 6 months old[a]

Treatment	Corticosterone level (ng/ml)		
	2-month-old	4-month-old	6-month-old
Saline	62.00 ± 6.17 (6)	68.00 ± 7.63 (7)	60.66 ± 8.51 (6)
DEX	11.2 ± 2.77 (8)[b]	37.75 ± 5.59 (8)[b,c]	68.00 ± 5.34 (7)

[a] 0.2 μg/100 g.b.w. of DEX (or saline) was injected sc at 9 AM. Blood was drawn at 1 PM. Number of observations in parentheses.
[b] $p < 0.01$ in comparison with saline-treated group.
[c] $p < 0.001$ in comparison with 2-month-old rats given DEX.
Source: Oxenkrug et al., Dexamethasone suppression test: experimental model in rats, and effect of age. Biological Psychiatry 19,413. Copyright 1984 by the Society of Biological Psychiatry.

populations). Chief among them is the difficulty in choosing comparable dexamethasone doses for young and aged rats when they differ considerably by size. Does one adjust the dose for body weight, for blood volume, or for metabolic rate? Furthermore, the half-life of dexamethasone in the bloodstream may differ by age. Thus, young and aged rats might differ in dexamethasone responsiveness not because their feedback sensitivities differ, but because differing amounts of dexamethasone reach feedback sites.

To get around these confounds, we studied feedback sensitivity in young and aged rats, using corticosterone as the glucocorticoid (to avoid the use of synthetic hormones) and monitoring the corticosterone concentrations achieved in the bloodstream by our treatment, ensuring they were matched in the two age groups. We observed that sensitivity of aged rats to both fast and delayed feedback inhibition was somewhat blunted (Sapolsky et al. 1986a).

Figure 3.7 demonstrates the blunting of delayed feedback regulation in the aged rats. Animals were infused with corticosterone in a way that achieved a steady plateau of the hormone in the circulation. One hour after, animals were stressed with histamine injections, and the corticosterone secretory response was monitored. In both young and aged rats, the higher the circulating corticosterone concentrations (produced by the infusion), the smaller the histamine stress-response (i.e., level-sensitive feedback occurred). However, the threshold for the feedback differed by age. In young rats, responsiveness to histamine was blocked by corticosterone concentrations of 26 μg/dl or higher.

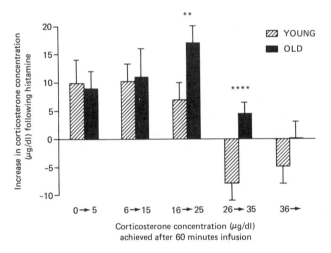

Figure 3.7. Higher concentrations of circulating corticosterone are required to elicit delayed feedback inhibition in aged than in young rats. The adrenocortical axis was stimulated with histamine 60 minutes after the beginning of corticosterone infusion. In young rats, as higher 60-minute concentrations of corticosterone are achieved, subsequent responsiveness to the histamine challenge becomes progressively damped. Similar delayed feedback inhibition occurs in old rats; however, higher concentrations of circulating corticosterone must be achieved before secretory responsiveness is damped. **, **** indicate significant age difference at that time point; $p < .025, .001$, respectively. (From Sapolsky et al., The adrenocortical axis in the aged rat: Impaired sensitivity to both fast and delayed feedback. Neurobiol Aging 7, 331. Copyright 1986, Pergamon Press plc.)

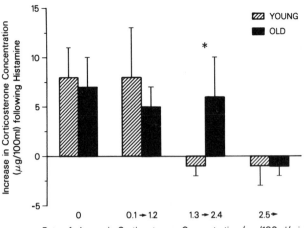

Figure 3.8. Old rats are less sensitive to rate-sensitive fast feedback. Data are presented as the change in corticosterone concentration following a histamine challenge 5 minutes into a period of corticosterone infusion. In young rats, as a greater rate of change of corticosterone concentration is induced during the 5-minute infusion period, animals become progressively less responsive to the histamine challenge. Similar regulation occurs in old rats; however, a greater rate of change of corticosterone concentration must be achieved in order to elicit fast feedback inhibition of histamine responsiveness. * indicates significant age difference at that time point; $p < .05$. (From Sapolsky et al., The adrenocortical axis in the aged rat: Impaired sensitivity to both fast and delayed feedback. Neurobiol Aging 7, 331. Copyright 1986, Pergamon Press plc.)

In contrast, this much of a feedback signal was insufficient to inhibit responsiveness in aged rats.

A similar pattern occurred with rate-sensitive fast feedback (figure 3.8). Corticosterone was infused and the histamine challenge was given 5 minutes later. Circulating corticosterone was monitored at the beginning and end of the 5-minute infusion (to determine the rate of change achieved), and then after the histamine challenge (to determine the responsiveness to histamine). Again, feedback inhibition occurred in both age groups, in that higher rates of change in corticosterone concentration inhibited responsiveness to histamine. However, as with the delayed feedback, the younger rats were more sensitive to the feedback signal, having their histamine responsiveness blocked at a rate that failed to do so in aged rats.

Collectively, these studies show that aged rats are somewhat less sensitive to inhibitory feedback signals. This might explain why there is hypersecretion of corticosterone basally and during the poststress recovery period. (It should be noted that the negative feedback literature has linked feedback resistance with basal hypersecretion far more so than with hypersecretion during the poststress recovery period; the latter phenomenon has become a focus of interest in the feedback literature much more recently. Thus, the poststress recovery problem may in fact not be related to a feedback problem at all. In addition, it remains puzzling to me why there is not also hypersecretion at the peak of the stress-response, although the system may be at a maximum at that

The Glucocorticoid Cascade Hypothesis

point.) The succeeding chapters detail the search for the site(s) within the brain at which feedback regulation fails. A final question before turning to that must be, What are the consequences, if any, of the glucocorticoid hypersecretion in the aged animals?

Given the literature reviewed in the previous chapter, they could be many and deleterious—theoretically, the hypersecretion could contribute to the atherosclerosis, osteoporosis, and glucose intolerance typical of aging. But is the hypersecretion (either basally or during the poststress recovery period) large enough to cause trouble? Because of the dynamics of glucocorticoid interactions with CBG, this is probably the case. As discussed, only the tiny free fraction of glucocorticoids are biologically active, and even a small rise in total glucocorticoid concentrations would greatly increase the free fraction. Thus, as reported (van Eekelen 1990; Sabatino et al. 1991), there is a considerable rise in the free corticosterone fraction with age. Given that many glucocorticoid effects on target tissues are turning out to be linear rather than all-or-none, the hypersecretion of the aged rat is likely to exert a heavy price.

This has been shown in two studies. In one, the consequences of the corticosterone hypersecretion after stress were assessed; the pathologic endpoint examined was tumor growth. Stress, at least in part through glucocorticoid secretion, promotes the establishment of tumors and accelerates tumor growth (Sklar and Anisman 1979; Riley 1981; Visintainer et al. 1982). This is probably due to a combination of the immunosuppressive effects of glucocorticoids, as well as their effects on tumorigenesis factors and metabolism. If aged rats secrete more corticosterone per stressor than do young subjects, will chronic stress be more permissive of tumor growth in aged rats? We injected rats with cells transformed with Fujinami sarcoma virus, stressed the rats repeatedly, and found that aged rats were vastly more vulnerable to stress-induced acceleration of the growth of these tumor-forming cells (figure 3.9). Replicating the aged pattern of corticosterone hypersecretion at the end of stress in young rats increased their vulnerability to tumor growth (figure 3.10) (Sapolsky and Donnelly, 1985).

A second study, to be discussed in more detail in chapter 6, examines the consequences of the glucocorticoid hypersecretion on neural plasticity. Following hippocampal damage, regrowth of some axonal projections occurs, allowing a certain degree of recovery of function. Such "compensatory sprouting" is normally less dramatic in aged than in young hippocampi. This was shown to be due to the high glucocorticoid concentrations in aged rats; as evidence, when basal corticosterone concentrations in young rats were raised to the levels seen in old rats, the young individuals had a similar defect in compensatory sprouting (figure 3.11; DeKosky et al. 1984).

Both of these studies are artificial in some ways, in that induced tumor growth and surgical lesioning of the brain do not represent typical pathologic insults. Nevertheless, they suggest that the hypersecretion of glucocorticoids in aged rats may have some deleterious pathophysiologic consequences. These observations gave impetus to figuring out the causes of the hypersecretion.

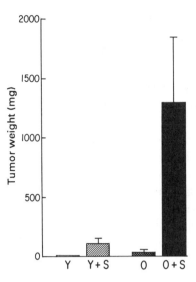

Figure 3.9. Stress-induced stimulation of tumor growth is accelerated in aged rats. Data are average tumor weight in subjects 2 weeks after injection of a threshold dose of Fischer fetal rats cells transformed with Fujinami sarcoma virus. Rats were either young and unstressed (Y), young and stressed repeatedly during the first postinjection week (Y + S), old and unstressed (O), or old and repeatedly stress (O + S). (From Sapolsky and Donnelly; Vulnerability to stress-induced tumor growth increases with age: Role of glucocorticoid hypersecretion. Endocrinology 117, 662–667, 1985. Reprinted with permission of Williams and Wilkins Publishers.)

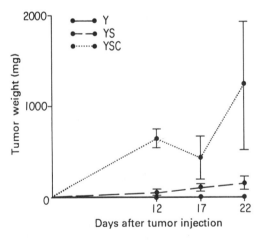

Figure 3.10. Time course of tumor growth in rats injected with Fischer fetal rat cells transformed with Fujinami sarcoma virus. Rats were either young and unstressed (Y), young and stressed (YS), or young, stressed, and receiving injections of 100 µg corticosterone at the end of each stressor (YSC). (From Sapolsky and Donnelly, 1985, Vulnerability to stress-induced tumor growth increases with age: Role of glucocortiocid hypersecretion. Endocrinology 117, 662–667. Reprinted with permission of Williams and Wilkins Publishers.)

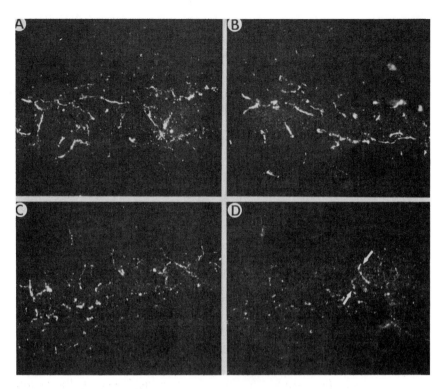

Figure 3.11. Glucocorticoids disrupt compensatory sprouting following injury to the hippocampus. Fluorescence histochemistry of the dentate gyrus 30 days after a lesion of the fimbria-fornix in adult male rats. Following this type of lesion, sympathetic fibers originating in superior cervical ganglion grow into the dentate gyrus. The response of a normal animal is observed in (a) and that of an adrenalectomized rat given cholesterol in (b). An animal that underwent steroid replacement therapy equivalent to that of young adult animals is shown in (c) while an animal with replacement equivalent to aged animals can be observed in (d). (From DeKosky et al., 1984, Neuroendocrinology 38, 33. Reprinted with permission of S Karger AG, Basel.)

CHAPTER SUMMARY

Aged rats appear to be quite capable of secreting glucocorticoids in response to various stressors, and this is commensurate with the picture of aging—the consequences of a failure to initiate glucocorticoid secretion during a major physical stressor are usually immediate and catastophic, whereas the normative picture of aging is one of decrement and gradual accumulation of damage.

The defect in the aged adrenocortical axis is one of excessive glucocorticoid secretion. This is seen basally, where there is an increase in basal corticosterone concentrations in aged rats; in particular, there is a marked increase in the free fraction of the hormone. Moreover, aged rats have a marked inability to terminate glucocorticoid secretion at the end of stress, and delayed habituation to mild stressors.

Potentially, the hypersecretion could be peripheral in origin, reflecting, for example, enhanced adrenal sensitivity to ACTH. However, the evidence suggests that the hypersecretion originates, at least in part, at the level of the brain. Moreover, the hypersecretion represents a failure of negative feedback inhibition of the adrenocortical axis by glucocorticoids. In this complex form of regulation, circulating glucocorticoids inhibit subsequent activity of the axis with differing time domains and dynamics of feedback, and with differing strengths depending on time of day, and whether there is a coincident stressor. Such regulation is impaired in aged rats. As evidence, the synthetic glucocorticoid dexamethasone does not inhibit adrenocortical secretion as readily as in young rats. As more direct evidence, the endogenous glucocorticoid, corticosterone, does not either, and aged rats demonstrate defects in both rate-sensitive fast feedback and level-sensitive delayed feedback.

This failure of feedback regulation and the resultant glucocorticoid hypersecretion appear to have a pathologic price for the aged rat. Therefore, it becomes important to identify what neural site(s) that normally mediates feedback inhibition fails with aging.

APPENDIX

As noted earlier, except for the final chapters, the bulk of the studies to be discussed were carried out on rats. This phylogenetic provincialism reflects the wealth of information available on this species. The mouse has been nearly as well studied when it comes to the endocrine issues to be considered, and far better studied in the genetic realm. However, the neurobiological and neuroendocrine literatures to be discussed are almost entirely derived from studies of the rat. The reader is referred to the recent work of Finch (1990) for an encyclopedic and masterly coverage of senescence throughout the animal and plant kingdoms.

When considering any studies regarding aging, it is important to dissociate aging itself from the diseases of aging. Fortunately, most gerontologists accept this, and most of the studies to be cited involve postmortem examination of animals and exclusion of those with pathologies that may have confounded the study. In the case of the Fischer 344 rat, which is the subject of a bulk of the aging studies to be discussed, the typical senescent pathologies of the adrenal include mononuclear cell leukemic infiltration (6% of male subjects in the 24 to 30 month range), nodular hyperplasia (2%), adenoma (2%), diffuse hypertrophy (2%), and pheochromocytoma (4%). Anterior pituitary lesions include chromophobe adenomas (17%) and colloid cysts (2%). Central nervous system lesions include vacuolization (12%), ischemic necrosis (2%), and focal hemorrhage (2%). Additional pathological features that may be of relevance include chronic interstitial nephritis (70%) and myocardial fibrosis (76%) (Coleman et al. 1977). In general, these rates of pathologies during aging are similar to those seen for other rat strains.

4   The Problem of Receptor Loss

SUMMARY OF THE BOOK SO FAR

The body responds to various somatic and psychogenic stressors with a set of convergent endocrine and neural adaptations, the stress-response. Central to the stress-response is the secretion of glucocorticoids by the adrenal gland. Glucocorticoid actions epitomize the two-edged nature of the stress-response. They are vital to surviving a short-term physical stressor, in that they help mobilize and deliver energy substrates to target tissues that need them, and they inhibit long-term anabolic physiology that cannot be afforded during the emergency. However, they are also at the center of the emergence of disease that sometimes occurs with repeated or chronic stress, and overexposure to glucocorticoids can cause a variety of stress-related disorders.

The critical need for glucocorticoid secretion during stress, coupled with the damaging consequences of glucocorticoid excess suggest that there should be tight regulation of the adrenocortical axis. This is brought about through a variety of complex regulatory mechanisms.

These features of the adrenocortical axis captured the attention of gerontologists who have wondered whether aged organisms can respond appropriately to stress and whether chronic stress over the lifetime can accelerate the rate of senescent degeneration.

In approaching these issues, a first question is whether aged rats appropriately initiate glucocorticoid secretion during stress. This appears to be the case. The problem, instead, is one of glucocorticoid excess, in that aged rats hypersecrete the hormone basally, particularly when considering the biologically active free fraction. Moreover, they also hypersecrete the hormone at the end of stress, and during habituation to mild stressors. Finally, aged rats are relatively resistant to glucocorticoid feedback inhibition, which may be related to these other instances of glucocorticoid hypersecretion. Critically, this overexposure to these catabolic hormones appears to carry a pathogenic price for aged rats. Finally, the hypersecretion of glucocorticoids appears to be driven, at least in part, at the level of the brain.

The subsequent chapter details the search for the site(s) within the brain that normally helps mediate glucocorticoid negative feedback inhibition, and which fails during aging.

A central concept of molecular endocrinology is that most hormone effects on target tissues are mediated by interaction with chemically specific receptors. Furthermore, a large change in the numbers of receptors in a tissue typically changes the sensitivity of that tissue to the hormone. The previous chapter demonstrated that aged rats tend to hypersecrete corticosterone basally and after the end of stress, and that this hypersecretion arises from a damped sensitivity to glucocorticoid feedback inhibition. This suggested that the loss of sensitivity could be derived from a loss of receptors for corticosterone in a brain region that mediates feedback inhibition. This chapter supports that idea. To appreciate that, it is necessary to review the workings of corticosteroid receptors (the term for receptors binding glucocorticoids and mineralocorticoids) and their regulation in the brain.

STEROID RECEPTORS AND THEIR MECHANISMS OF ACTION

Steroid hormones are now known to affect target tissues in a bewildering variety of ways. Because of their steroidal ring structure and lipophilic nature, they readily penetrate cell membranes and can *fluidize* them in the process, changing the affinity of membrane receptors, the coupling between receptors and ion channels, and so on. Nonspecific fluidization is usually inferred when the same effect is provoked by a broad range of steroids, including those not thought to be traditional hormones (such as cholesterol). Some evidence has also accumulated that steroid hormones can interact with *membrane-bound receptors*. Evidence for interaction with membrane-bound receptors arises from the demonstration of specific, saturable, competable binding to membrane fractions by the steroids (Towle and Sze 1983; Gametchu 1987; Quelle et al. 1988; Orchinik et al. 1991a, b). Such membrane-bound receptors could be specific for steroids (i.e., principally or exclusively binding some steroid hormone). Alternatively, the receptor could be for something else, and steroids may simply also bind to it or act as a binding cofactor. As an example of the latter, a class of progesterone-derived steroid metabolites bind to the GABA receptor in the brain, interacting with the site that also binds barbiturates. Much like barbituates, these steroids increase chloride influx into neurons. This discovery clarified the long-recognized ability of these particular steroids to act as anesthetics (Majewska et al. 1986; Lambert et al. 1987). Another recent report suggests that some steroids can bind to the sigma opioid receptor (Su et al. 1988). With either membrane fluidization, or interaction with membrane-bound receptors, the hormone effect can be demonstrated in membrane preparations, and occurs too rapidly to be explained by genomic interactions (reviewed in Maclusky, 1987; Hua and Chen 1989).

While these findings demonstrate the broad range of possible mechanisms of action of steroids, these collectively constitute a rather minor sideshow. The bulk of steroid hormone actions, however, are via the traditional route that has long been recognized: The hormones pass through the lipid membrane and bind to intracellular receptors. These receptors can be cytosolic or nuclear (and in the case of corticosteroid receptors, it remains controversial as to where precisely they are located within the cell [reviewed in Howell et al. 1990]). The unoccupied receptors can be dimerized in some circumstances, or bound to other molecules which can regulate their affinity (for example, the unoccupied glucocorticoid receptor is bound to and stabilized by the heat shock protein hsp90, and such binding is neccesary for the receptor to have its normal affinity [Picard et al. 1990; Pratt 1990], where unsaturated fatty acids bind to the receptor at a different site and inhibit its affinity for the steroid hormone [Vallette et al. 1991]). Once a hormone/receptor complex forms, the receptor is "activated" and translocates to the DNA. The translocation involves a conformational change which unmasks a domain that binds to specific DNA sequences known as *steroid hormone–responsive elements*. These are usually upstream from a gene whose transcription is then either increased or decreased by the hormone. Therefore, while peptide hormones, which bind to membrane receptors, typically change the activity of preexisting proteins (for example, by causing their phosphorylation), steroid hormones typically change the rate of transcription of new proteins. Consensus sequences for the responsive elements for most steroid hormones have been identified, and the affinity of the hormone/receptor complex for the responsive element can determine the efficacy of a hormone as much as does the affinity of the hormone for the receptor itself (Zeelan 1990).

Naturally, such gene regulation is quite complex. A single gene can have multiple responsive elements upstream, and the spacing between them can determine the efficacy of transcriptional control. The steroid-responsive elements tend to consist of two sequences which, in their idealized form, are perfect palindromes (which bind to the two zinc-containing peptide loops that form in the activated receptor complex); both the degree to which the two sequences match the idealized palindromic consensus sequence and the spacing between the two halves determine the affinity of the interaction with DNA (Luisi et al. 1991). Furthermore, there are interactions between glucocorticoid/receptor complexes and a variety of other transcriptional regulators, and these interactions can be additive, synergistic, or even antagonistic (reviewed in Beato 1989; Burnstein and Cidlowski 1989). In a further twist to this story, steroid hormones can apparently be either positive or negative regulators at the *same* DNA responsive element, depending on the presence of other binding cofactors (for example, oncogene protein products interacting with the glucocorticoid/receptor complex) (Diamond et al. 1990).

Why such complexity? In theory, it should not have to be this way. Suppose steroid hormone X modulates transcription of ten different genes in a particular cell type. Life would be so much simpler if those ten genes were arranged in series, with a single "X-responsive element" sequence upstream of them, turning them all on. Therefore, only a single copy of the receptor for hormone X would be needed. Or, if the clustering of those ten genes into a line would make life difficult for other factors that regulate only some of those genes, the genes could be separated, and the system would now require only ten copies of the receptor for hormone X. Why, instead, tens of thousands of copies of steroid receptors in a single cell, and the complexity of interactions at the genomic responsive elements?

The answer is clear when considering a consequence of such a simplified system: The cell would not be able to differentiate between ten and ten thousand copies of hormone X reaching it from the circulation. Therefore, the cell would no longer be responsive to different concentrations of hormone X in the bloodstream, but merely differentiate in an all-or-none way between the presence and absence of the hormone.

Instead, it is obvious that hormones have dose-related effects on target tissues (why, otherwise, raise glucocorticoid levels during stress?). Translated into genomic terms, there should be a *hierarchy* of steroid-induced responses: A low concentration of hormone reaching a target cell should first turn on a few highly responsive genes, while higher concentrations of the hormones should activate those genes further and/or recruit new genomic responses. How to build this hierarchy of sensitivities into the system? One possibility is to have not just one DNA sequence which forms the responsive element for that hormone/receptor complex, but a collection of related sequences with differing affinities for the complex. Therefore, the highly responsive genes would be downstream of the responsive elements with the greatest transcriptional affinity for the complex. While there are consensus sequences for responsive elements (rather than only a single sequence), and this may be a means of generating hierarchical sensitivities, it seems not to be the sole means of such regulation. Most probably, the complex interactions with other transcriptional elements is a means for generating these subtleties.

For example, one of these transcriptional cofactors might stabilize the hormone/receptor complex to its responsive element, increasing the likelihood of turning on the gene downstream. Genes that are highly responsive to a particular hormone may be those with such transcriptional stabilizers in the neighborhood of the hormone-responsive element. In addition, the interaction of the hormone/receptor complexes with other transcriptional factors allows for *conditional* gene regulation by the hormone (i.e., hormone X turns on a particular gene if and only if some other cellular event has occurred). Thus, the complexity of steroid hormone interaction with the genome affords the obvious advantage of far subtler endocrine control of events in the cell.

A central tenet of endocrinology is, of course, that the strength of endocrine communication will be changed by varying the amount of hormone reaching a target tissue. A consequence of the "receptorology" emphasis in recent decades has been the recognition that the strength of endocrine communication can also be shifted by varying the numbers of receptors. One of the most interesting examples of regulation of receptor number is *autoregulation*, where the numbers of a receptor are regulated by the amount of its ligand to which it is exposed. Typically, low levels of hormone (such as after removal of the gland from which it is secreted) lead to up-regulation (i.e., increases) of receptor number, while high concentrations of hormones down-regulate receptor number. This makes some sense, and can be viewed as an attempt by target tissues to compensate for abnormally strong or weak endocrine signals (by becoming less or more sensitive to the signal, respectively). In general, the magnitude of the shift in receptor number allows for only partial compensation for the changing hormonal signal (and in the case of up-regulation following removal of a hormone-secreting gland, obviously no amount of up-regulation can compensate for the loss of the hormonal signal). Importantly, autoregulatory changes have functional implications, such that, for example, when glucocorticoid receptors are down-regulated in the liver, glucocorticoids are less capable than normal of inducing tyrosine aminotransferase (Yi-Li et al. 1989).

The mechanisms underlying autoregulatory change are many. For example, for a few hours after exposing a target tissue to heavy steroid hormone concentrations, there are fewer available cytosolic receptors. This "down-regulation" is due to occupation and translocation of receptors from the unbound cytosolic pool. Even after the hormones dissociate from activated receptors, the latter can sometimes fail to bind new hormone for awhile (Chou and Luttge 1988). In either of these scenarios, there are fewer receptors available for binding more hormone. However, the total cellular concentration of receptors does not change. In contrast, with more sustained overexposure to hormone (perhaps 12 hours or more), true down-regulation occurs, in that the total cellular concentration of receptor declines. Such autoregulation can arise from changes in the rate of synthesis of receptors or in the stability (i.e., half-life) of preexisting receptors (Okret et al. 1986; Kalinyak et al. 1987; Dong et al. 1988; Rosewicz et al. 1988; Burnstein et al. 1991).

RECEPTORS FOR GLUCOCORTICOIDS

Glucocorticoid actions fit well within this general framework. Predictably, there are complications, in that receptors for these hormones, collectively known as *corticosteroid receptors*, are of two classes. While first characterized in peripheral tissue, they also coexist in the brain, as will be reviewed below.

The first receptor, termed the *Type I* corticosteroid receptor, binds both endogenous glucocorticoids such as corticosterone as well as mineralocorticoids such as aldosterone, thus accounting for its name, the *mineralocorticoid receptor*; in contrast, it does not bind synthetic glucocorticoids such as dexamethasone. (This has been challenged recently, in that the receptor does turn out to bind dexamethasone with a high affinity [Luttge et al. 1989a]; however, dexamethasone is not able to stimulate any Type I–typical responses in the brain, arguing against the biological relevance of the binding [Bohus and de Kloet, 1981; Nestler et al. 1981; Sumners and Fregley, 1989).

In contrast, the *Type II* corticosteroid receptor preferentially binds corticosterone and dexamethasone (with only a small affinity for aldosterone); for this reason, it is termed the *glucocorticoid receptor*. While this dichotomy in ligand specificity is not perfect, it is fairly accurate within the physiological range of hormone concentrations.

The two receptors also differ in affinity and distribution. The Type I receptor is of extremely high affinity for both aldosterone and corticosterone (Kd approximately 0.5 nM). In peripheral organs, the Type I receptor is restricted to the kidney (logically, given its mediation of mineralocorticoid effects), colon, and salivary glands. In contrast, the Type II receptor has an approximate order of magnitude lower affinity for corticosterone (2.5 to 5.0 nM). It is found in nearly every cell type throughout the body. Basically, in peripheral tissues, glucocorticoid actions are typically mediated by the Type II receptor. As will be seen, the distribution in the brain of the two receptors and their differing affinities has some important functional implications.

The dual role of the Type I receptor (i.e., it binds both mineralocorticoids and glucocorticoids) creates some interesting difficulties. In the kidney, it has a mineralocorticoid flavor, given its mediation of aldosterone effects on water balance. In contrast, in the hippocampus (which has plentiful Type I receptors), the bulk of the actions which it mediates are glucocorticoid (Bohus and de Kloet 1981; Micheau et al. 1985; Micco and McEwen 1980; de Kloet et al. 1982, 1986; Arriza et al. 1988), and aldosterone often functions as an antagonist to glucocorticoid action (de Kloet et al. 1990). How does the same receptor know which hormone to pay attention to? A quantitative analysis of hormone data raises an even more perplexing question. The Type I receptor has roughly equal affinities for both aldosterone and corticosterone. Yet, the latter circulates at a concentration an order of magnitude higher than the former under most circumstances. Therefore, one suddenly has the nagging quandary—how does aldosterone ever effectively compete with the corticosterone and manage to get to the receptor? Why isn't the kidney a glucocorticoid-responsive organ?

One can construct some models that would solve this problem. Traditionally, corticosteroid receptors (i.e., both Types I and II) were thought to float freely in the cytoplasm. This was due to their being measurable in a free, unbound state in cytosolic fractions prepared by ultracentrifugation of homogenized cells. More recent work suggests that the Type I receptor is, instead, somehow loosely bound to the nuclear membrane (from which it is sheared free during the ultracentrifugation, giving the mistaken impression that it is normally free in the cytoplasm). This mooring to the nuclear membrane led to the suggestion that, due to changes in the substratum to which it was attached, the binding preference of the receptor could be regulated. In one conformation, it would have the usual equal affinity for corticosterone and aldosterone (thus guaranteeing that only the more plentiful corticosterone would interact with it), while in a different conformation, there would be enough of a preference for aldosterone to guarantee a mineralocorticoid effect. In this scenario, when the receptor is sheared free of the mooring during ultracentrifugation, it reverts to the generic "aldosterone = corticosterone" form (Funder and Sheppard 1987). Some evidence for this model has been found (Arriza et al. 1988).

In another model, the Type I receptor always has an equal affinity for aldosterone and corticosterone. However, within the cell (specifically, in the area of the receptors) is found a degradative enzyme that breaks down glucocorticoids, allowing aldosterone to have access to the receptor. In this scenario, the geometry of receptor distribution allows glucocorticoids to still interact freely with the Type II glucocorticoid receptor (located throughout the cytoplasm, and thus more peripheral than the Type I receptor). However, the glucocorticoids are degraded before they reach the inner circle of Type I receptors. Such a degradative enzyme, 11-β-hydroxysteroid dehydrogenase, has been demonstrated in the kidney (Funder et al. 1988) and in the brain (including the hippocampus), where it may buffer neurons from some of the effects of glucocorticoids (Sakai et al. 1989; Moisan et al. 1990; Lakshmi et al. 1991; Seckl et al. 1991). One can postulate that the enzyme will only be found in some hippocampal neurons, and those will be aldosterone responsive. Such mapping studies have not yet been conducted.

When considering the tissues in which both Types I and II receptors are primarily concerned with binding glucocorticoids (i.e., the hippocampus), the obvious question is why two receptor types are needed. Two rather different ideas are currently being discussed in the field:

1. Two receptors with very different affinities for the same ligand is simply a convenient way to expand the range of responses to the single hormone, allowing responses to small changes in low basal levels of the hormone as well as to enormous changes at the ceiling of hormone secretion. This makes considerable sense when considering glucocorticoids, given that their secretion is tightly regulated basally (and small increases in basal secretion have deleterious consequences), while it is also a system that occasionally has to have explosive increases in secretion (i.e., during stress). In order to bring about the same flexibility with a single receptor system, one would need a vast number of those receptors, and extreme post-receptor sensitivity (in order to distinguish between small changes at the extremes of receptor occupancy). "We suggest that there is no single receptor system which can adequately accommodate such a dynamic change, but two receptors with high and low affinity could provide a continuum of control and thus expand the range of the physiological response" (Evans and Arriza 1989). This teleological argument for having two receptors for glucocorticoids generates the prediction that, at least in some ways, Types I and II receptor occupany should have qualitatively similar effects on the cell, but simply of different magnitudes. This has been shown in molecular studies in transfected cells expressing either receptor type; both receptor types, when interacting with their specific responsive element, were able to turn on the same luciferase reporter gene. Importantly, in support of this idea of an overlap, the Type I response was triggered by a lower glucocorticoid concentration, but its maximal magnitude of luciferase induction was smaller than were Type II responses (Arriza et al. 1987). As a physiological example of this (discussed in chapter 3), both Types I and II receptors appear to mediate glucocorticoid feedback inhibition of basal adrenocortical activity, but the former mediates the highly sensitive inhibition occurring during the circadian trough, while the latter contributes only to inhibition during the less sensitive circadian peak. In arguing against this idea of the two-receptor system forming a functional continuum, one should point out that the luciferase studies were conducted with a rather unphysiologic transfection system, and that just because both Types I and II receptors appear to mediate aspects of feedback inhibition, this does not imply a continuum of the cellular mechanisms bringing about such inhibition.

2. Two receptors with very different affinities for the same ligand afford very different ligand-mediated responses, depending on the concentrations of this ligand. This idea also makes considerable sense when considering gluco-

corticoids, in that it allows glucocorticoids to do very different things under basal and stressed circumstances (i.e., the former involves heavy occupancy of only the Type I receptors whereas the latter involves heavy occupancy of both) (de Kloet and Reul 1987; de Kloet et al. 1987), or during circadian trough versus circadian peak or stressed times. In an extension of this scenario, the two receptor types might even mediate opposite functions (de Kloet et al. 1990). This scenario would work so long as the Type II effects dominant when both Types I and II receptors are heavily occupied. There is evidence for the two receptor systems working in this way as well. For example, the glucocorticoid induction of the vesicular protein synapsin I is mediated only by Type I occupancy (Nestler et al. 1981). As another example, in hippocampal CA_1 neurons, Type I receptor occupancy mediates cellular excitability, while Type II occupancy does the opposite (Joels and de Kloet 1989a,b; Joels et al. 1991). A similar dichotomy occurs in Type I versus Type II regulation of some aspects of behavior, learning, and cardiovascular physiology (Bohus et al. 1982; Van den Berg et al. 1990). In a striking example of this in the metabolic realm of glucocorticoid actions, glucocorticoid concentrations in the range seen during the circadian trough are anabolic (in terms of weight gain and feeding efficiency), whereas all higher concentrations are catabolic. As a more explicit demonstration of the multiple receptor mediation of these opposing effects, the low-dose anabolism can be triggered by Type I agonists, whereas the higher-dose catabolism is triggered by Type II agonists (Devenport et al. 1989). No doubt each of these models of the workings of this two receptor system will prove valid in some instances, and this remains an area of very active research.

Once glucocorticoids bind to their receptor (either Type I or II), translocation to the DNA occurs. Both receptor types have been cloned recently (Arriza et al. 1987; Hollenberg et al. 1985), and it is understood which parts of the protein are essential for hormone binding, for nuclear translocation, and for binding to the DNA (Wolff et al. 1987; Evans 1988). Consensus sequences for glucocorticoid-responsive elements (GREs) in DNA have been recognized that overlap with responsive elements for other steroid hormone/receptor complexes (Moore, 1989). Once glucocorticoids and their receptors bind to the DNA, they can positively or negatively regulate genomic activity (i.e., increase or decrease transcription rates). Examples of positive regulation occur at the genes for glutamine synthetase, lipocortin, and calbindin; negative regulation is seen at the POMC (pro-opio melanocortin) gene (Yamamoto 1985). As noted above, the glucocorticoid/receptor complex interacts not only with the DNA, but with other transcriptional factors.

CORTICOSTEROID RECEPTORS IN THE BRAIN AND THEIR REGULATION

As noted, the brain contains both corticosteroid receptor types, but with differing distributions. Type I receptors are limited almost exclusively to the hippocampus and septum; within the hippocampus, they are widespread, but most plentiful in the CA_1, CA_3, and dentate regions (Reul and de Kloet 1985, 1986, as based on cytosolic binding assays and on autoradiography, respectively). In some of the receptor binding studies, an order of magnitude lower level of Type I receptors are found in additional brain regions such as the nucleus of the solitary tract, the paraventricular nucleus of the hypothalamus (containing the cell bodies for CRF- and vasopressin-containing neurons), and the cortex (Reul and de Kloet 1985; Luttge et al. 1989a,b). In more recent studies, levels of mRNA for the Type I receptor have been measured throughout the brain. Some investigators have found a pattern similar to that reported for receptor binding (i.e., relatively enormous levels of mRNA in the hippocampus and septum, but consistent amounts elsewhere [Chao et al. 1989]), while others have found mRNA only in the hippocampus and septum (Arriza et al. 1988). Whether the studies differ in their stringency of detection is not clear, but it is safe to conclude that the hippocampus and septum are vastly more important Type I sites than other brain regions.

The Type II receptor is far more evenly distributed than the Type I. It occurs in essentially every region of the brain to at least some extent, and in both neurons and glia. While studies differ as to the precise neuroanatomical distribution, the general consensus has been that the hippocampus (particularly the dentate), paraventricular nucleus, amygdala, cortex, and nucleus of the solitary tract are among the most pronounced of target sites (McEwen et al. 1986). These conclusions are based on receptor binding studies (cf. Reul and de Kloet 1985), immunocytochemical studies using antibodies against the receptor (Gustafsson et al. 1987; van Eekelen et al. 1987), and in situ hybridization work (Aronsson et al. 1988). (It should be noted that this dichotomy between the two receptor types, in terms of distribution and affinities for different steroids, was defined best in the rat. Studies of other species, such as the dog or hamster, have shown these differences to be less extreme [Reul et al. 1990; Sutanto and de Kloet 1987].)

This dichotomizing between the two receptor types is only recent, and was made possible by the development (through studies of peripheral corticosteroid receptors) of highly specific antagonists against each receptor (Reul and de Kloet, 1985). Much of the literature to be discussed below predates the distinction, and some interpretations of the data made at the time were wrong. For example, the earliest demonstrations of corticosteroid receptors in the brain involved qualitative autoradiography with ^{3}H-corticosterone (McEwen et al. 1968). With the development of quantitative autoradiographic techniques (Palacios et al. 1981), similar tracer doses of ^{3}H-corticosterone could be used to quantify receptor concentrations within individual cell fields (Sapolsky et al. 1983c). In both of the studies, the hippocampus and septum were far more heavily labeled than any other brain region. In contrast, when ^{3}H-dexamethasone was used as the ligand, labeling was lower and more evenly distributed throughout the brain (Rees et al. 1966; Stumpf 1971; Warembourg 1975; Sapolsky and McEwen 1985). In hindsight, it is apparent that the dexamethasone was labeling the ubiquitous Type II receptors, whereas the corticosterone was apparently of a low enough concentration to only label the high-affinity Type I receptors. At the time, however, the interpretation some-how evolved that the corticosterone labeled neurons, whereas dexamethasone only labeled glia. This interpretation depended on the idea that dexame-thasone (which is not transported by CBG) could only gain access to the brain through slow diffusion in from the ventricles, mostly reaching ependymal glia. This was thought to account for the broad distribution of its binding. There were many obvious problems with this interpretation, but it was accepted and oddly unquestioned at the time (see, for example, the now-embarrassing discussion in Sapolsky et al. 1983b).

Collectively, these studies show the hippocampus to be a major target tissue for glucocorticoids in the brain (along with the septum, amygdala, and hypothalamus). The original studies predating the Type I/II distinction and dismissing dexamethasone binding as "merely" glial, left the impression that the hippocampus and septum were the only sites in the brain to have substan-tial amounts of neuronal corticosteroid receptors. While the more recent studies have shown that this is untrue, the hippocampus still has more total corticosteroid receptors than any other brain site. Both receptor types are plentiful throughout the structure, although there is some disagreement about the precise distributions. Immunocytochemistry and in situ hybridization studies indicate that Type I receptors are most concentrated in the CA_3 cell field, while Type II receptors are densest in CA_1 and CA_2 (Arriza et al. 1988; Fuxe et al. 1985; Aronsson et al. 1988; van Eekelen et al. 1987, 1988; Herman et al. 1989a, Yang et al. 1988; Sousa et al. 1989). This contrasts with binding studies (using either autoradiography or assays of micropunches of tissue from different hippocampal regions), which show a fairly different pattern (Reul and deKloet 1985, 1986). This remains unresolved and reflects the not very surpris-ing fact that levels of mRNA, of protein for a receptor, and degree of binding by that receptor may not always change in parallel. In any case, there are plentiful amounts of both receptor types throughout the hippocampus, and numerous neurons probably coexpress both receptors (Arriza et al. 1988; van Eekelen et al. 1987, 1988; Herman et al. 1989a).

The autoregulation of receptor number discussed previously certainly ap-plies to corticosteroid receptors in the brain. Up-regulation occurs after adre-nalectomy (as first demonstrated by McEwen et al. 1974), and the process occurs to different extents in different brain regions (Turner 1986) (interest-ingly, the rise is transient, lasting approximately a week). From a physiological standpoint, it is even more interesting that sustained glucocorticoid exposure during stress can down-regulate neural corticosteroid receptors in some circum-stances. In the first demonstration of this (Sapolsky et al. 1983b), 3 weeks of varied stressors (e.g., cold, ether, histamine, immobilization) caused down-regulation without changing the affinity of corticosteroid receptors (this study predated the Type I/II dichotomy). Most interestingly, down-regulation was not induced in all brain regions; rather, there were approximately 50% declines of total cellular concentrations of receptors in the hippocampus and amygdala without changes in the pituitary or hypothalamus (although a biochemical study such as this [in contrast to an autoradiographic one] could not detect an autoregulatory change in a small nucleus within the hypothalamus, such as the PVN). This 50% figure appears to represent the limit to the down-regulation. As evidence, stress down-regulated receptors to that extent, whereas stress plus exogenous corticosterone administration caused no greater down-regulation. As further evidence, 50% down-regulation was achieved after about half a week of exogenous corticosterone administration (in the upper stress range of concentrations achieved), while additional weeks of administration caused no further down-regulation. Finally, the down-regulation is not permanent, and with the abatement of stress, receptor concentrations normalized within a week. That first study used a rather severe paradigm of stress (i.e., a minimum of three stressors per day). Subsequent studies have examined whether more subtle patterns of stressors will down-regulate receptors as well and, in general, the answer has been that the phenomenon is not all that readily elicited. Thus, daily exposure of rats to ethanol (which stimulates the adrenocortical axis—see chapter 14) for a period of weeks, while sufficient to cause some degree of adrenal hypertrophy and elevation of basal corticosterone, failed to down-regulate corticosteroid receptors (Spencer and McEwen 1990). Similarly, a series of electroconvulsive shocks as stressors raised basal corticosterone concentrations without down-regulating receptors (Young et al. 1990a), as did 2 hours of immobilization stress per day for 5 days (Lowry 1991). Collectively, these studies suggest that while chronic or repeated stressors can down-regulate neural corticosteroid receptors, it appears to take a rather severe stress paradigm. The implications of this will be discussed in chapter 6.

With the distinction made between Types I and II receptors, it became necessary to determine whether the autoregulation observed in the total corticosteroid receptor pool was due to changes in Types I and/or II receptors. This is somewhat of a mess at the moment. There is good consensus that there is robust autoregulation of Type II receptor number and mRNA for the receptor (Olpe and McEwen 1976; Okret et al. 1986; McEwen et al. 1986; Sapolsky and McEwen 1985; Stephenson and Funder 1987; Reul et al. 1987a,b, 1989; Brinton and McEwen 1988; Dong et al. 1988; Rosewicz et al. 1988; Eldridge et al. 1989; Herman et al. 1989; Luttge et al. 1989b; Chao et al. 1989; Luttge and Rupp 1990; Sheppard et al. 1990; Spencer et al. 1991). Within the hippocampus, Type II receptors are autoregulated far more readily in some cell fields than in others (CA_1 > dentate > CA_3, as measured by mRNA levels for the receptor) (Herman et al. 1989a). About the only point of confusion regarding autoregulation of the Type I receptor is how long there are changes in mRNA levels following manipulation of circulating glucocorticoid concentrations (cf. Reul et al. 1989; Herman et al. 1989a; McEwen, personal communication).

There is no consensus, however, as to whether there is autoregulation of Type I receptors. Some investigators report an increase in Type I receptors after adrenalectomy, and/or a decrease following prolonged occupancy of the receptors (with aldosterone, most frequently) (Stephenson and Funder 1987; Luttge et al. 1989a,b; Chao et al. 1989; Brinton and McEwen 1988; Spencer et al. 1991 showing the potential for down-regulation, but not up-regulation), while others report no autoregulation (Reul et al. 1987b, 1989). It seems reasonable that it is difficult to down-regulate Type I receptors with high ligand concentrations, since the receptors are usually heavily occupied anyway. Recent work has focused on levels of mRNA for the Type I receptor, and the story becomes even more of a mess. One group reports that adrenalectomy leads to an increase in levels of mRNA, but no up-regulation in numbers of receptors (Reul et al. 1989), another group merely reports that adrenalectomy leads to more mRNA for the receptor (Herman et al. 1989a), while another group reports an up-regulation in numbers of receptors with no increase in mRNA (Chao et al. 1989). The only point of agreement is the obvious one that this implies some sort of post-translational regulation of receptor number, or receptor-associated factors that confer functionality to the receptor (Funder 1991). Some of the Type I confusion might be due to rather different glucocorticoid dosages used in the various studies (discussed in Spencer et al. 1991). Nevertheless, at this stage one would have to conclude that the hippocampal Type II receptors are very sensitive to autoregulation, whereas Type I receptors are far less so. As will be seen below, Type I appears to be regulated by a number of neuropeptides instead.

These studies demonstrate that, for example, elevated glucocorticoid concentrations will down-regulate Type II receptors in hippocampal neurons. The unstated assumption when these findings first appeared was that this represented *autologous* regulation—that, for example, down-regulation of the Type II receptor was due to a corticosterone/Type II receptor complex binding to a responsive element upstream from the Type II receptor gene and negatively regulating it. Such autologous responsive elements do exist upstream from the genes. Just to make life more difficult, however, there is *heterologous* regulation as well: In cells in which both receptor types occur, occupation of one type of receptor can regulate the numbers of the other receptor type. Heavy occupancy of the Type I receptor (in this case, with aldosterone) will down-regulate both Types I and II receptors in the brain in both the rat and mouse (Brinton and McEwen 1988; Luttge et al. 1989a; the regions and magnitude of the down-regulation differed in these two reports, perhaps reflecting species differences).

As an odd twist, heavy occupation of Type II receptors (with dexamethasone) will cause an increase in Type I receptor concentrations and levels of mRNA for the Type I receptor (Reul et al. 1987a; 1989; Brinton and McEwen 1988). For example, we have observed that microinfusion of dexamethasone into the hippocampus (sufficient to occupy at least 90% of the Type II receptors, but which causes minimal occupation of the Type I receptor) causes more than a threefold increase in Type I receptor concentrations within a few hours (Stein and Sapolsky, unpublished). These observations imply that the gene for each receptor is downstream of response elements for both receptor types. The physiological relevance of such heterologous receptor regulation is a bit subtle. It appears quite convincing that heavy Type I occupancy does down-regulate the Type II receptor. Because the Type I receptor is usually heavily occupied (Reul and de Kloet 1985), this suggests that the "normal" concentrations of Type II receptors result, in part, from tonic inhibition from Type I occupancy. If heavy Type II occupancy up-regulates Type I receptor number (at the same time that down-regulation of the Type II receptor is occurring), then this should happen during response to major stressors. I do not think anyone can predict the consequences of this.

As a final complexity, corticosteroid receptor number can also be regulated by other factors, including neuropeptides such as ACTH, vasopressin, and centrally acting synthetic analogs of these peptides (Veldhuis and de Kloet 1982a,b; Felt et al. 1984; Sapolsky et al. 1984a). These effects have been most pronounced with Type I receptors (Veldhuis and de Kloet 1982a; Rigter et al. 1984; Reul et al. 1987a). In addition, Type II receptor numbers can be regulated by biogenic amines (Lowy 1990; Mitchell et al. 1990a,b), by antidepressants (Pepin and Barden 1991), by thyroid hormone (Meaney et al. 1987), or by tetrahydrocannabinol (THC; Eldridge and Landfield 1990). Importantly, many of these instances of regulation occur independently of changes in circulating glucocorticoid concentrations, and some of these nonsteroidal factors have been shown to interact directly with corticosteroid receptors (for example, THC; Eldridge and Landfield 1990).

CORTICOSTEROID RECEPTOR LOSS IN THE AGING BRAIN

With this background in steroid hormone action and neural corticosteroid receptors, one can begin to consider the aging adrenocortical axis. Does the aged brain become less sensitive to glucocorticoid feedback inhibition because it has lost some corticosteroid receptors? The remainder of this chapter documents the evidence for this loss and its regional specificity.

The first demonstations of this predated the distinction between Types I and II neural corticosteroid receptors. In a first report, Angelucci and colleagues (1980) reported a loss of cytosolic corticosteroid receptors in the aged hippocampus. A variety of studies soon replicated this, showing an approximate 50% loss of corticosterone receptors in the aged hippocampus (Sapolsky et al. 1983b, 1984a; Rigter et al. 1984; Reul et al. 1988; Patacchioli et al. 1989, Peiffer et al. 1991). We then observed that this loss of cytosolic receptors was associated with a decrease in the levels of nuclear-translocatable corticosteroid receptors in the aged hippocampus (figure 4.1; Sapolsky et al. 1983b). This is accomplished by injecting rats with saturating concentrations of ^{3}H-corticosterone, fractionating cells from the hippocampus, purifying nuclei, and determining the content of tracer (i.e., the amount of translocated hormone/receptor complexes). This study also indicated that the affinity of binding by corticosteroid receptors and the capacity to translocate were not changed in the aged hippocampus. In other words, the aged hippocampus lost cytosolic corticosteroid receptors (and thus, fewer hormone/receptor complexes were translocated to the nucleus), but the remaining receptors functioned in a fairly normal fashion. Importantly, the receptor loss is relatively specific to the hippocampus, with either no loss or inconsistent reparts of losses in the amygdala, hypothalamus, cortex, midbrain, or pituitary (Sapolsky et al. 1983b,

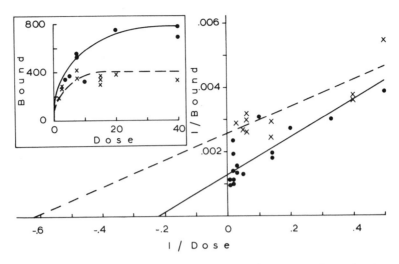

Figure 4.1. Loss of nuclear-translocatable corticosteroid receptors in the aged rat hippocampus. Dose-response analysis of binding capacity of nuclei of hippocampus of young (closed circles) and aged (X) rats, presented as bound versus dose (*inset*) and 1/bound versus 1/dose. Each point represents two pooled subjects. The dose of administered unlabeled corticosterone was injected as competition with 100 μCI of radiolabeled corticosterone. Note that the figure in the inset is extended only to the highest dose where counts were detectable in both age groups. (From Sapolsky et al., 1983, Brain Res 289, 235. Reprinted with permission from Elsevier Science Publishers.)

1984a; Rigter et al. 1984; Reul et al. 1988; Patacchioli et al. 1989; Peiffer et al. 1991; van Eekelen et al. 1991.) (As a foreshadowing, the next section will discuss one important study by Eldridge and colleagues [1989a,b] that seemingly negated these findings).

As noted, these studies predated the Type I/II distinction. Subsequent studies have demonstrated losses of both types (figure 4.2, Reul et al. 1988; see also Issa et al. 1990; Morano and Akil 1990; van Eekelen et al. 1991; Meaney et al. 1988a, 1990a, 1991; Lorens et al. 1990) (although in some of these cases, losses of both types are not reported in the same study; for a view opposing these conclusions, see Eldridge et al. 1989a,b, discussed below).

The hippocampus is neuroanatomicaly heterogeneous (figure 4.3), and corticosteroid receptors are not equally distributed throughout the structure. Autoradiographic work has shown that the receptor loss is more pronounced in some cell fields than others (Sapolsky et al. 1984a). In the subiculum, CA_4 region, and dentate gyrus regions, no receptor loss is observed; instead, the decline is most pronounced among the pyramidal neurons of Ammon's horn. In addition to this pattern indicating which neurons lose receptors, it underlines that the loss is neuronal, rather than glial. As noted, these studies predated the Type I/II distinction in the hippocampus, and autoradiographic clarification of where in hippocampal cell fields Type I versus II receptors are lost has not been carried out yet.

These observations raise important questions: Does the aged hippocampus have fewer such receptors per neuron, or are receptors lost because the

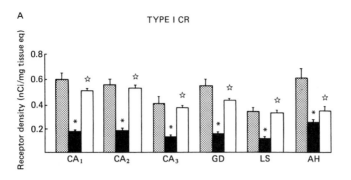

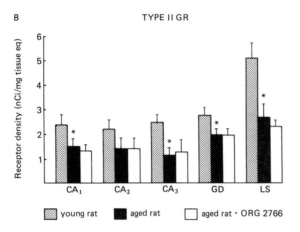

□ young rat   ■ aged rat   □ aged rat · ORG 2766

Figure 4.2. Density of Type I (A) and Type II (B) receptors in subregions of the hippocampus and lateral septum of young, aged, and ORG 2766–treated aged rats as measured autoradiographically. For the purpose of this book, this figure demonstrates a loss of both receptor types in the aged hippocampus. (From Reul et al., Neurotrophic ACTH analogue promotes plasticity of Type I corticosteroid receptor in brain of senescent male rats. Neurobiol Aging 9, 253. Copyright 1988, Pergamon Press plc.)

neurons in which they were contained have died, or both? To answer this, it was necessary to carry out high-resolution silver-grain autoradiography and count numbers of grains per neuron and numbers of neurons (Sapolsky et al. 1984a; Patacchioli et al. 1989). In our rather tedious study of this issue, we observed that (1) there was an approximate halving of the numbers of corticosteroid receptors in the aged Ammon's horn region, while there was only an approximate 20% loss of neurons themselves (a magnitude of loss documented frequently, as reviewed in Coleman and Flood 1987); (2) the percentage of Ammon's horn neurons that specifically bound corticosterone was approximately halved (from 49% to 23%); and (3) the remaining neurons that bound corticosterone had approximately half the number of binding sites. When putting these various pieces together, one must conclude that there is preferential loss of corticosterone receptor-rich neurons in the aging Ammon's horn region: Something about large numbers of such receptors predisposes neurons to senescent loss. This prefigures the demonstration in subsequent

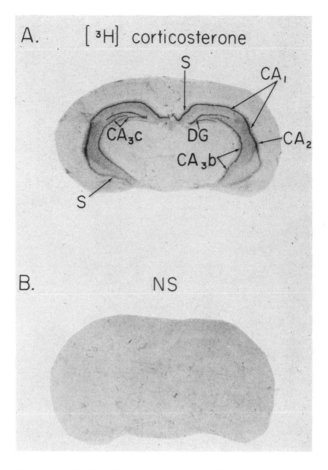

A.   [³H] corticosterone

B.   NS

Figure 4.3. LKB Ultrofilm autoradiogram of [³H]corticosterone uptake. (A) Total uptake, [³H] corticosterone alone. (B) Nonspecifc uptake; a vast excess of unlabeled corticosterone was given 30 minutes prior to injection of the [³H]corticosterone. S, subiculum; DG, dentate gyrus; NS, nonspecific uptake of tracer. Note that this study predated the distinction between Types I and II corticosteroid receptors in the brain. (From Sapolsky et al., 1983, Brain Res 271, 331. Reprinted with permission from Elsevier Science Publishers.)

chapters that glucocorticoids play a major role in bringing about the death of these aging neurons.

A POSSIBLE REINTERPRETATION OF THESE DATA

To summarize, the aging hippocampus loses both Types I and II cytosolic receptors, with the remaining ones having normal affinity. The loss is neuronal and concentrated in the Ammon's horn region. Moreover, the loss occurs most dramatically among the neurons containing high concentrations of corticosteroid receptors. Two recent papers demonstrated an additional functional deficit in corticosteroid receptors in the aged hippocampus; this finding initially casts doubt on the validity of all these conclusions. These papers reported that in the aging hippocampus, Type II receptors neither down-regulate (following stress), nor up-regulate (following adrenalectomy) as readily as do receptors in young hippocampi (Eldridge et al. 1989a,b).

This is interesting, in terms of suggesting a functional deficit in transcriptional or post-translational regulation of receptor number with aging. The authors suggested that this caused an important artifact in the literature cited above. In all of these measurements of corticosteroid receptor number (whether by cytosolic or nuclear translocation assay, or by quantitative or high-resolution autoradiography), it is neccesary to adrenalectomize rats. This allows the removal of endogenous glucocorticoids that would occupy the receptor and thus decrease the amount of radioactive binding to the receptor (giving spuriously low binding results). The trick is to find a time window in which the endogenous hormone has dissociated from the receptor (allowing measurement of 100% of the receptors present), but before there has been compensatory, postadrenalectomy up-regulation of receptor number (making it impossible to determine how much receptor there was before this perturbation). The authors of these recent reports argued that the aged hippocampus does not really lose receptors. Rather, they posit, everyone is measuring them under conditions where there is already postadrenalectomy up-regulation occurring. They theorize that both young and aged hippocampi start from the same point but, because the latter are impaired in up-regulation, by the time the rats are killed and receptors measured, they have fewer receptors; the incorrect conclusion is then reached that the aged hippocampus normally has fewer receptors. Following up on this idea, the authors then show that under different measurement conditions, there is no loss of Type II receptors in the aged hippocampus.

This is an important observation, and one which potentially changes the thinking outlined above. However, I am unconvinced of this revisionism for three reasons:

1. In some demonstrations of corticosteroid receptor loss in the aged hippocampus, the postadrenalectomy interval was up to 7 days (for example, the demonstration of decreased nuclear translocation [Sapolsky et al. 1983b]). The revisionist view is correct in critiquing this, as this is sufficient time for compensatory up-regulation to have occurred (McEwen et al. 1974, 1980). However, at least two of the demonstrations of receptor loss (the demonstration of decreased cytosolic number [Sapolsky et al. 1983b, 1984a] and the quantitative and high-resolution autoradiography data [Sapolsky et al. 1984a]) were carried out 12 hours after adrenalectomy, an interval at which there is little evidence of up-regulation occurring in young hippocampi (McEwen et al. 1974). Therefore, the age difference observed at that point cannot be a function of different speeds of up-regulation.

2. There are rather considerable technical problems in interpreting the reports by Eldridge et al. (1989a,b) in which this revisionism was proposed (the reader should be forewarned: This next section will be stultifying to all but the most ardent fans of steroid receptor assay methodology). In order to get around the problem of deciding when postadrenalectomy up-regulation has occurred (and thus when animals of different ages begin to differ arti-

factually), the authors did not adrenalectomize the rats. Therefore, endogenous glucocorticoids are still binding to the receptor. Under such conditions, if the cytosolic fraction is incubated with the tritiated glucocorticoids for the minimal amount of time it takes for binding equilibrium to occur, only receptors that were unoccupied at the time of death will bind radioactive hormone (i.e., there will not have yet been time for the previously occupied receptors to dissociate). If the cytosolic fraction is, instead, incubated for the length of time it requires for all of the endogenous hormone to dissociate and be replaced by radioactive hormone (i.e., "exchange conditions"), the technique yields a measure of the total number of receptors at the time of death. In theory, such exchange assays are possible with corticosteroid receptors, but they have proven to be far less effective in practice, mainly because the Type II receptors, once transformed, do not rebind steroid very readily (Chou and Luttge 1988). Thus, the data derived by the authors was not likely to be comparable to those of the previous studies that they purported to negate—it is not really possible to conduct an exchange assay that will give accurate measures of total corticosteroid receptors, and if the authors were merely measuring the unoccupied fraction, this would be a different endpoint than utilized by the previous investigators. Moreover, since the authors ran their incubations "overnight" (Eldridge et al. 1989a), it is difficult to evaluate whether they were even measuring the unoccupied fraction accurately in the absence of any exchange occurring.

(There were additional problems in these studies. The authors note [Eldridge et al. 1989b] that under their conditions of measuring unoccupied Type II receptors in young intact rats, they find the same quantity of receptors as when they measured total receptor number in young rats adrenalectomized 2 days earlier—thus, either their measures in the first case are incorrectly large, or else the robust postadrenalectomy up-regulation of receptors in young rats that is the center of their previous paper [Eldridge et al. 1989a] does not occur. As a second problem, in their demonstration that the chronic stress of a repeated shock paradigm does not down-regulate Type II receptors in the aged hippocampus very readily, the authors do not document the concentrations of circulating corticosterone achieved by the stressor, but mention in passing that "plasma CORT [corticosterone] concentrations in rats chronically trained in this apparatus, or in similar tasks, have been found to be even *lower* than in unstressed controls [italics added]." [Eldridge et al. 1989b] Therefore, it is not surprising that they do not see glucocorticoid-induced down-regulation of receptors, if glucocorticoid concentrations are not elevated).

3. Recent molecular evidence supports the picture of receptor loss in the aged hippocampus. Amid the confusions of trying to infer the total number of receptors by binding kinetics, it would be quite helpful to simply measure total receptor number immunocytochemically (i.e., independent of binding status). This has been done recently, and the aged hippocampus was shown to sustain a loss of Type II immunoreactivity (Zoli et al. 1991a). Another way of getting around the confusion of receptor binding studies would come from measuring levels of mRNA for the receptors instead. Such levels (while certainly not

correlating exactly with numbers of receptors) gives some indirect sense of numbers of receptors, independent of issues of occupancy and adrenalectomy-induced autoregulation. The molecular tools for such an analysis have become available recently, and aged hippocampi were shown to sustain a substantial loss of mRNA for Type II receptors, with no decline elsewhere in the brain (Morano and Akil 1990; Reiffer et al. 1991; van Eekelen et al. 1991).

Given these data, I would come down in favor of there being a pronounced loss of corticosteroid receptors in the hippocampus during aging.

CHAPTER SUMMARY

Chapter 2 established that the aged rat hypersecretes glucocorticoids and is less sensitive to glucocorticoid feedback inhibition. Because such feedback is mediated by interactions with receptors for glucocorticoids, and a marked decrease in the numbers of such receptors could cause a desensitization of feedback regulation, the obvious question is raised—Is there a loss of receptors for glucocorticoids in some area of the aged brain that could explain the feedback insensitivity?

To appreciate the answer, it is necessary to review steroid hormone receptorology, with a particular emphasis on receptors for glucocorticoids in the brain. The bulk of steroid hormone action is attributable to binding to intracellular receptors; following the binding, the hormone/receptor complex translocates to the DNA and binds to specific sequences—responsive elements—which are upstream from genes under the transcriptional control of that hormone. The hormone/receptor complex can either increase or decrease genomic transcription, and this regulation occurs in consort with a bewildering variety of other transcriptional factors.

Glucocorticoid action fits within this framework but is complicated somewhat by the occurrance of two classes of receptors that bind this hormone. The high-affinity Type I receptor also binds aldosterone; in the periphery, it is limited to the kidney and is primarily concerned with mineralocorticoid, rather than glucocorticoid effects. The lower-affinity Type II receptor binds both endogenous and synthetic glucocorticoids (but aldosterone only at a far lower affinity) and is distributed in essentially every cell type throughout the body. In the brain, both Types I and II receptors occur. Again, the latter are ubiquitous throughout the brain, whereas the former are mostly limited to the hippocampus and septum. Various physiological studies have shown the hippocampal Type I receptor, despite its capacity to also bind aldosterone, to be primarily a mediator of glucocorticoid actions. Therefore, the hippocampus contains both a low- and high-affinity system of glucocorticoid-binding receptors, and the convincing argument has been made that this allows for a greatly expanded range of responses. This makes sense in considering that glucocorticoid concentrations must be tightly regulated with the basal range (given the pathologic consequences of slight glucocorticoid excess), yet must increase dramatically during stress. The restriction of this dual receptor system in the brain to the hippocampus (and septum) and the fact that the hippocampus has more corticosteroid receptors than any other brain region suggest that this is among the major neural targets for glucocorticoid action.

Receptors for glucocorticoids are subject to autoregulation, in that extremely low glucocorticoid concentrations (after adrenalectomy) cause upregulatory increases in receptor number; of greater physiological significance, high concentrations of glucocorticoids (during stress) will down-regulate such receptors. Of considerable importance in coming chapters, it is the hippocampus in which such autoregulation most readily occurs, with the Type II receptors being more sensitive than the Type I pool.

With this background, it is possible to consider the age-related changes in corticosteroid receptors in the brain. There is a marked (approximately 50%) decline in such receptors in the aged hippocampus, with losses of both Types I and II receptors. This can be demonstrated by a decline in receptor binding, in levels of the receptor protein, and in mRNAs for the receptor. A smaller and less consistent loss of receptors occurs in the aged amygdala, but not elsewhere in the brain. Remaining receptors appear to function properly, insofar as their affinity is not changed. The receptor loss within the hippocampus occurs in neurons, but not glia, and is most pronounced in the Ammon's horn pyramidal neurons. Finally, and of considerable significance, the receptor loss is probably secondary to loss of neurons themselves: There is a smaller (approximately 20%) loss of neurons in the aging hippocampus, and the neurons lost are those with disproportionately high concentrations of corticosteroid receptors (i.e., those neurons with, arguably, the greatest sensitivity to glucocorticoid action).

The loss of corticosteroid receptors (and the neurons that contained them) in the aging brain suggests that this might underly the loss of sensitivity to glucocorticoid feedback and might cause the glucocorticoid hypersecretion. The fact that the loss is so concentrated in the hippocampus focuses attention on that structure as a potential mediator of glucocorticoid negative feedback regulation. The next chapter documents this endocrine role for the hippocampus.

5 The Hippocampus as a Mediator of Glucocorticoid Feedback Regulation

SUMMARY OF THE BOOK SO FAR

The body responds to a variety of stressors with a set of neural and endocrine adaptations, the stress-response. Glucocorticoids are central to both the adaptive and pathogenic nature of the stress-response, in that an inability to secrete glucocorticoids in response to stress can be fatal, while overexposure to these highly catabolic hormones can cause a variety of stress-related diseases.

It is this two-edged nature of glucocorticoid secretion which has attracted the attention of gerontologists interested in stress. Two themes that have permeated gerontology—Can aged organisms deal with stress normally, and can a history of excessive stress accelerate aspects of aging?—are easily framed in the context of glucocorticoids. Is glucocorticoid secretion regulated properly in aged organisms? Can overexposure to glucocorticoids over the lifetime accelerate features of senescent degeneration?

The previous two chapters examined the workings and parts of the adrenocortical axis in aged rats in pursuit of the answer to these questions. Two broad classes of defects were uncovered.

While aged rats have no difficulty secreting glucocorticoids in response to stress, they tend to terminate the stress-response at the end of a stressor more slowly than do younger rats. This is but one symptom of a larger syndrome of glucocorticoid excess, in that aged rats hypersecrete the hormone basally (this is particularly pronounced when considering the biologically active free fraction), and their glucocorticoid secretion habituates slowly to mild stressors. These instances of hypersecretion are driven, at least in part, at the level of the brain, are associated with a failure of sensitivity of glucocorticoid feedback inhibition, and appear to exert a pathogenic price for the aged rat.

These findings prompted the search for the site(s) within the brain at which glucocorticoid feedback regulation fails during aging. Because the bulk of glucocorticoid actions are mediated through corticosteroid receptors, it was hypothesized that the loss of feedback sensitivity might be due to a loss of such receptors. Therefore, corticosteroid receptor levels in the aged brain were studied, uncovering a second class of defects. The aged brain sustains a loss of corticosteroid receptors, and in a site-specific manner, in that the loss is concentrated in the hippocampus (a principal neural target site for glucocorticoids, with the highest concentrations of such receptors in the brain). There is a loss of both the high-affinity Type I and lower-affinity Type II receptors, while remaining receptors appear to function normally. The loss is most pronounced in the pyramidal neurons of the Ammon's horn region of the hippocampus. Most importantly, the receptor loss is accompanied by neuron loss, and it appears that there is preferential loss of corticosterone receptor-rich neurons with age.

The present chapter begins to connect two broad defects in the aging adrenocortical system: (1) the problem of corticosterone hypersecretion (and associated with that, the blunting of negative feedback regulation), and (2) the loss of hippocampal corticosteroid receptors (and associated with that, the loss of hippocampal neurons). I will review the literature showing that the hippocampus is an important mediator of glucocorticoid negative feedback regulation, and that the damage that it sustains during aging (both the loss of the corticosteroid receptors and of the neurons) impairs the efficacy with which it inhibits the adrenocortical axis; the corticosterone hypersecretion in aged rats thus ensues.

THE ANATOMY OF GLUCOCORTICOID FEEDBACK INHIBITION

Two chapters ago, I reviewed the literature concerning how glucocorticoid negative feedback works—the different time domains (rapid versus delayed feedback), the differing dynamics of the feedback signal (rate- versus level-sensitive feedback; square waves versus sigmoidal waves of feedback signals), and the effects on release of preexisting stores of hormones versus effects on hormone synthesis. Obviously, this is a brutally complex subject. However, that review did not consider an additional question in understanding this feedback regulation. Collectively, all of those data imply that there is a feedback "brake," or brakes, that monitor glucocorticoid concentrations and inhibit subsequent secretion of adrenocortical hormones. A critical question is where are these brakes? This paves the way for asking which one fails during aging.

On first thought, the pituitary would be ideal for mediating feedback inhibition. Varied stressors are perceived via the brain, triggering the secretion of various combinations of hypothalamic secretagogs, which all converge on the pituitary to stimulate ACTH release. Given the presence of corticosteroid receptors in the pituitary (and particularly in its corticotroph cells), it seems logical and efficient for glucocorticoids to be inhibiting at the pituitary, regulating pituitary sensitivity to the hypothalamic secretagogs. Numerous studies have confirmed this. This can be shown in vitro, where pituitary secretion of ACTH in response to secretagogs is blunted by glucocorticoids. Experimental preparations have included dispersed pituitary cells or entire anterior pituitary explants; tissue could be placed in static cultures (containing secretagogs plus or minus glucocorticoids), or in superfusion systems; the pituitary tissue could be stimulated with purified hypothalamic secretagogs or (predating the isolation of CRF) with hypothalamic extracts containing relatively undefined amounts of secretagogs (Arimura et al. 1969; Russell et al. 1969; Sayers and Portanova 1974; Mulder and Smelik 1977; Buckingham 1979; Roberts et al. 1979; Phillips and Tashjian 1982; Vale et al. 1983; Bilezikjian and Vale 1983; Widmaier and Dallman 1984; Mahmoud et al. 1984; Abou-Samra et al. 1986a;

Shipston and Antoni 1991). Some studies have also examined this issue in vivo (Ganong and Hume 1955; de Wied 1964; Dunn and Critchlow 1973; Yates et al. 1971; Stark et al. 1973; Jones et al. 1977; Rivier et al. 1982; Mahmoud et al. 1984). In these cases, the hypothalamus is destroyed (to remove the source of endogenous secretagogs) or the release of secretagogs is blocked pharmacologically; the pituitary is then challenged with exogenous secretagogs, with or without glucocorticoids. Finally, the recent literature has examined the molecular biology of glucocorticoid feedback inhibition at the pituitary. Glucocorticoids can down-regulate the number of CRF receptors (Childs et al. 1986; Hauger et al. 1987) and uncouple the CRF receptor from its second messengers (Bilezikjian and Vale 1983; Abou-Samra et al. 1986a; Bilezjikjian et al. 1987), as well as inhibit transcription of the POMC gene (the gene from which ACTH is derived) (Roberts et al. 1979; Bilezikjian and Vale 1983).

Collectively, these studies have shown that both fast and delayed feedback occur at the level of the pituitary. Is the pituitary the negative feedback "brake" that fails during aging? This cannot be. The simplest test of this is to give the pituitaries of young and aged intact rats an identical CRF challenge. If the pituitary accounts for the feedback problem in aged rats, glucocorticoids should exert less of a feedback signal on the aged pituitary, and the CRF challenge should therefore provoke greater ACTH secretion. Instead, as discussed previously, the opposite occurs; the aged pituitary is hyporesponsive to CRF (Hylka et al. 1984). Thus, as concluded in chapter 2, the hypersecretion must occur at the level of the brain. This implies that there must be neural mediators of glucocorticoid feedback in addition to the pituitary.

The evidence for such a neural role has existed for some time. The original demonstrations predated the isolation of CRF and were extremely arduous studies. At that period, since it was not possible to directly assay CRF (and the role of the other secretagogs was not yet recognized), one had to assay "CRF-like bioactivity" in hypothalamic tissue. The hypothalamus would be excised, ground, and an extract of it applied to an explanted pituitary; the amount of ACTH secreted would be used as an indirect assay of how much secretagog was contained in the hypothalamus. These studies showed that glucocorticoids decreased hypothalamic secretagog bioactivity, implying feedback inhibition at the level of the brain.

Another pre-CRF strategy for confirming feedback at the level of the brain was physiological in nature. First, one would demonstrate some feature of feedback regulation in an intact rat (for example, that glucocorticoid administration blunted stress-induced ACTH release). Then, the mediobasal hypothalamus would be lesioned (to remove endogenous secretagogs) and the rat administered glucocorticoids and challenged with a CRF extract. Now, if ACTH were secreted (as it was, in these studies), it would prove that the previous blockade of ACTH secretion was due to feedback regulation at the level of the brain, rather than the pituitary (Mahmoud et al. 1984).

With the purification of CRF and the recognition of the role of the other secretagogs, it was possible to examine glucocorticoid feedback regulation at the brain more directly. Following surgical or chemical adrenalectomy, concentrations of CRF and vasopressin, and of mRNA for those peptides, increase in the hypothalamus, whereas glucocorticoid treatment reverses this pattern (Antoni et al. 1983b; Swanson et al. 1983; Suda et al. 1983; Merchenthaler et al. 1983; Bugnon et al. 1983; Kiss et al. 1984; Sawchenko et al. 1984; Wolfson et al. 1985; Kovacs et al. 1986; Young et al. 1986; Plotsky and Swachenko, 1987; Sawchenko, 1987a,b; Schafer et al. 1987; Watson et al. 1989). Elevated glucocorticoid concentrations decrease hypothalamic levels of mRNA for CRF, vasopressin, and oxytocin, as well hypothalamic content of the peptides themselves. The latter was shown by extraction studies, in which the hypothalamus was ground, hormones were extracted and then measured by radioimmunoassay or by immunocytochemical studies, in which secretagog content in relevant hypothalamic regions (such as the paraventricular nucleus or the median eminence) could be quantified. The ultimate measure of the brain as a neuroendocrine organ is, of course, the levels of hormones that wind up in the hypophysial portal circulation. With the refinement of surgical techniques for cannulating such vessels and the development of radioimmunoassays sensitive enough to measure secretagogs in the minute quantities of portal blood obtained, it became possible to demonstrate that glucocorticoids decrease portal concentrations of CRF, vasopressin, and oxytocin (Plotsky and Vale, 1984; Plotsky et al. 1985a,b, 1986; Fink et al. 1988; Sheward and Fink 1991).

In summary, both the brain and pituitary are mediators of glucocorticoid negative feedback. Which is the more important, sensitive site for feedback? It seems plausible that it be the brain, given that it, and not the pituitary, contains large amounts of the high-affinity Type I corticosteroid receptors. An extremely elegant study has confirmed that it is the brain which is the more sensitive feedback site (Levin et al. 1988). Rats were adrenalectomized and therefore hypersecreted ACTH. When an exogenous glucocorticoid feedback signal was imposed (which produced circulating corticosterone concentrations of 4 to 7 μg/dl), the ACTH hypersecretion was reversed. The neural component of feedback was then "subtracted" by lesioning the mediobasal hypothalamus (to eliminate secretagog release), and rats were infused with CRF in a pattern to replicate the rise in ACTH in normal adrenalectomized rats. With this approach, 30 μg of corticosterone/dl were required to suppress ACTH. This implies that the smaller amounts of corticosterone (the 4 to 7 μg/dl in the first part of the study) were being inhibitory at the level of the brain, demonstrating that the brain is more sensitive to steroid feedback than the pituitary.

In another model of study, a systemic glucocorticoid feedback signal is imposed which is the minimum necessary to inhibit ACTH secretion. One then assesses whether such a regimen blocks pituitary responsiveness to secretagogs; if not, then the previously demonstrated inhibition has occurred at the level of the brain, rather than the pituitary. This has been reported (although in that study, the only secretagog tested was CRF) (Nicholson et al. 1986).

In summary, the brain is the most sensitive mediator of feedback inhibition. Where are the feedback brakes within the brain? The most logical place to look is at the hypothalamus itself, and numerous studies support its role as a mediator of both rapid and delayed feedback. In in vitro studies, hypothalamic explants, median eminence explants, synaptosomal preparations, or monolayer cultures consisting of neurons and glia are made, and either secretagog content in the hypothalamic tissue or secretagog release into the media can be monitored. Addition of glucocorticoids to the media inhibit secretagog levels and release (Jones et al. 1977; Buckingham and Hodges 1977; Vermes et al. 1977; Suda et al. 1985; Spinedi et al. 1991).

In vivo studies have demonstrated a role for the hypothalamus as well. In the most direct of these, glucocorticoids are microimplanted into the hypothalamus (or into relevant subregions, such as the median eminence or paraventricular nucleus), and concentrations of secretagog mRNA or peptide, ACTH and/or glucocorticoid concentrations are measured. In such studies, one must be certain that the steroid implants do not leak into other brain regions (and thus influence other potential brakes), or leak out of the brain and reach the pituitary. Careful studies have shown that the hypothalamus is one of the loci of feedback (Kovacs et al. 1986; Sawchenko 1987b; Kovacs and Mezey 1987). In an interesting twist on this approach, in one recent study, the Type II corticosteroid antagonist RU 38486 was implanted into the paraventricular nucleus, causing glucocorticoid hypersecretion (de Kloet et al. 1988a). As additional, supportive evidence, we have recently observed that the extent of hypothalamic corticosteroid receptor occupation by glucocorticoids is a significant predictor of portal concentrations of CRF under prestress and stress conditions; the more the hypothalamic receptors are occupied, the less CRF is released (Sapolsky et al. 1990a).

All of this suggests that the hypothalamus mediates glucocorticoid feedback regulation. However, it is not the sole brake within the brain. As evidence, hypothalamic deafferentation (i.e., surgical isolation) disrupts sensitivity to glucocorticoid feedback inhibition, and rats become resistant to the inhibitory effects of dexamethasone (Feldman et al. 1973). Therefore, when the hypothalamus is isolated, other brakes are no longer being felt.

THE HIPPOCAMPUS AS A SUPRAHYPOTHALAMIC BRAKE

(This section will consider only the rodent and rabbit literature; the primate and human literature is considered in the final chapter. For a far more exhaustive exploration of this topic, see Jacobson and Sapolsky [1991b]. I thank Lauren Jacobson, a postdoctoral fellow in my laboratory, for the superb scholarship that went into that review and star with asterisks the ideas in the following sections that are exclusively the result of her insights.)

The best documented of these suprahypothalamic brakes is the hippocampus. A priori, this makes sense. If a structure is going to serve as an important mediator of a hormone's feedback signal, it must be extremely sensitive to that hormone, and such sensitivity is aided by large concentrations of receptors for the hormone. Therefore, the atypically high concentrations of corticosteroid receptors in the hippocampus suggest this negative feedback role. The evidence for such a role predated even the first demonstrations of neural corticosteroid receptors.

It is useful to first review the sort of experimental approaches utilized. The most direct test of a hippocampal role comes from lesion studies. In these, either the hippocampus is destroyed or its major route for communicating with the hypothalamus, the fornix and the accompanying striae terminalis, is severed. The latter approach is usually favored, given the traumatic nature of the lesion required to destroy the entire hippocampus.

A second model of study involves electrical stimulation of the hippocampus. If a lesion represents destruction of a putative brake, stimulation should represent putting one's metaphorical foot down on the brake, and adrenocortical activity should thus be inhibited.

Some studies have explored another version of "pressing down" on the hippocampal brake. Rather than stimulating the structure, glucocorticoids are microimplanted directly into the structure. Finally, some studies have disinhibited the hippocampus from glucocorticoid feedback regulation by implanting glucocorticoid receptor antagonists.

In terms of the endpoints utilized, very early studies (predating even radioimmunoassays for glucocorticoids) used adrenal ascorbic acid depletion as an indirect measure of glucocorticoid secretion. Later studies used circulating glucocorticoid concentrations as an endpoint, and, still later, ACTH concentrations. In the post-CRF era, it has been possible to study directly which secretagogs are under hippocampal control, examining either levels of mRNA for, or portal concentrations of various secretagogs.

Collectively, these approaches have shown that the hippocampus can inhibit the adrenocortical axis basally, during stress, and during the recovery period after stress (table 5.1). *In terms of the basal inhibition, initial studies suggested that this was either strongest during, or exclusive to the circadian trough, in that hippocampal lesion or fornix transection would raise the trough of secretion (Mason 1958; Nakadate and DeGroot 1963; Lengvari and Halasz 1973; Moberg et al. 1971; Fischette et al. 1980) while failing to do so to the peak (Nakadate and DeGroot 1963; Lengvari and Halasz 1973; Moberg et al. 1971; Fischette et al. 1980). This could be because the hippocampus truly does not inhibit peak secretion, or because the inhibitory effect of the elevated trough on peak secretion offsets the stimulatory effects of the hippocampal damage. The latter is clearly the case. When circulating corticosterone concentrations are controlled (by subcutaneous implantation of pellets secreting glucocorticoids at a constant rate), implantation of a glucocorticoid receptor antagonist into the hippocampus causes ACTH hypersecretion during the circadian peak (Bradbury and Dallman 1989). This shows that the hippocampus inhibits the axis throughout the circadian cycle.

Therefore, the evidence is pretty solid that the hippocampus can inhibit the adrenocortical axis. Is this inhibition a manifestation of feedback inhibition? In

Table 5.1. Summary of studies implicating the hippocampus as an inhibitor of the adrenocortical axis

| Intervention | Adrenocortical secretion monitored during | | | |
	Basal conditions	Stress	Poststress	Dexamethasone
Lesion	Mason 1958; Nakadate & DeGroot 1963; Lengvari & Halasz 1973; Moberg et al. 1971; Fischette et al. 1980; Herman et al. 1989a; Wilson et al. 1980; Margarinos et al. 1987; Knigge 1961; Sapolsky et al, 1984a	Wilson et al. 1980; Feldman & Conforti 1979, 1980; Fendler et al. 1961; Sapolsky et al. 1984a; Knigge & Hays 1963	Sapolsky et al. 1984a; Kant et al. 1984	Margarinos et al, 1987; Feldman & Conforti 1976, 1980; Wilson 1975; Wilson & Critchlow 1973a
Stimulation	Mason 1958; Slusher & Hyde 1961	Porter 1954; Dupont et al. 1972; Kawakami et al. 1968		
Implantation of glucocorticoids	Kovacs et al. 1986			
Implantation of corticosteroid receptor blocker	Bradbury et al. 1989			

other words, does the hippocampus put the brake down all on its own (tonic inhibition), or does it do so only under the prompting of glucocorticoids (feedback inhibition)? At least some of it is as feedback inhibition. The studies showing the inhibitory effects of implanting glucocorticoids and the stimulatory effects of implanting glucocorticoid receptor antagonists support this. Furthermore, hippocampal damage causes resistance to the feedback effects of the synthetic glucocorticoid dexamethasone (table 5.1). In another study, ACTH secretion was shown to increase after hippocampal lesion. The difference between lesioned and nonlesioned rats then disappeared after adrenalectomy—everyone hypersecreted ACTH to equal extents. This suggests that the ACTH hypersecretion after hippocampal lesion arises from disinhibition from feedback (Wilson et al. 1980). Therefore, the hippocampus helps mediate glucocorticoid feedback regulation. As will be discussed below, it is far less clear whether it also plays a tonic inhibitory role, independent of glucocorticoids.

All of this looks pretty good for the hippocampus. *However, the data are not all unanimous about it being inhibitory. Some investigators have found that hippocampal electrical stimulation can *increase* adrenocortical activity (Casady and Taylor 1976; Feldman et al. 1982, 1987), or that the intensity of stimulation determines whether the adrenocortical axis is stimulated or inhibited (Endroczi and Lissak 1962). This may be due to stimulation of different hippocampal cellfields in different studies. For example, CA_1 stimulation appears to have different effects on the adrenocortical axis than stimulation elsewhere in the hippocampus (Kawakami et al. 1968; Dunn and Orr 1984).

*Further contradictions appear in the literature. While most lesion studies suggest an inhibitory role for the hippocampus, this has not been shown in all studies, or the increases have been only trends, rather than reaching statistical significance (Kim and Kim 1961; Knigge 1961; Revzin and Maickel 1966; Kawakami et al. 1968; Coover et al. 1971; Lengvari and Halasz 1973; Wilson and Critchlow 1973a; Kearley et al. 1974; Lanier et al. 1975; Wilson 1975; Conforti and Feldman 1976; Feldman and Conforti 1976, 1979; Margarinos et al. 1987). The most likely explanation for this is the time lag between the hippocampal damage and the assessment of adrenocortical status; importantly, there is plasticity in the system, such that in the rat, by about 2 weeks post surgery, many of the features of the adrenocortical hypersecretion abate (Fischette et al. 1980). Critically, of the 14 studies cited immediately above showing no hypersecretion after hippocampal damage, all but the last three were performed at least 2 weeks post surgery. The mechanisms underlying this plasticity are not known, but imply that other neural sites influence the axis, and that following hippocampal damage, their strengths can change, producing partial recovery of function. We have recently observed a similar plasticity in the primate following hippocampal lesions, with glucocorticoid secretion normalizing over months, rather than weeks (see chapter 14).

In summary, a large, but not entirely consistent literature suggests that the hippocampus can inhibit secretion by the adrenocortical axis under a number of different circumstances. I emphasize that while the hippocampus is not the sole brake or perhaps even the most important one quantitatively, it is of interest because it is the most readily damaged of any of the putative brakes (see chapter 9), and it is the one most damaged in the case of normal aging.

HOW DOES THE HIPPOCAMPUS WORK AS A FEEDBACK INHIBITOR?

In this section, a number of questions will be considered. These reflect the recent progress in understanding this neuroendocrine role of the hippocampus.

1. *Which part of the hippocampus contributes to feedback inhibition?* Given the heterogeneous nature of the hippocampus, it is appropriate to ask whether the entire structure is involved in feedback inhibition. This focuses on two dimensions of hippocampal structure: whether all the lamellae over the dorsal or ventral extent of the hippocampus are involved, and whether all the neurons within any given lamella are involved.

It is relatively easy in the rat to lesion only the dorsal or ventral hippocampus. Such studies have generally shown that it is the dorsal portion which contributes to glucocorticoid feedback regulation (Feldman and Conforti 1980; Herman et al. 1989a; this is also shown indirectly in the failure of Tannahill et al. [1991] to inhibit secretagog concentrations in the portal circulation with ventral hippocampal stimulation). It has been much harder to determine whether, for example, CA_3 neurons within any given lamella contributes to feedback while CA_4 neurons do not. This is because it is difficult to lesion only one cell type (despite the existence of some neurotoxins which have a certain degree of selectivity for different cell types). Moreover, it is not possible to implant glucocorticoids into the hippocampus such that the steroids will reach the broad extent of, for example, CA_4 neurons without influencing dentate neurons. Therefore, it has not been possible to ascribe the inhibitory role to a subset of hippocampal neurons. My guess, however, is that if one had the techniques to selectively remove only certain hippocampal neurons, the answer at the end would be that nearly all the neurons within any dorsal lamella contribute to feedback. This is because of the circular nature of connections in the hippocampus, in which dentate neurons project to CA_4 and CA_3 neurons which, in turn, project to CA_1 neurons. My bias is that asking which neuron type is most critical to feedback regulation is like asking which one point in a rubber band is most critical to it working as a rubber band. The sole electrophysiological study in which individual cell fields were stimulated also supports the view that most hippocampal sites inhibit adrenocortical function (Dunn and Orr 1984).

2. *By which neuroanatomical pathway does the hippocampus send its inhibitory information to the hypothalamus?* If the hippocampus is going to be an inhibitor of the adrenocortical axis, it must have some means of influencing events in the paraventricular nucleus (or to the axon terminals arising from the PVN). This is shown in the demonstration that hippocampal stimulation inhibits activity of PVN neurons projecting to the median eminence (Saphier and Feldman 1987). By which route does the hippocampus influence PVN events? The only way in which the hippocampus can directly (i.e., monosynaptically) project to the medial parvocellular portion of the paraventricular nucleus is from the ventral subicular region (Berk and Finkelstein 1981; Silverman et al. 1981, Sawchenko and Swanson 1985). This is a rather weak projection. Moreover, as noted above, the ventral hippocampus appears to be far less of an adrenocortical brake than is the dorsal hippocampus. Not surprisingly, then, lesioning of the connection between the ventral subiculum and the paraventricular nucleus (the medial corticohypothalamic tract) fails to alter adrenocortical profiles (Herman et al. 1989b).

The hippocampal input, instead, appears to be multisynaptic. The most direct routes would be either via the fimbria fornix, which then connects to paraventricular projections either via the lateral septum or via the bed nucleus of the stria terminalis. Lesion and neuroanatomical tracing studies indicate that the bed nucleus pathway is most involved in the inhibitory effects of the hippocampus (Herman et al. 1989b; Cullinan et al. 1991).

3. *Which neurotransmitters mediate the inhibitory actions of the hippocampus on glucocorticoid secretion?* In the sole study focusing on this question, somatostatin was implicated in this role. As evidence, microinfusion of somatostatin antibodies into the hippocampus of rats produced feedback resistance (Ferrara et al. 1991).

4. *Which hypothalamic secretagogs are under the control of the hippocampus?* As outlined above, hippocampal lesion leads to increased concentrations of

mRNA for CRF and vasopressin in the hypothalamus (Herman et al. 1989a). Morever, after fornix transection, there are elevated portal concentrations of CRF, oxytocin, and vasopressin (Sapolsky et al. 1989). Therefore, all of these secretagogs appear to be regulated, in part, by the hippocampus. At present, it is not clear if other secretagogs, such as the catecholamines or angiotensin, are regulated as well. The state of knowledge about putative CIFs (i.e., corticotropin *inhibiting* factors) is far too tentative to begin to examine regulation of their release (this is most unfortunate, as I suspect that the minute CIF is isolated and characterized with some certainty, half of the studies discussed in this chapter will have to be repeated in order to factor in its role).

As a complication, while the hippocampus regulates CRF, oxytocin, and vasopressin secretion into the portal circulation, it regulates each differently (Sapolsky et al. 1989). In this study, we had to control the strength of the glucocorticoid feedback signal reaching the brain. Adrenalectomized rats are too fragile to survive portal surgery; instead, rats were given the adrenal steroidogenesis inhibitors metyrapone and aminoglutethimide to greatly reduce (although not entirely eliminate) glucocorticoid synthesis. Rats were then either infused with saline (low glucocorticoid feedback) or 2 hours of corticosterone in the mid-physiological range (high glucocorticoid feedback). Portal blood was collected before and during hypotensive stress.

Fornix transection did not affect prestress values of CRF, with or without glucocorticoid feedback (figure 5.1A, columns 1, 3, 5, and 7). Nor did it effect the size of the hypotensive stress-response in the absence of feedback (columns 2 and 6). In intact rats, a glucocorticoid feedback signal blocked the stress-response (3 versus 4). In contrast, fornix-transected rats were resistant to such feedback (7 versus 8). Therefore, the hippocampus mediates aspects of feedback inhibition, and does so via CRF.

The regulation of vasopressin differed. Fornix transection caused a rise in initial and stressed vasopressin concentrations in the absence of feedback (figure 5.1B, columns 5 and 6 versus 1 and 2). Vasopressin does not increase in response to hypotension stress (Plotsky et al. 1986); thus, there was no rise in intact or fornix-transected rats made hypotensive. The transected rats were still sensitive to a heavy glucocorticoid feedback signal (7 and 8 versus 5 and 6), implying participation of other feedback sites. Therefore, the hippocampus mediates aspects of initial, prestress inhibition, and does so via vasopressin.

Finally, the regulation of oxytocin was a mixture of that for CRF and vasopressin. There, transection led to initial hypersecretion, as well as feedback resistance (figure 5.1C)

These findings have an important implication. *There are multiple domains by which the hippocampus inhibits the adrenocortical axis.* It can regulate the magnitude of initial, prestress secretion, the size of the stress-response, and the efficacy of glucocorticoid feedback inhibition. Moreover, it plays each of these roles with different patterns of secretagog inhibition. The hippocampus appears to mediate inhibition of initial vasopressin and oxytocin secretion under low feedback conditions, and contributes to sensitivity of CRF and oxytocin to feedback in response to hypotension stress (as a caveat, the reader must be

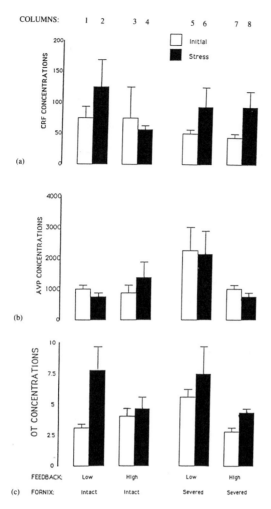

Figure 5.1. Hypersecretion of secretagogs following fornix transection. Hypophysial portal concentrations of CRF, vasopressin (AVP), and oxytocin (OT) in rats with and without hypotensive stress, with either low or high glucocorticoid feedback, with or without fornix transection. (A) In intact rats with low feedback, stress caused a significant rise in CRF concentrations (compare columns 1 and 2; $p < .05$). A high feedback signal blocked this stress response (column 3 vs. 4; not significant). In fornix-severed rats with low feedback, there was a stress response (5 vs. 6; $p < .05$). A heavy feedback signal, however, was not able to block this stress response (7 vs. 8; $p < .05$). Thus, fornix transection made the CRF stress response resistant to feedback. (B) AVP concentrations did not rise in response to stress. However, fornix severing caused an increase in AVP concentrations in low feedback rats (5 vs. 1; 6 vs. 2; both $p < .05$). Thus, fornix transection caused hypersecretion of AVP but did not alter sensitivity of secretion to a heavy feedback signal. (C) There was a significant rise in OT in response to stress in intact rats with low feedback (1 vs. 2; $p < .05$), which was blocked in high feedback rats (3 vs. 4; not significant). In contrast, both groups of fornix-severed rats (low or high feedback) responded significantly to stress (5 vs. 6; 7 vs. 8; $p < .05$). Thus, as with CRF, OT secretion was made resistant to feedback by fornix transection. Fornix transection also caused basal hypersecretion of OT in low feedback rats (5 vs. 1; $p < .02$). Thus, as with AVP, OT was hypersecreted basally in fornix rats. (From Sapolsky et al., 1989, Endocrinology 125, 2881. Reprinted with permission of Williams and Wilkins Publishers.)

The Hippocampus as a Mediator of Glucocorticoid Feedback Regulation reminded that these findings were obtained using the very invasive and unphysiologic preparation of cannulating the hypophysial portal circulation).

This suggests that individual hippocampal neurons differ in their feedback roles. They will differ as to which secretagog they inhibit in response to different amounts of glucocorticoids, with or without coincident stress. From the perspective of trying to study how this works, the prospect of having to conduct single-cell neuroendocrinology in as inaccesible a structure as the hippocampus is appalling. We are, at present, still spared the techniques that would make such an Herculean task feasible.

5. *Is the hippocampus a tonic inhibitor as well as a mediator of feedback inhibition?* As noted, the hippocampus could be a tonic brake (i.e., inhibiting secretagog release under some conditions independently of what circulating glucocorticoid concentrations are), and/or a mediator of glucocorticoid feedback. The evidence is relatively convincing that it contributes to steroid feedback. A tonic role, however, is less clear. Upon initial reading, one study (Sapolsky et al. 1989; figure 5.1) suggests that there is a tonic role for the hippocampus. For example, vasopressin was shown to be hypersecreted after fornix transection even in the absence of high glucocorticoid feedback (figure 5.1B, column 5 versus 1). If fornix transection causes hypersecretion, even in the absence of glucocorticoid feedback, that implies that the hippocampus is at least somewhat inhibitory irrespective of being prompted by glucocorticoids. However, the alternative to high feedback was not zero feedback in that study, but merely low feedback. This was because the steroid synthesis blockers administered reduced, but did not eliminate secretion. Therefore, it is not clear if transection, in this case, released secretion from tonic hippocampal inhibition or from mediation of a low feedback signal.

One study (Wilson et al. 1980) suggests that the hippocampus does not play a tonic feedback role. In that report, already discussed, hippocampal lesion produced ACTH hypersecretion. Then, lesioned and nonlesioned rats were adrenalectomized (ADX). If the lesioned/ADX rats still hypersecreted ACTH, when compared to nonlesioned/ADX rats, then a tonic role for the hippocampus independent of glucocorticoid status is indicated. However, in this study, both groups were equally hypersecretory after adrenalectomy (Wilson et al. 1980).

In summary, only one study suggests that the adrenocortical inhibition by the hippocampus is purely a manifestation of feedback inhibition. Obviously, this issue needs to be studied in more detail, examining a number of questions. For example, the strength of feedback inhibition shifts dramatically over the circadian cycle. Does the hippocampus become more sensitive to glucocorticoids at some points in the cycle? Does that represent adding on of a tonic component of inhibition? Does circadian fluctuation involve a change in hypothalamic sensitivity to an inhibitory hippocampal input? These will not be easy questions to answer.

6. *Does the hippocampus contribute to delayed or fast feedback?* To the extent that the hippocampus mediates feedback inhibition, is it rapid or delayed feedback? The following sections will detail a number of studies involving

protocols in which animals were infused with glucocorticoids for a number of hours. These implicate the hippocampus in delayed feedback. In contrast, one study suggests that the hippocampus (or at least its Type II receptors) is not involved in rapid feedback, in that hippocampal microimplantation of a Type II antagonist did not increase corticosterone secretion 30 minutes later (de Kloet et al. 1988a).

7. *Which hippocampal corticosteroid receptors are involved in the inhibition*? Both Types I and II corticosteroid receptors have been implicated in glucocorticoid feedback inhibition. In an indirect indication of this, we infused corticosterone or dexamethasone into chemically adrenalectomized rats. We then quantified the extent of corticosterone receptor occupancy in hypothalamus, amygdala, and hippocampus, and determined which best predicted the extent of se- cretagog inhibition. As would be expected from the many studies implicating the hippocampus as a feedback brake, hippocampal corticosteroid receptor occupancy (of either Type I or II) was the best predictor of inhibition of basal and stressed CRF concentrations, of basal vasopressin concentrations, and of basal and stressed oxytocin concentrations (table 5.2). In some cases, multiple regression analysis showed that the extent of hypothalamic receptor occupa- tion added significantly to the predictiveness of the model, but in all the cases just cited, hippocampal receptor occupancy was the best predictor. In another study, hippocampal Type I occupancy was predictive of basal ACTH concen- trations (Cascio et al. 1989). (It should be noted that in the experimental design of these two studies, this does not *prove* that the hippocampus is a brake or that either receptor type is involved. Because glucocorticoids were infused systemically, receptors throughout the brain were occupied, and this study merely analyzed where receptor occupancy was the best correlative predictor. Therefore, these studies only suggest roles for both Types I and II receptors in this hippocampal function.)

One style of study argues indirectly for a hippocampal Type I effect. In these studies, rats are adrenalectomized, producing ACTH hypersecretion,

Table 5.2. Correlation between extent of occupancy of Types I and II hippocampal corticosteroid receptors and concentrations of portal secretagogs under initial and hypotensive stress conditions

	Initial	Stress
CRF	Hippocampal Type II Hypothalamic Type II	Hippocampal Type I Hypothalamic Type II
Vasopressin	Hippocampal Type II	
Oxytocin	Hippocampal Type I Hippocampal Type II	Hippocampal Type II

Boxes contain the receptor population(s) in which occupancy was significantly correlated with secretagog concentration. In all cases, the correlation was inverse (i.e., increasing occupancy was associated with inhibition of secretagog concen- trations. In boxes in which two receptor populations are listed, the first one was more significantly correlated to concentration in a step-wise regression analysis.

increased hypothalamic secretagog content, and so on. Then, very low levels of corticosterone are shown to normalize the endpoint (ACTH hypersecretion, elevated hypothalamic content, etc.) (Dallman et al. 1985, 1987, 1989; Levin et al. 1987, 1988; Beyer et al. 1988). Such exogenous steroids produced free circulating corticosterone concentrations in the range of the Kd for the Type I receptor and far below the Kd for the Type II receptor. One can then argue that if feedback is caused by such tiny amounts of corticosterone, it must be via the Type I receptor, and if it is via that receptor type, it must be via the hippocampal-septal system. In a similar vein, doses of corticosterone that are too small to involute the thymus (a purely Type II tissue) are sufficient to inhibit ACTH release, implying a Type I, hippocampal-septal effect (Akana et al. 1985b; Levin et al. 1987). One can see the problems with this argument. The feedback could have been mediated by very low levels of occupancy of the Type II receptors. Moreover, some investigators (Reul and de Kloet 1985; Luttge et al. 1989a) (although not all [Arriza et al. 1988]) find small quantities of Type I receptors in other than the hippocampal-septal region.

A more direct approach supports a Type I role, in that local infusion of a Type I antagonist causes corticosterone hypersecretion during the circadian trough (Ratka et al. 1989).

Data also support a Type II hippocampal role in feedback. Since dexamethasone binds almost exclusively to the Type II receptor in vivo, any dexamethasone-induced feedback inhibition is presumed to be Type II mediated. Therefore, if hippocampal Type II receptors contribute to feedback inhibition, hippocampal lesion or fornix transection should cause dexamethasone resistance. This has been observed (Feldman and Conforti 1976). The one problem with this view is the report that dexamethasone can also bind to the Type I receptor in the hippocampus after all (Luttge et al. 1989a); as noted, however, it is not clear if such binding has biological significance.

As more direct evidence for a Type II role, implantation of a Type II antagonist causes hypersecretion during the circadian peak (Bradbury and Dallman 1989).

In summary, both receptor types appear to be involved in regulating the adrenocortical axis, and their differing affinities predict that they should be involved in different aspects of feedback regulation. A few years ago, as evidence for the Type I involvement emerged, it appeared to fly in the face of the prevailing dogma playing a rather boring rate-limiting role in this system. In the original demonstration of the two receptor types in the brain, Reul and de Kloet (1985) reported that the high-affinity Type I receptors were approximately 90% occupied even during the circadian trough. Therefore, occupancy could not be increased much by a stressor. In contrast, the Type II receptors were occupied only 5% to 50% basally, and heavy occupancy did not occur until circumstances of major stress. This suggested a functional dichotomy: The Type I receptors should carry information about circulating glucocorticoid concentrations, but in a permissive, all-or-none way (since even the lowest physiological concentrations of circulating glucocorticoids would cause nearly as much occupancy as the highest concentrations)—thus, the Type I receptors could only indicate *whether* there were circulating glucocorticoids or not. They would serve, in effect, as rate-limiting factors, where the Type I "signal" heard by the cell would not particularly increase in response to higher circulating hormone concentrations, but only in response to an increase in the amount of Type I receptor available. In contrast, the Type II receptor should carry information about how much glucocorticoids are circulating, since the degree of occupancy of these receptors would be sensitive to a wide range of glucocorticoid concentrations.

Despite the initial attractiveness of this dichotomy, it seems a bit illogical. Why should the Type I system exist if it can only really differentiate between being adrenalectomized and being intact? Moreover, it ran counter to the ideas and data presented in chapter 4, suggesting that at least in some cases, Types I and II receptors regulate a similar set of genes, forming a continuum of effects (Arriza et al. 1988; Evans and Arriza 1989). This problem is resolved with the recognition that the original estimates of the extent of basal Type I receptor occupancy were probably overestimated. One subsequent abstract reported that basal occupancy over the circadian cycle ranges only from 12% to 45% (Cascio et al. 1989). Methodologically, the two studies differed in an important way. In the study of Reul and de Kloet, adrenalectomized rats were injected with corticosterone and circulating levels were measured a few hours later. In such rats, even those with extremely low circulating concentrations at the point of measurement had heavy Type I occupancy. However, steroid injection caused a transient (approximately 30-minute) pulse of circulating hormone concentrations; therefore, the heavy occupancy due to low circulating concentrations (at time of assessment) were probably due instead to far higher (and unmeasured) levels earlier. In contrast, in the latter study showing far less occupancy, corticosterone secreting pellets were implanted, which do not cause as pronounced an initial pulse of release. Another recent study (Spencer et al. 1990) reports that basal occupancy of the Type I receptors in the hippocampus fluctuates between 65% and 95% of the circadian cycle.

These findings have freed the Type I receptors to play a more dynamic role in adrenocortical function—they are no longer simply all-or-none reporters of the presence of glucocorticoids but can differentiate between different amounts of circulating glucocorticoids. Therefore, the view has emerged that the Types I and II receptors sometimes represent a functional continuum (obviously, this would apply only to cells containing both receptor types). Type I receptors are likely to mediate information about the circadian trough, while a combination of both are involved in the circadian peak and during stress (Dallman et al. 1987, 1989; Bradbury et al. 1992). As further evidence, blockade of the Type I receptor in the brain causes ACTH hypersecretion during both the circadian trough and peak (Bradbury et al. 1992).

8. What is the relationship between the extent of occupancy of these receptors and the magnitude of inhibition? An important issue concerns the relationship between occupancy and inhibition. How much do the receptors have to be occupied before one of the secretagogs is inhibited? Moreover, if even more

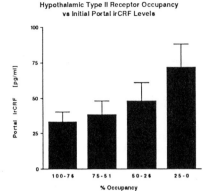
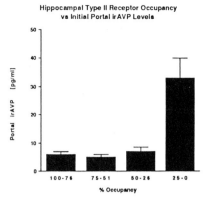

Figure 5.2. Hypophysial portal concentrations of CRF (*left*) and vasopressin (AVP, *right*) as a function of level of occupancy of hippocampal type II corticosteroid receptors. (From Sapolsky et al., 1990a, Neuroendocrinology 51, 328. Reprinted with permission of S. Karger AG, Basel.)

receptors are occupied, is the brake depressed further, or is it depressed once in an all-or-none manner?

It appears that the hippocampus not only regulates the different secretagogs under different conditions, but with differing strengths. This was observed in the study described above (Sapolsky et al. 1990a), in which corticosteroid receptor occupancy in different brain regions was correlated with extent of inhibition of secretagog concentrations. As noted, those data agreed with the fornix transection study, in that the hippocampus was implicated in regulating CRF, vasopressin, and oxytocin—the more occupancy, the less secretion. However, the shapes of these occupancy curves differed (figure 5.2). For CRF, the relationship was linear, with approximately 50% of receptor occupancy associated with 50% inhibition of CRF, and successively greater occupancy associated with greater inhibition. In contrast, the relationship for vasopressin was nonlinear. Only 12% of receptor occupancy was needed to inhibit 50% of vasopressin release; the profile looks much more like an all-or-none step function. Inhibition of oxytocin was also nonlinear, although at a higher level of occupancy.

This suggests that the hippocampus regulates vasopressin more tightly than it does CRF—it only takes a tiny glucocorticoid feedback signal to inhibit the former. While this study should be evaluated with the usual caveat that it utilized the unphysiologic portal cannulation approach, other studies using other methods suggest the same conclusion. Following adrenalectomy, there is a far greater increase in vasopressin than in CRF. This is seen when the endpoint measured is mRNA for the secretagogs, in hypothalamic content of the peptides, or in portal concentrations (Schafer et al. 1987; Davis et al. 1986; Watson et al. 1989; Plotsky and Sawchenko 1987; Holmes et al. 1986. Data showing equal increases in vasopressin and CRF: Fink et al. 1988). Moreover, it then takes less replacement corticosterone or dexamethasone to normalize the postadrenalectomy rise in vasopressin content than to normalize CRF content (Fink et al. 1988) or, for the same levels of corticosterone, vasopressin immunostaining is more suppressed than is that for CRF (Akana and Dallman 1987).

When considering the consequences of hippocampal damage, these occupancy/feedback relationships imply that it takes more hippocampal damage to disinhibit vasopressin than CRF secretion: Only a moderate decrease in receptor occupancy is needed to disinhibit CRF secretion, whereas a profound decrease is required for the nonlinear disinhibition of vasopressin secretion. Therefore, in cases of moderate hippocampal damage, any hypersecretion of adrenocortical hormones should be driven principally by CRF. As more damage occurs, oxytocin hypersecretion joins in. Only with very large amounts of damage should there be hypersecretion of vasopressin (Sapolsky and Plotsky 1990). The possible relevance of this to the hippocampal damage and glucocorticoid hypersecretion in Alzheimer's disease is discussed in chapter 14.

This allows one to hypothesize an immensely complicated picture. The data discussed regarding the differing domains of hippocampal feedback inhibition suggest that individual hippocampal neurons differ in their feedback roles. They might differ as to which secretagog they inhibit in response to different amounts of glucocorticoids, with or without coincident stress. These new data suggest that, in addition, the neurons might be "tuned" differently as to their threshold and shape of inhibition—some will be linear, others all-or-none.

9. *Do changes in the numbers or affinity of hippocampal corticosteroid receptors alter the efficacy with which feedback works?* The previous section suggests that for every incremental increase in hippocampal corticosteroid receptor occupancy, there is greater inhibition of CRF secretion. What happens, then, if there is a decrease in the number of such receptors? The hippocampus could be sensitive to either *percentage change* in levels of occupancy or to *absolute change* in levels of occupancy. If the hippocampus is sensitive to the former, a loss of receptors should make no difference: Suppose the hippocampus has a rule that, for example, CRF secretion is inhibited 80% when 80% of the receptors are occupied. Therefore, even if there is a decrease in total receptor number, it is still possible to inhibit secretion 80% under some circumstance. In contrast, if the system is sensitive to absolute levels of receptor occupancy, a loss of receptors should blunt feedback efficacy: Suppose the hippocampus has a rule that, for example, there is 80% inhibition of CRF secretion when there is 220 fmole of glucocorticoids bound to receptors per milligiam of protein. Therefore, if receptors are lost to the point where maximal receptor occupancy drops below 220 fmole hormone bound per milligram of protein, the brake can never be triggered enough to inhibit 80% of CRF secretion; there will be hypersecretion.

I know of no circumstance where the response of a target tissue to a hormonal signal is sensitive to percentage change in occupancy. Instead, endocrine systems appear to be sensitive to absolute changes in levels of hormone occupancy (cf. Yi-Li et al. 1989). Thus, when the hippocampus loses corticosteroid receptors, the efficacy of feedback regulation is damped, and hypersecretion occurs.

This is most commonly seen with the down-regulation of corticosteroid receptors that follows chronic stress and chronic glucocorticoid overexposure. As discussed in chapter 4, some circumstances of sustained stress can preferentially deplete the hippocampus of corticosteroid receptors in rats. The previous sections on the relationship between receptor occupancy and feedback efficacy suggest that such animals should then be feedback resistant and should hypersecrete glucocorticoids. This is observed. Chronically stressed rats are unable to terminate corticosterone secretion promptly at the end of stress, exactly as is seen with aged rats (figure 5.3; Sapolsky et al. 1984b; Bhatnagar et al. 1991). Furthermore, they become resistant to both fast and delayed glucocorticoid feedback (Vernikos et al. 1982; Young et al. 1990a). After the end of stress, the hippocampus recovers from its down-regulation within a week, and when receptor concentrations normalize, the ability to shut off the stress-response normalizes as well (figure 5.3). (One could argue that these instances of hypersecretion are merely correlates of the hippocampal changes, and may, in fact, not even be driven at the CNS level. For example, it could all be due to chronic stress making the pituitary resistant to glucocorticoid feedback, and thus more responsive to secretagogs. However, the opposite is observed [Hauger et al. 1988], showing that the feedback resistance must be driven at the level of the brain).

A second model of depletion of hippocampal corticosteroid receptors offers the same conclusion. The Brattleboro rat strain is congenitally deficient in vasopressin. The peptide serves its classic role as an antidiuretic hormone peripherally, as an ACTH secretagog, and as a neurotransmitter or neuro-modulator in the brain. Neural vasopressin can apparently regulate hippo-campal corticosteroid receptors, as Brattleboro rats are deficient in cortico-steroid receptors; a loss does not occur elsewhere in the brain and it is corrected by administration of vasopressin or a centrally acting vasopressin analog (Veldhuis and de Kloet 1982; Sapolsky et al. 1984b). While these studies predated the Type I/II distinction, the neuroanatomical pattern of loss

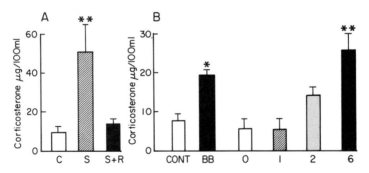

Figure 5.3. Corticosterone concentrations 1 hour into recovering from 1 hour of immobilization stress. (A) Subjects were Long-Evans control subjects (C), subjects exposed to 1 week of daily stressors (S), and stressed subjects allowed 1 week to recover from the stress regimen (S + R). (B) Subjects were Long-Evans controls (C), untreated Brattleboro rats (B), and Brattleboro rats treated for 1 week with a vasopressin analog and tested either 0, 1, 2, or 6 weeks after the suspension of such treatment. (From Sapolsky et al., 1984b, Proc Natl Acad Sci USA 81, 6174.)

(Sapolsky et al. 1984b) suggests that it is the Type I receptors which are deficient (McEwen et al. 1986). The Brattleboro rat hypersecretes corticosterone at the end of stress, just as with the aged rat or the chronically stressed rat (figure 5.3). Furthermore, normalization of the receptor deficit with a vasopressin analog normalizes corticosterone secretion. Finally, after suspension of the vasopressin analog therapy, receptor concentrations decline over 6 weeks to pretreatment levels, and corticosterone hypersecretion reemerges in parallel.

This can also be shown in rats in whom diabetes mellitus has been induced with the drugs streptozotocin or alloxan. Such animals show a small reduction in hippocampal corticoteroid receptor number and, accompanying that, a neurally driven syndrome of glucocorticoid hypersecretion that includes basal hypersecretion, an enhanced and prolonged stress-response, and feedback resistance (reviewed in Scribner et al. 1991). Another example of this is seen with the demonstration that, following manipulation of social setting in rats, a reduction in hippocampal Type I receptor number was associated with a sluggish habituation of glucocorticoid secretion to novelty stressors (Maccari et al. 1991a). In another example of this relationship, although a more purely correlative one, rats with lower affinities of both Types I and II hippocampal corticosteroid receptors were reported to show the same problem with habituating secretion to a novelty stressor (the stressor of a novel environment) (Maccari et al. 1991b).

These models indicate that hippocampal feedback efficacy is sensitive to concentrations of or affinities of receptors. Among these various models, the common neural site at which a change in number or affinity occurs is the hippocampus, and in no case is the receptor loss accompanied by neuron loss (Sapolsky et al. 1984a; Sapolsky et al. 1985). (Glucocorticoids and vasopressin appear to regulate hippocampal corticosteroid receptor number independently. Autoradiographic analysis demonstrates differing hippocampal cell fields sensitive to each of the substances [Sapolsky et al. 1984a]. Furthermore, glucocorticoid-induced autoregulation of such receptors is not mediated by vasopressin [Felt et al. 1984]). In these models, the common deficit of depletion or altered affinity of hippocampal corticosteroid receptors is accompanied by syndromes of corticosterone hypersecretion and feedback resistance. Which secretagogs are hypersecreted in these models? This is not yet known; however, some predictions are possible. As discussed above, the relationship between Type II receptor occupancy in the hippocampus and inhibition of CRF is linear; in contrast, inhibition of oxytocin is stepwise, with the step occurring around the point of 50% occupancy of receptors, while inhibition of vasopressin is stepwise, around the point of 12% occupancy. Therefore, mild amounts of stress (producing, for example, 25% down-regulation of receptors) is likely to disinhibit only CRF secretion. Around the maximal point of down-regulation achievable (approximately 50%), hypersecretion should be driven by both CRF and oxytocin. Finally, down-regulation should never be sufficient to cause vasopressin hypersecretion. Given the magnitude of receptor loss normally seen in the Brattleboro rat, one might speculate that hypersecretion is driven by both oxytocin and CRF (obviously, it can never be driven by vasopressin, as the peptide is congenitally absent in that strain). In chapter 14, I consider the relevance of these observations to the glucocorticoid hypersecretion in humans with major depression.

THE HIPPOCAMPUS AS A FEEDBACK BRAKE IN THE AGING RAT

An extensive literature suggests that the hippocampal damage of aged rats might be partially responsible for the corticosterone hypersecretion and resistance to negative feedback inhibition. Most explicitly, this is supported by the observation that after hippocampal lesion or fornix transection, rats hypersecrete corticosterone both basally and after the end of stress, just as do aged rats. However, these are more severe insults than occur in aged rats, who do not have fornix transections, nor damage in large percentages of the hippocampus. Instead, they typically lose around 15% to 20% of the hippocampal neurons, with the damage concentrated in the Ammon's horn region. Does more subtle hippocampal damage of this magnitude produce hypersecretion as well?

One way of testing this would be to produce small hippocampal lesions and examine subsequent adrenocortical function. It would not be enough to mimic the 15% to 20% neuron loss by lesioning entirely a hippocampal cell field that accounts for 15% to 20% of all hippocampal neurons. The problem there, obviously, is that the neuron loss in the aging hippocampus is distributed among different cell fields. Replicating this sort of damage has not been attempted. A number of studies, however, provide strong correlative evidence that the relationship between hippocampal damage and glucocorticoid hypersecretion is linear and that even relatively small amounts of neuron loss are disruptive.

In one such study, the hippocampi of aged rats were examined and ranked according to severity of hippocampal neuropathologic degeneration; rats with more severe degeneration were those who also had more severe hypersecretion of corticosterone (Landfield et al. 1978). An equivalent correlation has emerged in humans suffering from Alzheimer's disease, in which there is diffuse damage to, and isolation of, the hippocampus. The more severe the hippocampal atrophy, the more cortisol hypersecretion (De Leon et al. 1988). Finally, the data concerning the relationship between the extent of corticosteroid receptor occupancy in the hippocampus and extent of inhibition of secretagog release make the same point: If progressive decreases in hippocampal corticosteroid receptor occupancy are associated with progressive increases in CRF concentrations, then every little bit of hippocampal neuron loss should be associated with CRF hypersecretion as well.

These studies suggest that the relatively subtle hippocampal neuron loss in aged rats is enough to cause the hypersecretion and that the relationship is at least somewhat linear. The data concerning the different domains of hippocampal feedback function have an interesting implication for the aged rat. In a collection of aged rats, even if all have lost (for example) 20% of their hippocampal neurons, they are unlikely to have the identical pattern of neuron loss, and this should produce individualistic profiles of corticosterone hypersecretion—individual aged rats should differ as to whether they hypersecrete basally or following a stressor, how sensitive they are to different feedback signals, and so on. This may also explain some of the variability in glucocorticoid hypersecretion in Alzheimer's disease. In that syndrome, approximately 50% of patients hypersecrete cortisol; in some cases, there is basal hypersecretion, in others, dexamethasone resistance, and in others, both. Such individual differences may arise from differing patterns (although of similar magnitudes) of hippocampal neuron loss. These ideas are considered in chapter 14.

The data concerning the functional consequences of receptor down-regulation suggest that if the aged hippocampus lost only corticosteroid receptors, instead of both receptors and neurons, there would still be corticosterone hypersecretion and feedback resistance. (Because both receptor types appear to mediate feedback and the aged hippocampus loses both receptor types, it is not clear which is responsible for the hypersecretion). Therefore, the rat is impaired both because of its loss of neurons and from the loss of receptors (figure 5.4).

Which secretagogs mediate the hypersecretion of aged rats? As noted, the difficult portal cannulation studies have not been carried out, mostly because of the fragility and expense of aged rats. The data reviewed here, however, allow for some informed speculations. As rats age and the extent of neuron and/or receptor loss becomes more pronounced, adrenocortical hypersecretion should be driven first by CRF, then CRF and oxytocin, and perhaps only in the most extreme cases of damage by all three secretagogs.

To finish, it is worth trying to relate the role of the hippocampus in glucocorticoid regulation, as reviewed in this chapter, to its much more established role in learning and memory. As should be familiar to most readers, the hippocampus is critical in cognition, particularly in memory consolidation, and both experimental and neuropathologic damage to the structure, in both humans and other species, produces profound cognitive impairments and dementias (Squire 1986). Does it make any sense that the hippocampus should be involved in both cognition and adrenocortical regulation? The neuro-

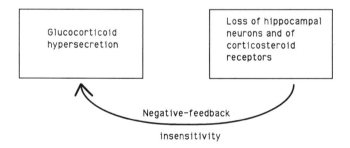

Figure 5.4. Schematic representation of the possible contribution of senescent hippocampal degeneration to the glucocorticoid hypersecretion typical of aged rats.

biologist interested in learning and memory might ask, Why should a structure so critical to cognition be so sensitive to glucocorticoids (i.e., have so many receptors for them)? The neuroendocrinologist might ask, Why should this structure, which is involved in regulating adrenocortical activity, be so sensitive to cognitive states?

This intersection of roles makes some sense. To begin with, it is not really surprising that the hippocampus, concerned with learning and memory, should be so sensitive to glucocorticoids—cognition is altered during extreme stress or arousal. Most of us know of anecdotal evidence for this. In an oft-cited example, everyone remembers where they were when John Kennedy was shot, but no one can tell you what they were doing 24 hours before that. As another example, if you have ever been mugged or physically threatened, you no doubt can remember an astonishing array of sensations and impressions about those 30 seconds. Ethologists have studied a similar phenomenon in cases of "prepared learning" or "one-trial learning," in which, during times of emotional arousal, certain types of learning can occur faster than predicted according to the standard operant rules of trial and error. This makes some sense—in certain emergencies, it is adaptive for associations to be learned very rapidly, without the delay of trial and error learning. While a role for glucocorticoids in these phenomena has not been established, a connection seems plausible. As an alternative piece of teleology, there are also circumstances where, if things are sufficiently stressful and traumatic, it may be adaptive to forget the situation. Again, there is no evidence to link glucocorticoids with traumatic amnesia, but a link is conceivable.

Why might it make sense for the hippocampus, with its role in inhibiting glucocorticoid secretion, to also be sensitive to memory? One does not need any access to memory in order to decide whether or not a major hemorrhage is stressful. However, memory is neccesary for many cognitive stressors. For example, one must be able to remember what is the norm in a situation in order to decide that the present case is not normal (and to thus have a stress-response triggered by novelty and discrepancy). One must be able to remember some awful previous event in order to recognize that the same distressing scenario is unfolding again (and thus have a conditioned stress-response). A number of studies have shown that while hippocampal damage does not influence the stress-response to somatic stressors, it will influence responsiveness to conditioned stressors. In conclusion, it strikes me that the intersection of the hippocampus as a structure near and dear to the hearts of both neuroendocrinologists and neurobiologists concerned with learning is not as surprising as at first glance.

CHAPTER SUMMARY

In the aged rat, there is hypersecretion of glucocorticoids (associated with resistance to feedback regulation) and a loss of hippocampal corticosteroid receptors (related to a loss of hippocampal neurons). This chapter begins to link these two deficits in showing that the glucocorticoid hypersecretion in the aged rat is most likely a consequence of the hippocampal degeneration.

An extensive literature is reviewed implicating the hippocampus as a mediator of glucocorticoid feedback regulation. While such regulation occurs at both the level of the pituitary and the brain, the latter is a more sensitive mediator of the inhibition. And while neural feedback regulation certainly occurs in the hypothalamus, suprahypothalamic structures contribute as well. Of these, the hippocampus has often been implicated in the neuroendocrine role.

1. Lesions of the hippocampus, or of its efferent projections cause glucocorticoid hypersecretion. This can occur basally, during stress and during the poststress recovery period, as well as in the form of resistance to glucocorticoid feedback signals. This can be shown by measuring glucocorticoids, ACTH, and the hypothalamic secretagogs (either their concentrations in the portal circulation, their levels in the hypothalamus, or the levels of mRNAs for these peptides).

2. Stimulation of the hippocampus, conversely, inhibits the adrenocortical axis.

3. Microimplantation of glucocorticoids into the hippocampus can inhibit the adrenocortical axis.

4. Microimplanation of glucocorticoid antagonists into the hippocampus disinhibits the adrenocortical axis.

While there are some exceptions to these reports (some of which can be explained by there being some degree of recovery of function after hippocampal lesions), this literature collectively demonstrates that the hippocampus helps mediate glucocorticoid feedback regulation (and again I emphasize that it is not the sole or probably even the most important such regulator. It is simply the one damaged most readily during aging).

Recent studies have revealed some of the workings of the hippocampus as a feedback site.

1. The dorsal hippocampus appears to play a larger role in this than the ventral hippocampus.

2. The hippocampal projection to the mediobasal hypothalamus via the bed nucleus of the striae terminalis appears to be the pathway that contributes to feedback information.

3. While the hippocampus can inhibit the secretion of CRF, vasopressin, and oxytocin, it regulates each in a different manner. The hippocampus can regulate the magnitude of initial prestress secretion, the size of the stress-response, and the efficacy of glucocorticoid feedback inhibition, all by inhibiting different combinations of secretagogs. As a caveat, these data were derived with the invasive and unphysiologic portal cannulation technique.

4. While it seems clear that at least part of the inhibition of the adrenocortical axis by the hippocampus represents glucocorticoid feedback inhibition, it is not clear whether it also plays a tonic inhibitory role (i.e., whether it inhibits independently of a glucocorticoid feedback signal).

5. There is more evidence that the hippocampus is involved in delayed, rather than fast feedback.

6. Both types I and II hippocampal corticosteroid receptors appear to be involved in glucocorticoid feedback inhibition.

7. The hippocampus not only regulates the secretion of different secretagogs, but with differing strengths. CRF is inhibited in a linear manner, such that increasing degrees of occupancy of corticosteroid receptors are associated with progressively greater inhibition of CRF release. In contrast, vasopressin and oxytocin are regulated in an all-or-none manner. Only minimal amounts of receptor occupancy are needed before there is maximal inhibition of vasopressin release, whereas only moderate amounts of occupancy are needed for maximal inhibition of oxytocin. In effect, the hippocampus regulates vasopressin the most tightly of the secretagogs, and CRF the least.

8. A reduction in the numbers of hippocampal corticosteroid receptors (as during stress-induced down-regulation) will blunt the efficacy with which the hippocampus mediates glucocorticoid feedback inhibition.

These findings suggest that the aged rat hypersecretes glucocorticoids and is feedback resistant because of the loss of hippocampal neurons and hippocampal corticosteroid receptors that are a normal part of aging. The heterogeneous nature of hippocampal regulation of the adrenocortical axis (e.g., regulation of different secretagogs, of basal, stress or poststress situations) predicts that individual aged rats will differ as to the precise circumstances under which they are hypersecretory, as a function of their distribution of neuron and receptor loss. Moreover, while not yet demonstrated, it is possible to make some informed speculations as to which secretagogs are hypersecreted in the aged rats.

6   Glucocorticoid Neurotoxicity

SUMMARY OF THE BOOK SO FAR

A variety of stressors will trigger the endocrine and neural adaptations that constitute the stress-response. The adrenal secretion of glucocorticoids is central to the stress-response and typifies its two-edged quality: While glucocorticoid secretion is vital to surviving short-term physical stressors, over-exposure to glucocorticoids in the face of chronic or repeated stress can be highly deleterious, causing a variety of stress-related diseases.

This suggests that glucocorticoid secretion is tightly regulated and that a failure of this regulation carries a price. These features of the adrenocortical axis have attracted the attention of gerontologists interested in whether aged animals can appropriately respond to stress, and whether prolonged exposure to stress over the lifetime can accelerate some degenerative features of stress.

So far, we have examined the workings of the aged adrenocortical axis and have uncovered two deficits. First, aged rats tend to hypersecrete glucocorticoids. While they can appropriately turn on glucocorticoid secretion with the onset of stress, they have difficulties turning off secretion during the recovery period. Furthermore, they hypersecrete the hormone basally and during habituation to mild stressors. Finally, aged rats are relatively resistant to glucocorticoid feedback inhibition. These instances of hypersecretion appear to be driven, at least in part, at the level of the brain.

In addition, aged rats sustain a loss of corticosteroid receptors in the hippocampus. The structure is a major target tissue in the brain for glucocorticoids, and it loses approximately half of both the high- and low-affinity corticosteroid receptors with aging. Most importantly, there is neuron loss in the aged hippocampus as well, and it appears that the loss preferentially occurs among the corticosterone receptor-rich neurons.

The previous chapter suggested a first connection between these two defects. It reviewed the extensive evidence that the hippocampus helps mediate glucocorticoid feedback inhibition. Therefore, hippocampal damage leads to feedback resistance and glucocorticoid hypersecretion. Conversely, stimulation of the hippocampus inhibits adrenocortical activation, as does micro-implantation of glucocorticoids in the hippocampus. Logically, the inhibitory effects of glucocorticoids in the hippocampus involve interaction with corticosteroid receptors; a depletion of such receptors has been reported to damp the ability of the hippocampus to serve as a negative feedback "brake." The chapter reviewed the emerging story as to which corticosteroid receptors contribute to such feedback, how the hippocampus might influence basal, stress, and poststress adrenocortical activity, and which hypothalamic secretagogs are sensitive to hippocampal regulation. Most importantly, this extensive literature suggests that the loss of neurons and the loss of corticosteroid receptors combine to impair the ability of the aged hippocampus to inhibit glucocorticoid secretion. The feedback resistance and the glucocorticoid hypersecretion in the aged rat ensue.

The present chapter examines why the aged hippocampus loses neurons and corticosteroid receptors, and the rather unexpected punchline is the basis for the remainder of the book.

The previous chapter linked the two deficits outlined, suggesting that the loss of corticosteroid receptor-rich neurons in the aging hippocampus gives rise to the glucocorticoid hypersecretion and feedback resistance. The critical question now becomes, What is the cause of the hippocampal neuron loss?

When considering neurodegeneration, it is natural to consider the usual likely suspects—autoimmune attack, environmental toxins, even slow viruses. However, none of these is the cause of the degeneration in the present case; instead, a major pacemaker of hippocampal neuron loss appears to be the extent of cumulative exposure to glucocorticoids. More than two decades after the first evidence for glucocorticoid neurotoxicity, it still seems surprising that hormones, which are essential for life, can damage the brain.

The first evidence for this was the demonstration that glucocorticoids damaged the brain of guinea pigs, with the hippocampus being preferentially vulnerable (Aus der Muhlen and Ockenfels 1969). In retrospect, the study was basically ignored. It was published (in the opinion of this Anglocentric reader) in an obscure German journal, the dosages were pharmacologic, and the species was not common to either gerontological or neurobiological research. Probably most important, there was no reason to find the preferential hippocampal damage to be particularly interesting—the publication came around the same time as the first demonstration of corticosteroid receptors in the brain, in which the hippocampus and corticosteroids were forever linked (McEwen et al. 1968).

The subject lay dormant for a decade until a series of studies emerged; none was, by itself, quite waterproof, but they collectively showed that glucocorticoids play a central role in the normal senescent loss of hippocampal neurons.

The first study was a purely correlative one; Landfield and colleagues (1978) replicated the observation that basal glucocorticoid concentrations rose with age in the rat. They then showed that the more severe the hypersecretion, the more hippocampal degeneration, as assessed by astrogliosis, a measure of neuronal degeneration (figure 6.1; see also Issa et al. 1990). Then, in an important followup study (Landfield et al. 1981a), they adrenalectomized rats at mid-age (12 months) and replaced them with very low levels of corticosterone. Therefore, for the remainder of their lives, the rats were spared the progressive elevation in basal glucocorticoid concentrations and the intermittent bursts of secretion in response to stress. Critically, in their old age (approximately 2 years), these rats had not sustained the typical hippocampal degeneration, nor did they have the typical cognitive deficits (impaired reversal learning) (figure 6.2).

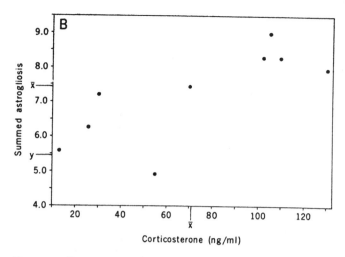

Figure 6.1. Demonstration that among aged rats, there is a positive correlation between the extent of basal hypersecretion of corticosterone and extent of degenerative astrogliosis in the hippocampus. (From Landfield et al., 1978, Hippocampal aging and adrenocorticoids: A quantitative correlation. Science 202, 1098, copyright, AAAS.)

We then performed a complementary study, showing that high but physiologic concentrations of glucocorticoids could accelerate hippocampal degeneration. Young rats (3 to 5 months of age) were exposed for either 2 weeks or 3 months to concentrations of injected corticosterone that were continuously in the range seen during major stressors (Sapolsky et al. 1985). After 2 weeks exposure to the high glucocorticoids, there was a marked down-regulation of corticosteroid receptors in the hippocampus (figure 6.3). This agreed with the time course and magnitude of the down-regulation observed earlier (Sapolsky et al. 1984c). And, in agreement with that prior study, by a week after the end of the glucocorticoid exposure, receptor concentrations had normalized. Rats exposed to 3 months of corticosterone, however, were much different. Essentially, we had produced a picture like that of the aged hippocampus. A similar extent of receptor loss was observed as in the rats exposed to only 2 weeks of steroids (figure 6.3). This agreed with our prior demonstration that corticosteroid receptors in the hippocampus could only be down-regulated a maximum of approximately 50%, and this was achieved after a week of glucocorticoid exposure. However, the receptor loss did not normalize even 4 months after the hormone exposure stopped. We then did a morphometric analysis of their hippocampi. While overall hippocampal size did not change, there was a 25% loss of neurons in Ammon's horn, particularly the CA$_3$ region. We then did a size analysis on the soma of each cell in the CA$_3$ region (figure 6.4) from controls, 2-week hormone exposure ("acute"), 3-month exposure ("chronic"), and normal aged rats. The chronic and aged rats shared three traits. Each had approximately 25% fewer cells than in young controls. Both had a substantial loss of the largest cells which, by morphological and cytological criteria, were the pyramidal cells, the principal neurons of the CA$_3$ region. In addition, in both groups, there was more of the smallest class of cells; on

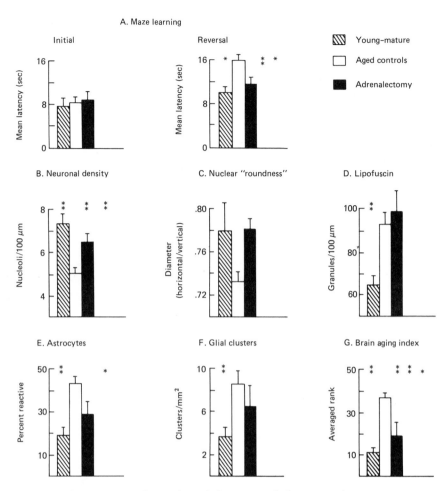

A. Maze learning

Initial   Reversal

Mean latency (sec)

Young–mature
Aged controls
Adrenalectomy

B. Neuronal density   C. Nuclear "roundness"   D. Lipofuscin

E. Astrocytes   F. Glial clusters   G. Brain aging index

Figure 6.2. Demonstration that prolonged diminution of glucocorticoid exposure prevents some of the degenerative features of hippocampal aging. (A) The age-dependent behavioral impairment, indicated by elevated latency, is confined to the reversal phase. (G) A composite index incorporating the morphologic variables shown individually in graphs B, C, E, and F. Rats were either young-mature, aged controls (approximately 2 years of age), or aged rats adrenalectomized at 1 year of age and maintained on minimal replacement corticosterone concentrations into old age. (Modified from Landfield et al., 1981, Brain aging correlates: Retardation by hormonal-pharmacological treatments. Science 214, 581, copyright AAAS.)

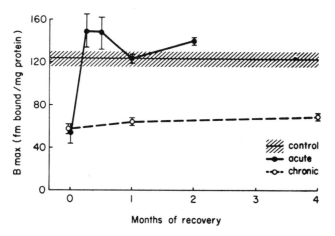

Months of recovery

Figure 6.3. Three months of daily corticosterone exposure, rather than 2 weeks of exposure, causes a persistent depletion of hippocampal corticosteroid receptors. Maximal binding receptor binding capacity (as measured by binding of [³H]dexamethasone) from control, acute, and chronic subjects. Acute subjects received daily corticosterone injections for 2 weeks; chronic subjects received injections for 3 months. Subjects were then allowed to recover from such treatment and a subset of them were culled at each time point during the recovery period for receptor assay. Both acute and chronic subjects had significantly diminished binding capacity relative to controls (shading represents 95% confidence intervals) at the beginning of the recovery period. Acute subjects recovered to at least control levels within a week, whereas no recovery occurred among chronic subjects even 4 months during the recovery period. (From Sapolsky et al., 1985, J Neurosci 5, 1221. Reprinted with permission of Oxford University Press.)

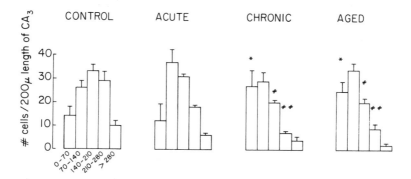

Figure 6.4. Histograms of the distribution of cell body sizes in the CA3 pyramidal cell region of hippocampi of control, acute, chronic, and aged subjects. Treatment groups were as defined in figure 6.3. The area of all cell bodies in the first 200 μm of the CA_3 region (moving from the CA_2/CA_{3a} boundary) containing nuclei was determined. Cell body areas were then grouped into the categories of 0–70, 70–140, 140–210, 210–280, and >280 μm² of area. Asterisk indicates significantly greater number of cells, relative to controls, $p < .05$; #, ## indicate significantly fewer number of cells relative to controls, $p < .05, .01$, respectively. (From Sapolsky et al., 1985, J Neurosci 5, 1221. Reprinted with permission of Oxford University Press.)

morphologic grounds, these were the darkly staining reactive microglia that proliferate and invade into neural tissue in response to neuronal degeneration (Wisniewski and Terry 1973; Scheibel and Scheibel 1975). Thus, if there was an overall loss of approximately 25% of the cells *despite* a significant increase in the microglial population, this implies an even greater than 25% loss of neurons (for example, there was an approximate 70% loss of cells in some of the larger size classes).

Finally, we did high-resolution autoradiographic analysis of hippocampal corticosteroid receptors and found that there was a preferential loss of neurons that had contained high concentrations of such receptors (figure 6.5).

This study showed that prolonged glucocorticoid exposure produced hippocampal degeneration resembling that seen during normal aging: (1) There was a marked loss of corticosteroid receptors that was apparently permanent; the same occurs during aging, as reviewed in chapter 2. (2) There was a greater than 25% depletion of pyramidal neurons, with damage most pronounced in Ammon's horn and least pronounced in the CA_1 and dentate regions. The same is seen during aging (Landfield et al. 1977, 1981a; Brizzee and Ordy 1979; Coleman and Flood 1987). (3) There was preferential loss of neurons that contained high concentrations of corticosteroid receptors, much as during aging (Sapolsky et al. 1984a). (4) The neuronal degeneration was accompanied by glial infiltration and proliferation, as seen during aging (Ling and Leblond 1973; Vaughan and Peters 1974; Landfield et al. 1981b).

Shortly after that, Meaney and colleagues (1988a) studied *neonatal handling*, a developmental phenomenon in which daily handling of rats for the first few weeks of life produces adults with lowered basal glucocorticoid concentrations. The mechanisms of this effect will be discussed in chapter 12. For the present, the most important consequence of that study was the observation that neonatally handled rats, who secreted less cumulative glucocorticoids over their lifetimes, had decelerated hippocampal aging. Aged handled rats had more hippocampal neurons, more hippocampal corticosteroid receptors, and better spatial-learning skills than control aged rats.

Most recently, prolonged stress was shown to accelerate hippocampal aging as well (Kerr et al. 1991). The stressor in this study was 6 months of training in a two-way shuttle box; in this paradigm, rats are exposed to relatively low levels of footshock but to sustained anxiety. Both electrophysiological and morphometric indices of aging were accelerated by the chronic stress, although rats of different ages were differentially sensitive to alterations of the different parameters. Sustained stress made young hippocampi (those of 10- or 18-month-old rats) resemble aged ones from an electrophysiological standpoint—reduced thresholds for population spikes and for field excitatory postsynaptic potentials, and reduced frequency potentiation. The chronic stress paradigm did not worsen the electrophysiologic parameters in aged (24-month-old) rats, which were already as bad in control rats as in any of the young stressed animals. Conversely, the chronic stress paradigm did not change neuron density in the hippocampi of the younger two ages, but did cause an approximate 25% decrease in pyramidal cell density in the oldest rats.

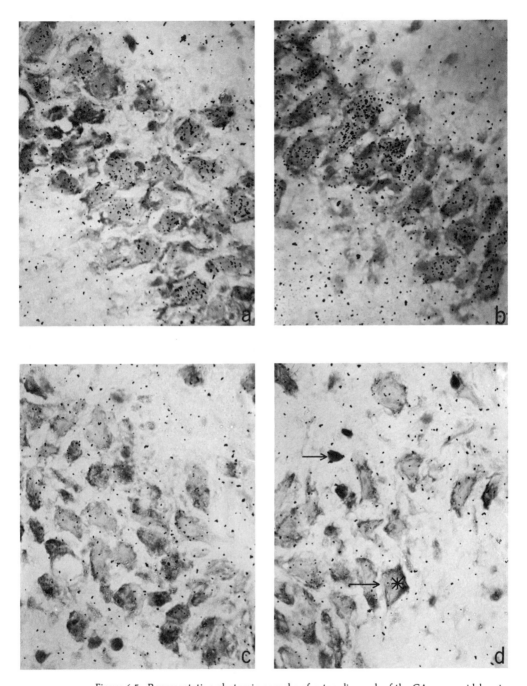

Figure 6.5. Representative photomicrographs of autoradiograph of the CA_{3a} pyramidal region of hippocampus in control (A), acute (B), chronic (C), and aged (D) subjects. The upper arrow in D indicates a representative cell of the $0-70\ \mu m^2$ size class; the arrow pointing to the asterisk indicates a representative cell of the $140-180\ \mu m^2$ size class. Magnification × 400. (From Sapolsky et al., 1985, J Neurosci 5, 1221. Reprinted with permission of Oxford University Press.)

Each of the studies has its weaknesses, which are generally compensated for in one of the other studies. The study by Landfield and colleagues (1981a) showed that something that came out of the adrenal glands served as a major pacemaker of the rate of normal hippocampal neuron loss, but it was not possible to tell if it was glucocorticoids, mineralocorticoids, catecholamines, or any of a number of other possible humoral factors. Our subsequent study (Sapolsky et al. 1985) showed that it was indeed the glucocorticoids. The neuropathological analysis done in the Landfield et al. study was also somewhat problematic. For example, the relative densities, rather than absolute numbers of neurons were measured. Therefore, it is possible that there was an increase in overall size of the hippocampus, decreasing the density of neurons (the effect reported) without actually changing the numbers of neurons. Actual neuron counts and total hippocampal size was measured in subsequent studies, however (Sapolsky et al. 1985; Meaney et al. 1988a). Moreover, the somewhat unorthodox measure of nuclear "roundness" was used in the Landfield et al. study, which the authors have argued is a characteristic of nonsenescent hippocampal neurons.

In our study showing that sustained glucocorticoid overexposure accelerated hippocampal degeneration (Sapolsky et al. 1985), we emphasized that our report differed from the first report of glucocorticoid neurotoxicity in the guinea pig (Aus der Muhlen and Ockenfels, 1969) in that we carefully assured that the circulating concentrations of glucocorticoids generated were in the upper physiologic range (i.e., that seen during stress), rather than in the pharmacologic range (Hauger and colleagues [1987] have also demonstrated that this treatment paradigm produces physiologic levels of glucocorticoids). However, the rats were exposed to such levels constantly for 3 months, which is certainly unphysiologic. This made it unclear whether real patterns of intermittent stressors would also be neurodegenerative. This was shown to be the case in the subsequent study by Kerr and co-workers (1991). That study's strength was, naturally, that it showed that something as "real" as sustained stress could be neurodegenerative, as opposed to the artifical condition of exogenous hormone administration. The obvious weakness was that it was not clear which of the many hormonal shifts stimulated by the stressors was the proximally damaging agent. In addition, as a minor problem, the study would have been strengthened by data regarding a decrease in absolute neuron number, rather than neuron density. In the study by Meaney and associates (1988a) showing the neuroprotective effects of the behavioral manipulation, it was not clear if the proximally protective effect was truly the lowered circulating glucocorticoid concentrations or some other factor not even considered or measured.

Nevertheless, these studies collectively implicate glucocorticoids as pacemakers of hippocampal aging. Prolonged exposure to glucocorticoids, whether due to exogenous hormone administration or to repeated stressors, accelerates hippocampal aging. Conversely, prolonged diminution of glucocorticoid exposure, whether due to surgical or behavioral interventions, decelerates hippocampal aging.

A recent study reinforces this picture of glucocorticoid neurotoxicity. Rats were administered the same high concentrations of daily glucocorticoids as in our prior study (Sapolsky et al. 1985). At the end of 3 weeks, while there was not yet overt hippocampal neuron loss, there were signs of degeneration. Golgi staining revealed that corticosterone-treated hippocampal neurons had fewer apical dendritic branch points and decreased length of apical dendrites; in addition, pyknotic neurons were noted. Importantly, this degeneration was noted only in the CA_3 region (Woolley et al. 1990). This represents, in effect, a snapshot of the hippocampus when neurons are beginning to be damaged by glucocorticoid overexposure.

THE PRECEDENT FOR GLUCOCORTICOID NEUROTOXICITY

Although initially the idea of hormones, which are essential for life, being potentially neurodegenerative is hard to accept, there are precedents for neurodegeneration induced by sustained overexposure to an endogenous ligand. The female rodent loses the capacity to ovulate with age, and such reproductive failure arises from loss of the triggering surge of luteinizing hormone (LH) before ovulation. Degenerative changes in the senescent hypothalamus (in particular, the arcuate nucleus) appear to underlie the failure of the LH surge, and an extensive and elegant body of studies showed that cumulative exposure of mice and rats to estrogen, accelerated the hypothalamic dysfunctions in gonadotropin regulation (Finch et al. 1984).

Thus, sustained steroid exposure was already recognized as accelerating brain aging. In addition, and more directly, a literature already existed demonstrating the catabolic effects of glucocorticoids in the brain: *Stress and/or glucocorticoids can be neurodegenerative in other situations.* Stress can damage the retina, decreasing the numbers of photoreceptor and bipolar neurons, and this toxicity can be prevented by adrenalectomy (O'Steen and Donnelly 1982; O'Steen and Brodish 1985).

Stress and/or glucocorticoids can disrupt normal aspects of neural development. The adverse effects of perinatal glucocorticoid exposure have long been recognized. Rats treated neonatally with glucocorticoids have permanently reduced adult brain weights, RNA, DNA content, protein synthesis, and fewer neurons and glia (Howard 1965, 1968; Winick and Coscia 1968; Balazs and Cotterrell 1972; Cotterrell et al. 1972; Gumbinas et al. 1973; Oda and Huttenlocher 1974; Howard and Benjamin 1975; Ardeleanu and Sterescu 1978). The reduced DNA content is due to suppression of cell division, rather than to the death of existing cells, as shown by ^{3}H-thymidine–incorporation studies. Therefore, the effect is most profound in those regions where there is extensive postnatal mitosis, such as the cerebellum and the dentate gyrus of the hippocampus (Bohn 1980; Bohn and Lauder 1978; Weichsel 1974; Gutierrez and Meyer 1988). Conversely, adrenalectomy leads to heavier brain weight, more myelin deposition, and more cell proliferation, and it is the loss of glucocorticoids which is critical to this enhancement (Devenport and Devenport 1983, 1985; Meyer 1985; and Yehuda et al. 1985).

Neonatal glucocorticoid treatment also disrupts neural morphogenesis, as evidenced by reduced numbers of dendritic spines and branches, and less synaptogenesis in various brain regions. Prenatal stress in rats (i.e., to the mother while pregnant) results in offspring with a mild reduction (10% to 20% reduction in 75% of animals) in numbers of hippocampal pyramidal neurons and poor development of dendritic processes (Uno et al. 1989a). As possible mechanisms mediating these disruptive effects of glucocorticoids, the steroids suppress expression of growth-associated protein-43 (GAP-43) in PC12 cells and block NGF-induced increases in GAP-43 (Federoff et al. 1988). GAP-43 plays an important role in neuronal growth and remodeling. Moreover, gluco-corticoids reduce mRNA for insulin-like growth factor, which normally stimulates neuronal thymidine incorporation (Adamo et al. 1988). Glucocorticoids reduce mRNA for the nerve growth factor receptor both in vivo and in vitro (Yakovlev et al. 1990). Finally, heavy perinatal exposure to glucocorticoids causes prolonged cognitive deficits, including deficits in passive and active avoidance learning (de Kloet et al. 1988b). Therefore, there is considerable precedent for glucocorticoids having adverse effects during development. It has been suggested that this is the reason for the *stress hyporesponsive period* seen in neonatal rats. Fetal rats have a surprisingly mature adrenocortical axis, in terms of capacity to secrete hormones in response to stressors, presence of corticosteroid receptors, sensitivity to feedback regulation, and so on. Shortly after birth, the system involutes, and the stress-response either disappears entirely or is damped. Mechanistically, this is brought about by postnatal changes in receptor concentrations (reviewed in Sapolsky and Meaney 1986). It has been suggested that the stress hyporesponsive period is logical and adaptive, in that it represents a means to minimize glucocorticoid secretion at a time of life at which it would be profoundly and permanently catabolic to the brain. In effect, the neonatal rat gambles that it need not have a stress-response of its own, in the hopes that mom will be able to take care of the problem instead. As support for this bit of anthropomorphism, when neonatal rats are separated from their mothers, the stress hyporesponsive period wanes and pups quickly reattain the capacity to have an adrenocortical stress-response (Stanton et al. 1988). Therefore, I suppose that glucocorticoids are so potentially damaging to the developing brain that there has evolved a dramatic developmental phenomenon to protect against their catabolic effects.

Glucocorticoids impair the capacity of nervous tissue to recover from injury. Following damage to the brain, there is often elaboration and growth of surviving neurons in the area of the injury. This phenomenon of compensatory sprouting is particularly common when certain pathways into the hippo-campus are severed, and can be viewed as a partially successful compensation by the brain to respond to the injury (given that no new neurons can be made). Glucocorticoids inhibit compensatory sprouting in the hippocampus, and the progressive rise in basal glucocorticoid concentrations with age accounts for the impaired capacity of aged rats to undergo compensatory sprouting following injury (DeKosky et al. 1984; see figure 3.11). There are some clues as to how this works. Glucocorticoids inhibit the rate of clearing of debris and of degenerating neurons following the initial injury (Scheff et al. 1986). This delay is, in part, due to decreased microglial proliferation following the injury. Glucocorticoids inhibit their proliferation, probably via inhibition of their monocyte precursors (Vijayan and Cotman 1987), and such proliferation is essential for clearing of debris. Moreover, glucocorticoids may make the microglia less effective during this time. The microglia are thought to secrete interleukin-1, which stimulates astrocyte proliferation; astrocytes are then thought to secrete NGF, which mediates aspects of regeneration (Fagan, personal communication). Glucocorticoids are robust inhibitors of interleukin-1 in peripheral tissues (Munck et al. 1984) and are likely to do so in the brain as well. Finally, the glucocorticoid inhibition of GAP-43 expression (Federoff et al. 1988) may also play a disruptive role.

All of this makes for the rather convincing argument that excessive exposure to glucocorticoids damages both the developing and the adult brain and disrupts the capacity of the brain to recover from injury. This gives more precedence to the finding of glucocorticoid neurotoxicity in the aging hippocampus. As an important, but not too surprising twist to this story worth reviewing briefly, pathologic *underexposure* to glucocorticoids can also damage the brain. In the adult, elimination of glucocorticoids (due to adrenalectomy) will also retard compensatory sprouting (Scheff et al. 1986), much as does an overabundance of the hormones. In the developing brain, adrenalectomy disrupts myelinization, and changes the epinephrine-norepinephrine ratio in the sympathetic nervous system (reviewed in Sapolsky and Meaney 1986). In perhaps the most dramatic example, adrenalectomy can also lead to neuron death in the dentate gyrus in rats 3 to 4 months later (Sloviter et al. 1989; McNeill et al. 1990; Roy et al. 1990; Sapolsky et al. 1991b; Woolley et al. 1991), and as little as 3 days after adrenalectomy, pyknosis of cells can already be detected (Gould et al. 1990). Intriguingly, there has even been a recent case report regarding granule cell necrosis in a human with rapidly progressive adrenocortical insufficiency due to Addison's disease (Maehlen and Torvik 1990). These observations regarding the deleterious effects of long-term glucocorticoid elimination have been somewhat controversial. First, it appears to be the chronic absence of Type I receptor occupancy which is neurotoxic, such that the effect can be prevented by very small amounts of circulating glucocorticoids, or by Type I agonists such as aldosterone or RU28362 (Woolley et al. 1991). Therefore, if adrenalectomies are not complete, if auxillary adrenal tissue (which can secrete corticosteroids) is not entirely removed, or if small doses of replacement maintenance glucocorticoids are given, the effect is missed (cf. Landfield et al. 1981a; Hashimoto et al. 1989). Thus, before the stringency of this requirement for the complete absence of glucocorticoids was recognized, there was an impression that the effect had not been replicated by other investigators. This stringency also explains a feature of the phenomenon, namely that the neuron loss is observed only in the subset of rats with attenuated weight gain and electrolyte imbalances (i.e., those with complete elimination of corticosteroids). As a second point of controversy, the original report by Sloviter and colleagues suggested that long-term adrenalectomy caused "nearly complete" destruction of the dentate gyrus. Subsequent reports, however, have generally shown that the magnitude of neuron loss is far less severe. Finally, the original reports of the phenomenon emphasized the restriction of damage to the dentate (Sloviter et al. 1989; Gould et al. 1990; McNeill et al. 1990; Roy et al. 1990); however, there appears to be subtle, but significant neuron loss in other hippocampal regions as well (Sapolsky et al. 1991b). The basis for this phenomenon is not yet known.

AN INTEGRATED MODEL

In summary, pathologic glucocorticoid over- and underexposure can damage areas of the brain with pronounced sensitivities to these hormones. For the purposes of this chapter, the most striking effect is, of course, the degenerative consequences of overexposure. The careful reader will have noted that these findings combine with those of the previous chapter in a rather insidious way (figure 6.6). The separate features of the aging adrenocortical axis—the glucocorticoid effects on the hippocampus, and the hippocampal regulation of glucocorticoid secretion—combine to form a feedforward cascade of senescent degeneration. Short periods of stress and of excessive glucocorticoid secretion (of perhaps up to a month or so), down-regulate the number of corticosteroid receptors per hippocampal neuron without damaging the neurons themselves. This down-regulation is sufficient to disrupt feedback sensitivity, as discussed previously, and further hypersecretion ensues. If the stressor abates, the system can normalize—the receptor down-regulation at this stage is not permanent, and when normal receptor number returns, feedback sensitivity normalizes as well. With longer overexposure to glucocorticoids, however, hippocampal neurons themselves are finally damaged. This dampens feedback regulation as well, but in a irreversible manner, and the subsequent glucocorticoid hypersecretion becomes permanent. This leads to further neuron loss and further hypersecretion. Figure 6.6H lists a number of pathologies that both are more common with aging and arise as a consequence of glucocorticoid overexposure.

Encompassed in figure 6.6 are the answers to the questions that dominated the beginning chapters, at least as narrowly defined in the context of glucocorticoids. Do aged organisms handle stress as well as do younger individuals? The answer, with respect to the adrenocortical axis, is clearly no, given the instances of glucocorticoid hypersecretion in aged rats and the pathologic price paid by these animals. Can a lifetime of stress accelerate some of the degenerative correlates of aging? With respect to stress-induced glucocorticoid secretion and senescent hippocampal degeneration, the answer appears to be a guarded yes.

The *glucocorticoid cascade* hypothesis represents the main purpose of part I of this book. In its simplest form, it merely posits that over the lifespan of the rat, there is a tendency for glucocorticoids to damage the hippocampus and a tendency for hippocampal damage to provoke excessive glucocorticoid secretion, and that these two self-reinforcing pieces may contribute to some of the dysfunctions of aging. The remainder of this chapter will consider some of the dynamics of this proposed cascade, air some caveats, note some unanswered questions about it, and recant some of the details about it that have not been validated since this model was originally proposed (Sapolsky et al. 1985).

How physiologically relevant is this proposed cascade? In the original presentation of the model, I envisioned repeated stressors playing a critical role in bringing about the initial corticosteroid receptor down-regulation in the hippocampus and, ultimately, the hippocampal damage. However, there are two problems with this. First, it is a rather rare and unphysiologic circumstance for a rat to be exposed to a continuous array of repeated stressors. Second, even in the face of such an event, it is rare for an organism to respond to that with continuous glucocorticoid secretion (rather than to undergo some degree of habituation, hormone depletion, etc.). Thus, it is not surprising that, as reviewed in the last chapter, corticosteroid receptor down-regulation appears to occur only in circumstances of very sustained and extreme stressors. Therefore, I have come to believe that if this cascade occurs during normal aging in most rats (at least of the strains studied), repeated stressors and resultant down-regulation cannot be a prerequisite. Instead, I think that the elevated basal glucocorticoid concentrations may play a more important role than I had originally thought.

If that were the case, three features must be clarified.

1. The hippocampal damage should probably precede the change in adrenocortical function and would arise for reasons other than from glucocorticoid excess. This is because if one eliminates the possibility of many external stressors as being physiologic, the only place to begin the circle of dysregulation is with hippocampal damage. Implicit in this is the idea that this cascade model does not predict that *all* senescent hippocampal damage is due to glucocorticoid excess (and for the majority of neurogerontologists who think about hippocampal neuron loss without worrying about the ideas in this book, there is no shortage of other mechanisms for the hippocampus sustaining neuron loss during aging).

2. If one deemphasizes repeated stressors as the driving force on the cascade and instead views basal glucocorticoid hypersecretion as the thing that accelerates hippocampal aging, the step of receptor down-regulation is deemphasized as well. This is because there is little evidence that I know of that a small rise in basal glucocorticoid concentration will down-regulate such receptors. Interestingly, syndromes of elevated basal glucocorticoid concentrations are associated with a problem with terminating the stress-response, even in instances where the rat has not been exposed to repeated stressors. This is seen in streptozotocin-diabetic rats (Scribner et al. 1991).

3. This emphasis on basal glucocorticoid hypersecretion requires that such hypersecretion (in the absence of numerous stressors) is sufficient to damage hippocampal neurons. I believe two studies indirectly suggest this. In the demonstration by Landfield and colleagues (1981a) that adrenalectomy protected the hippocampus from senescent neuropathologies, the control group was undisturbed rats, rather than repeatedly stressed rats. Thus, protection

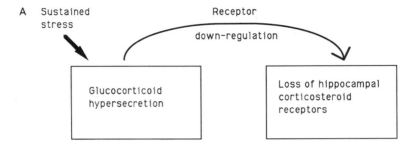

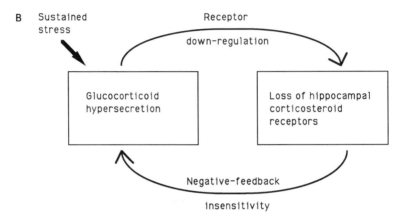

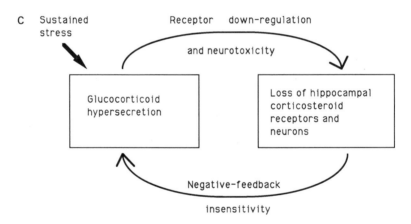

Figure 6.6. Schematic representation of the glucocorticoid cascade. In one scenario, the cascade can be initiated by periods of sustained stress (*A–C*). In a second scenario, the cascade can be initiated by senescent hippocampal neuron loss (*D–E*). In either case, the eventual version of these interrelationships is shown in (*F*). (*F* from Sapolsky et al., The neuroendocrinology of stress and aging: the glucocorticoid cascade hypothesis. Endocr Rev 7, 284–306, 1986. Reprinted with permission of Williams and Wilkins Publishers.)

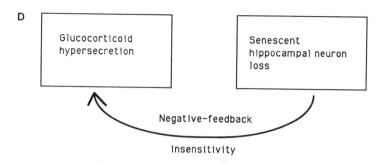

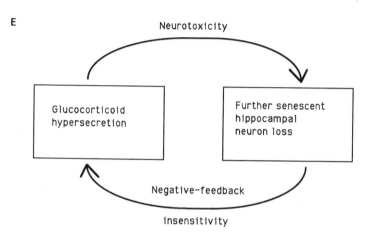

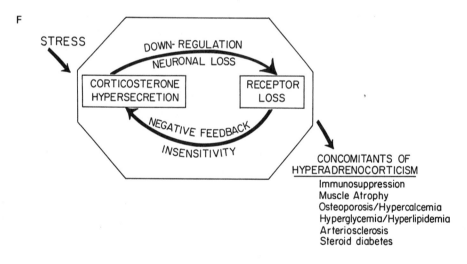

from prolonged exposure to basal concentrations of glucocorticoids was associated with hippocampal protection. In the study of Meaney and colleagues (1988; to be reviewed in more detail in chapter 12), two groups of rats that differed only in life-long patterns of basal glucocorticoid secretion (i.e., the rats were not stressed) differed in rates of hippocampal neuron loss.

These various findings and ideas lead me to believe that the cascade is most likely related, under physiological circumstances, to the abnormalities in basal glucocorticoid secretion, rather than in poststress secretion.

Which components of the cascade model are neccesary for it to be valid? There seems to be a number of general components to the model: (1) Chronic or repeated stress will down-regulate corticosteroid receptors in the hippocampus. (2) Sufficient exposure to glucocorticoids will eventually damage hippocampal neurons. (3) Hippocampal receptor down-regulation leads to glucocorticoid hypersecretion. (4) Hippocampal neuron loss leads to glucocorticoid hypersecretion. (5) Glucocorticoid hypersecretion includes basal hypersecretion. (6) Glucocorticoid hypersecretion includes a sluggish termination of the stress response.

It seems to me that not all of these components are critical to the model.

1. Chronic or repeated stress will down-regulate corticosteroid receptors in the hippocampus. The phenomenon of such down-regulation is reasonably well documented in the hippocampus for Type II receptors, and far less so for the Type I receptor (see chapter 4). However, those studies mostly involved exogenous glucocorticoid administration, and it remains less clear how readily physiological stressors cause such down-regulation. Thus, this component of the model is far from certain. However, as just discussed, I suspect that basal glucocorticoid hypersecretion, rather than chronic stress, plays the major role in this cascade, deemphasizing the importance of such putative down-regulation.

2. Sufficient exposure to glucocorticoids will eventually damage hippocampal neurons. This component strikes me as absolutely essential to the validity of this cascade model.

3. Hippocampal receptor down-regulation leads to glucocorticoid hypersecretion. This aspect of hippocampal function has been explored in only a few studies (see chapter 5) and is by no means well established. However, as just detailed, the role of repeated stressors causing receptor down-regulation (and subsequent glucocorticoid hypersecretion) is probably less important than I originally theorized.

4. Hippocampal neuron loss leads to glucocorticoid hypersecretion. This component, which I feel has been rather well established (see chapter 5), is probably essential to this cascade model. I reiterate a point that I tried to underline in chapter 5: This emphasis on the hippocampus as an inhibitor of glucocorticoid secretion does not imply that it is the *sole* neural inhibitor or, at an extreme, even one of the more important ones. It is simply the one damaged most readily during normal aging.

5. Glucocorticoid hypersecretion includes basal hypersecretion. This is probably essential for the model, given the emphasis on the basal hyper-

secretion driving subsequent hippocampal damage and the physiological rarity of rats being exposed to repeated stressors.

6. Glucocorticoid hypersecretion includes poststress hypersecretion. This component, which has been studied by only a few investigators (see chapter 3), is probably not essential to the model. This is because of the rarity of frequent stressors (and thus frequent problems with poststress recovery), and because of the studies of Landfield et al. (1981a) and Meaney et al. (1988a), just discussed, showing the pathogenic potential of basal glucocorticoid hypersecretion in the aging rat.

Are there nonlinearities in the cascade model (i.e., are the various components progressive with time)?

1. In instances where the cascade is being driven by chronic or repeated stressors, should hippocampal damage emerge progressively with each bout of stress? This is almost certainly not the case. As will be reviewed in coming chapters, glucocorticoid endangerment of hippocampal neurons appears to be, at least in part, receptor mediated. Therefore, if glucocorticoids down-regulate the numbers of such receptors, this predicts that such down-regulation should actually *protect* the hippocampus from the toxic effects of the steroids. This is probably the case, but does not go on indefinitely. This is because the down-regulation is finite—after about a week or so of heavy stress and/or heavy glucocorticoid exposure, the maximal 50% extent of down-regulation is reached. Therefore, if overexposure continues at that point, the hippocampus has exhausted its compensatory mechanism. Metaphorically, during the initial period of glucocorticoid exposure, the hippocampus can back away from the hormones; however, within a short time, it has been backed into a wall and must endure the ravages of the steroids. This predicts that the relationship between glucocorticoid overexposure in instances of many stressors (or during exogenous glucocorticoid administration) and hippocampal damage should be nonlinear, which it is—neuron loss does not emerge with the first instance of hormone overexposure, but instead requires weeks or months to occur.

2. In instances where the cascade predominately involves basal glucocorticoid hypersecretion, should hippocampal damage worsen with each unit of time of basal hypersecretion? This is almost certainly not the case either. This is because the neuron loss, as noted, takes a long period to emerge, even in instances of constant high glucocorticoid concentrations (mimicking constant stress).

3. Should basal hypersecretion and hypersecretion during the poststress recovery period worsen in parallel? It strikes me that this need not be the case (although it does appear to happen [Meaney et al. 1988a; Sabatino et al. 1991])—this might represent two different and dissociable forms of neuroendocrine regulation.

4. Is there a limit to how many hippocampal neurons are damaged by glucocorticoids with age? Stated differently, does the neuron loss progressively worsen with age, once it has first begun? I believe that most studies of multiple ages of rats show that the neuron loss continues to emerge with age, rather than asymptotes (reviewed in Coleman and Flood, 1987). However, I do

not think the model requires that all of these instances of neuron death be glucocorticoid-mediated; every hippocampal neuron need not neccesarily be fatally vulnerable to these hormones.

5. Is there a limit to the severity of the instances of glucocorticoid hypersecretion that emerge with age? Stated differently, will, for example, the basal hypersecretion of glucocorticoids worsen progressively with age, once it emerges? At present, I am fairly confused about this issue. Potentially, the glucocorticoid hypersecretion might even abate somewhat in aged rats. In the review of the role of the hippocampus in glucocorticoid feedback regulation (chapter 5), it was emphasized that the glucocorticoid hypersecretion after hippocampal damage is not necessarily permanent. In rats and primates, secretion tends to normalize over weeks and months, respectively. This is almost certainly not due to the hippocampus recovering from its injury, but from other mediators of feedback in the brain changing the strength of their regulation. Therefore, one might predict that there should be similar recovery of function in the aging rat and thus, there should not be permanent instances of glucocorticoid hypersecretion. However, that would be expected only if the senescent neuron loss occurred in the hippocampus all at once (i.e., like an experimental lesion). Instead, the progressive neuron loss over time means, most likely, that the other compensating neural feedback sites cannot keep pace with the emerging dysfunction.

What about the other side of this question: If the glucocorticoid hypersecretion is unlikely to abate with age, is it likely to worsen progressively? In the original presentation of the glucocorticoid cascade model (Sapolsky et al. 1986b), this prediction was somewhat implicitly made, and I am no longer sure if that is the case. Even if hippocampal damage emerges progressively with age, it is not neccesarily the case that glucocorticoid hypersecretion should also worsen progressively. I think that that depends on whether every hippocampal neuron is involved in regulating (i.e., inhibiting) glucocorticoid secretion. Were that the case, with every additional neuron lost past a certain threshold, there should be worsening hypersecretion. It is not known whether every such neuron serves such a neuroendocrine role, but I would be surprised if that were the case. (The single study using the rather unphysiologic preparation of portal cannulation in which hippocampal corticosteroid receptor occupancy was correlated with inhibition of hypothalamic secretagog release [Sapolsky et al. 1990a] suggested that a fairly large percentage of such receptors are involved in regulating secretagog release. However, receptors do not equal neurons.) If it is unlikely that every hippocampal neuron has something to say about glucocorticoid secretion, at some point glucocorticoid hypersecretion will have gotten as bad as it is going to get due to hippocampal damage, and further damage should have little impact. In support of this prediction, the maximal or near-maximal extent of glucocorticoid hypersecretion appears to already have been achieved in rats by around 16 to 19 months of age (Meaney et al. 1988a; Sabatino et al. 1991).

Do all aged rats have to demonstrate this putative cascade? As discussed, even the parameters considered to most reliably represent biomarkers of aging show vast amounts of variability, and I do not believe that this model need show any less interindividual variability to be judged valid. As will be discussed in chapter 12, in at least two instances, rats seemed spared the rubric of dysfunctions that I am terming the glucocortiocid cascade. One is in rats defined by cognitive and learning criteria to be "successful agers," and the other is in rats neonatally handled. These will be discussed in more detail in that chapter, as will likely strain differences in the emergence of this cascade (also see van Eekelen et al. 1991.)

For the same cumulative glucocorticoid exposure, is more damage caused by a single square wave of glucocorticoids or by multiple pulses? This issue is important, as it concerns what *patterns* of stressors are most likely to be neurodegenerative. However, the answer is not known.

Is the cascade model positing anything about lifespan? The model does not, so far as I can tell. In a recent study, Sabatino and colleagues (1991) demonstrated that in food-restricted rats, in whom lifespan is extended, there is increased cumulative glucocorticoid exposure over the lifetime. The authors felt that this study weighed in against the cascade model in part because the rise in basal glucocorticoids that they observed in their aged rats did not emerge progressively with age. As discussed in a preceding section, I do not think that progressive worsening is a prerequisite at all for the validity of this model. In addition, I sensed a somewhat tacit thread in their paper suggesting that the cascade model was also argued against because the food-restricted rats, despite their enhanced cumulative glucocorticoid exposure, nevertheless lived longer (and I apologize here to the authors if I was reading more of a critique into their paper than they intended). I do not think that the cascade model implies anything about longevity. I believe it is most relevant to some senescent dysfunctions that arise from hippocampal damage (glucocorticoid excess and, more important I suspect, some learning and memory impairments), or from moderate glucocorticoid excess and its pathogenic consequences throughout the body.

How do glucocorticoids kill hippocampal neurons? This is, obviously, a tremendous number of questions incorporated into one. A considerable amount has now been learned about the cell biology of glucocorticoid neurotoxicity; this is the subject of part II of this book.

CHAPTER SUMMARY

In the aging rat, there is hypersecretion of glucocorticoids and a loss of hippocampal corticosteroid receptors (and, associated with that, a loss of hippocampal neurons). Chapter 5 linked these two deficits, showing that corticosteroid receptor loss and/or overt hippocampal damage can lead to the feedback resistance and glucocorticoid hypersecretion. This shifts the focus to why aging hippocampal neurons die.

The surprising answer is that a major pacemaker of hippocampal neuron loss appears to be the extent of glucocorticoid exposure over the lifetime; excessive glucocorticoids can be neurotoxic to the hippocampus. The first evidence for this, in 1969, was that pharmacologic levels of glucocorticoids damage the guinea pig brain, with damage preferentially occurring in the hippocampus. This finding had little impact, in part because there was no framework in which to find the preferential hippocampal damage to be interesting—the publication predated the demonstration of the vast numbers of corticosteroid receptors in the hippocampus.

A decade later, a body of studies established that glucocorticoids play a major role in the normal physiological aging of the hippocampus. Such aging (as assessed by neuron loss, reactive microglial infiltration, and electrophysiological impairments) is accelerated by chronic stress or by chronic exposure (3 months) to the high concentrations of glucocorticoids caused by major stressors. As little as 3 weeks into such exposure to high glucocorticoid concentrations, hippocampal neurons already have fewer apical dendritic branch points and shorter apical dendrites. The glucocorticoid-induced hippocampal damage is most pronounced in the CA_3 cell field, just as is the normative hippocampal degeneration during aging.

Conversely, prolonged diminution of glucocorticoid exposure over the lifetime slows down hippocampal senescence (as assessed by less neuron loss and associated neuropathologic changes, and by sparing of memory function). Such protection can be brought about by surgical reduction in glucocorticoid exposure (adrenalectomy at mid-age followed by replacment with low glucocorticoid concentrations) or by behavioral means which lower basal glucocorticoid concentrations chronically.

Collectively, these studies suggest that glucocorticoids can damage hippocampal neurons over the lifetime. Such neurotoxicity, while surprising, is not without precedent. An extensive literature demonstrates that stress and/or glucocorticoids can be neurodegenerative in other situations; they can disrupt normal aspects of neural development, including damaging developing neurons. Furthermore, glucocorticoids impair the capacity of nervous tissue to recovery from injury.

The findings also demonstrate that this glucocorticoid toxicity plays the important physiological role of pacing the rate of hippocampal neuron loss during aging. This feature, combined with the effects of the hippocampus upon glucocorticoid secretion, form a feedforward cascade of senescent degeneration, referred to as the *glucocorticoid cascade* (figure 6.6). In one version of this model, senescent hippocampal neuron loss (arising for any of a variety of reasons) leads to glucocorticoid hypersecretion which, in turn, exacerbates the hippocampal neuron loss. In an alternative and probably rarer scenario, short periods of stress and of excessive glucocorticoid secretion (of perhaps up to a month) down-regulate the number of corticosteroid receptors per hippocampal neuron without damaging the neurons themselves. This down-regulation disrupts feedback sensitivity, and further hypersecretion ensues. When the stressor abates, the receptor number normalizes, as does the hypersecretion. However, with longer periods of glucocorticoid exposure, hippocampal neurons themselves are finally damaged, and the hypersecretion problem is now irreversible. This leads to further neuron loss and further hypersecretion. In either scenario, once the feed-forward cascade of receptor and neuron loss and of glucocorticoid hypersecretion emerge, each exacerbates the other.

Part II of this book explores the cellular and molecular mechanisms by which glucocorticoids are neurotoxic.

II How Does a Neuron Die?

7   Glucocorticoids Endanger Hippocampal Neurons

SUMMARY OF THE BOOK SO FAR

Part I of this book explored the relationships between stress and aging, specifically examining how aged organisms deal with stress and whether prolonged lifelong stress can accelerate some degenerative features of aging. The focus has been on a class of adrenal steroid hormones that are central to the stress-response, glucocorticoids. In many ways, glucocorticoids typify the two-edged nature of the stress response: While glucocorticoid secretion is vital to surviving short-term physical stressors, overexposure to this hormone (either in the face of exogenous administration or in some instances of chronic or repeated stressors) can be highly deleterious, causing a variety of stress-related disorders. Of necessity, then, the secretion of glucocorticoids is tightly regulated to protect the organism from the pathologic consequences of glucocorticoid under- or overexposure. This tight and complex regulation makes it a candidate to become dysfunctional with age.

In examining the regulation of glucocorticoid secretion in the aged rat, two broad classes of deficits were uncovered:

1. While the aged rat can appropriately secrete glucocorticoids in response to stress, it is impaired in its capacity to terminate glucocorticoid secretion at the end of stress. Furthermore, aged rats hypersecrete glucocorticoids basally and when habituating to mild stressors. These instances of glucocorticoid excess exact a pathologic price for the aging animal. The hypersecretion also manifests itself as a resistance to glucocorticoid feedback inhibition.

2. Within the brain, there is a loss of receptors for glucocorticoids (collectively called corticosteroid receptors). The loss is nearly exclusive to the hippocampus, which is a principal neural target site for glucocorticoids, with extremely high concentrations of such receptors. The aging hippocampus loses approximately half of such receptors (losing both receptor subtypes); remaining ones appear to function normally. The loss is predominately in neurons and in the pyramidal cell region of the hippocampus. Most importantly, the receptor loss is accompanied by a loss of hippocampal neurons as well, and it is corticosteroid receptor-rich neurons that are lost. Apparently, it is hippocampal neurons that had the highest concentrations of corticosteroid receptors which are most vulnerable to dying.

These two deficits—the glucocorticoid hypersecretion (and feedback failure) and the receptor loss (and neuron death)—are intertwined.

1. The degenerative changes in the hippocampus can cause the hypersecretion. The hippocampus has long been recognized for its role in glucocorticoid negative feedback. Circulating glucocorticoids are sensed by the

numerous hippocampal corticosteroid receptors; this causes the hippocampus to inhibit hypothalamic release of the peptides that ultimately cause glucocorticoid release from the adrenal. Thus, hippocampal damage blunts one of the CNS contributors to feedback efficacy, producing glucocorticoid hypersecretion. Even more subtly, mere loss of corticosteroid receptors in the hippocampus, without overt neuron loss, also blunts the efficacy with which the hippocampus works as a glucocorticoid feedback "brake." Experimental replication of the receptor and neuronal deficits of the aging hippocampus produces glucocorticoid hypersecretion very similar to that of the aging rat.

2. The degenerative changes in the aging hippocampus can be caused by excessive lifelong exposure to glucocorticoids. Short periods of stress and/or glucocorticoid overexposure can transiently down-regulate (i.e., decrease) the number of corticosteroid receptors in the hippocampus. With even more prolonged exposure to glucocorticoids, hippocampal neurons themselves will be destroyed. The recent literature concerning glucocorticoid neurotoxicity in the hippocampus suggests that the extent of lifetime exposure to glucocorticoids acts as a major determinant of the extent of hippocampal neuron loss during aging.

These pieces of dysregulation combine to form a feedforward cascade of senescent degeneration termed the glucocorticoid cascade (summarized in figure 6.6). Such degeneration can be initiated through a number of different routes. As the hippocampus begins to lose neurons as a normative part of aging (for reasons unrelated to glucocorticoids), the efficacy of feedback regulation is blunted, leading to glucocorticoid hypersecretion and feedback resistance. This, in turn, exacerbates the hippocampal damage, leading to further hypersecretion. As an alternative route to such dysregulation, during periods of sustained stress, the glucocorticoid-induced down-regulation of hippocampal corticosteroid receptors might blunt the efficacy of hippocampal feedback regulation, causing further hypersecretion. If stress abates at that point, the receptor depletion and the hypersecretion can normalize. But with more prolonged glucocorticoid overexposure, hippocampal neurons themselves are gradually lost, causing the pattern of hypersecretion to become permanent. The further glucocorticoid overexposure causes more hippocampal damage and further hypersecretion; pathologic consequences result throughout the body.

In part II of this book, the cellular mechanisms underlying the glucocorticoid neurotoxicity are explored.

Even nearly a decade after first beginning to think about this glucocorticoid cascade, the single component that seems most striking, most distressing, is the capacity of glucocorticoids to damage the hippocampus. It is at the center of the model, the means by which transient dysfunction can become permanent. How can glucocorticoids be neurodegenerative? The general features of the glucocorticoid neurotoxicity will be described in this chapter, as they begin to give clues as to how the steroid is damaging. In subsequent chapters, I will review how neurons are known to die—under conditions of controlled, programmed cell death, and during the energetic crises of neurological insults. This will then allow a synthesis of the current knowledge as to how glucocorticoids fit into the known mechanisms of neuron death.

In considering neurological disorders, certain likely suspects come to mind immediately—toxins, autoimmune attacks, metabolic disasters, and slow viruses. We do not immediately think of neurons being killed by hormones that are essential for life. When I began to consider the possible mechanisms of glucocorticoid neurotoxicity, the first question was whether the steroids really did kill neurons. It occurred to me that this was not actually necessary; glucocorticoids might only need to endanger neurons in some way to, in effect, put them near the edge of some sort of fatal cliff. If nothing else challenged the neurons at that time, the period of glucocorticoid exposure would pass, and the neurons would recover without any undue consequences. However, if during this period of glucocorticoid exposure the neurons were challenged with some additional insult, the latter might be less readily survived. In effect, if someone shoves you from behind such that you lurch 2 feet forward, that need not be a particularly damaging event—unless you are standing 1 foot from the edge of a cliff. Thus, if neurons are placed on the edge of some hypothetical metabolic cliff by glucocorticoids, various insults that should normally be survived now become more damaging.

This "threshold" model of glucocorticoids being not so much toxic as endangering predicted that various neurological insults should become more damaging as the hippocampus is exposed to more glucocorticoids. Considerable evidence now supports this idea. The first insult for which this was demonstrated was kainic acid (Sapolsky 1985a, 1986a,b; Theoret et al. 1985). The compound is an analog of the excitatory neurotransmitter glutamate (which will be discussed at length in chapter 9). In rats, kainic acid produces something resembling human status epilepticus (Ben-Ari 1985). When microinfused into Ammon's horn of the hippocampus, it preferentially damages CA_3 pyramidal neurons, the hippocampal region with the highest concentrations of kainic acid receptors. Because kainic acid causes an extremely discrete lesion of this linear cell field, it is possible to measure the length and width of cell deletion within any one coronal section, yielding a measurement of the area of damage (figure 7.1; Stein and Sapolsky, 1988); by combining those measures in consecutive sections, one can determine the volume of damage. In the initial study of the effects of glucocorticoids on kainic acid damage, the toxin was microinfused into the hippocampus of rats. Three different groups were compared: normal intact rats administered kainic acid; rats adrenalectomized and kept glucocorticoid-free for a week before and after the kainic acid exposure; and rats given exogenous corticosterone, such that they had circulating concentrations in the upper stress range for a week before and after the kainic acid exposure. Total hippocampal damage and damage within specific hippocampal cell fields was least in adrenalectomized rats and most in corticosterone-treated rats (table 7.1). Importantly, the reader should recall that 2 weeks of corticosterone treatment is insufficient to damage the hippocampus on its own (Sapolsky et al. 1985). Thus, the glucocorticoids, while not damaging on their own, were somehow exacerbating the excitotoxic kainic acid damage.

A similar pattern occurs with the antimetabolite 3-acetylpyridine (3AP). This compound uncouples electron transport and deprives the cell of its main source of energy (Hicks 1955). Thus, as an insult, it is somewhat similar to hypoglycemia. When 3AP is microinfused into Ammon's horn, it preferen-

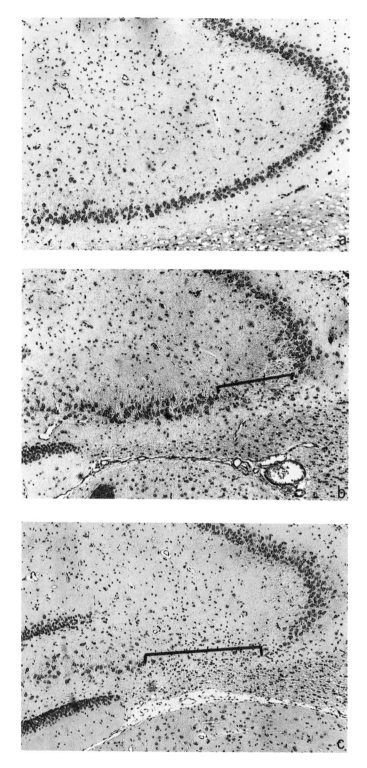

Figure 7.1. Representative photomicrographs of the CA_3 region of the hippocampus showing kainic acid–induced damage. (A) Control subject brain with no damage. (B) Mild damage. Bars demarcate extent of CA_3 damage, approximately 200 μ in length. (C) Severe damage; approximately 325 μ in length. (From Stein and Sapolsky, 1988, Brain Res 473, 175. Reprinted with permission from Elsevier Science Publishers.)

Table 7.1. Effects of corticosterone treatment on kainic acid–induced hippocampal damage ($\mu m^3 \times 10^5$)

Cell Field	ADX ($n = 7$)	INT ($n = 7$)	CORT ($n = 15$)
CA1	8 ± 5	4 ± 2	8 ± 3
CA2	0	0	0
CA3a	22 ± 2	30 ± 8	32 ± 6
CA3b	55 ± 10	107 ± 24	119 ± 11[a]
CA4	6 ± 3	18 ± 11	14 ± 5
DG	31 ± 18	40 ± 27	54 ± 18
Total damage	122 ± 31	199 ± 34	227 ± 43

Subjects were either adrenalectomized for 1 week before surgery (ADX), left intact (INT), or injected subcutaneously daily with 5 mg of corticosterone in sesame oil (CORT), treatments were continued for 1 week after surgery. Subjects were surgically infused with 0.035 μg of KA unilaterally into the hippocampus.
[a] Significant at the 0.05 level, Sheffe test following one-way analysis of variance (as compared with ADX subjects). Values are mean $\pm$ SE.
From Sapolsky (1985a).

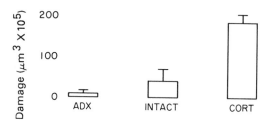

Figure 7.2. Glucocorticoids exacerbate the neurotoxicity of an antimetabolite. Volumes of hippocampal damage induced by 3AP microinfusions in adrenalectomized rats kept glucocorticoid free for 1 week before and after 3AP exposure and in intact rats and after administration of high physiological concentrations of corticosterone for a week before and after infusion. (From Sapolsky, 1985, J Neurosci 5, 1228. Reprinted with permission of Oxford University Press.)

tially damages dentate gyrus neurons. The reason for this vulnerability is not clear but hypoglycemia also preferentially damages these neurons (see chapter 9). As with kainic acid, the more glucocorticoids present, the more 3AP-induced damage (Sapolsky 1985a,b, 1986b; figure 7.2). With kainic acid, damage increased most dramatically when comparing adrenalectomized with intact animals; the transition from intact to corticosterone-treated did not cause much more exacerbation of damage. With 3AP, it was instead the transition from intact to corticosterone-treated rats in which there was the greatest exacerbation of damage.

A third model in which glucocorticoids exacerbate hippocampal damage is hypoxia-ischemia. When blood flow to the brain ceases (for example, following cardiac arrest), the first neurons to be damaged are CA_1 pyramidal neurons of the hippocampus. This selective vulnerability can be replicated with the four-vessel occlusion model of hypoxia-ischemia in the rat, in which the vertebral arteries are cauterized, and the carotids can be quickly and reversibly closed under pressure. With hypoxia-ischemia, there is usually not a discrete deletion of all the neurons within measurable stretches of hippocampal cell fields, as with kainic acid or 3AP exposure. Instead, damaged cells are typically scattered throughout the neurons of a particular cell field (usually CA_1). Thus, damage is assessed by blind scoring on a scale of severity of damage, rather than volume measurements as with the prior insults. With such a scoring system, we observed that following hypoxia-ischemia, corticosterone administration worsened damage, whereas adrenalectomy reduced damage (figure 7.3; Sapolsky and Pulsinelli, 1985); this glucocorticoid sensitivity has been replicated subsequently (Koide et al. 1986; Morse and Davis 1990b; Hall 1990; and Miller and Davis 1991, for the gerbil). In addition, a recent paper demonstrates that antagonism of CRF action protects against ischemic hippocampal injury in the rat (Lyonsm et al. 1991); however, the study does not clarify whether it is the antagonism of the neuroendocrine function of CRF (i.e., its

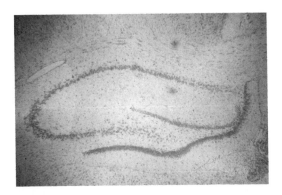

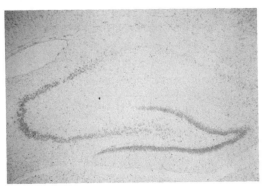

Figure 7.3. Glucocorticoids exacerbate hypoxic-ischemic damage to the hippocampus. Representative low-power photomicrographs of dorsal hippocampus from animals either adrenalectomized (*top*) or treated with corticosterone (*bottom*) immediately after 20 minutes of forebrain ischemia and killed 72 hours after reperfusion. Neurons were mostly preserved in the CA1 zone in adrenalectomized rats, but were completely lost in corticosterone-treated animals. (From Sapolsky and Pulsinelli, 1985, Glucocorticoids potentiate ischemic injury to neurons: Therapeutic implications. Science 229, 1397. Copyright AAAS.)

ability to stimulate the adrenocortical axis) or of its neuromodulatory role within the brain that is critical to the protection.

Finally, two recent abstracts suggest that glucocorticoids will also exacerbate the toxicity of the cholinergic neurotoxin ethylcholine aziridinium in the hippocampus (Hortnagl et al. 1991), and the cognitive deficits due to traumatic brain injury (Gbadebo et al. 1991).

In summary, glucocorticoids *synergize* with various neurological insults—under conditions where glucocorticoids are not, themselves, damaging hippocampal neurons, they are impairing the capacity of the neurons to survive insults. What is most striking is the potency of the glucocorticoid effect. In the models in which damage is quantifiable (kainic acid and 3AP), the volume of damage increased as much as an order of magnitude in some regions when comparing adrenalectomized and corticosterone-treated rats. In the qualitative scoring system for hypoxia-ischemia, shifting from zero to high glucocorticoid treatments shifted the predominant finding from no damage to severe damage. Thus, whatever the steroids are doing, it is a powerful effect.

These observations raised a number of questions, and in recent years, progress has been made in answering some of them. They clarify features of this glucocorticoid endangerment of the hippocampus.

DO GLUCOCORTICOIDS ENDANGER NEURONS IN OTHER BRAIN REGIONS?

Are the endangering effects of glucocorticoids limited to the hippocampus? In the first demonstration of a glucocorticoid/insult synergy (Sapolsky 1985a), I focused on this question. I examined whether the synergy occurred in a region that is vulnerable to kainic acid but has little sensitivity to glucocorticoids (the cerebellum, with plentiful kainic acid receptors, but few for corticosteroids), and one area in which there is marked sensitivity to glucocorticoids, but little to kainic acid (the hypothalamus, with plentiful corticosteroid receptors, but few for kainic acid). In the cerebellum, kainic acid microinfusion caused damage that was not affected by glucocorticoid manipulation. In the hypothalamus, no kainic damage was observed in any group. As will be discussed shortly, glucocorticoids also exacerbate kainic acid damage in vitro in primary hippocampal cultures. The steroids do not exacerbate kainic acid damage in cultures from cerebellum or hypothalamus (Packan and Sapolsky 1990). In summary, of the regions examined both in vivo and in vitro, the glucocorticoid/kainic acid synergy is restricted to the hippocampus.

With hypoxia-ischemia, additional brain regions known to be sensitive to the insult were also examined. In the neocortex, which has moderate numbers of corticosteroid receptors, severity of damage was modulated by glucocorticoid manipulation (Sapolsky and Pulsinelli 1985; Koide et al. 1986). In the striatum/caudate, which has lower concentrations of receptors, one study noted a moderate degree of exacerbation of damage by glucocorticoids (Sapolsky and Pulsinelli 1985), while another saw protection (Koide et al. 1986).

As another example of the anatomical specificity of this effect, glucocorticoids do not exacerbate monosodium glutamate—induced toxicity in the hypothalamus in the neonatal rat (Zoli et al. 1991b). Finally, in the studies in which the rate of hippocampal senescence was modulated by glucocorticoids, little attention was paid to whether senescent damage in other brain regions was altered by the manipulation.

Collectively, these findings suggest that, of the brain regions examined to date, the glucocorticoid/insult synergy is either exclusive to, or most dramatic in the hippocampus.

DO GLUCOCORTICOIDS ENDANGER HIPPOCAMPAL GLIA AS WELL?

As will be reviewed in chapter 9, a characteristic neuropathologic feature of the insults made worse by glucocorticoids is the selective vulnerability of neurons to them; typically, glial damage is only minimal except in the face of truly severe insults. Thus, our attention has mostly focused on the ability of glucocorticoids to endanger neurons. However, we have observed recently that glucocorticoids will impair the capacity of hippocampal astrocytes to survive hypoglycemia, hypoxia, and a combination of the two (Virgin et al. 1991; Tombaugh et al. 1992). These studies were done with in vitro monolayer cultures, and their relevance is not clear to the in vivo picture, given the rarity of astrocytic damage during these insults. However, they suggest that even under circumstances where glucocorticoids are not enhancing overt glial death, they may be impairing glial function. Chapter 11 explores some of the implications of this idea, given the numerous ways in which glia can aid neuronal survivorship during neurological insults.

DO GLUCOCORTICOIDS INCREASE THE TOXICITY OF THE INSULTS OR DECREASE THE RESILIANCE OF THE NEURONS?

Initially, this seems a rather abstract, even undefined question. It is helpful to state it more concretely. Kainic acid is more damaging to the hippocampus when more glucocorticoids are present. Is this because the excitotoxin has somehow been made more intrinsically toxic? Potentially, glucocorticoids could increase the diffusion of kainic acid throughout the hippocampus, or increase its half-life in the synapse, or increase the numbers of its receptors. All of these would be the biochemical equivalents of kainic acid now pushing the neuron harder. Alternatively, kainic acid could push with the same forcefulness that it always has, but the neurons may be less capable of resisting the pushing (i.e., they are already closer to the edge).

These are difficult questions, and in a rather simplistic first approach, I found that glucocorticoids do not increase the hippocampal diffusion of ^{3}H-kainic acid, nor do they increase the binding of a single concentration of ^{3}H-kainic acid in the hippocampus (Sapolsky 1985a). This suggests that the steroids are not changing anything about the kainic acid pharmacokinetics. Moreover, should the excitotoxin somehow be made intrinsically more toxic by gluco-corticoids, then there should also have been a glucocortiocid/kainic acid synergy in the cerebellum. Thus, glucocorticoids are probably not altering the excitotoxic potency of kainic acid. There is some disagreement as to whether they alter the excitatory potency of kainic acid. One report found that gluco-corticoids potentiated the functional indices of kainic acid–induced seizures (Lee et al. 1989), while another showed that glucocorticoids do not alter the EEG indices of kainic acid-induced seizures (Stein and Sapolsky 1988). Glucocorticoids also appear not to make hypoxia-ischemia more damaging by making the insult itself intrinsically more disruptive. As evidence, gluco-corticoids, under conditions where they exacerbate ischemic damage, do not alter the electrophysiological responses to ischemia (Koide et al. 1986).

Little additional work has been done to answer this question, but I think it unlikely that glucocorticoids somehow increase the intrinsic toxicity of kainic acid, 3AP, and hypoxia-ischemia. These insults are so varied in some of their specific mechanisms of action that, instead, it seems more plausible that the steroids make the neurons more vulnerable to a broad range of insults.

ARE GLUCOCORTICOIDS THEMSELVES THE ENDANGERING AGENTS, OR DO THEY ENDANGER SECONDARILY THROUGH OTHER ACTIONS?

The previous section suggests that, as a result of glucocorticoid exposure, hippocampal neurons are made vulnerable in some manner (as opposed to the steroids increasing the intrinsic toxicity of the insults themselves). But are the neurons made more vulnerable as a result of the glucocorticoid molecules working directly on them, or does the endangerment arise secondarily through some glucocorticoid action elsewhere? A priori, either scenario seems plausi-ble. On one hand, glucocorticoids have such vast numbers of actions through-out the body that there are endless ways in which they could affect the hippocampus indirectly—changes in cerebral blood flow, changes in circu-lating glucose, insulin, free fatty acid concentrations, so on. For example, a recent abstract suggests that glucocorticoids exacerbate hypoxic-ischemic damage in the hippocampus by raising temperature (which, in chapter 9, will be discussed to be a means of enhancing ischemic damage) (Morse and Davis 1990a; a view not supported by Sapolsky and Pulsinelli 1985, Koide et al. 1986, and a subsequent study by the same authors, Miller and Davis 1991). As a contrasting view, the fact that it is the hippocampus—with its uniquely high concentrations of corticosteroid receptors—in which the hormone/insult synergy is most likely argues that this results from a direct effect of gluco-corticoids on the hippocampal neuron.

The best evidence that the steroid effect is direct, rather than secondary to peripheral effects, is to eliminate the periphery—that is, to study the phenom-enon in tissue culture. As methodological background, cultured neurons can be damaged by excitotoxins, antimetabolites, and anoxia (cf. figure 7.4, show-ing time-lapse photographs of a cultured hippocampal neuron exposed to

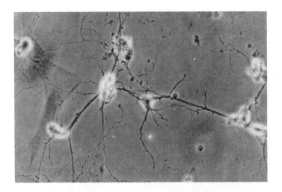

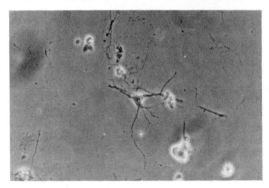

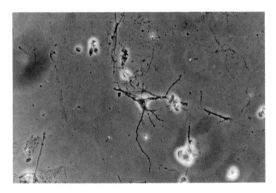

Figure 7.4. Time-lapse photographs showing primary cultures of hippocampal neurons undergoing kainic acid-induced degeneration. (A) Time zero, prior to exposure. (B) Three hours later, neighboring neurons have disintegrated, the central pyramidal neuron has lost processes, and the nucleus is becoming chromolytic. (C) After 6 hours, the cell body is bursting.

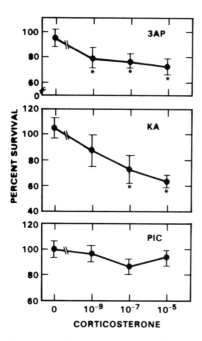

Figure 7.5. Glucocorticoids exacerbate neurotoxicity in cultured hippocampal neurons. Cultures were pretreated with indicated concentrations of corticosterone for 24 hours prior to exposure to kainic acid (KA) for 24 hours. (From Sapolsky et al., 1988, Brain Res 453, 367. Reprinted with permission from Elsevier Science Publishers.)

kainic acid). Damage can be quantified by measuring the media concentrations of an enzyme that is ubiquitous to all cells in roughly equal amounts, and is stable in media. Lactate dehydrogenase (LDH) meets these requirements (Koh and Choi 1987), and its efflux into the media represents dying cells lysing; one then determines if such cell loss is neuronal by immunocytochemically staining against a neuron-specific antigen. Finally, cultured hippocampal neurons and glia contain both types of corticosteroid receptors (Sapolsky et al. 1988; Bing et al. 1989; Vielkind et al. 1990).

Using this system, we have observed the same synergy as in vitro (Sapolsky et al. 1988; figure 7.5; Tombaugh et al. 1992). Again, as with the in vivo picture, the steroids exacerbate damage under conditions where they themselves are not damaging. We have now observed the synergy with kainic acid, 3AP, hypoglycemia, anoxia (the in vitro equivalent of hypoxia), the combination of anoxia and hypoglycemia, and the oxygen radical generator paraquat (Sapolsky et al. 1988, Tombaugh et al., submitted). These findings certainly suggest that the glucocorticoids work directly on the hippocampal neurons to endanger them.

An opposing view has been voiced. Landfield and colleagues (1981a) have suggested that at least some of the glucocorticoid toxicity in the aging hippocampus is secondary to glucocorticoid effects on ACTH. Their work demonstrated that long-term dimninution of glucocorticoid exposure protects the hippocampus from the neuron loss typical of aging (Landfield et al. 1981a).

Given the workings of negative feedback regulation, the diminished glucocorticoid concentrations will lead to ACTH hypersecretion, and the authors hypothesized that the salutary effects of low glucocorticoid exposure arose not so much from the hippocampus being exposed to *less* glucocorticoids, but to *more* ACTH. The rationale for this was the known stimulatory effects of ACTH, especially with respect to hippocampal electrophysiology. This idea predicted that prolonged exposure of the aging hippocampus to ACTH (or an ACTH analog) would have the same salutary effects as diminishing glucocorticoid exposure itself. This was demonstrated (Landfield et al. 1981a); in addition, similar protective effects were shown using a nonendocrine hippocampal stimulant (pentylenetetrazol).

These findings suggest that it is the ACTH molecule which is directly acting on the hippocampus to influence neuron death, rather than the glucocorticoid molecule. This suggests, for example, that under circumstances where sustained corticosterone overexposure damages the hippocampus (as in normal aging [Landfield et al. 1981a], chronic exogenous corticosterone administration [Sapolsky et al. 1985], or chronic stress [Kerr et al. 1991]), that it is not so much the high glucocorticoids, but the low ACTH concentrations that are the problem. The difficulty here is that the data fit with only one of three of those models. In the case of exogenous corticosterone administration, those high levels of glucocorticoids should indeed drive down endogenous ACTH release (via feedback regulation), making this scenario feasible. However, during aging, as reviewed, endogenous corticosterone concentrations are elevated *because* of elevated ACTH concentrations (reviewed in chapter 2). Likewise, in cases of chronic stress, the elevated corticosterone concentrations must be driven by ACTH. Therefore, while it is possible that the salutary effects of adrenalectomy are directly due to high levels of ACTH reaching the hippocampus, the damaging effects of high glucocorticoids cannot be due to inhibition of ACTH secretion. Furthermore, ACTH secreted by the pituitary does not readily cross the blood-brain barrier to reach the hippocampus, and there is little evidence for glucocorticoids regulating ACTH synthesized in the brain (Liotta and Krieger 1983). Collectively, these data, along with the tissue culture data lead me to think that the glucocorticoid endangerment is predominately direct, rather than secondary. By direct, I mean that the glucocorticoid molecule interacts with hippocampal cells to endanger them. This is somewhat simplistic; as will be seen in chapter 11, at least part of the endangerment of hippocampal neurons is due to glucocorticoids impairing the capacity of hippocampal astrocytes to aid neurons during neurological insults.

WHAT IS THE STEROID AND RECEPTOR SPECIFICITY OF THE GLUCOCORTICOID EFFECT?

Are glucocorticoids the only steroids that endanger the hippocampus? Before exploring that issue, do all glucocorticoids endanger the hippocampus? There are a number of naturally occurring glucocorticoids and vast numbers of synthetic ones. To date, only three have been examined. Corticosterone was the one utilized in most of the studies discussed. In addition, we find that cortisol and dexamethasone also exacerbate kainic acid damage in vitro. In agreement with this, dexamethasone exacerbates hypoxic-ischemic hippocampal damage in vivo (Koide et al. 1986). Another synthetic glucocorticoid, methylprednisolone, exacerbates hypoxic-ischemic damage in the gerbil (Hall 1991). Thus, at least a number of different glucocorticoids can endanger the structure. The effect appears limited to glucocorticoids, however, since neither estrogen, progesterone, testosterone, nor aldosterone exacerbate kainic acid damage in vitro (Packan and Sapolsky 1990; Tombaugh and Sapolsky, submitted).

If various glucocorticoid and nonglucocorticoid steroids exacerbated damage, it would suggest some generic steroidal effect, perhaps involving membrane fluidization. Instead, the limitation of the effect to glucocorticoids suggests mediation by one or both corticosteroid receptor types. Supporting this view, the corticosterone synergy with kainic acid in vitro is prevented with the Type II glucocorticoid receptor antagonist RU 38486 (Packan and Sapolsky 1990).

Finally, in at least one case, steroids protect neurons from injury, showing further that the glucocorticoid endangerment is not a generic steroid phenomenon. Excitotoxic injury to cultured neurons is decreased by the new 21-aminosteroid compounds (Monyer et al. 1990). This class of steroids does not have any glucocorticoid action.

In summary, the glucocorticoid endangerment appears to be specific to glucocorticoids, and to be glucocorticoid receptor-mediated. Returning to the question of whether glucocorticoids endanger directly or secondarily via ACTH, the glucocorticoid receptor mediation of the phenomenon in vitro certainly strengthens my conviction that it is direct hormone effect.

WHAT IS THE DOSE DEPENDENCY OF THE EFFECT?

How much corticosterone does it take to endanger the hippocampus? It is clear that the levels achieved during stress are capable of damaging—the studies with exogenous corticosterone administration produced circulating concentrations equivalent to those seen during stress. But can even basal concentrations of corticosterone endanger the hippocampus? Three sets of data suggest that to be the case; however, all three have some problems:

1. In the in vivo studies with the various insults, damage could be increased by exogenous corticosterone administration and decreased by adrenalectomy. The former finding suggests that the levels of corticosterone seen during stress can exacerbate injury. Initially, the latter finding seems to suggest that even basal concentrations of corticosterone can impair survivorship during those insults. The problem here, of course, is that corticosterone concentrations are not basal in rats undergoing excitotoxic seizures, hypoxia-ischemia, so on. This is shown in figure 7.6 (see Rao et al. 1989; Daniels et al. 1990; Farah et al. 1991), in which corticosterone concentrations soar to the upper physiological limits in rats undergoing hours of status epilepticus convulsions following

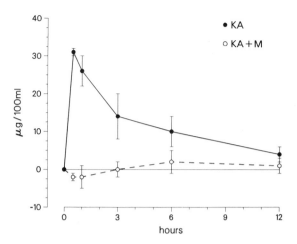

Figure 7.6. Kainic acid-induced seizures represent a robust stressor that stimulates glucocorticoid secretion. Circulating corticosterone concentrations are shown for control rats (exposed to sham microinfusion of kainic acid), rats microinfused with kainic acid (KA), or rats microinfused with kainic acid and then injected peripherally with the adrenal steroidogenesis inhibitor metyrapone (KA + M). (From Stein and Sapolsky, 1988, Brain Res 473, 175. Reprinted with permission from Elsevier Science Publishers.)

kainic acid administration. Thus, adrenalectomy in these cases is preventing the brain from being exposed to stress levels of corticosterone, rather than basal.

2. Adrenalectomy at 12 months of age prevents the hippocampal neuron loss that would typically occur in intact controls over the remaining year of life (Landfield et al. 1981a). Since the control rats were simply housed, undisturbed, in their home cages, they were probaby not exposed to a high frequency of stressors. Thus, the protective adrenalectomies were seemingly removing basal rather than stressed secretion. Initially, this seems strong evidence for even basal concentrations contributing to damage. However, a footnote in that report indicates that adrenalectomized rats were given low maintenance levels of corticosterone to help keep them alive for that period, and the circulating glucocorticoid concentrations produced by this treatment were not reported. Thus, it is not clear if that was sufficient to reinstate basal values of circulating corticosterone.

3. The in vitro studies showed that as little as 1 nM corticosterone exacerbates damage, while damage is exacerbated further when corticosterone concentrations are increased to the micromolar range (see figure 7.5). Basal corticosterone concentrations are certainly in the low nanomolar range; however, as is always the case with in vitro studies, one must be extremely cautious about extrapolating from there to the in vivo, physiologic situation.

In summary, at this stage, while there is some evidence that even basal concentrations of corticosterone can be endangering, it is far from settled. The reader should be reminded of the literature (reviewed in chapter 6) showing that prolonged absence of glucocorticoids (i.e., after adrenalectomy) can also damage the hippocampus (cf. Sloviter et al. 1989).

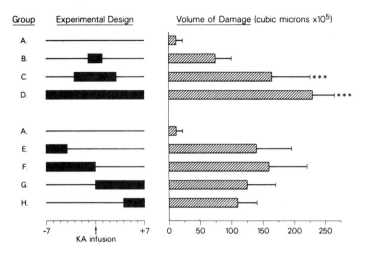

Figure 7.7. Time windows of corticosterone exposure exacerbating kainic acid-induced damage. (*Left*) Schematic representation of experimental design. Solid black bars indicate times during the 7 days prior to and following kainic acid (KA) infusion into the hippocampus during which adrenalectomized rats were injected daily with 10 mg corticosterone. Thin lines indicate times when rats were maintained free of corticosterone. (*Right*) Total hippocampal damage in rats of different experimental groups. (From Sapolsky 1986, Neuroendocrinology 43, 440. Reprinted with permission of S, Karger AG, Basel.)

WHAT IS THE TIME DEPENDENCY OF THE EFFECT?

The studies showing that stress and/or elevated corticosterone concentrations accelerates hippocampal aging involved months of treatment (Sapolsky et al. 1985; Kerr et al. 1991). The studies showing glucocorticoids exacerbating neurological insults involved days of exposure. In the case of the synergies with kainic acid or 3AP, steroid concentrations were manipulated for a week prior to and following the insult. For hypoxia-ischemia, manipulations were made for 72 hours following the insult. What is the minimal amount of time needed for endangerment? This was examined for the kainic acid synergy (figure 7.7 and table 7.2). As shown before, animals kept corticosterone-free for a week before and after the kainic acid infusion (group A) had minimal damage; rats with exposure to high concentrations for the week before and after (group D) had a significant increase in damage. Reduction of the period of corticosterone exposure to 3 days prior to and following the insult still augmented CA_3, CA_4, and total hippocampal damage (group C); as little as 24 hours of elevated steroid bracketing the insult augmented damage in CA_3 (group D). It is not known if even shorter periods of glucocorticoid exposure will also endanger. In chapter 11, I will argue that glucocorticoids endanger hippocampal neurons, at least in part, via inhibition of glucose transport in the hippocampus. We have shown that this effect takes a minimum of 4 to 8 hours of corticosterone exposure to occur. My bias at this point is that approximately 8 hours is probably the shortest time interval of corticosterone exposure that could be endangering.

Glucocorticoids Endanger Hippocampal Neurons

Table 7.2. Volumes of damage ($\mu m^3 \times 10^5$) following kainic acid infusion into the hippocampus

Group	n	CA3a	CA3b	CA4	Dentate gyrus
			Hippocampal region		
A	8	1 ± 1	6 ± 4	6 ± 6	0 ± 0
B	8	2 ± 1	$63 \pm 24^*$	30 ± 19	5 ± 5
C	8	7 ± 2	$96 \pm 34^{***}$	$66 \pm 34^*$	3 ± 3
D	18	$34 \pm 5^{****}$	$112 \pm 10^{***}$	46 ± 15	13 ± 5
A	8	1 ± 1	6 ± 4	6 ± 6	0 ± 0
E	8	9 ± 5	34 ± 14	68 ± 29	12 ± 9
F	8	1 ± 1	16 ± 5	94 ± 31	0 ± 0
G	8	4 ± 2	$55 \pm 24^*$	57 ± 24	0 ± 0
H	8	9 ± 3	$112 \pm 33^{***}$	37 ± 34	5 ± 5

$*$, $***$, $****$ significant difference from group A rats at the 0.05, 0.01, and 0.001 levels of significance, respectively; Newman-Keuls test following one-way analysis of variance; mean values $\pm$ SE.

Thus, whatever the glucocorticoids are doing, it is rapid. This is, of course, a relative term. This observation allowed the elimination of some potential mechanisms of endangerment. Glucocorticoids can nonenzymatically form adducts with proteins, which can impair protein function or lead to destructive cross-linked protein aggregates. This mechanism has been proposed for glucocorticoid-induced cataract formation (Bucala et al. 1982). As another mechanism, sustained glucocorticoid exposure, with its subsequent increase in steroid-receptor interaction with DNA, might increase the possibility of modifications of nucleic acids with damaging addition products. This was one of the mechanisms proposed to underlie some of the damaging effects of chronic estrogen exposure (Finch et al. 1984). Both of these mechanisms require weeks to months to occur. In contrast, most of the known catabolic effects of glucocorticoids on glucose transport and on macromolecular synthesis and degradation occur within a day. These will be considered in chapter 11.

The second part of the experiment shown in figure 7.7 examined another feature of the time dependency. In groups G and H, corticosterone concentrations were elevated only *after* the insult; in the case of H, with a 3-day delay. In both cases, damage was augmented. This implies that neuronal degeneration following kainic acid exposure emerges gradually, and its course can be influenced by glucocorticoids even after days. This delayed program of degeneration agrees with the known cell biology of these neurological insults (see chapter 9). In groups E and F, rats were exposed to corticosterone only *prior* to the insult. In the case of group E, this occurred even days before the infusion. In both cases, there was a manyfold increase in damage, as compared to group A (although these increases were not significant, because of large amounts of variability). These findings suggest that whatever the steroids are doing, they leave residual effects on the neurons, for up to days afterward.

In summary, fairly brief exposure to corticosterone can be endangering, and both a history of overexposure prior to an insult, as well as overexposure in its aftermath can exacerbate damage. Similar results have emerged in studying the synergy between corticosterone and 3AP (Sapolsky 1985b).

WHICH HIPPOCAMPAL CELL FIELDS ARE MOST VULNERABLE TO THE SYNERGY?

Data already presented suggest that glucocorticoids endanger the hippocampus via the type II glucocorticoid receptor. As a dogma of endocrinology, there is a rough correlation between the numbers of hormone receptors in a cell and its sensitivity to that hormone. This suggests that whichever hippocampal cell field has the highest concentration of glucocorticoid receptors should be the most vulnerable to the endangering effects of the hormone. This cannot be the case. Chapter 4 reviewed the distribution of corticosteroid receptors in the hippocampus and noted some controversy as to the relative concentrations in different cell fields, but regardless of the pattern, there cannot be a strict covariance between sheer numbers of receptors and vulnerability to the glucocorticoid synergy. In the case of aging, CA_3 neurons are most vulnerable to the toxic effects of glucocorticoids. In the case of kainic acid exposure, CA_3 neurons are most vulnerable to both the excitotoxin alone and to the kainic acid/glucocorticoid synergy. With hypoxia-ischemia, in contrast, it is the CA_1 region that is most sensitive to the insult alone and to the synergy, whereas with 3AP, it is the dentate gyrus.

All of these regions have high concentrations of glucocorticoid receptors relative to the rest of the brain. Where they differ is in their vulnerabilities to the insult themselves. This suggests that plentiful glucocorticoid receptors are neccesary, but not sufficient to explain the synergy. Instead, the glucocorticoid/insult synergy must arise from a neuron being both vulnerable to that particular insult and having a marked sensitivity (i.e., plentiful receptors) to glucocorticoids.

ARE THERE ANY HIPPOCAMPAL INSULTS THAT ARE NOT EXACERBATED BY GLUCOCORTICOIDS?

If an insult damages hippocampal neurons, yet does not synergize with glucocorticoids, the steroids and the insult might work via independent mechanisms. Thus, such a case would be of considerable heuristic value. There appears to be no synergy between corticosterone and the organometals trimethyl-lead and trimethyl-tin (which preferentially damage the hippocampus) (Theoret, Krigman, and Sapolsky, unpublished; O'Callaghan, personal communication). Unfortunately, this observation has not been of much use, as far less is known about the mechanisms of organometallic injury than about the neurological insults that synergize with glucocorticoids.

While global ischemic damage (i.e., cessation of blood flow to the entire brain) is clearly worsened by glucocorticoids, it is not clear whether infarct stroke damage (i.e., closure of single cerebral vessels in the brain) is also worsened. In one such study of infarct in neonatal rats, mortality was increased at least some of the time by glucocorticoids (Altman et al. 1984) while in another report, there was no increase in mortality but a decrease in damage (Barks et al. 1991). It is not clear whether this contrasts with the literature reported above because of the global/local ischemia contrast, or the adult/neonatal difference. As further support that the age difference might be of importance, excitotoxic damage to the neonatal rat hippocampus is not exacerbated by glucocorticoids (Barks 1991). Finally, as will be discussed later in this chapter, glucocorticoids reduce edema associated with brain tumors including, presumably, those in the hippocampus.

IMPLICATIONS AND CONCLUSIONS

Mechanisms of the Glucocorticoid Endangerment

This chaper reviews a considerable amount of data concerning glucocorticoid neurotoxicity. The most important finding is that the steroids need not directly kill the neurons, but merely endanger them. In numerous models, a synergy between glucocorticoids and an insult is generated under conditions where the hormones themselves are not damaging. This occurs with as little as 24 hours of high glucocorticoid exposure bracketing kainic acid infusion in vivo, or with as little as 1 nM corticosterone exposure in vitro. In summary, the hormones need not be toxic, only catabolic.

Whatever the catabolic, endangering actions of glucocorticoids are, they are very broad and general in nature. Hypoxia-ischemia and hypoglycemia halt substrate delivery to the brain; 3AP uncouples electron transport and disrupts oxidative phosphorylation; excitotoxins increase the level of neuronal excitation to pathologic levels; oxygen radicals cause uncontrolled cascades of cross-linking reactions and damage membranes. These are insults whose basic features are quite different; yet all synergize with glucocorticoids. The steroids probably do not interact directly with any of the insults, but instead place the neuron on the metaphorical edge of a very general cliff, such that varied insults are now more likely to push it over the edge.

Some of the mechanics of the endangerment are apparent from the data. Basically, the endangerment seems to work along the lines of the known features of glucocorticoid action in peripheral tissues. The steroid appears to act directly upon the target cell (as most strongly suggested by the in vitro data) in a classic, receptor-mediated fashion. Given the involvement of receptors, it is not surprising that there is steroid specificity, in that only glucocorticoids trigger a synergy with insults. Nor is it surprising that there is tissue specificity, as the effect is either exclusive to or most pronounced in the hippocampus, with its atypically high concentrations of corticosteroid receptors.

It is the Type II, lower-affinity, higher-capacity glucocorticoid receptor that seems to mediate the endangerment. As evidence, endangerment is caused by the Type II agonist dexamethasone and blocked by a Type II antagonist. In contrast, endangerment is not affected by a Type I agonist (aldosterone) or antagonist. The endangerment is triggered in vitro by nanomolar concentrations of corticosterone, suggesting that even low levels of Type II receptor occupancy are sufficient for endangerment. This suggests that even basal concentrations of glucocorticoids may be endangering; as discussed above, however, the current data do not support or exclude this possibility.

The data also suggest that glucocorticoid endangerment is not merely a function of how many receptors a neuron has. Instead, it appears that large numbers of receptors are neccesary, but not sufficient to cause a synergy between glucocorticoids and an insult—the cells have to be particularly vulnerable to the insult as well. In summary, in each model studied, the synergy is most pronounced in the hippocampal region in which the insult is, itself, most damaging.

Relevance to Neurology

The most important implication of this chapter concerns the insults worsened by glucocorticoids. Part I of this book is about glucocorticoids and hippocampal aging. With the introduction of these insults, the second half shifts to issues of glucocorticoids and hippocampal neurology. The synergy with the insults shows that glucocorticoids can endanger and, perhaps, kill outright; the variety of the insults testifies to the broadness of the glucocorticoid endangerment, while the existence of insults that do not synergize with glucocorticoids might suggest ways in which the steroids do *not* endanger. Should any of this apply to the primate or human (see chapter 14), these findings have some potential clinical relevance, in that some of the most common neurological insults to the hippocampus may be exacerbated by stress.

These results have some potential implications for neurology. The first concerns the use of exogenous glucocorticoids. If a rat has sustained a seizure or a hypoxic-ischemic crisis and is given exogenous glucocorticoids afterward, these data show that hippocampal damage will be increased. That might suggest that administration of glucocorticoids following such insults is contraindicated. Yet, there is a long-standing neurological tradition of administering glucocorticoids following hypoxia-ischemia or brain trauma. This is for one of two reasons: First, steroids are administered to prevent the edema (brain swelling) often induced by these insults. Glucocorticoids are quite efficacious in reversing the edema caused by tumors, and this has promoted their use to treat a broad range of edemas. Despite this reflex, a large literature derived from animals and humans shows that glucocorticoids are not particularly good at reversing the edema produced by global ischemia, focal ischemic stroke, and seizure (reviewed in chapter 11). As will be discussed in that chapter, a likely explanation is that glucocorticoids mostly protect against vasogenic edema, while seizures and hypoxia-ischemia mostly cause cellular edema.

Second, Megadoses of glucocorticoids are also used to decrease the pathologic consequences of spinal trauma (Young and Flamm 1982; Braughler and Hall 1985a; Bracken et al. 1990). This is most likely due to the ability of glucocorticoids to stabilize the membrane against peroxidative oxygen radical attack (see chapter 11). Thus, to the extent that glucocorticoids influence vascular permeability and oxygen radical damage, they can be helpful; to the extent that they are metabolically disruptive to neurons (to give away the punchline of a later chapter), they are endangering. Imagine the scenario of a traumatic insult affecting numerous brain regions, including the hippocampus. Do you administer the megadoses of glucocorticoids? I do not know the answer, but fortunately, this clinical choice probably is not neccesary. This is because there are substitutes available for glucocorticoids that more than match their protective potential. In the case of edema, mannitol is at least as efficacious, while in the case of spinal trauma, a number of nonglucocorticoid steroids are just as protective. This has been shown for progesterone (Betz and Coester 1990), and for the new 21-aminosteroids (aptly named "lazaroids") developed by the Upjohn Company (Hall et al. 1987). This subject will be discussed at greater length in chapters 11 and 14. For the present, the main point is that glucocorticoids can probably be dispensed with in those circumstances, and safer alternatives used (Sapolsky and Pulsinelli 1985).

But the data in this chapter have an even more striking potential neurological implication. At the time of these insults, not only can exogenous glucocorticoids make things worse, but adrenalectomy can decrease hippocampal damage. This implies that endogenous glucocorticoid secretion during these insults is sufficient to endanger the neurons and add to damage. Glucocorticoid secretion equal to that following major physical stressors can be provoked by kainic acid seizure (figure 7.6), hypoxia-ischemia (Pulsinelli and Sapolsky, unpublished) and, in the human, focal brain ischemia (Feibel et al. 1977). This has a critical implication: What is now viewed as "normal" hippocampal damage following one of these neurological insults may in fact be normal damage being worsened by the coincident adrenocortical stress response. Obviously, should this apply to humans, there will be the constraint that humans cannot be adrenalectomized following one of these neurological insults. Chapter 13 reviews data concerning the feasibility of transient, pharmacological adrenalectomy to reduce hippocampal damage after these insults. The data in figure 7.7 show that elevated glucocorticoid secretion occurring even before these insults may worsen damage. Whether this can be extrapolated to mean that even a history of stress prior to an insult can be endangering will also be considered in chapter 13.

All of this strikes me as rather alarming—the data in this chapter begin to suggest that neurological damage might need to be considered a stress-related disorder. These observations raise a fairly glaring question: Why should the adrenocortical axis be mobilized in response to a seizure or a stroke anyway? Chapter 1 suggests the adaptive logic of adrenocortical responsiveness in the context of acute physical demands—the logic again of the fleeing gazelle and the persuing lion. There seems no handy teleology that would explain why one should inhibit reproduction or divert glucose to quadriceps in response to hypoxia-ischemia. The only explanation that I can see is a fairly obvious one: There is no real reason why this response should be logical. Throughout evolution, there has been no selective pressure against mobilizing the adreno-cortical axis at that stage. Up until only the most recent of times, a hominid undergoing status epilepticus or hypoxia-ischemia would not survive. The deleterious consequences of the endocrine response to these insults have only recently been experienced for the first time. Seemingly, some features of these neurological crises trigger, in effect, the same alarms as would various physical and psychological stressors. For us, that convergent neuroendocrine wiring may well be maladaptive, but on an evolutionary time scale, that has been far too recent a development for there to have been any selection against that convergence.

For the neuroscientist concerned with neurological disorders and with neuron death, the overriding fact of the hippocampus is its profound vulnera-bility to neurological insult. It is either the primary, or among the primary brain regions damaged by global ischemia, various forms of sustained epileptic seizures, Alzheimer's disease, hypoglycemia, organometal toxicity, and alco-holic dementia (Siesjo, 1981). A variety of different theories have held sway over the years to explain why the hippocampus should be so fragile a struc-ture. These have focused on the microvasculature of the structure, the electro-physiological properties of individual hippocampal neurons, the distribution of excitatory amino acid neurotransmitter receptors, and so on. Chapters 9 and 10 will review current thinking about the issue. The present chapter's data suggest that an additional factor may add to the vulnerability of the hippocampus to injury—its marked sensitivity to glucocorticoid actions. Chapter 11 will examine what those critical actions may be.

Relevance to Aging

Before departing into the realm of the hippocampus and neurological injury, what do this chapter's data have to say about hippocampal aging? The studies reviewed earlier show that glucocorticoids have the potential to kill hippo-campal neurons over the lifetime, and that this appears to play an important role in hippocampal aging. Does this arise from the glucocorticoid endan-germent reviewed in this chapter? In other words, is it possible that gluco-corticoids lead to accelerated hippocampal aging merely by making the neu-rons more vulnerable to neurological insults? Figure 7.8 presents a schematic version of the two possibilities. On the left, the steroids kill the neurons outright, and glucocorticoid exposure leads to a gradual loss of hippocampal neurons. On the right is the scenario in which glucocorticoids are not actually killing, but exacerbate the damage due to external insults. In this case, damage is punctate, with the steroids increasing the size of the steps downward. This is a dichotomy central to gerontology: The left represents intrinsic degenera-tion, the right represents degeneration as a function of the rate of external insults. The question here, of course, is, What external insults? Epileptiform

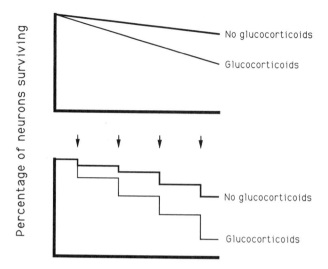

Figure 7.8. Schematic representation of the means by which glucocorticoids accelerate hippocampal neuronal senescence. On top is the scenario in which there is progressive and intrinsic neuron loss, with the slope of the decline being increased by glucocorticoids (GC). On the bottom is the scenario in which neuron loss is punctate, resulting from discrete and extrinsic insults (arrows); in this scenario, glucocorticoids enhance the extent of damage caused by individual extrinsic insults.

discharges, hypoxia-ischemia, and so on, are not normal everyday events just waiting to be exacerbated by glucocorticoids. Potentially, however, with prolonged glucocorticoid overexposure, hippocampal neurons become so endangered, so close to the edge, that they are pushed off by tiny external insults. The beleagured hippocampal neuron, awash in glucocorticoids, might be unable to survive even the brief hypoxia due to transient vasospasm or the mild hypoglycemia due to the animal being fed a few hours late.

This reminds me of a dichotomy that arises in depression research, where there is often the attempt to distinguish between "reactive" and "endogenous" depressions, with the former being depressions in response to an external trauma, and the latter occurring for no obvious external reason. In effect, all depressions are endogenous until the outside observer can find an event to which the depression can be viewed as being a reaction. There appear to be genetic propensities toward depression that lower the "threshold" for the triggering of reactive depressions (or, to insert our metaphor, which place the individual close to the edge of a depressive cliff). In effect, the genetic vulnerability can be great enough to trigger reactive depression in response to minor traumas; these may be too subtle to be discerned by the outside observer, and the depression will appear to be endogenous. Analogously, the glucocorticoid-induced vulnerability might be so great that even minor external insults damage; to the outside observer, these might be too subtle to be discerned, and the neuronal degeneration will be viewed as intrinsic.

At present, it is not clear whether glucocorticoids accelerate hippocampal aging through intrinsic killing or endangering—one can see how difficult it

would be to conduct these years-long studies in which every external perturbation would have to be controlled. However, this dichotomy between glucocorticoids killing neurons outright versus making them vulnerable during
aging seems somewhat academic. Basically, if glucocorticoids endanger neurons to the point that over the lifetime they are blown over by every little
gust of wind, that strikes me as a pretty close approximation to intrinsic aging
anyway.

CHAPTER SUMMARY

This chapter is the first in a series that seek to explain how glucocorticoids kill
hippocampal neurons. It introduces the idea most central to part II of this book:
Glucocorticoids need not necessarily kill the neurons outright. Instead, this
chapter reviews the evidence that glucocorticoids *endanger* the neurons. The
metaphor used throughout is that the steroids place the neurons close to the
edge of a cliff, and that any of a variety of insults are now more likely to push
the neuron over the proverbial edge. Thus, glucocorticoids *synergize* with a
number of neurological insults to the hippocampus, in that under conditions
where the steroids are not themselves damaging, they enhance the toxicity of
the insults. These insults include hypoxia-ischemia, seizure, hypoglycemia,
antimetabolites, and oxygen radical generators. Abruptly, this shifts the focus
of the book from the role of glucocorticoids in normative hippocampal aging
to their role in neurological disorders of the hippocampus.

The chapter then reviews the features known about this glucocorticoid
endangerment.

1. The synergy between glucocorticoids and these insults is either exclusive
to, or most pronounced in the hippocampus, of the brain regions tested
(hypothalamus, cortex, cerebellum, striatum). Nonglucocorticoid steroids (such
as estrogen, progesterone, aldosterone, testosterone, and steroid anesthetics)
do not endanger hippocampal neurons.

2. Potentially, the glucocorticoids could be enhancing the toxicity of these
insults (i.e., the insults now push harder), or they could be compromising the
ability of the neurons to survive the insults (i.e., the neurons cannot withstand
the usual degree of pushing). As an example of the former, glucocorticoids
might increase the binding of an excitotoxin to its receptor. A small amount
of data, plus teleological reasoning, suggest that glucocorticoids are compromising the abilities of neurons to survive these extremely varied insults.

3. Potentially, glucocorticoids could endanger by working directly on the
hippocampal neuron or secondarily through the many glucocorticoid actions
throughout the body. As examples of the latter, this could include changes in
blood glucose or insulin concentrations, cerebral blood flow, and so on. While
there has been at least one report to the contrary, the bulk of findings suggest
that the effects are direct. As the strongest evidence, glucocorticoids synergize
with these insults in vitro (with primary monolayer cultures of hippocampal
neurons), and the endangerment can be blocked by antagonizing Type II
corticosteroid receptors.

4. While there is a receptor mediation of the endangerment, sheer numbers of receptors does not guarantee a synergy. Instead, a reasonably high concentration of receptors is necessary but not sufficient; in addition, the neuron must be particularly vulnerable to the neurological insult as well.

5. Fairly low concentrations of corticosterone (in the low nanomolar range) endanger the neurons in vitro. While this suggests that even basal glucocorticoid concentrations might be endangering in vivo, this has not been tested.

6. As little as 24 hours of glucocorticoid exposure bracketing an insult will exacerbate damage. This eliminates a number of possible mechanisms of endangerment, including the slow, nonenzymatic formation of steroid/nucleic acid adducts. Moreover, glucocorticoid exposure in the period prior to the insult will exacerbate damage (suggesting that a recent history of glucocorticoid overexposure can worsen neurological insults) as will steroid exposure only following an insult.

7. At present, the sole insults to the hippocampus which are not exacerbated by glucocorticoids are the organometallic toxins and tumor-associated edema (in which glucocorticoids are protective).

Collectively, these data suggest that glucocorticoids act in a direct manner in the hippocampus to induce a very broad vulnerability in neurons. These findings have implications for both neurology and gerontology:

Neurological Implications

The most striking point is that stress and/or glucocorticoids might, perhaps, have to now be considered as exacerbators of neurological insults to the hippocampus. These data show that glucocorticoid administration around the time of numerous insults will increase hippocampal damage; this paves the way for the discussion in chapter 11 as to when exogenous glucocorticoid administration is still useful in clinical neurology. Just as importantly, these data show that diminishing endogenous glucocorticoid secretion at the time of these insults is protective. These insults are sufficiently stressful to provoke considerable amounts of glucocorticoid secretion, and this suggests that what is viewed as "normal" neurological damage after, for example, hypoxia-ischemia, might be normal damage exacerbated by the coincident glucocorticoid stress-response. Chapter 13 explores some possible clinical interventions to subtract out endangering glucocorticoids at the time of neurological insults.

Gerontological Implications

In returning to the glucocorticoid neurotoxicity presented in part I, the present findings bring up the question of whether glucocorticoids really do directly kill hippocampal neurons during aging, or simply make them so endangered that extremely small and subtle insults are now toxic. The answer to this is not known.

In summary, this chapter shifts the emphasis from glucocorticoid toxicity to glucocorticoid endangerment, and from gerontology to neuron death during neurological disorders. The next three chapters review the mechanisms of neuron death during neurological crises and during programmed cell death. This paves the way for understanding the cellular biology by which glucocorticoids endanger hippocampal neurons and makes some of these neurological crises more damaging.

8   A Brief Interlude: Programmed Cell Death

SUMMARY OF THE BOOK SO FAR

Various stressors will trigger the endocrine and neural adaptations that form the stress-response. The adrenal secretion of glucocorticoids is central to the stress-response, and typifies its two-edged quality: While glucocorticoids are essential for surviving short-term physical stressors, overexposure to these hormones can cause varous stress-related diseases.

Part I of this book examined how glucocorticoid secretion is regulated during aging, as well as whether excessive exposure to glucocorticoids over the lifetime can accelerate aspects of brain aging. Chapter 3 documented how aged rats hypersecrete glucocorticoids under a number of circumstances— basally, during habituation to mild stressors, and when recovering from stressors. Moreover, aged rats are resistant to glucocorticoid feedback inhibition. This suggested that a site in the brain involved in such feedback loses its sensitivity to glucocorticoids during aging. A plausible site is the hippocampus—it contains the highest concentrations of receptors for glucocorticoids of any brain region and has long been recognized for its role as a mediator of glucocorticoid feedback inhibition. Chapter 4 reviewed how the aged hippocampus loses a substantial percentage of receptors for glucocorticoids; in addition, it loses neurons, and those lost are particularly rich in corticosteroid receptors. This suggests that the senescent degeneration of the hippocampus contributes to the hypersecretion of glucocorticoids. The senescent loss of hippocampal neurons unexpectedly turns out to be, at least in part, due to cumulative exposure to glucocorticoids. Chapter 6 reviewed the evidence for such glucocorticoid neurotoxicity.

These features of glucocorticoid actions and regulation combine to form a feedforward cascade of degeneration, termed the *glucocorticoid cascade*. In its simplest form, this model incorporates the fact that glucocorticoids can damage the hippocampus and impair its capacity to function as a glucocorticoid negative feedback "brake." This leads to glucocorticoid hypersecretion which, in addition to its other deleterious effects, damages the hippocampus further. The end of chapter 6 elaborated on this model and emphasized some caveats about its likely validity.

Part II of the book explores how glucocorticoids damage hippocampal neurons. Chapter 7 reviewed how the steroids need not neccesarily be toxic. Instead, glucocorticoids appear to *endanger* hippocampal neurons, making them less capable of surviving coincident metabolic insults. Such insults include hypoxia-ischemia, seizure, hypoglycemia, exposure to antimetabolites, and oxygen radical generators. Therefore, glucocorticoids may not only play a role in accelerating hippocampal aging but might also augment the toxicity of some of the most common neurological insults to the hippocampus. The coming chapters examine how glucocorticoids endanger the hippocampus and increase the toxicity of these insults. In order to appreciate this, it is useful to review how neurons die, both in cases of pathologic insults and in cases of programmed cell death.

The previous chapters have outlined the evidence that glucocorticoids can be neurotoxic in the hippocampus and the features of this neurotoxicity. The critical point is, perhaps, that the steroids need not be directly toxic, but may well merely act in some catabolic fashion to endanger the neurons, impairing their capacity to survive other coincident insults. Recent work has uncovered what may be the mechanisms of the glucocorticoid endangerment. To appreciate which cascades of degeneration are exacerbated by the hormones, it now becomes necessary to devote the next few chapters to reviewing how neurons are thought to die.

The two chapters following this examine how energetic insults kill neurons. They will focus on the three neurological insults of hypoxia-ischemia, seizure, and hypoglycemia. Recall that all of them are worsened by glucocorticoids. The general theme throughout is one of chaos: a primary insult leading to oxygen radical production, abnormal movement of ions, neurotransmitters, and protons. Potentially, such perturbations can be contained but with a large energetic cost. During these crises, energetic defenses are eventually breached and the dysfunctions spiral out of control. Each point of perturbation can potentially exacerbate many of the others, and neurons eventually die. The hallmark characteristics of such *necrotic cell death* are the broad range of cell processes that become deranged, the idiosyncratic and individualistic paths by which the cells can reach the point of dying, and the (relatively) delayed time course.

In contrast to this picture of cells dying during an energetic crisis, cells are often killed as a feature of normal physiology, rather than pathophysiology. These represent instances of *programmed cell death*, or *apoptosis*. In programmed cell death, the cascade of damaging events is usually more linear than in necrotic cell death, involving less obvious global derangements until just before the cell dies. Thus, the process is less idiosyncratic, and instead is more stereotypical—a large percentage of the cells die with a similar time course and similar degenerative features, with the death occurring in an active fashion. At least three systems of apoptosis have been studied in some detail. As a first example, neurons may die during development, not because they are dysfunctional or because a major neurological crisis has occurred, but rather because they have become expendable in the normal developmental process. Second, the immune system attacks and lyses virally infected or tumorous cells as a requisite component of immune defenses. Finally, glucocorticoids destroy lymphocytes and thymocytes as a means by which the stress-response suppresses immune function. This chapter reviews what is known about the mechanisms underlying these instances of apoptosis and reviews how, in the one case tested, an apoptotic model does not explain how glucocorticoids endanger hippocampal neurons.

NEURAL DEGENERATION DURING DEVELOPMENT

The neurologist thinks of neuron death as a central feature of disease and dysfunction. However, for the developmental neurobiologist, resorting to the sort of platitude that festers at commencement ceremonies, neuron death is not so much an end as a beginning. Massive amounts of neuronal "die-off" are required for normal CNS development (Hamburger and Oppenheim 1982; Cowan et al. 1984). In some cases, neurons are needed only transiently during development. Such neurons may form perfectly adequate synapses and seem destined for long, rewarding lives but may, in fact, die during development. Recent work suggests that these cells resemble some of the trappings of construction sites, serving as the neuronal equivalents of scaffolding, porto-toilets, or worksheds. When the neural ediface has reached a certain stage of completion, these neurons are removed by apoptotic mechanisms (Chun et al. 1987). As an even more common feature of neural apoptosis, there is considerable overproduction of the primary neurons of the nervous system. As a result of this, there emerges a competition for synaptic connections with neighboring neurons, and those less connected are eliminated. Such developmental pruning is viewed as an adaptive means of shaping, selecting for optimal wiring of the nervous system, and correcting errors (Hamburger and Oppenheim 1982). As an extension, there is overproduction and pruning of synapses as well (Rakic et al. 1986).

This system of neuronal competition and elimination during development requires that something about making a neuronal connection be life saving. It may be the synaptic activity that is essential or a "life-factor" that is encountered as a result of contact. Various trophic factors appear to serve the second role. The most plausible of these is nerve growth factor (NGF), the first such trophic factor isolated (Levi-Montalcini 1987). For example, sympathetic neurons of the superior cervical ganglion of rats encounter NGF when they form synaptic contacts during fetal development, and such NGF is essential for survival. Therefore, sympathetic neurons die within 24 to 48 hours when deprived of NGF in vitro. Recent work has focused on why NGF deprivation is toxic. One might assume that in the absence of a critical trophic factor, the neuron simply collapses in some manner, undergoing passive attrition. However, in this case, the death is instead an active process, actually involving turning on of a suicide switch. It requires RNA and protein synthesis, and it can be prevented with synthesis inhibitors. Inhibitors such as cycloheximide must be applied before the first morphologic signs of degeneration (at around 18 hours), implying that the process has become independent of protein synthesis at that point (Martin et al. 1988). Moreover, at least 80% of protein synthesis must be inhibited in order to be protective (Martin et al. 1990). Currently, a number of issues are not yet settled. First, it is not clear how turning on this suicide switch kills. It does not appear to involve rampant proteolysis, since the programmed death cannot be prevented with protease inhibitors. Little information is available beyond that, except that death is not prevented by phorbol esters, polyamines, kinase inhibitors, or drugs that alter the cytoskeleton, but is prevented by interferon (Chang et al. 1990). It is also not clear how NGF suppresses the suicide switch. There is evidence that agents which elevate intracellular cAMP levels prevent the cell death. However, it is not clear whether elevated cAMP prevents the activation of the suicide mechanism, inactivates the protein(s) synthesized, or promotes the repair of whatever damage the protein(s) causes. Moreover, this appears to be a pharmacological, rather than physiological effect, since NGF deprivation does not cause a drop in intracellular cAMP (Martin et al. 1990). As a final hint, flunarizine, a calcium channel blocker, prevents the death; however, the dose of flunarizine required is far in excess of that which blocks channels, and other channel blockers are not efficacious, suggesting that the protection arises from some as yet unrecognized additional mechanism of action of the drug (Rich and Hollowell 1990).

Work from this group has also shown that in the absence of NGF, neuronal depolarization can also save the neuron. This is seen with the salutary effects of high potassium concentrations in the medium. The critical consequence of the potassium appears to be opening of voltage-dependent L-type calcium channels, as the protective effects of potassium are prevented by removing calcium from the medium, or by blocking such channels (Koike et al. 1989). It is not known how the depolarization-induced influx of calcium saves the cell or whether this route interacts with the route of the genomic suicide switch.

In my view, the most important finding from these studies is that NGF suppresses the expression of a genomic suicide switch, which would otherwise produce a fatal protein(s). A similar picture occurs in the dorsal root ganglion of the developing chick. Apoptotic death is, again, an active process requiring protein synthesis. Death can be enhanced by blockade of ganglionic transmission, suggesting dependency on activity. Again, the final cascade does not appear to involve proteolysis (Maderdrut et al. 1988; Oppenheim and Prevette 1988). Along the same lines, there is some suggestion that cGMP also prevents motoneuron death (Weill and Greene 1984), although this view is not unanimous (Oppenheim 1985).

For sheer magnitude of transformation of organisms during development, nothing can rival the metamorphosis of insects. Elegant research has focused on the mechanisms of programmed motoneuron death in the moth, *Manduca sexta*, and the fly, *Drosophila melanogaster*, in which individual neurons can be identified and followed over time (Truman 1984; Truman and Schwartz 1984; Weeks and Truman 1985, 1986; Booker and Truman 1987; Fahrbach and Truman 1987). In these cases, the signal is not withdrawal of NGF but rather from ecdysteroid hormones. Ecdysteroid levels gradually rise over days during development. Around the time of eclosion, hormone concentrations begin to drop, and within a day, degeneration in motoneurons destined to die begins. The endoplasmic reticulum becomes disrupted, ribosomes are released, the nucleus is ruptured, and neuronal remains are phagocytosed by glia. Cells are dead by 72 hours. Neurons that lack ecdysteroid receptors are insensitive to the phenomenon and survive this period.

Thus, both exposure to and withdrawal from ecdysteroids are required for neuron death. If the initial rise does not occur or, once having occurred, the withdrawal is prevented, no death occurs. This has been shown in vitro, where the pattern of cellular vulnerability in these identified neurons is identical to the in vivo situation. It is during the period of withdrawal that an active suicide process is initiated. Up to 12 hours after withdrawal, reexposure to ecdysteroids can save the cells. Beginning approximately 12 hours after withdrawal, the cells lose ecdysteroid receptors and become insensitive to the hormone. During that period, the cells can be saved by inhibition of RNA synthesis. Shortly after that, they can only be saved by inhibition of protein synthesis. Ultimately, the cell becomes insensitive to any of these manipulations. There is also a transneuronal component of dying: The ecdysteroid-induced death requires some sort of signal from the neighboring neurons. As evidence, if vulnerable neurons are isolated by crushing connections to them and destroying neighboring ganglia, the target cell survives the ecdysteroid withdrawal. Isolation like this is protective even up to 50 hours after hormone withdrawal.

The nature of the induced death protein(s) and of the transneuronal communication is not known. What seems most interesting to me is the necessity for both exposure to and withdrawal from ecdysteroids for death to occur. In effect, the insect nervous system becomes fatally "addicted" to ecdysteroids. Several models can be constructed explaining these data. All must explain why there is no death prior to or during ecdysteroid exposure and why killing is protein synthesis dependent during withdrawal. In one such model, ecdysteroids induce the synthesis of proteins A and B. Protein C is constitutively made at all times. A and C combine to form a toxic complex. B, in contrast, can bind to the toxic A/C complex and inactivate it. The only assumption needed to explain the data is that A has a longer half-life than either B or C. Thus, prior to ecdysteroid exposure, only C is made, which is benign on its own. During ecdysteroid exposure, A, B and C are all made, and the nontoxic

Table 8.1. Necessary features to explain ecdysteroid "addiction" among insect motoneurons

Time period	Ecdysteroid-induced products	Constitutive products	Result
Pre-ecdysteroid secretion	None present	Factor C	Survival
Ecdysteroid secretion	Factors A and B; A is longer lasting	Factor C	A/B/C complex; survival
Ecdysteroid withdrawal	Persistence of factor A	Factor C	Fatal A/C complex dependent on continued synthesis of C

A/B/C complex is formed. Following ecdysteroid withdrawal, preexisting B and C molecules are eliminated, but the A molecules persist. No new B proteins are made (because of the ecdysteroid withdrawal), but new constitutive C is formed. A and C can now form a toxic complex—so long as protein synthesis is not inhibited (table 8.1). A number of other models can be constructed along similar lines. In each case, the ecdysteroids produce two signals that neutralize each other yet differ in their half-lives, and the longer-lasting one must interact with something made during the withdrawal period. (I am grateful to Desta Packan, Geoff Tombaugh, and Charles Virgin for brainstorming about some of these models.)

CELL-MEDIATED KILLING BY THE IMMUNE SYSTEM

A major task of the immune system is to destroy bacteria or native cells that have become virally infected, senescent, or transformed and tumorous. Two types of immune "killer cells" exist and mediate this destruction—cytotoxic T cells and natural killer cells. The killer cell binds tightly to a targeted cell, and the targeted cell begins to die within minutes, with degeneration being dependent on the presence of calcium. Somehow, the binding initiates a fatal cascade that continues even after the killer cell has separated from the targeted cell. In recent years, a number of apoptotic mechanisms have been identified that are relevant to this cell-mediated killing.

The mechanism that has received, perhaps, the most attention involves the formation of pores in the cell membrane of the targeted cell. This is caused by the insertion into the membrane of the protein perforin, contained in secretory granules in killer cells (Masson and Tschopp 1985; Podack et al. 1985; Young et al. 1986). As the killer cell approaches the targeted cell, the granules are reoriented in the cytoplasm near the binding site between the cells. Binding itself triggers a massive calcium influx into the killer cell, causing perforin release.

The perforin enters the membrane of the targeted cell. The protein is single-chained, and as a monomer, cannot form a pore. Instead, when calcium is present around the membrane, polymers of perforin form, producing ringlike pores. Prior to the isolation of perforin, electron microscopy demonstrated such pores on targeted cells after contact with killer cells (Dourmashkin 1980; Podack and Dennert 1983). The role for calcium in allowing perforin release and polymerization is the basis for the calcium dependency of killing. In addition, since perforin can enter the membrane only as a monomer, any secreted perforin that somehow becomes free in the extracellular space and is polymerized by calcium will be unable to pass through a membrane and form a damaging pore. This is thought to be a protective mechanism to insure that neighboring nontargeted cells are not inadvertently destroyed by errant perforin (Young and Cohn 1986). As an outsider to this area of research, I am confused as to what happens after the pore formation. Some authors have emphasized that the pores now allow the indiscriminate *outward leakage* of critical ions and molecules, killing the cell. Others have emphasized that the pores allow the indiscriminate *entry* of water and salts into the cell, leading to profound osmotic disequilibrium and bursting (reviewed in Young and Cohn 1986; Stanley and Luzio 1988).

Thus, pore formation appears to be an important mechanism underlying cell-mediated killing. It may also be involved in humoral-mediated killing. In this instance, bacterial cells become targeted as a result of being labeled by antibodies. This triggers an attack on the cell by the complement cascade. It has been known for some time that complement-induced killing also involves pore formation on the membrane of the target cell (Humphrey and Dourmashkin 1969). It turns out that the final step in the complement cascade is the production of a protein that polymerizes in the target membrane and forms pores. Not surprisingly, there is considerable sequence homology between this protein (the C9 component of the complement membrane attack complex) and the perforin of killer cells (Shinkai et al. 1988). As further evidence for the ubiquity of this mechanism in immune defenses, a pore-forming protein found in human eosinophils induces damage in the membranes of target cells (Young et al. 1986).

Perforin insertion, however, is not the sole mechanism for killer cell-induced apoptosis (Ostergaard et al. 1987). Another mechanism involves fragmentation of DNA in the targeted cell. This has been reported, based on cytological observation. Recently, cytotoxic T lymphocytes were shown to fragment the DNA of targeted cells (Ucker 1987). At this stage, it is not clear how this is accomplished, although it is assumed that the killer cell either injects an endonuclease into the targeted cell or induces the expression of an endonuclease by the targeted cell itself.

As described, the immune system has at least two different mechanisms for bringing about the rapid killing of target cells. Perforin works within minutes, while DNA fragmentation takes hours. Collectively, they form an extremely efficient pair of weapons in the immune armamentarium. As will be seen, this is not the only instance in which programmed cell death is brought about by the fragmentation of DNA. Ironically, the other example is in the ability of glucocorticoids to kill lymphocytes during stress.

IMMUNOSUPPRESSION BY GLUCOCORTICOIDS DURING STRESS

Since the time of Selye, stress has been recognized to suppress the immune system. Immune tissues such as the thymus and lymph nodes atrophy; circulating lymphocyte counts decline, immunocompetence is impaired, and various pathologic challenges to the body become more damaging (Krieger 1982). Glucocorticoids are central to this suppression, reducing the production of new lymphocytes, lysing preexisting lymphocytes or thymocytes and blocking the release of and sensitivity to a variety of lymphokines (reviewed in Cupps and Fauci 1982; Munck et al. 1984; Bateman et al. 1984). It remains somewhat unclear whether this is a pharmacological or physiological effect of the steroids. Most psychoimmunologists are betting on the latter, namely, that a relatively small change in glucocorticoid concentrations (for example in response to psychological stressors) actually does change immune function. Finally, it remains unclear just why it makes sense to suppress immune function during stress. As discussed in chapter 2, it is currently a matter of much discussion whether glucocorticoid-induced immunosuppression represents mediation of the stress-response or recovery from it. As noted, whichever the case, there is probably some adaptive purpose to this immunosupression, rather than it being a mere epiphenomenon. As evidence, the glucocorticoid-induced immunosuppression appears to be so useful to the immune system that the latter, in effect, *asks* the brain to trigger that response during stress— during immune challenge by a pathogen, stimulated macrophages and monocytes release interleukin-1, which can trigger hypothalamic release of CRF and thus initiate an adrenocortical cascade (Sapolsky et al. 1987; Berkenbosch et al. 1987).

Among the immunosuppressive actions of glucocorticoids, the one most relevant to this chapter is their lysing of lymphocytes. Such apoptosis occurs within 6 to 12 hours for murine lymphocytes and after 20 to 24 hours for those of humans (Burton et al. 1967; Munck and Crabtree, 1981; Compton and Cidlowski 1986). As an early morphologic sign of cellular degeneration, chromatin condenses; in retrospect, this was an important clue to the mechanism of the killing. The lymphocytolysis is triggered by low nanomolar concentrations of essentially all glucocorticoids but not by nonglucocorticoid steroids (Compton and Cidlowski 1986). As a measure of the physiological relevance of the apoptosis, the killing can also be caused by acute stress or ACTH (Compton and Cidlowski 1986; Masters et al. 1989).

Initially, researchers thought that glucocorticoids killed lymphocytes merely by being as catabolic as they are in most other tissues. Glucocorticoids decrease glucose transport into lymphocytes (Munck and Crabtree 1981), inhibit their macromolecular and lipid synthesis (Makman et al. 1966, 1968; Rosen et al. 1972; Foley et al. 1980), accelerate RNA and protein degradation (Cidlowski 1982; MacDonald et al. 1980), and inhibit polyamine synthesis and block cell growth (Harmon et al. 1979; Russell et al. 1981; Bradshaw and Vedeckis 1983; Bittner and Wielckens 1988). While these are certainly unpleasant things to happen to a cell, the consensus in the field is that the magnitude of these effects is insufficient to kill. These are, instead, thought to cause the "cytostatic" (arresting of cell growth) effects of glucocorticoids on lymphocytes (Bittner and Wielckens 1988).

Instead, the lysis occurs through a much more discrete, selective mechanism. Much as with the examples of neuronal killing, the lymphocytolysis involves an active genomic suicide switch. As evidence, the lysis can be blocked with RNA and protein synthesis inhibitors (Wyllie et al. 1984; Cohen and Duke 1984). Moreover, mutant lymphocyte cell lines exist which are resistant to the lysis (Gehring 1986). Much as with one of the mechanisms of cell-mediated immune killing, the steroid-induced killing involves DNA fragmentation. The steroids induce the synthesis of at least one endonuclease which cleaves the DNA at multiple sites; a candidate nuclease has been identified (Compton and Cidlowski 1987). Not surprisingly, this proves fatal to the cell. As a distinctive feature of this model, cleavage occurs at internucleosomal sites. When visualized on an agarose gel, this produces a distinctive "ladder" of DNA fragments that are multiples of about 180 base pairs (Wyllie 1980; Umansky et al. 1981; Wyllie et al. 1984; Cohen and Duke 1984; Compton and Cidlowski 1986, 1987; Compton et al. 1988; figure 8.1). The DNA fragmentation precedes death and appears to trigger attempts by the cell at DNA repair: Poly(ADP-ribosyl)ation is activated, NAD concentrations fall, and glucocorticoid toxicity is exacerbated by the poly(ADP-ribose)synthetase inhibitor, benzamide (Wielckens and Delfs 1986; Wielckens et al. 1987). Some researchers have viewed the cell death as arising not from the DNA fragmentation but from the energetic costs (i.e., the NAD depletion) of repairing the DNA (Bittner and Wielckens 1988). However, this is a distinctly minority view, and I know of no study that shows that the lymphocytolytic effects of glucocorticoids can be reversed by

DNase Sensitivity

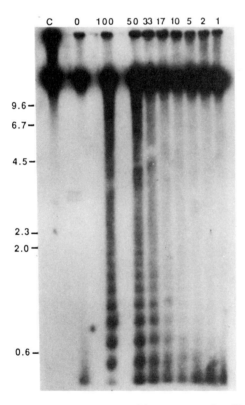

Figure 8.1. Fragmentation of thymic DNA induced by glucocorticoids. Samples of thymic DNA from adrenalectomized rats treated with oil (lane C) or dexamethasone (DEX) at concentrations of 100, 50, 33, 17, 10, 5, 2 or 1 ng. (Modified from J. Masters, C. Finch, R. Sapolsky. Glucocortiocid endangerment of hippocampal neurons does not involve DNA cleavage. Endocrinology l24, 3083–3088, 1989. Reprinted with permission of Williams and Wilkins Publishers.)

supplementing the cells with excess energy. Instead, the massive DNA fragmentation itself seems the most likely cause of death.

As noted, the same mechanism can be triggered by cytotoxic T cells (Uckers 1987), and it may be part of the normal armamentarium of the immune system. In addition, it appears to be the same mechanism by which diphtheria toxin and the dioxin TCDD are cytotoxic (McConkey et al. 1988; Chang et al. 1989). Moreover, calcium-dependent DNA cleavage has also been observed in the apoptosis that occurs in the postcastration prostate (English et al. 1989) and in uterine epithelium (Rotello et al. 1989). These observations imply that this glucocorticoid-inducible suicide switch might exist in all cell types. Could glucocorticoids be damaging the hippocampus by this route? We examined this issue recently. We first replicated the glucocorticoid-induced DNA fragmentation in thymocytes (figure 8.1). In contrast, under conditions where glucocorticoids exacerbate kainic acid—induced cell loss in primary hippocampal cultures, we did not detect any DNA fragmentation (figure 8.2). Furthermore, benzamide did not worsen the glucocorticoid/kainic acid toxicity, implying that there was no active DNA repair occurring at this time; this contrasts with the picture in lymphocytolysis (Wielckens and Delfs 1986).

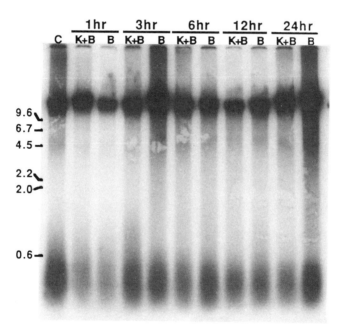

Figure 8.2. DNA blot analysis showing lack of DNA fragmentation in hippocampal cultures under conditions where corticosterone increases kainic acid toxicity. DNA blots of samples of DNA (1 μg) from cells treated with 10 μ mol KA (K) or 10 μ mol KA plus 100 nmol corticosterone (K + B) for indicated times were hybridized to nick-translated rat DNA. C, control. The numbers on the left represent the sizes and positions of the molecular weight markers. (From J. Masters, C. Finch, R. Sapolsky. Glucocorticoid endangerment of hippocampal neurons does not involve DNA cleavage. Endocrinology l24, 3083–3088, 1989. Reprinted with permission of Williams and Wilkins Publishers.)

Therefore, we concluded that glucocorticoids do not endanger the hippo-campus by causing DNA fragmentation (Masters et al. 1989).

GENERAL FEATURES OF APOPTOTIC MECHANISMS

The present chapter reviews the mechanisms known to underlying some of the better-understood examples of apoptosis. This has been, by no means, exhaustive, and several interesting examples of the phenomenon have been omitted (see Lockshin and Zakeri 1990, for discussions of the genetics of apoptosis in *Caenorhabditis elegans*, the calcium-dependent transglutaminases that trigger cross-linking reactions in proteins in involuting liver cells, or the emergence of antigenic markers in senescent red blood cells that target them for immune attack). Nevertheless, the examples reviewed—lymphocytolysis, neuronal pruning, and immune attack—demonstrate well the basic themes of apoptosis which contrast with necrotic neuron death following energetic insults (to be reviewed in the next chapters). In these cases of apoptosis, there is some *active* turning on of a genomic suicide switch, rather than the mere passive attrition of the cell. This is seen with the nuclease induction in cytotoxic T cell attack and lymphocytolysis, and with the RNA-synthesis dependency of the pruning. In addition, the killing is relatively *rapid*. Some of the apoptotic mechanisms occur over the course of minutes to hours (e.g., killer cell attacks, lymphocytolsis). In contrast, glucocorticoid-induced neurotoxicity (i.e., where glucocorticoids directly damage the hippocampus, rather than exacerbate the toxicity of a coincident neurological insult) requires months, and the neurological insults whose toxicities are worsened by glucocorticoids damage over the course of days. In addition, the apoptotic mechanisms are more *complete* than the necrotic insults. By this I mean that, for example, all neurons with ecdysteroid receptors die after eclosion; that any cell with its DNA cleaved, or whose membrane is indiscriminately perforated, dies. In contrast, a theme to be emphasized in the next chapter is the "selective vulnerability" of neurons to the energetic necrotic insults. As such, the entire brain can be equally hypoxic, equally depleted of ATP or phosphocreatine, accumulate lactate and acidity to equal extents, yet only certain classes of neurons are destined to die days later.

As a final contrast between apoptotic and necrotic cell death, I would emphasize the degree of *stereotypy* of apoptotic mechanisms. One single thing appears to go extremely wrong. For example, having DNA fragmented into little pieces or undergoing a massive influx of extracellular fluid certainly qualifies as something going extremely wrong. In contrast, as will be reviewed, necrotic injury to neurons often involves many things going a little wrong—a bit too much excitatory neurotransmitter malingering in the synapse, an increase in acidosis or oxygen radical generation, a sluggishness in clearing free calcium from the cytoplasm. This contrast is probably best appreciated in considering the glucocorticoid-induced lymphocytolysis. The mechanism that is most accepted at this point—the DNA fragmentation—is a fine example of a discrete, stereotypical cascade of damage. The earlier, and now rejected model—damage resulting from some inhibition of glucose transport, of RNA, protein and lipid synthesis, and some acceleration of RNA and protein degradation—seems a case of a lot of things going somewhat wrong. This is closer to the mechanisms of necrotic neuronal death. Apoptosis seems a case of a linear route of destruction, while necrotic insult resembles more a web of dysregulation where it is never clear which precise point of dysregulation will finally kill the cell.

In this regard, it does not seem surprising that glucocorticoids do not endanger the hippocampus via the one apoptotic mechanism tested so far. The fact that it was a route by which glucocorticoids killed immune cells made it attractive, initially. However, in retrospect, it does not fit the pattern of the glucocorticoid actions in the hippocampus. The steroids need not directly kill the neurons—my gut feeling is that they in fact never do that. They instead endanger, disrupt, make the neuron less robust, less able to withstand varied insults. The following chapters review the web of dysregulation that occurs with energetic insults that produce necrotic neuronal death. Following that, I will argue that glucocorticoids do not exacerbate these insults by making one thing very wrong but, rather, make many points in the web a little bit worse.

CHAPTER SUMMARY

In order to understand how glucocorticoids might endanger hippocampal neurons, it is neccesary to review how neurons are known to die. The following two chapters consider instances of *necrotic* neuronal death, in which there is a pathologic insult that causes an energetic crisis. This triggers a web of ultimately fatal dysregulation to occur. The present chapter considers cases of *programmed cell death,* or *apoptosis,* in which there is a linear, stereotypical, and rapid progression of events leading to death. In effect, a single suicide switch is thrown. Three of the better-studied examples of apoptosis are reviewed.

1. Neural degeneration during development. Such cell death represents a normal, rather than pathologic event. Massive neuron death occurs during development—some neurons become expendable after a certain point of development, others fail to make proper connections to other cells and are pruned. The mechanisms of the pruning are best studied. Neurons that fail to make proper connections are not exposed to local trophic factors (such as NGF) released by their target cell. These factors normally suppress a "death program" whose nature is not fully understood but which requires protein synthesis. Therefore, strikingly, this apoptosis requires *active* killing rather than mere attrition. In an interesting elaboration on this general theme, in the insect nervous system undergoing metamorphic pruning, neurons develop, in effect, an "addiction" to the ecdysteroid hormones. When hormone levels decline, this activates a protein synthesis-dependent killing process.

2. Cell-mediated killing by the immune system. A major task of the immune system is to destroy bacteria, or native cells that have become virally infected, senescent, or transformed and tumorous. Attention has focused on how a subclass of immune cells, natural killer cells, causes apoptosis. When attacking

a targeted cell, they secrete a protein, perforin, which inserts itself in the membrane of the target cell, polymerizes, and forms pores. At that point, critical ions and molecules can leak out, and water and salts can enter; the cell dies. Similarly, during humoral-mediated immune killing, the final step in the complement cascade of apoptosis is to insert a pore-forming protein into the targeted cell. This protein is highly homologous to perforin.

In addition to killing cells through this route, the natural killer cells can also destroy targeted cells by fragmenting their DNA. This is most probably accomplished by the insertion of a nuclease into the target cell.

3. Immunosuppression by glucocorticoids during stress. As discussed in chapter 2, while glucocorticoids have long been recognized for their ability to suppress the immune system, it is still debated what role this serves during the stress-response. Regardless of the teleology, a cornerstone of the suppression is the ability of glucocorticoids to kill lymphocytes. Glucocorticoids can kill cells of the immune system by fragmenting their DNA. This is accomplished by induction of a protein, presumably an endonuclease, which attacks the DNA at internucleosomal sites. This produces a distinctive "ladder" of fragments, comprising multiples of 180 base pairs, when the DNA is run on an agarose gel.

This mechanism of DNA fragmentation immediately brings the hippocampus to mind. As noted, DNA fragmentation can be triggered by the immune system in targeted cells; thus, potentially, cells throughout the body contain this suicide switch. Furthermore, glucocorticoids are able to throw this switch in lymphocytes and thymocytes. Do hippocampal neurons contain this suicide switch, and is it triggered by glucocorticoids? We have tested this possibility and find no evidence that this occurs.

In retrospect, it is not really surprising that this apoptotic mechanism is not caused by glucocorticoids. In apoptosis, one thing goes very wrong. In contrast, in the necrotic cell death arising from an energy crisis, many different threads in a web go a bit out of kilter. In the latter case, it is never clear a priori which precise point will prove fatal; instead, it is the overall disruption of the web that is fatal. Glucocorticoids do not actually kill but instead endanger and thus increase neuronal vulnerability to a broad array of insults. This suggests that they do not turn on a single suicide switch in the hippocampal neuron, or even make it more likely to be turned on. Instead, it is most likely that they exacerbate the dysregulation occurring at multiple points in the web of necrotic neuronal death, causing an overall increase in vulnerability.

The next two chapters review the mechanisms of necrotic neuronal death, as a prelude to reviewing how glucocorticoids interact with them.

9 Metabolic Chaos I: The Mediators of Necrotic Neuronal Injury

SUMMARY OF THE BOOK SO FAR

A variety of stressors stimulate the endocrine and neural adaptations known as the stress-response. This set of responses is dominated by the adrenal secretion of glucocorticoids. These hormones typify the two-edged quality of the stress-response: While glucocorticoids are needed for surviving short-term physical stressors, overexposure to these hormones (either with sustained exogenous administration or in some cases of chronic or repeated stressors) can cause numerous stress-related diseases.

Part I of this book examined how glucocorticoid secretion is regulated during aging, and whether excessive glucocorticoid exposure over the lifetime can accelerate aspects of brain aging. Chapter 3 reviewed how aged rats secrete excessive glucocorticoids under a variety of conditions, and sustain a failure of glucocorticoid feedback inhibition. This suggested that some neural site that contributes to feedback inhibition loses its sensitivity to glucocorticoids during aging. As reviewed in chapter 5, a likely site is the hippocampus, which has long been recognized for its role in glucocorticoid feedback inhibition. Chapter 4 documented how the aged hippocampus loses a substantial percentage of its receptors for glucocorticoids; associated with this is a loss of neurons as well and, in particular, it is corticosteroid-receptor rich neurons that are lost. This suggests that the hypersecretion of glucocorticoids in the aged rat arises from the senescent degeneration of the hippocampus. Chapter 6 reviewed the surprising evidence that the most likely cause of the hippocampal degeneration (i.e., the neuron death) is cumulative lifelong exposure to glucocorticoids.

These features of glucocorticoid actions and regulation combine to form a feedforward cascade of degeneration, termed the *glucocorticoid cascade*. In its simplest form, this model incorporates the fact that glucocorticoids can kill hippocampal neurons and impair the capacity of the hippocampus to function as a glucocorticoid negative feedback "brake." This leads to glucocorticoid hypersecretion which, in addition to its other damaging consequences, causes further neuron death in the hippocampus.

Part II explores the mechanisms of glucocorticoid neurotoxicity. Chapter 7 reviewed how the steroids need not actually be toxic. Instead, glucocorticoids appear to endanger hippocampal neurons, impairing their ability to survive coincident neurological insults such as hypoxia-ischemia, seizure, hypoglycemia, antimetabolites, and oxygen radical generators. Therefore, glucocorticoids may not only play a role in accelerating hippocampal aging, but might augment the toxicity of some of the most common neurological insults to the hippocampus. Chapter 8 began the process of exploring the mechanisms of neuron death, in order to understand how glucocorticoids exacerbate the process. Specifically, the chapter focused on instances of apoptotic, or programmed, cell death (for example, during neural development). Glucocorticoids were shown not to be endangering via the one apoptotic mechanism tested, and I suggested that they are not likely to endanger through any apoptotic route of damage. Thus, the focus of the next two chapters shifts to understanding the mechanisms of necrotic neuron death during metabolic insults, in order to understand their sensitivity to glucocorticoid actions.

(*Note:* The following is an extremely long and detailed chapter; it is clearly not everyone's idea of fun reading. For that reason, the summary at the end is the most extensive of any chapter. I would suggest skipping immediately to the summary for those readers who are principally interested in continuing the thread being developed in this book regarding glucocorticoids and who would be satisfied with merely a primer on some of the most prominent mediators of neuron death. For those readers seeking, instead, a rather detailed entree to the current literature regarding those mediators, I would recommend the main text of this chapter.)

This and the next chapter are the ones that I most dreaded writing since first contemplating this book. This trepidation was particularly acute after finishing the previous chapter. One of its two main themes was the elegance, the simplicity, with which some apoptotic mechanisms have evolved for killing cells. Unfortunately, the other main theme was that, in my estimation, none of those attractive mechanisms will tell us how glucocorticoids endanger the hippocampal neuron. To do so, it is neccesary to review a far messier problem—how various neurological insults are thought to kill the hippocampal neuron. A fair amount is known, and amid the chaos of dysregulation, the first hints of a common cascade by which these various insults converge in producing damage are beginning to surface. This sets the stage for chapter 11, where I examine how glucocorticoids might exacerbate this cascade.

Two concepts must be emphasized regarding necrotic cell death in the hippocampus. The first is *selective neuronal damage*. During the neurological insults to be discussed, neurons are far more readily damaged than are glia. (Some confusion has arisen with in vitro models of these insults, as relative glial and neuronal vulnerability appears to depend heavily on culturing conditions [cf. Tombaugh and Sapolsky 1990a,b; Giffard et al. 1990b]). Moreover, not only are neurons more vulnerable, some sets of neurons are far more so than others. It should be apparent by now that numerous neurological insults damage the hippocampus. This borders on an understatement; the hippocampus is notorious for its neurological vulnerability. It is among the most vulnerable of brain regions when it comes to damage induced by hypoxia-ischemia (secondary to cardiac arrest), hypoglycemia, epilepsy, alcoholic damage, Alzheimer's disease, and organometal toxicity. In approaching the vast question of "How does a neuron die?" a more manageable first pass must be, "Why do some neurons die so much more readily than others?" The entire brain may be equally deprived of oxygen following cardiac arrest or equally deprived of glucose during hypoglycemia, yet it is hippocampal neurons that are among the most likely to succumb. Why the preferential vulnerability? Early researchers considered the hippocampus to be at an unfortunate vascular crossroads in the brain, in a "watershed" at a relatively vast distance between sparse vascular beds. According to this view, there is nothing intrinsically wrong with the hippocampal neuron that some more generous vascularization wouldn't cure. While there is some empirical support for this view (cf. Imdahl and Hossmann, 1986), it has not held up for a number of reasons. First, as one moves further to the tips of this supposedly inadequate vascular tree (i.e., more anteriorly and dorsally in the hippocampus), neuronal vulnerability should increase; this cline of damage is not observed. Moreover, the hippocampus is also preferentially vulnerable in in vitro slice systems, where this vascular disadvantage should be canceled out. Most tellingly, the extent of metabolic perturbation in the hippocampus during neurological insults is not necessarily worse than in more resistant regions—it need not be that these neurons become more acidotic, more glucose-deprived, more depleted of ATP, and so on. Rather, in some cases, they appear intrinsically less capable of withstanding the same degree of energy deprivation. Therefore, the emphasis has switched from systemic explanations of hippocampal vulnerability, such as poor vascularization, to cellular (often called "parenchymal") explanations. There is something inherently vulnerable about hippocampal neurons (cf. Pulsinelli 1985b).

This is shown clearly in a study by Pulsinelli and Duffy (1983), which examined regional energy balance in the rat after hypoxia-ischemia. Comparison was made between the hippocampus and the paramedian neocortex. After 30 minutes of hypoxia-ischemia, both regions have nearly identical depletion of phosphocreatine, ATP, and glucose, and increases in lactate concentration. Moreover, these values return to normal at the same speed in both regions following reperfusion. Yet, days later, it is hippocampal neurons that die, while the neocortical cells are extremely resistant. The same pattern occurs in a latter study by Arai and colleagues (1986) comparing vulnerable and resistant regions in the gerbil brain after ischemia. This mystery surrounding the nature of the vulnerability is deepened by the observation (as will be detailed shortly) that all hippocampal cell fields are not equally vulnerable; different insults preferentially damage different cell types.

The second theme that must be reckoned with is of *delayed neuron death* (Kirino 1982; Pulsinelli et al. 1982b; Kirino and Sano 1984; Kirino et al. 1984; Petito et al. 1987). If a neuron is put through a severe challenge (e.g., 10 minutes of hypoxia or of hyperexcitation) it is reasonable that it might die during that insult. This, however, is not the pattern observed. Typically, neurons show at least partial recovery, as assessed by electrophysiology, energetic profiles or neurochemistry. Neuron death emerges days later. For example, McIntosh and co-workers (1987) examined alterations in pH following traumatic brain injury. As will be discussed, acidity is a frequent consequence of various neurological insults and is thought to damage cells. Therefore, it is not surprising that within minutes of the brain trauma, lactic acid concentrations rose, while pH declined. However, some 90 minutes after the insult, both measures had normalized, and damage was not apparent until hours afterward. Another example of this is seen with experimental hypoxia-ischemia in the rat and gerbil (Pulsinelli and Duffy 1983; Arai et al. 1986). In these studies, phosphocreatine, ATP, and glucose concentrations fell during the hypoxia, whereas lactate concentrations rose. After reperfusion, all values had returned to baseline in vulnerable brain regions within 6 hours. It is only days later that damage emerged (or in some cases, even weeks afterward [Nakano et al. 1990]). Similar themes of delayed and selective neuron death emerge when looking at patterns of inhibition of protein synthesis after ischemia. In general, synthesis declines throughout the brain immediately after the insult, generally recovers to at least near-normal levels during the hours afterward, and then declines precipitously in the brain regions destined to die (Johansen and Diemer 1990; Widmann et al. 1991). This implies that the insults are not immediately fatal, but activate a cascade that is eventually damaging, even if critical cellular parameters have normalized. This is heuristically impor-tant, as it suggests that the cell biology of this type of neuron death is complex. This time lag might be of clinical importance, as it may allow for intervention before cell death occurs. Any candidate mechanism for mediating hippocampal neuron death must make sense in the context of this time delay.

In summary, the mystery of hippocampal neuron death revolves around preferential and delayed vulnerability. During the course of an insult, a particu-lar hippocampal neuron may become as acidotic or energy depleted as, say, a thalamic neuron. After the end of the insult, both neurons may return to homeostatic balance with equal rapidity, such that a naive neurobiological observer coming on the scene hours later might find no immediate indication that anything had gone wrong. Yet, 48 to 72 hours later, the hippocampal neuron dies. To begin to understand this, it is necessary to first describe the most common neurological insults that preferentially damage the hippocampus.

HYPOXIA-ISCHEMIA, SEIZURES, AND HYPOGLYCEMIA

Hypoxia-Ischemia

Each year, approximately one million Americans sustain cerebral damage due to impaired blood flow that leads to impaired oxygen delivery (hypoxia) and nutrient delivery (ischemia) to the brain. It can take a variety of forms, with there being a broad dichotomy between a local infarct—a stroke—arising from the occlusion of a particular vessel(s) in the brain, and global ischemia, arising from cardiac arrest and cessation of blood flow to the entire brain. The latter provides an ideal example of the principles of selective and delayed hippocampal vulnerability. During the course of transient hypoxia-ischemia in a rat (in this case, not from cardiac arrest, but from experimental occlusion of the vertebral and carotid arteries), metabolism is disrupted throughout the brain. Electrical activity and neural transmission are silenced, there are massive declines in levels of phosphocreatine, ATP, and glucose; pH drops; and lactate accumulates.

As another measure of the collapse of normal function in the cell at that time, neuronal protein synthesis (as typically assayed by incorporation of tagged amino acids into protein) is inhibited throughout the brain (Kleihues and Hossmann 1971; Yanagihara, 1976; Cooper et al. 1977; Dienel et al. 1980; Thilmann et al. 1986; Kieslling et al. 1986; see Raley-Susman and Lipton 1990 for a similar phenomenon in the anoxic hippocampal slice). (It should be noted that a subset of proteins are synthesized at that time. Some of these are neuronal in origin and are heat-shock proteins [Vass et al. 1988], while others are glial and endothelial [Nowak 1985; Dienel et al. 1986; Jacewicz et al. 1986; Kiessling et al. 1986; Raley-Susman and Lipton, 1990] and probably reflect the microglial infiltration that occurs in response to ischemic injury to neurons [Kirino 1982; DeLeo et al. 1987]. Other studies suggest that they are neuronal, and their induction correlates with resistance to injury [Nowak 1991]).

During this period, there is neuronal hyperexcitation in the hippocampus; as will be reviewed, this is probably due to increased trafficking of the excitatory neurotransmitter glutamate, as well as impaired activity of Na-K-ATPase.

The severity of the metabolic and functional changes are roughly similar in different hippocampal regions and the striatum. With reperfusion, these parameters normalize within hours, and degeneration emerges gradually over subsequent days in vulnerable regions (Pulsinelli and Duffy 1983). Chief among these regions is the CA_1 cell field of the hippocampus, which is astonishingly vulnerable to hypoxic-ischemic damage (for example, see the selectivity of CA_1 damage in figure 7.3). Marked vulnerability also occurs in the hilus of the dentate gyrus, in pyramidal cells in layers 3, 5, and 6 of the neocortex, cerebellar Purkinje cells, and neurons of the caudate/putamen (Brierley, 1976). Some damage occurs within a day in somatostatin-positive neurons in the hilus of dentate gyrus (Benveniste and Diemer 1988). However, the most characteristic neuropathologic feature of hypoxia-ischemia is the delayed damage to CA_1 neurons; as a possible correlate of this, the transmission failure that occurs during anoxia (in the tissue slice) is also most pronounced in CA_1 (Kass and Lipton 1986). With more sustained hypoxia-ischemia, generalized infarction occurs, in which there is pannecrosis, involving a broader array of neurons and glia as well.

The cellular neuropathology of hypoxic-ischemic damage is well characterized. Within minutes, there is *microvacuolation* within the cell body and *dendritic swelling*. The former arises from swelling of mitochondria; this is probably due to sequestration of calcium (see below). The dendritic swelling is a reversible marker of damage; its ionic basis will also be discussed. Following that, *ischemic cell changes* develop; these include shrinking and darkening of the cell body. This leads, over hours or days, to *homogenizing cell changes*, in which distinctive intraneuronal cytoarchitecture is lost and the nucleus becomes granular and fragmented (Brierly and Graham 1984).

The clinical picture of hypoxic-ischemic damage contains a paradox that offers an important clue to the mechanisms of damage. Partial cessation of blood flow ("trickle phenomenon") is more damaging to the hippocampus than is complete cessation; moreover, preloading neurons with plentiful amounts of glucose (e.g., postprandially) also *increases* damage. This is thought to reflect increased acidotic damage. Preloading with glucose allows for more anaerobic metabolism during the hypoxia-ischemia, resulting in more lactic acid production. Partial blood flow during the hypoxia may not provide enough oxygen to support aerobic metabolism, but may provide enough substrate to fuel more lactate production. These observations suggest that hippocampal neurons succumb during hypoxia-ischemia not for lack of energy, but for having generated energy via too damaging a route. I will return to this later and suggest that this model is more complex than presented here.

Seizures

Seizures are among the most common of neurological disorders; a conservative estimate is that approximately one million Americans will experience repeated seizures (Hauser and Kurland 1975). Epileptic brain activity can be defined as frequent and rhythmic electrical discharges. The disorder is very heterogeneous in its clinical manifestations, underlying etiology, and neurophysiology.

Sustained or repeated seizure activity is neurotoxic. Brain damage is noted on postmortem examination in chronic epileptics. In earlier years, it was doubted that the damage was a consequence of the seizures and was, instead, thought to be a cause. Neuronal damage was theorized to arise from head trauma, infantile fever, or hypoxia-ischemia and that this damage led to disinhibition and seizure activity. The most reasonable explanation for this would be if the neurons lost had been inhibitory (GABAergic) interneurons, leading to loss of recurrent inhibition, which produces hyperexcitation. This idea remains controversial, as some investigators have found preferential damage to GABAergic neurons in epilepsy (Balcar et al. 1978; Bakay and Harris 1981; Houser et al. 1986; Ribak et al. 1979, 1986; Romijn et al. 1988), while others observe that GABAergic interneurons (or neurochemical markers for such neurons) are surprisingly resistant to various forms of damage, including epilepsy (Francis and Pulsinelli 1982; Frotscher and Zimmer 1987; Sloviter 1987; Selander et al. 1988). This issue remains unresolved. Another early hypothesis of how brain damage could lead to seizure was that glial scarring after damage could impair the capacity of glia to take up potassium (one of their most vital ionic roles in the brain), leading to a more excitatory ionic environment for neurons (Kimelberg and Norenberg 1989). Regardless of mechanism, most early investigators felt that the damage was more likely a cause rather than a consequence of the seizures.

The best evidence that seizures can cause neuronal damage, as well as result from such damage, came with the development of experimental animal models for inducing epilepsy, both pharmacologically and electrophysiologically. Under those conditions, damage that was characteristic of chronic human epilepsy arose following the seizures. Again, the hippocampus is preferentially vulnerable, with pyramidal neurons of Ammon's horn being most damaged (predominately CA_3 and CA_4); preferential vulnerability also occurs in the neocortex, cerebeller Purkinje cells, and among thalamic and amygdaloid nuclei (Corsellis and Meldrum 1976). In a neuropathological picture similar to that of hypoxia-ischemia, ischemic cell changes are noted, with pyknosis and microvacuolization, dendritic swelling, and glial infiltration (Spielmeyer 1922). This similarity in neuropathology led to the early suggestion that epileptic damage was, in fact, a version of hypoxic-ischemic damage. As initially theorized, such hypoxia was thought to arise either from apnea due to systemic convulsions, or from cerebral vasoconstriction during seizure. The development of animal models of seizure in which damage occurred in paralyzed/ventilated animals (i.e., without convulsions or apnea) eliminated the first possibility (Meldrum et al. 1973). The second possibility was eliminated by the demonstration that seizure induces cerebral vasodilation, rather than constriction. More recent speculations about seizure as a form of hypoxia-ischemia have concentrated on the idea that, as a result of seizure-induced edema, there is compression on local vessels within the brain, producing local hypoxia. Recent studies, detailed below, argue against the possibility of seizure damage to the hippocampus being hypoxic-ischemic in nature.

Some of the features of seizure-induced damage are similar to those of hypoxia-ischemia. With the onset of seizure activity, rates of oxygen and glucose utilization rise dramatically. Blood pressure and cerebral blood flow increase, and cerebrovasculature vasodilates to increase the delivery of these substrates to the brain to compensate for the pathologic demands. With sustained seizure, however, a "mismatch" occurs; the compensatory mechanisms fail, and glucose and ATP levels plummet (see below). It should be noted that the decline in energy stores during seizures is never severe enough to cause isoelectricity; that is, seizures do not cease for lack of energy to sustain them. Epileptic seizures demonstrate the principles of selective and delayed vulnerability. Metabolism is disrupted to roughly equal extents in hippocampal and nonhippocampal tissues. With the cessation of seizures, profiles return to normal within hours, and hippocampal damage emerges only days later.

As noted, seizures can be induced pharmacologically by drugs that fit into two classes—those that stimulate excitatory neuronal processes, and those that inhibit inhibitory ones. In either case, the consequence is hyperexcitation. A member of the former class is kainic acid, an analog of the excitatory neurotransmitter glutamate. When given systemically to the rat, its electrophysiological, clinical, and neuropathological sequelae closely resemble status epilepticus, a particularly severe form of human epilepsy (Ben-Ari 1985). Within an hour, seizure activity begins in the hippocampus; it then spreads to limbic seizures and hours of generalized seizures. The seizures are paralleled by initial wet-dog shakes and facial tremor, progresses to clonic-tonic limb movements, and then on to generalized convulsions. Neuropathologically, damage is most dramatic in the CA_3/CA_4 region (with its copious quantities of kainic acid receptors [Cotman et al. 1987]); CA_1 cells also sustain damage with higher kainic acid concentrations. Damage can also be evoked with direct microinfusion of kainic acid into the hippocampus or into connecting limbic structures such as the amygdala. In those instances, the seizure activity tends to be more localized and the clinical profile less severe. The neurotoxicity is due to the seizure rather than to the kainic acid molecule itself. As evidence, when kainic acid is microinfused into the brain, damage can occur at distant sites (that are presumably driven by seizure activity); the distant damage can be prevented by compounds that inhibit seizures, such as benzodiazepines (Ben-Ari et al. 1980).

The seizure-inducing drugs that inhibit inhibitory interneurons generally antagonize the GABAergic synapse. Among them are bicuculline, pentylenetetrazol, and picrotoxin, which seem to be good models for grand mal seizures. They will be considered in less detail in this chapter than will the glutamatergic excitotoxins. Finally, seizures and seizure-typical hippocampal damage can be induced electrophysiologically by stimulating the hippocampus itself, the perforant path leading into the structure, or other limbic sites that send projections into the hippocampus (such as the amygdala).

Hypoglycemia

In a clinical setting, hypoglycemia most frequently arises from insulin overdose. Experimental models can involve induction of hypoglycemia with insulin. Other models are less similar to hypoglycemia, in that they involve selective disruption of only components of energy metabolism. For example, drugs such as 3-acetylpyridine disrupt oxidative phosphorylation by uncoupling electron transport (Hicks 1955) while iodoacetic acid inhibits glycolysis (Raffin et al. 1988). Despite species differences, damage typically occurs when glucose concentrations are lower than 1 μM/gram of tissue. As a tighter correlation, damage generally occurs whenever the hypoglycemia is sufficient to block spontaneous EEG activity (i.e., isoelectricity) (Auer et al. 1984a,b). Upon return to normoglycemia, there is a characteristic period of neuronal hyperexcitability.

Again, the hippocampus is most vulnerable to damage. Dentate gyrus neurons (and to a lesser extent, CA_1 neurons) are most vulnerable; neocortical layers 2 and 3, and the caudate/putamen are also markedly vulnerable. There are some disagreements regarding the nature of the resulting neuropathology. Earlier investigators have noted tendencies toward microvacuolization and ischemic cell changes, thus emphasizing the similarity with hypoxia-ischemia and seizure (Brierley and Graham 1984). More recently, there has been an emphasis on the differences (Auer and Siesjo 1988). These will be considered at the end of chapter 10.

The pattern of damage induced by hypoglycemia provides insight into the workings of selective vulnerability. With the development of methods for measuring regional glucose utilization, it was found that utilization during hypoglycemia was heterogeneous, with areas more resistant to damage receiving more glucose (such as the cerebelleum) (Abdul-Rahman and Siesjo 1980). This appeared to be due to systemic factors, such as the efficacy of vascular autoregulation in different brain regions (Siesjo et al. 1982). This suggested that the selective vulnerability does not arise from some intrinsic and mysterious features of different cells, but simply from the fact that glucose was delivered to some areas longer than others during hypoglycemia (Agardh et al. 1981). However, the notion that at least part of selective vulnerability is intrinsic within the cell is reinstated by the observation that after 30 minutes of hypoglycemia, there is complete energy collapse in a resistant area like the cerebellum—yet even as much as 60 minutes of profound hypoglycemia usually does not damage its neurons (Agardh and Siesjo 1981).

While other insults also damage the hippocampus, hypoxia-ischemia, hypoglycemia, and seizure are the three that have most dominated neurological progress in recent years. Furthermore, all three are exacerbated by glucocorticoids. Their similarities and differences in suspected mechanisms of damage are also the most relevant to understanding where glucocorticoids fit into the picture.

SUSPECTED MECHANISMS MEDIATING HIPPOCAMPAL NEURON DAMAGE

With the first demonstrations of the selective vulnerability of the hippocampus came hypotheses to explain that vulnerability; since then, there has been no shortage of alleged villains at whom suspicious fingers have been pointed. The current excitement in the field arises from a number of these villains looking sufficiently plausible that some protective interventions can be made. Excitement also arises from the recognition that these different mechanisms interact, exacerbating each others' potentials for damage. Slowly, the hint of a final common pathway has become discernable. The remainder of this chapter examines the evidence for each of the leading suspects. The next chapter outlines their interactions and the role of energy failure in these interactions.

Excitatory Amino Acids

The belief that excitatory amino acid (EAA) neurotransmitters are central to neuron death is currently at a frenzied pitch, with papers on the subject near to inundating the journals. Fortunately, the belief seems quite justified.

Physiological Functions of EAAs   The EAAs are amino acids diverted from their more traditional metabolic and structural roles and used for communicatory purposes in the nervous system. Their excitatory potential has been long recognized (Curtis and Watkins 1960), and they fulfill many of the criteria to qualify as neurotransmitters. They are now recognized to be among the most ubiquitous of excitatory neurotransmitters, particularly in the hippocampus (Cotman et al. 1987, 1989). It remains unclear whether a related dipeptide, N-acetylaspartylglutamate, is also an endogenous neurotransmitter (Bernstein et al. 1985; Blakely et al. 1988). The regulation of EAA secretion has a number of interesting qualities. For example, there is negative feedback regulation of its release. EAAs will induce the release of adenosine (through both receptor-dependent and independent mechanisms [Hoehn and White 1990a,b]); adenosine, in turn, acts as an neuromodulator, preferentially decreasing the release of excitatory neurotransmitters such as EAAs (Fredholm and Dunwiddie 1988; Greene and Haas 1991; Yoon and Rothman 1991). With sustained EAA release, a positive feedback component emerges. The EAAs cause generation of arachidonic acid, which can diffuse as a retrograde messenger back to the presynaptic neuron, where it can either enhance further EAA release (cf. Lynch and Voss 1990) or inhibit it (Freeman et al. 1991; Herrero et al. 1991), depending on the biochemistry of the processing of the arachidonic acid. The positive-feedback component has been speculated to play a role in EAA-induced plasticity, such as long-term potentiation (see below). Some recent studies suggest that EAAs can also stimulate formation of nitric oxide in postsynaptic neurons, which then diffuses back to the presynaptic neuron and regulates subsequent EAA release (Garthwaite 1991). Such regulation may be critical for long-term potentiation (Schuman and Madison 1991). Nitric oxide will be considered at greater length in chapter 11).

The EAAs interact with a class of receptors that include the N-methyl-D-aspartate (NMDA) receptor, and non-NMDA receptors (the kainate, quisqualate/AMPA, L-AP4, and ACPD receptors) (reviewed in Cotman et al. 1989). Such receptors are particularly plentiful in the hippocampus, although with different neuroanatomical distributions within that structure. Just to add to the complexity, there appear to be different isoforms of the various receptors, with different functional properties (Cotman et al. 1989; Sommer et al. 1990).

It is the NMDA receptor that is most relevent to hippocampal neuron death. (However, it should be noted that non-NMDA EAA receptors play a role in neuron death as well [cf. Kaku et al. 1991]). This receptor is heavily concentrated in the CA_1 region (this being its highest concentrations in the brain), with moderate amounts in the CA_3 and dentate gyrus, and minimal amounts in the axon terminals of the mossy fiber system (Cotman et al. 1987). The bulk of the receptors are thought to be postsynaptic.

The receptor itself is extremely complex in a way central to its normal and pathologic roles. It has an association with a glycine receptor, which probably serves an allosteric role, facilitating NMDA receptor activation by increasing the frequency of channel opening (Johnson and Ascher 1987). Recent studies suggest that glycine is not only facilitative of, but essential for EAA transmission (Huettner 1989). Zinc also interacts with the receptor complex, noncompetitively reducing NMDA-evoked currents (Westbrook and Mayer 1987; Christine and Choi 1990). Moreover, receptor function can be inhibited by low extracellular pH (Grantyn and Lux 1988; Tang et al. 1990; Traynelis and Cull-Candy 1990; Vyklicky et al. 1990) and by an oxidized redox state (Aizenman et al. 1989) (or at least by some, but not all reducing agents [Majewska et al. 1990]). The receptor itself can be antagonized by a class of compounds, while the channel to which it is coupled can be blocked by an additional class.

This channel has several relevant features. It allows the flow of calcium, sodium, and potassium. Once these diverse ions enter, there is obviously the potential for a vast array of effects on the cell, including ionically mediated changes in membrane potentials, activation of inositol-dependent cascades, protein phosphorylation, and so on (cf. Bading and Greenberg 1991, and Scholz and Palfrey 1991). The broad array of ions that enter through the channel suggests a rather nonspecific permeability to various cations. As a critically important exception, however, physiologic concentrations of magnesium block the channel and prevent NMDA-typical responses (Mayer et al. 1984; Nowak et al. 1984; Ogura et al. 1988). The blockade is voltage dependent; release from the magnesium blockade occurs with depolarization. Therefore, there is an important nonlinearity built into the NMDA receptor. Progressively stronger activation of the receptor does not neccesarily lead to progressive ionic consequences. Rather, past a certain threshold of depolarization, the receptor-gated channel suddenly carries an explosively strong ionic signal. This appears to occur when the membrane potential is slightly negative (Randall et al. 1990; Alford et al. 1991)—in other words, requiring somewhat less depolarization than is needed to trigger an action potential.

This nonlinearity fits nicely with the evidence that the NMDA receptor is involved in learning and memory. The hippocampus is vital to memory consolidation; it strikes me that such plasticity can very readily emerge from nonlinearities in cellular function in hippocampal neurons. Associative learning itself seems to exemplify nonlinearity, in that a continuous barrage of input (e.g., repeated experience, repeated stimulation) suddenly triggers a discontinuous, long-lasting response (i.e., learning has occurred—in effect, aha! and the proverbial light bulb goes on). Possible reductionistic underpinnings to learning might encompass some of this nonlinearity. Therefore, some models concerning the molecular basis of learning focus on molecules that, when sufficiently phosphorylated into an active state, will suddenly autophosphorylate in a persistent manner (Kennedy 1989). At the electrophysiological level, similar nonlinearities have been searched for along the lines of patterns of stimulation that will suddenly induce long-lasting enhancement of neuronal communication. Long-term potentiation (LTP) at hippocampal synapses appears to be one such reductionistic component of learning. LTP in the CA_1 region depends on NMDA receptor activation, as LTP there is disrupted by NMDA receptor antagonists (Collingridge and Bliss 1987). In addition, kindling, another form of hippocampal electrophysiological plasticity that might have some relationship to learning, also is NMDA receptor dependent (Mody and Heinemann 1987). It is the sudden excitatory potential of the NMDA receptor, its nonlinearity, which makes it so logical for use in a phenomenon of plasticity like LTP; however, this is a two-edged sword, as this is also the root of neurotoxic vulnerability.

EAA Neurotoxicity   The neurotoxic potential of the EAAs has been recognized since 1957, with the demonstration that glutamate causes neuronal degeneration in the retinas of neonatal mice (Lucas and Newhouse 1957).

Glutamate and aspartate are also neurotoxic within the CNS; in sensitive neurons, exposure to high concentrations leads to dilation of the ER and dispersion of polyribosomes within 30 minutes. This is followed by clumping of nuclear chromatin, swelling of dendrites and their spines, and perikaryal pyknosis (Olney et al. 1971, Hajos et al. 1986). In addition, N-acetylaspartyl-glutamate is also neurotoxic (Pai and Ravindranath 1991).

I will shortly review the literature suggesting that EAA neurotoxicity and the NMDA receptor play roles in experimental and pathologic instances of hypoxia-ischemia, seizure, and hypoglycemia. In addition, some rather rare neurological disorders might have EAA components. In one, a degenerative disorder of motor systems called olivopontocerebellar atrophy, there is a deficiency in glutamate dehydrogenase activity. This leads to impaired EAA catabolism and elevated plasma glutamate concentrations (Plaitakis et al. 1982). As a second example, Guam amyotrophic lateral sclerosis/parkinsonian dementia, a disorder endemic to the island of Guam, involves a broad spectrum of neurological symptoms, including the muscle weakness and spasticity of ALS, the rigidity of Parkinson's disease, and dementia. A dietary source of EAAs (the EAA βN-methylamino-L-alanine, derived from a cycad plant) has been strongly implicated as a cause of the disorder (Kurland 1988). In addition, elevated plasma EAA concentrations are found in ALS patients (Plaitakis and Caroscio, 1987). As another case, a recent fatal outbreak of food poisoning in which victims had diffuse CNS lesions was found to come from the eating of mussels infected with toxic levels of domoic acid, an EAA analog (discussed in Olney 1990).

There is now considerable evidence that the pathogenesis of Huntington's disease involves excessive EAAs. Preferential loss of EAA receptor–bearing neurons is found in both symptomatic and presymptomatic cases (Young et al. 1988; Albin et al. 1990). Moreover, striatal and cortical lesions induced by EAAs reproduce neuropathological and neurochemical features of the disease (Coyle and Schwarcz 1976; McGeer and McGeer 1976; Beal et al. 1986, 1991b) (It should be noted that some investigators have not found support for this generalization [Beal et al. 1985; Davies and Roberts 1988; Boegman et al. 1987]; however, this may reflect the particular EAA used [Kowall et al. 1987]). Recent evidence suggests that toxicity of the "parkinsonian" compound MPTP is NMDA receptor–mediated (Turski et al. 1991). Finally, in a disorder that, tragically, is anything but rare, there is emerging evidence that EAAs might even play some role in the pathogenesis of Alzheimer's disease (Greenamyre and Young 1989). As evidence, EAAs can cause the accumulation of some of the antigenic markers of such filaments (Mattson 1990), and cause degradation of the amyloid precursor protein (Siman et al. 1990).

The threads of experimental and clinical evidence regarding the potential CNS neurotoxicity of EAAs gave rise to the *excitotoxic* theory of neuronal damage, namely, that excessive levels of endogenous glutamate could mediate various syndromes of neural degeneration (Olney et al. 1971). Impetus was given to the excitotoxic theory with the development of glutamate analogs and the demonstration that, generally, the most excitatory compounds tend to be the most toxic (Olney et al. 1971). (As will be discussed below in the section on the chloride hypothesis of damage, this parallelism is not as good as originally thought. Currently, the consensus is that toxicity is best predicted by how much calcium an analog mobilizes, rather than by how excitatory it is.)

In summary, earlier work established the excitatory and neurotoxic potential of glutamate and of glutamatergic analogs. As specific antagonists were developed against the different EAA receptor subtypes, attention focused on the NMDA receptor as the mediator of neurotoxicity. It was shown that the toxicities of glutamate and NMDA are blocked with NMDA-receptor antagonists (Choi 1987b; Choi et al. 1988; Michaels and Rothman 1990). (As a confusing complication, at least some kainic acid toxicity can also be blocked with NMDA receptor antagonists [Clifford et al. 1990; Sucher et al. 1991]. Since kainic acid binds to the kainic acid receptor and at least some of its toxicity is mediated in this way [Koh et al. 1990a], how can it also be toxic via the NMDA receptor? [1] Kainic acid might also interact nonspecifically with the NMDA receptor; there is some electrophysiological evidence for this [Cull-Candy and Usowicz 1987], as well as some against [Sucher et al. 1991]. [2] Kainic acid receptors may be presynaptic and, when binding kainic acid, may cause the release of glutamate and/or aspartate which then binds to postsynaptic NMDA receptors [Collins et al. 1983; Ferkany and Coyle 1983; Coyle 1983; Pastuszko et al. 1984; Gannon and Terrian, 1991]. [3] Kainic acid may block glutamate and aspartate reuptake into presynaptic terminals or into glia, thus exacerbating their actions to the point of toxicity [Lakshamanan and Padmanaban 1974; McGeer et al. 1978; Johnston et al. 1979; Krespan et al. 1982; Pastuszko et al. 1984; Pocock et al. 1988]. As evidence supporting either or both of these last two possibilities, kainic acid neurotoxicity in the hippocampus [as well as other brain regions] depends on intact glutamatergic inputs [Kohler et al. 1978; Nadler and Cuthbertson 1980; Coyle 1983], [4] Astrocytes respond to kainic acid by secreting glutamate, and thus may be the source of EAA release [Lehmann and Hansson 1988]. [5] Most straightforwardly, some neurons that have postsynaptic kainic acid receptors may release EAAs as a result of kainic acid stimulation.)

A vast literature now suggests that EAAs and the NMDA receptor play a role in the three neurological insults discussed above. As correlative evidence, hypoxia-ischemia, seizure, and hypoglycemia all cause elevated EAA concentrations in the synapse. This is probably due to both increased release from the axon terminal and inhibition of uptake back into that neuron or into neighboring glia. In seizure and hypoxia-ischemia, the excessive EAAs released are probably derived from neurotransmitter pools (i.e., EAAs that have either been packaged into secretory granules or may be in the process of being packaged following reuptake into the axon terminal), whereas in hypoglycemia, the suggestion has been made that the EAAs are mostly derived from the metabolic pool (Auer and Siesjo 1988). The excessive extracellular levels of EAAs can be shown with tissue slices or dispersed cultured cells, in which EAA concentrations rise in the media, or in vivo, as measured by dialysis perfusion of the extracellular space (Dodd and Bradford 1976; Dodd et al. 1980; Bosley et al. 1983; Benveniste et al. 1984; Chapman et al. 1985; Schiff and Somjen 1985; Drejer et al. 1985; Hagberg et al. 1985; Sandberg et al. 1986; Korf et al. 1988). As further correlative evidence, genetically seizure-prone rats release excessive amounts of aspartate both basally and in response to depolarization; no differences in levels of GABA, norepinephrine, or taurine are found (Lehmann et al. 1986).

If all of these insults cause excessive synaptic concentrations of the highly excitatory EAAs, they should also cause electrophysiological hyperexcitation. This occurs during the period following these insults (Madison and Niedermeyer 1970; Watanabe et al. 1980; Suzuki et al. 1983; Schiff & Somjen, 1985; Ben-Ari and Cherubini 1988; Franck et al. 1988; Urban et al. 1989; Furukawa et al. 1990; Hori et al. 1991. It should be noted that this is generally not the case with hypoglycemia; if this insult is severe enough, there is, in fact, a period of isoelectric silence [Fan et al. 1988]. Also, not all investigators have noted such excitability in ischemic models of injury [Armstrong et al. 1989; Buzsaki et al. 1989; Furukawa et al. 1990; Jensen et al. 1991] or the necessity for such excitability for damage to occur [Imon et al. 1991]). Obviously, this hyperexcitability could be due to the enhanced EAA concentrations, and as direct evidence for this, NMDA receptor antagonists block such postischemic excitability (Urban et al. 1990). Shortly, I will discuss how this could not be due entirely to the excessive EAAs, and review some other possible reasons for the hyperexcitation. There is a feedforward feature to this excitation, in that elevated extracellular potassium concentrations (which would be produced by the excitation) increase the activity of the NMDA receptor, in an undefined manner (Poolos and Kocsis 1990), causing further excitation. (One might wonder how this hyperexcitation ever stops. Some of the brake is provided by traditional inhibitory neurotransmitter, such as GABA, which is released by inhibitory interneurons throughout the hippocampus. Some additional sources of inhibition are coming to be recognized. As will be reviewed in the next chapter, these insults cause profound energy depletion, and the balance between ATP hydrolysis and resynthesis is upset in favor of the former. AMP, once produced, is readily dephosphorylated to adenosine, which is a potent neuromodulator that inhibits glutamate release and neuronal activity and alters vacular permeability [Dolphin and Archer 1983; Williams 1989; Fowler 1989]. Therefore, as adenosine accumulates, the hyperexcitation is eventually halted.)

As the most direct evidence that EAAs mediate the neurotoxicity of these insults, a vast but recent literature now demonstrates that blocking the NMDA receptor or silencing the NMDA synapse protects against these insults. This has been demonstrated with hypoxia-ischemia or focal ischemia in vivo, with anoxia in cultured neurons or slices, with excitotoxic seizures (of both the type involving hyperexcitation of EAA synapses as the primary effect, or inhibition of GABAergic synapses), with hypoglycemia and electron transport uncouplers, and with brain and spinal trauma. As strategies to silence the NMDA synapse, EAA release can be blocked with stimulation of adenosine A1 receptors. Alternatively, the NMDA receptor can be blocked with antagonists such as APV or APH, or with noncompetitive antagonists that block the receptor-gated channel (such as MK-801, opioids such as dextrorphan, or dissociative anesthetics such as phencyclidine or ketamine [Kemp et al. 1987]). Finally, it can be brought about by destruction of excitatory projections to the hippocampus (e.g., lesion of the perforant path, the entorhinal cortex) or within the hippocampus (mossy fibers, Schaffer collateral, or cell fields themselves). With these varied paradigms, there is usually protection (as measured by the numbers or volume of neurons lost, by biochemical or electrophysiological markers of injury, or by functional indices of damage). This is seen in various species (rodents, rabbits, cats, primates) within several age ranges. (Protection against hypoxia-ischemia, focal cerebral ischemia, or in vitro anoxia: Simon et al. 1984a; Rothman 1984; Pulsinelli 1985a; Wieloch et al. 1985a,b; Onodera et al. 1986; Lodge et al. 1986; Weiss et al. 1986; Goldberg et al. 1987, 1988; Johansen et al. 1987; Jorgensen et al. 1987; Clark and Rothman 1987; McDonald et al. 1987; Duverger et al. 1987; Germano et al. 1987; Rothman et al. 1987; Boast et al. 1987, 1988; Gill et al. 1987; Andine et al. 1988b; Sauder et al. 1988; Marcoux et al. 1988; Evans et al. 1988; von Lubitz et al. 1988; Goldberg et al. 1988; Swan et al. 1988; Church et al. 1988, Oxyurt et al. 1988; Kochhar et al. 1988; George et al. 1988; Prince and Feeser 1988; Steinberg et al. 1988; Raley and Lipton 1988; Kaplan et al. 1989; Lanier et al. 1990; Buchan and Pulsinelli 1990a) (Protection against seizure: Balding et al. 1986; Jones 1988; Wong et al. 1988) (Protection against hypoglycemia and antimetabolites: Wieloch 1985; Goldberg et al. 1988; Westerberg et al. 1988; Monyer and Choi 1988; Monyer et al. 1989; Armanini et al. 1990) (Protection against trauma: Faden and Siman, 1988; Faden et al. 1989) (A recent paper also shows that EAA antagonists protect against spontaneous neuronal death in primary cortical cultures [Drian et al. 1991].)

Limits to the EAA Hypothesis of Neurotoxicity   Despite this ocean of encouraging results, some reasons for caution have become apparent. One group reports that the protective effect of the antagonists against ischemic injury is secondary to the basic effect of lowering body temperature (which is a well-known route to reduce ischemic damage) (Buchan and Pulsinelli 1990a; see Boast and Hoffman 1991 for an opposite conclusion) (Just to complicate things, some have reported that neuroprotective doses of MK-801 *increase* body temperature [Pechnick et al. 1989; Ikonomidoua et al. 1989]). Just to throw a bit more water on the EAA party, some studies have failed to find protection by blocking the NMDA receptor. This has been most common with global ischemia (Block and Pulsinelli 1987; Jensen and Auer 1988, 1989; Aitken et al. 1988; Wieloch et al. 1989; Buchan and Pulsinelli 1990a; Lanier et al. 1990). In another study, antagonists were protective against moderate ischemia only at doses that were themselves toxic (Warner et al. 1991). In one recent study, a particular dose of ketamine was even reported to worsen postischemic CA_1 damage (Church and Zeman 1991).

In a careful review, Buchan (1990) considers these contradictions and the possible role of differences in species, experimental models, and adequacy of doses of antagonists in explaining them. Some of the contradictory findings are probably due to the nature of the insults themselves. The sense in the field is that EAA-mediated damage is the predominant route of damage in many of these insults, such as hypoglycemia, some forms of seizure, and in the more moderate ischemic crises (as in the perifocal areas surrounding a stroke lesion, in which antagonism of the NMDA receptor is consistently protective [Germano et al. 1987; Ozyurt et al. 1988; Steinberg et al. 1988]). However, in instances of more severe ischemic disasters, such as global ischemia, EAAs are but one of the many contributing routes of damage; the others, when activated during such a major insult, are more than capable of damaging even with the EAA component removed (Wieloch et al. 1989). This idea of EAAs playing a role, but not the sole role, is quite reasonable, and will be returned to. (This section suggests that NMDA anatagonists are more effective against local infarct than against global ischemia because the latter represents a more *severe* insult, and there is only so much you can do by blocking the NMDA receptor; in effect, MK-801 or the like is never going to substitute for a chestful of oxygen being delivered to the brain.

As an alternative view, some have emphasized [Choi 1990] that this difference arises because local infarct is more "NMDA-ish" in flavor than is global ischemia. As speculated, this is particularly the case in the "penumbra" in local infarct [the area in which there is partial compromise of neuronal function, rather than the complete compromise in the core of the infarct]; some of the evidence for this credible view will be noted shortly.)

In summary, a mass of evidence implicates EAAs and the NMDA receptor in mediating neuron death during these neurological insults, but it is not likely to be the sole mediator in each of these pathologies. We have recently uncovered an interesting way in which the EAA role in neuron death is only partial. As discussed, there are two components to hypoxic-ischemic damage in vivo. Moderate insults cause selective neuronal necrosis, preferentially damaging CA_1 neurons, while sparing dentate gyrus neurons and glia. With more sustained hypoxia-ischemia, pan-necrotic infarct damage occurs in glia and a broader range of neurons (Auer and Siesjo 1988). Numerous studies, referenced above, suggest a component of hypoxic-ischemic damage which is NMDA-mediated. Another literature, to be discussed below, emphasizes that damage arises from acidosis (generated by the lactic acid produced from anerobic metabolism during the hypoxia-ischemia). We studied anoxic damage with primary hippocampal cultures and found that these two mechanisms of damage can be dissociated from each other. When extracellular pH was greater than 6.0, anoxic damage involved NMDA receptor activation and was limited to neurons. Moreover, damage was energy dependent; elevating glucose concentrations in the media prior to or during the anoxia was protective (this contrasts with the probably incorrect but entrenched idea that glucose loading before or during this insult *always* exacerbates damage. This is discussed in the next chapter). In contrast, below pH 6.0, damage resembled the pan-necrotic picture seen at low pH in vivo, in that astroglial damage also occurred. Moreover, this component of damage was independent of NMDA receptor activation as well as of energy profile (Tombaugh and Sapolsky 1990a; Giffard

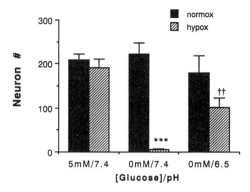

Figure 9.1. Demonstration of the ability of low pH to protect cultured neurons against hypoxic/aglycemic conditions. (*Left*) When incubated in 5 mM glucose at pH 7.4, hypoxia failed to cause neuron damage relative to normoxic conditions. (*Center*) 0 mM glucose plus hypoxia at pH 7.4 caused complete destruction of neurons. *Right*, In contrast, under the same hypoxic/aglycemic conditions, pH 6.5 caused significant protection. (Tombaugh and Sapolsky, unpublished.)

et al. 1990a). Therefore, while EAAs and the NMDA receptor play a role in hypoxic-ischemic damage, this in vitro study suggests that they are not the only mechanism.

This study uncovered an additional and important wrinkle in the NMDA/hypoxia-ischemia story. As noted, at pH 7.4, anoxic damage is selective and NMDA-dependent, whereas at 6.0 or lower, it is pan-necrotic and NMDA independent. As pH was dropped from 7.4 to 6.5, cultures were *protected* from anoxic damage—somehow, the NMDA-dependent component of vulnerability was removed (figure 9.1; Tombaugh and Sapolsky 1990a,b; Giffard et al. 1990a). This was explained with the demonstration that protons decrease the probability of the NMDA receptor–gated ion channel opening, such that the channel is shut by pH 6.6 (Tang et al. 1990; Traynelis and Cull-Candy 1990; Vyklicky et al. 1990). Therefore, moderate acidity can actually protect neurons from NMDA-mediated anoxic damage. More severe acidity, obviously, begins to damage on its own via the pan-necrotic route discussed.

This protective effect of mild acidity has an important clinical implication. As discussed, dialysis-perfusion studies have shown that there is a considerable increase in EAA concentrations in the synapse during hypoxia-ischemia. During reperfusion, EAA concentrations approach or reach preischemic values. The NMDA/pH interaction in figure 9.1 suggests that during the hypoxia-ischemia, EAAs, even at their high concentrations, are not likely to be damaging via the NMDA receptor. This is because the extracellular space is probably sufficiently acidic to shut down the channel gated to the NMDA receptor. In contrast, it is probably the lower, near-normal concentrations of EAAs in the reperfusion period that are damaging, as they are occurring when the pH has normalized and the NMDA receptor is functional. This fits nicely with the observation that administration of NMDA receptor antagonists or deafferentation during the reperfusion period *following* the hypoxia-ischemia can be protective (Boast et al. 1987; Johansen et al. 1987; McDonald et al. 1987; Gill et al. 1988; Park et al. 1988, Steinberg et al. 1988; George et al. 1988). The question, of course, becomes how these normal or, at worst, only mildly elevated EAA concentrations can be damaging. In some way, the postsynaptic neuron has had to become sensitized and vulnerable to these only moderate amounts of EAAs.

There are a number of possible mechanisms to explain this. (1) Following hypoxia-ischemia, activity of the Na-K-ATPase declines (Palmer et al. 1985, 1988; Goldberg et al. 1984) for a variety of reasons (see below). If the activity of this critical pump declines, neurons will depolarize, releasing the NMDA receptor-gated channel from its voltage-dependent magnesium blockade. This would make NMDA-mediated currents stronger, and even moderate NMDA receptor activation can be endangering during this vulnerable time. (2) Following hypoxia-ischemia, the redox systems tend to be in a reduced state (see below), and this can increase current flow through the NMDA receptor (Aizenman et al. 1989) as well as the toxicity of NMDA receptor agonists (Levy et al. 1990). (3) The initial NMDA receptor activation might cause a sustained increase in sensitivity of non-NMDA EAA receptors to stimulation. As evidence, non-NMDA receptor antagonists can be quite potently protective during the postischemic period (Sheardown et al. 1990). (4) The long-term potentiation induced by NMDA receptor activation under physiologic conditions involves both pre- and postsynaptic changes (cf. Cotman et al. 1989). The latter would cause enhanced sensitivity to even normal quantities of EAAs. Some authors have speculated that the burst of NMDA receptor activation during neurological insults such as hypoxia-ischemia induces similar changes (Choi 1990). (4) There could be decreased release of or sensitivity to inhibitory GABAergic input, biasing the system toward damaging hyperexcitation. At least one study suggests that this is not a component (Johansen et al. 1991). Regardless of the mechanism, the NMDA component of hypoxic-ischemic damage is probably at its most endangering during the reperfusion period, rather than during the hypoxic-ischemic period itself.

This paradoxical protective effect of mild acidity probably also helps to explain why, as noted above, local infarct damage might be more "NMDA-ish" and more readily protected by NMDA antagonists than is global ischemia. Infarction typically causes a pH of 6.7, while pH is typically 6.4 in the ischemic core (Hakim 1987; Siesjo 1988). Therefore, the lower pH in the latter case might damp the NMDA component.

In summary, numerous hippocampal insults cause exposure of neurons to damaging levels of the powerfully excitatory EAAs, whose proximal effects are mediated by their interaction with the NMDA receptor. As a caveat, this is not the sole route of damage in these insults. The precise mechanisms that lead to these damaging levels of EAAs will be discussed in the next chapter, and are intertwined with the energy crises induced by these insults. How does excessive activation of the NMDA receptor cause neuronal damage? The dominant feeling in the field is that a critical consequence is the subsequent exposure of the neuron to damaging concentrations of free cytosolic calcium.

Calcium

In many ways, the intracellular actions of calcium have a similar flavor to that of EAAs and their explosive, nonlinear activation of the NMDA receptor. Calcium is a dazzling intracellular transducer, both from the standpoint of the sheer number of cellular events that it can regulate, and the forcefulness with which it can do it—some of the most potent of cellular processes can be activated and amplified by calcium. Given its potential for altering cellular events, its regulation is efficient, complex, and multitiered. The need for this tight regulation can be appreciated in light of the fact that calcium has most of its intracellular effects in the mid-nanomolar range, whereas extracellular concentrations are three to four orders of magnitude higher. Therefore, given the potential torrents of calcium that could enter a cell and the potential consequences, the initial influx as well as the subsequent containment, sequestering, and efflux of the cation is very tightly regulated, and perhaps 0.1% to 1.0% of calcium entering neurons remains unbuffered (McBurney and Neering 1987).

A Role for Calcium Excess in Neuron Death A considerable amount of evidence suggests that under conditions of pathologic overactivation of the NMDA receptor, calcium mobilization overwhelms the normal system of containment, and damage ensues. First, EAAs increase calcium conductance (Ozawa et al. 1988; Crowder et al. 1987) and decrease extracellular calcium concentrations (Heinemann and Pumain 1980; Pumain and Heinemann 1985; Hamon and Heinemann 1986; Ashton et al. 1986; Lazarewicz et al. 1986, 1987; Butcher et al. 1987b). (The decline in extracellular calcium is presumably due to the ion moving into neurons, as kainic acid does not decrease extracellular calcium concentrations in pure glial cultures, but does in synaptosomal preparations [Lazarewicz et al. 1986].)

As more direct evidence, EAAs cause intracellular calcium accumulation (Berdichevsky et al. 1983; Price et al. 1985; Lazarewicz et al. 1986; Crowder et al. 1987; Carpenter et al. 1988; Burgoyne et al. 1988; Tanaka et al. 1989), which can be blocked with NMDA receptor antagonists. Early versions of these studies either used histological techniques for visualizing intracellular calcium or examined movement of calcium 45. More recent studies have taken advantage of the calcium indicator dyes such as fura-2, to demonstrate NMDA-induced increases in free cytosolic calcium concentrations in neurons (figure 9.2; Kudo and Ogura 1986; MacDermott et al. 1986; Murphy et al. 1989; Conner et al. 1988).

The most powerful evidence, of course, is that NMDA-dependent events can be blocked by eliminating this calcium response. For example, an increase in postsynaptic free calcium concentrations is a prerequisite for LTP (Dunwiddie and Lynch 1979), and NMDA-induced LTP can be blocked by intracellular loading of neurons with the calcium chelator EGTA (Lynch et al. 1983). Furthermore, calcium mediates EAA neurotoxicity, as proven when calcium is removed from culture media (Choi 1985, 1987a,b; Hori et al. 1985; Garthwaite

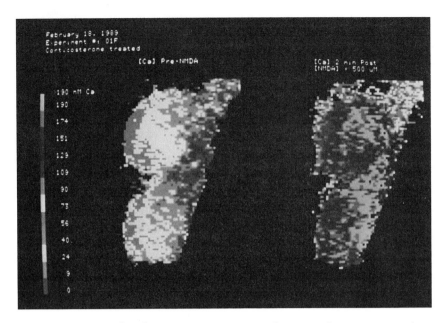

Figure 9.2. Free cytosolic calcium concentrations in two hippocampal neurons in monolayer cultured before (*left*) and after (*right*) stimulation with NMDA, as assessed by imaging with the calcium-sensitive dye fluo-3. (Courtesy of Elicia Elliott.)

and Garthwaite 1986; Garthwaite et al. 1986; Goldberg et al. 1986; Ogura et al. 1988; Hahn et al. 1988).

Moving back one step, if EAAs cause toxicity via calcium, then the various neurological insults that damage via EAAs should also be calcium dependent. As purely correlative evidence, the insults cause a fall in extracellular calcium concentrations and/or accumulation of neuronal calcium (reviewed in Simon et al. 1986). This occurs with seizure (Mody and Heinemann 1986), hypoxia-ischemia or anoxia (Nicholson et al. 1977; Hansen and Zuethen 1981; Hansen, 1985; Ashton et al. 1986; Martins et al. 1988), and hypoglycemia or antimetabolite exposure (Harris et al. 1984; Kauppinen et al. 1988a; Knopfel et al. 1990). The correlation is made tighter in hypoxia-ischemia, where both the defining CA_1 damage and CA_1 calcium accumulation emerge over days. However, a small subset of dentate gyrus somatostatin-staining neurons die during the first day, and calcium accumulation is similarly accelerated in these cells (Benveniste and Diemer 1988); in CA_3, there is neither much damage nor calcium accumulation (Martins et al. 1988). Even when calcium has not yet accumulated in CA_1, there is already something wrong in calcium trafficking. For example, calcium uptake evoked by electrical stimulation is enhanced postischemically at that time (Andine et al. 1988a).

As a second piece of evidence linking these insults to calcium, their toxicities are calcium dependent. For example, some of the disruptive effects of hypoxia-ischemia on ATP levels or electrophysiological activity can be prevented with calcium channel blockers (Yanagihara and McCall 1982; Dienel 1984; Simon et al. 1984a; Hori et al. 1985; Ashton et al. 1986; Christie-Pope and Palmer 1986; Fujisawa et al. 1986; Mabe et al. 1986; Deshpande et al. 1987); in in vitro studies with hippocampal slices, the blockade of neural transmission and of protein synthesis following anoxia is calcium dependent (Kass and Lipton 1982, 1986; Raley-Susman and Lipton 1990); microinjection of dentate gyrus neurons with calcium chelators protects the neurons from toxicity resulting from excessive glutamate excitation (Scharfman and Schwartzkroin 1989).

Thus, considerable evidence supports the cascade of various insults producing EAA overflow and, subsequently, calcium overload. To dampen the enthusiasm a bit, the extent of calcium mobilization is not a very good predictor of damage on a cell-by-cell basis. For example, following prolonged ischemia, essentially all cells examined accumulate calcium, yet only some die (Hossmann et al. 1983, 1985). On a more quantitative level, some investigators have seen a good correlation between the amount of calcium accumulated and the likelihood of a particular neuron dying (Ogura et al. 1988; Mattson et al. 1989), while others do not (Michaels and Rothman 1990). The answer here is the same as the one that runs throughout any discussion of selective neuronal vulnerability—all neurons may become equally depleted of energy, equally acidotic or, in this case, equally overloaded with calcium, but only some die. Clearly, the vulnerability involves both how bad the insult is, and how much trouble you are in when the insult is that bad. This will be a focus of the next chapter.

Sources of Excessive Free Cytosolic Calcium During Neurological Insults NMDA receptor activation can enhance a calcium signal by many routes. Most obvious is the calcium channel coupled to the NMDA receptor. As noted, with sufficient depolarization (probably via simultaneous activation of the non-NMDA receptors as well), the voltage-dependent magnesium blockade of that calcium channel is relieved, and calcium enters (Nowak et al. 1984; MacDermott and Dale 1987). An additional source of influx is opening of voltage-gated calcium channels during the depolarization. Both electrophysiological and pharmacological evidence suggests that this is the L subtype of the voltage-gated channels. Calcium can also enter via the plasma membrane sodium/calcium exchanger; flow in that direction is enhanced by sustained depolarization and increases in intracellular sodium concentrations. Finally, the increased cytosolic calcium concentrations could arise from release of the cation from intracellular organelles such as mitochondria or the endoplasmic reticulum. Release of calcium from mitochondria could occur due to reversal of the uniport calcium transporter, which normally transports calcium inwardly because of the large negative potential inside the mitochondrion. This potential is rapidly dissipated when electron transport fails during ischemia (Duchen et al. 1990). Alternatively, release can occur via a sodium/calcium exchanger, triggered by sodium influx during depolarization (McBurney and Neering 1987). Release of calcium from endoplasmic reticulum could occur due to failure of the ATP-dependent calcium accumulation pump (allowing for rather slow calcium leakage out of the endoplasmic reticulum). In addition, the inositol second messenger IP3 may also release stores of calcium from the endoplasmic reticuluum (Nahorski 1988; Seren et al. 1989; Schoepp and Johnson 1989).

How much does each of these potential sources of calcium contribute to the toxic overload during these neurological insults? This is not clear. Some authors have emphasized the role of the *NMDA-gated channel*. For example, calcium still enters neurons after EAA exposure or anoxia even if the voltage-gated channel is silenced (either by voltage clamping the cell, administration of tetrodotoxin [Lazarewicz et al. 1986], manipulating the resting potential by altering potassium concentrations or use of voltage-gated channel blockers [Lazarewicz et al. 1986; Holler et al. 1986; Peters 1986; Bouchelouche et al. 1989]). Furthermore, NMDA receptor antagonists block the neurotoxic actions of EAAs, while only partially blocking their excitatory actions (Rothman et al. 1987; Choi et al. 1988). All of this argues for the NMDA-gated calcium channel's being a primary route for the calcium mobilization.

Others emphasize the role of the *voltage-gated channels*, in that some of the neuropathologic consequences of hypoxia-ischemia can be blocked with L-channel blockers (Mabe et al. 1986; Ogura et al. 1988). One recent paper showed that such blockade is particularly effective against sustained exposure to low concentrations of NMDA (but not to acute exposure to high concentrations) (Weiss et al. 1990). In contrast, other investigators have observed that reduction in extracellular calcium or increases in free intracellular calcium following EAA exposure still occurs despite blockade of the L-type channel (Lazarewicz et al. 1987; Parks et al. 1991).

Others, in turn, have implicated the mobilization of calcium from intracellular stores (Bouchelouche et al. 1989). Some evidence suggests the importance of calcium mobilization via *sodium/calcium exchange*, particularly such exchange as a means to release calcium from mitochondria. For example, in studies of cultured basal ganglia, hypoxic-ischemic damage was dependent on the presence of either calcium or sodium in the medium. The authors suggested that sodium was needed as a means to release calcium from intracellular stores (Goldberg et al. 1986). Similarly, calcium-dependent neuron damage in the in vivo hippocampus post ischemia was decreased by blockade of sodium channels with tetrodotoxin (Yamasaki et al. 1991). As another example, NMDA mobilization of calcium in hippocampal cultures was blocked by drugs that antagonize the release of calcium from smooth endoplasmic reticuluum (SER) (Mody et al. 1988). As more evidence, in the in vitro hippocampal slice model of anoxia, damage is prevented with the NMDA receptor antagonist ketamine and zero calcium in the medium, but not either alone (Raley and Lipton 1990). This implies that even with the presence of ketamine, extracellular calcium can enter (via a non-NMDA route) and damage, and that even in the absence of extracellular calcium, NMDA receptor activation can lead to release of damaging intracellular calcium stores. In another report, dantrolene, a drug that supposedly blocks mobilization of intracellular calcium, decreased EAA toxicity in cortical cultures (Frandsen and Schousboe 1991). Finally, in a recent review, Siesjo and Bengtsson (1989) emphasized how the *phosphoti-*

dylinositol route of calcium mobilization could be more important than currently recognized.

I do not feel that these data implying which route(s) may account for the excessive calcium are in any way conflicting. No doubt, more than one route can contribute (as shown explicitly in the work of Ogura et al. 1990, or Milani et al. 1991), but do so to differing extents depending on the insult, the neuron type involved, and the neuron's immediate metabolic history. These ideas will be considered in the final section of the next chapter, concerning individual differences in neuronal vulnerability.

These findings emphasize that toxicity can occur because too much calcium is mobilized (from whatever source). However, the toxicity can also arise from too little removal of the calcium (i.e., a normal amount may be mobilized, but it may linger dangerously). Some studies, analyzing the kinetics of Ca^{2+}-45 movement during insults such as hypoxia in the hippocampal slice, emphasize that calcium accumulates because of *failure of efflux*, particularly of the Ca-ATPase route of efflux (Kass and Lipton 1986). Therefore, it becomes important to understand how calcium, once mobilized, is removed from the cytosolic compartment and how this regulation can fail during these insults.

Predictably, this is a hierarchy of steps for containment of calcium (Blaustein 1988). The first is its binding by any of a variety of cytosolic calcium-binding proteins (e.g., calmodulin, parvalbumin, or calcineurin). Sometimes, these proteins are the mediators of the intracellular calcium signal. Sometimes, they serve a negative feedback role in regulating subsequent calcium influx (for example, binding of calcium by calcineurin triggers its phosphatase activities; specifically, it dephosphorylates the voltage-gated calcium channel, leading to less calcium influx. Therefore, a heavy calcium influx signal inhibits subsequent calcium influx [Armstrong 1989]). In some cases, the binding proteins appear to serve mostly as a sponge. These proteins are generally high-affinity, forming the first means of containing a calcium signal; yet, they are also low-capacity, meaning that they are readily saturated.

Next in the hierarchy of containing calcium is its sequestration into storage sites such as the mitochondria and SER. These are the same sites from which they may have been released in the first place. The SER and (even more so) mitochondrial compartments bind calcium with a lower affinity but a higher capacity than do the cytosolic binding proteins. In both cases, sequestering is either ATP dependent or dependent on a sodium gradient. Mitochondria are thought to sequester little, if any calcium under normal, nonpathologic conditions because of this low affinity. However, their high capacity allows them to store calcium at orders of magnitude higher concentrations than in the surrounding cytoplasm. This is accomplished, in part, through the presence of various calcium-binding proteins within the mitochondria, and by the conversion of calcium to a calcium-phosphate precipitate. The latter allows the storing of that much calcium without causing osmotic damage to the organelle. As will be seen, that defense is breached in many pathologic circumstances.

Following binding and sequestration of calcium comes efflux out of the cell. One possible route is via an ATP-driven calcium pump in the plasma membrane, which seems to be of a different type than that found in the SER. This is a relatively high-affinity, low-capacity route of efflux, which can be enhanced by calmodulin. In addition, there is an electrogenic sodium/calcium exchanger. Under normal resting conditions, calcium efflux is favored. As noted, this is a point of vulnerability for neurons because, under circumstances of pathologic depolarization, high concentrations of intracellular sodium will reverse the direction of the exchanger, not only impairing calcium efflux, but actually promoting influx.

In summary, a multitiered system of calcium containment exists. The cytosolic binding proteins serve as the first line of containment, with binding half-times of perhaps 1 ms. Following that is sequestration over the course of tens of milliseconds, followed by efflux, over the course of seconds. To complicate the system further, the activity of various channels or transporters of calcium are regulated by calcium-binding proteins, in a way suggesting feedback regulation—for example, binding of calcium to calcineurin inhibits calcium influx through the calcium channel. As another example, binding of calcium to calmodulin increases the affinity of the ATP-dependent calcium efflux molecule (Kuo et al. 1979; Hakim et al. 1982). As another complication, calcium trafficking within a neuron can be compartmentalized (Hernandez-Cruz et al. 1990).

Just as the different routes of calcium influx probably contribute differentially to calcium mobilization by neurological insults, the differing routes of calcium containment and removal probably contribute differentially as well. This is poorly understood, and will be considered in the next chapter.

This system of calcium containment is costly, given that most of the routes of sequestration or of efflux are either directly dependent on ATP hydrolysis or on the maintenance of steep ionic gradients. For example, the efflux component alone is estimated to consume 3% of neuronal ATP under resting conditions, when the calcium challenge is quite small (Erecinska and Silver 1989). In the next chapter, I review how the decline in substrate availability during these neurological crises will disrupt this containment system and overwhelm the cell with free cytosolic calcium.

What Are the Pathologic Consequences of Too Much Calcium for the Neuron? Once extremely high cytosolic concentrations of calcium are reached, a vast number of cellular events can potentially become deranged, essentially guaranteeing cell damage; proteases, lipases, and nucleases can be activated (cf. Cheung et al. 1986). As one nonneural example of the consequences of elevated calcium, in the mdx strain of mice with a dystrophy resembling Duchenne muscular dystrophy in humans, there is pathologic proteolysis in muscle cells. This has recently been shown to be due to the elevated free calcium levels typical of the strain (Turner et al. 1988). As another example, excessive calcium can fragment DNA in rat liver cells (Jones et al. 1989).

In the brain, the first hints of "what happens after too much calcium" are emerging. Among the enzymes that can be activated are the protease calpain

I, phospholipase A2, protein kinase C, CaM kinase II, and calcineurin (reviewed in Choi 1990). Some understanding is emerging about the consequences of the normal physiologic activation of these enzymes by calcium (for example, during LTP) and how overactivation during these insults is pathologic. For example, the phospholipase A2 activation during LTP may indirectly contribute to enhanced glutamate release by release of arachidonic acid (i.e., this may be a mechanism for the potentiation seen during LTP); overactivation of this step during neurological insults might lead not only to even more EAA release, but also to oxygen radical formation (see below for discussion as to the role of arachidonic acid in oxygen radical generation). As another example, there is some suggestion that the protein kinase C activation can lead to enhanced presynaptic EAA release during LTP (Choi 1990). Perhaps, then, overactivation of protein kinase C leads to further pathologic release of EAA during the insults; as evidence, protein kinase C inhibitors can protect against hypoxic injury (Favaron et al. 1988; Komatsumoto et al. 1988; Kogure 1990).

One of the most interesting consequences of the calcium mobilization is the activation of calpain I. Among its substrates, it degrades the cytoskeletal protein spectrin (Siman and Noszek, 1988); this effect may underlie the remodeling of dendritic spines during LTP. Calpain activation also leads to proteolysis of the amyloid protein precursor (Siman et al. 1990). It is plausible that the overactivation of calpain I during these insults contributes to the neuron death. Neurons in susceptible brain regions contain relatively high concentrations of calpain I (Siman et al. 1985). Calpain I is induced by EAAs and by the neurological insults discussed here (cf. Arai et al. 1991). Furthermore, its induction precedes most neuropathological markers of neuron death and the insults produce the same sort of proteolysis as caused by calpain. Finally, antagonism of calpain I action can preserve some aspects of hippocampal function following hypoxia-ischemia or EAA exposure (Siman et al. 1989; Seubert et al. 1989; Lee et al. 1991; Bartus et al. 1991; Kent et al. 1991; Ton et al. 1991). (Although one recent study shows that fodrin proteolysis by EAAs can occur independently of neurotoxicity [Di Stasi et al. 1991], implying that cytoskeletal degredation, not surprisingly, is not the sole toxic consequence of calcium excess. However, in that study, the authors were not able to demonstrate any marked toxicity due to NMDA, in contrast to most other published reports).

As another potential route of damage, calcium excess will lead to phosphorylation of the microtubule-associated protein tau (in both rodent and human cultures neurons) (Mattson 1990; Mattson et al. 1991a). While a direct pathogenic consequence of such phosphorylation has not been identified, the similar phosphorylation of tau as a distinctive marker of Alzheimer's disease has lead to the assumption that this is, at least, not a healthy pattern for a neuron. As a different potential source of damage, the enzyme xanthine dehydrogenase is irreversibly converted to xanthine oxidase in the presence of high calcium concentrations; the latter enzyme is a potent generator of damaging oxygen radicals (McCord 1985). The excessive calcium influx following anoxia in hippocampal slices also appears to play a role in the collapse of protein synthesis typically seen (Raley and Lipton 1990; Raley-Susman and Lipton 1990).

In summary, these are all ways in which a marked excess of calcium can cause pathology. In some scenarios of damage, the calcium signal can be contained successfully, but at a damaging price. As visualized, the mitochondria might have to use more and more of their ATP to sequester the calcium, depriving the cell of energy and forcing it to function more anerobically. This point has been estimated to occur when cytosolic calcium concentrations reach the 10 μM range (McBurney and Neering 1987). Moreover, many mitochondrial enzymes are calcium regulated, and the entry of so much calcium into the mitochondria might disrupt mitochondrial function. For example, in cerebrocortical mitochondria, excessive calcium inhibits the activity of the pyruvate dehydrogenase complex (Lai et al. 1988). Or at a greater extreme, the mitochondria may become osmotically swollen and damaged by the sequestering of calcium. This is thought to be the cause of the mitochondrial microvacuolization that is a hallmark of hypoxic-ischemic and seizure damage to neurons.

Therefore, it is fairly clear that too much calcium can damage neurons, and there is no shortage of mechanisms by which this can occur. Determining *which* consequences of calcium excess are most damaging will be extremely difficult. I suspect also that, to some, it will be rather frustrating. This is because of the very satisfying convergence and linearity that seems to link various neurological insults to excessive EAAs, excessive NMDA receptor activation, and excessive free cytosolic calcium concentrations. Once that final step is reached, the clean linearity likely disappears. Calcium-dependent proteases, lipases, and endonucleases can be activated, with ever-broadening ripples of dysfunction being triggered. This will be a formidable task to unravel.

Acidosis

Acid-base balance is obviously tremendously important to a neuron; a profound alkalosis or acidosis is one of the most broadly endangering events that can happen to a cell, given the fairly narrow pH range at which most biochemical processes occur. Not surprisingly, numerous regulatory steps exist in neurons to maintain pH, and under normal circumstances, for each free hydrogen ion in the cytoplasm, approximately 20,000 protons are buffered (Moody 1984). The cellular regulators of pH include Na^+/H^+ exchangers and Cl^-/HCO^{3-} cotransporters, Na^+/H^+ exchangers on mitochondria, and complex shuttling of protons between neurons and glia (Kraig et al. 1985c, Chessler, 1990). *Acidosis*, rather than alkalosis, is most often considered in the context of neuron death, particularly following hypoxia-ischemia.

In this scenario, pH drops in neurons because metabolism is purely anaerobic, generating lactic acid. The interstitial space is also acidified, due to some efflux of the lactic acid (or the protons produced by it). As initial, correlative support for the acidotic model, tissue pH drops in hypoxia-ischemia, and lactate concentrations soar (Pulsinelli and Duffy 1983). Earlier studies demonstrated this with measurements of whole tissue pH, or extracellular pH; more recent techniques allow for measurement within cells, by way of nuclear magnetic resonance spectroscopy or pH-sensitive dyes. As more strongly correlative evidence, conditions that exacerbate the acidosis in hypoxia-ischemia exacerbate the damage. The most interesting and important example of this is one with profound clinical implications in hypoxia-ischemia. As discussed above, glucose preloading prior to hypoxia-ischemia worsens the insult (Myers and Yamaguchi 1977; Myers 1979; Ginsberg et al. 1980; Kalimo et al. 1981; Rehncrona et al. 1981; Pulsinelli et al. 1982a). This is thought to occur because the glucose preloading allows for more anaerobic metabolism and generation of lactic acid during the ischemia (Ljunggren et al. 1974). Intracellular pH, in turn, varies with the amount of lactic acid generated (Corbett et al. 1988), or with glucose concentrations preischemia (Combs et al. 1990). This predicts that damage should be worse when hypoxia-ischemia occurs postprandially, rather than preprandially, or when a trickle-flow of blood during the hypoxia allows the delivery of sufficient glucose to further fuel the production of lactate. These predictions are generally borne out in both experimental studies of animals and the clinical literature (Nordstrom et al. 1976; Steen et al. 1979; Longstreth et al. 1983; Pulsinelli et al. 1983; Levy et al. 1985). (In one seeming exception, the experimental model for producing incomplete ischemia did not cause more damage than complete ischemia, nor did it generate particularly high cerebral lactate concentrations [Dietrich et al. 1987]).

As the most powerful support for an acidotic route of damage, normal brain tissue can be damaged by exposure to the concentrations of lactate generated during hypoxia-ischemia in the presence of glucose (15 to 25 $\mu mol/g$; Kraig et al. 1987). The same occurs in vitro, but with more lactate required to cause damage, probably because of the buffering capacity of the vast extracellular space in monolayer cultures (Goldberg et al. 1986; Goldman et al. 1989; Nedergaard et al. 1991). It appears to be the *intracellular*, rather than extracellular acidification which is damaging (Goldman et al. 1989). This fits well with a careful study by Kraig and colleagues (1985b) showing that during ischemia, it is the intracellular compartment that becomes progressively more acidic. The authors showed that during complete ischemia, the interstitial space acidifies as lactate concentrations in whole tissue accumulate. This makes sense, given that a certain amount of the lactate or associated protons are pumped into the interstitial space. Critically, this interstitial acidification saturates, such that above a certain, mildly endangering level, further lactate accumulation does not acidify the interstitial compartment further. Therefore, if there is more lactate accumulating in the tissue as a whole and it is not being reflected in a further interstitial acidification, this implies that the intracellular compartment is becoming progressively more acidic (note that this study predated current techniques for measuring intracellular pH directly).

In summary, the evidence seems pretty good that hypoxia-ischemia damages, at least in part, via a drop in pH. In addition, seizure, and any other insult that causes a large increase in free cytosolic calcium, causes a certain degree of intracellular acidosis as well (Chesler 1990). This, in part, reflects the means of trafficking in calcium: With sufficiently increased calcium concentrations, the neuron must choose between using the sodium gradient for running the Na^+/Ca^{2+} exchanger, or the Na^+/H^+ exchanger, and it appears to choose the former, allowing protons to accumulate (Ahmed and Conner 1980). In addition, the increase in intracellular calcium might cause acidification due to Ca^{2+}/H^+ exchange at mitochondria (Chance 1965; although I am not aware of evidence for this happening in the brain). At the more extreme version of this picture, seizure could lead to even more extreme acidosis. This is because mitochondria, and oxidative metabolism, might ultimately be eliminated by the calcium challenge. This could be via so much calcium being sequestered into mitochondria as to cause them to microvacuolate and burst. Alternatively, the mitochondria may survive the sequestering of the calcium but may divert all their ATP to the task of sequestering the calcium (Ingvar et al. 1987). In either scenario, energy must increasingly be derived via anaerobic lactate production, with damaging acidotic consequences.

Once neurons become very acidotic, there will be disruption of mitochondrial enzymes (Mela et al. 1972; Rehncrona et al. 1981) and glycolytic enzymes (where, for example, a change of 0.1 pH unit drastically alters phosphofructokinase activity [Trivedi and Danforth 1966]). Furthermore, the neuron could get into even more trouble in the process of trying to pump out the H^+. Theoretically, large amounts of proton efflux via the Na^+/H^+ exchanger could lead to more depolarization and further disruption. Emphasizing this point, this exchanger appears to be the primary route of proton efflux in hippocampal neurons (Raley-Susman et al. 1991).

Some Limitations to the Acidotic Model   The most interesting implication of the acidotic model is that neurons die not for *lack* of energy, but because of the nature of the energy produced. While the model is almost certainly relevant to some instances of neuron death, there are limitations. In my mind, the strongest way to test whether acidosis plays a major role in mediating a particular instance of neuron damage is to determine whether the damage is worsened by glucose preloading—in effect, are the salutary aspects of giving a neuron more energy outweighed by the potential for generating acidosis with the glucose? As will be discussed, this is not the case with seizure. Therefore, I feel that the potential route of calcium shutting down oxidative metabolism and producing acidosis during seizure is not of great clinical relevance.

Many also feel that acidosis is only one of the routes of damage in hypoxia-ischemia. In a review of the subject, Auer and Siesjo (1988) dichotomize between selective neuronal vulnerability and pan-necrotic damage. Both can occur after hypoxia-ischemia. The former occurs with milder hypoxia-ischemia and involves NMDA receptor activation rather than severe acidosis. Glia are spared. The problem is on a cellular, rather than tissue level, and the relatively selective mechanism not only does much to explain "Why just neurons" but "Why only some neurons" as well. With pan-necrosis following severe hypoxia-ischemia (i.e., an infarction), the problem is more generalized, where axons are damaged at least as readily as dendrites and somas, glia as readily as neurons. In such cases, the problem is one of generalized tissue acidosis, rather than a problem of selective cellular vulnerability.

If this dichotomy is correct (i.e., acidosis does not account for all of hypoxic-ischemic damage with there being, instead, a separate energy-dependent component), there should be cases where glucose preloading protects against hypoxia-ischemia or anoxia. As discussed, our work with hippocampal cultures supports this. We found that within the pH range of 7.4 to 6.0, anoxic damage depends on NMDA receptor activation; glucose preloading protects against the damage, and it is neurons that are selectively damaged. At pH 6.0 or lower, damage is pan-necrotic and NMDA independent; moreover, glucose preloading is no longer protective (Tombaugh and Sapolsky 1990a). As further challenge to a strict anaerobic/acidotic route of anoxic damage, glucose preloading *helped* survivorship and recovery of electrophysiological function during reoxygenation in hippocampal slices (Schurr et al. 1987; Okada et al. 1988) and in basal ganglia cultures (Goldberg et al. 1986). In another such case, the transmission failure induced by anoxia in hippocampal slices could be prevented with energy substrates, and the likelihood of failure did not correlate with the extent of acidity generated (Lipton and Whittingham 1979, 1982; Kass and Lipton 1982). In an in vivo example of this dissociation, barbiturates can decrease ischemic damage in the brain (reviewed in the next chapter) without preventing ischemic acidosis (Nemoto and Frinak 1988).

As more evidence against a strictly acidotic model of damage, lactate accumulation during hypoxia or anoxia need not always be bad (Boakye et al. 1991), as it can be used during reperfusion as an energy substrate, via the tricarboxylic acid cycle (Schurr et al. 1988). Finally, as discussed, even acidosis itself is not always bad, since moderate acidity can shut down the conductance of the NMDA receptor and be partially protective (Tombaugh and Sapolsky 1990b; Giffard et al. 1990a). Therefore, acidosis generated by anaerobic lactate production seems not to be the mechanism for hippocampal damage following seizures, and not the sole mechanism for hypoxic/anoxic damage either.

An additional possible source of acidosis occurs during these varied insults that is independent of the lactic acid scenario. In cells, the biggest source of protons is the hydrolysis of ATP (Krebs et al. 1975). Normally, protons are consumed by oxidative phosphorylation and the transfer of high-energy phosphate groups from phosphocreatine to ADP; that is, normal energy metabolism balances acid production and consumption. When energy declines and ATP hydrolysis outstrips synthesis, there could be a major acidosis generated. As will be discussed in the next chapter, all three insults cause the hydrolysis of large quantities of ATP. However, the three insults differ dramatically as to how much ATP levels decline (ranging from approximately 95% for hypoxia-ischemia to 5% to 10% for seizure), and there is not a rank order relationship between the extent of ATP hydrolysis and the amount of acidity generated during the insult (i.e., hypoxia-ischemia and seizure, involving the most and least ATP hydrolysis, respectively, both produce acidoses, whereas hypoglycemia, with intermediate amounts of ATP hydrolysis, does not). (This argument is complicated by the fact that hypoxia-ischemia involves cessation of blood flow, so that potential source for clearing some protons out of the brain is lost. Nevertheless, stated in the simplest way, in comparing hypoglycemia and seizure, the latter involves more ATP hydrolysis yet more acidosis.) Therefore, while the ATP hydrolysis that accompanies these insults could theoretically lead to acidosis, it is probably not a major, damaging source of protons.

In summary, acidosis probably plays some role in mediating brain damage, particularly in explaining the glial damage that occurs during the pan-necrosis following major infarcts (cf. Giffard et al. 1990a). However, its role in the selective neuronal loss in milder hypoxic-ischemic injury is becoming less convincing, and it probably plays little role in damage during seizure or hypoglycemia. Furthermore, there is the emerging possibility that mild acidosis can even be somewhat protective. (In light of this restrained enthusiasm for the acidotic hypotheses, a recent paper suggests a nonacidotic route to explain why [under some circumstances] glucose preloading can exacerbate hypoxic damage. The authors showed that hyperglycemia reduces the posthypoxic extracellular accumulation of adenosine [Phillis et al. 1990]. This probably occurs because there is less breakdown of ATP to adenosine [i.e., less of an energy crisis]; as was discussed, adenosine can be neuroprotective, perhaps through its vascular actions or by inhibition of EAA release.)

Oxygen Radicals

There is a long-established belief that many forms of tissue damage can arise from the overproduction and/or impaired containment of oxygen radicals. Some researchers have suggested that oxygen radical generation underlies neuronal damage in response to neurological insults, especially hypoxia-ischemia; others have suggested a role of oxygen radicals in Alzheimer's disease (Volicer and Crino 1990).

Oxygen radicals are atoms or groups of atoms that are usually short-lived and that have an unpaired electron, which can form covalent bonds. The odd electron makes the atom highly reactive in an indiscriminate manner. Under normal circumstances, oxygen radicals are generated in cells as a part of oxidative phosphorylation; however, an array of protective mechanisms exist to prevent their becoming damaging. Oxidative damage arises from the promiscuous, uncontrolled tendency of oxygen radicals to cause chain reactions with a vast array of molecules, frequently impairing their function in the process.

Normally, oxygen radicals are generated during the reduction of oxygen, for example, in the cytochrome chain reaction. Oxygen is converted to the oxygen radical superoxide (O_{2-}), subsequently to hydrogen peroxide (H_2O_2) and to the highly reactive hydroxyl radical ($OH^.$), before being converted to water. While superoxide and, even more so, the hydroxyl radical can be highly toxic, these are normally tightly bound to the enzymes of oxidative phosphorylation. Furthermore, there are enzymes to inactivate the radicals, should they become free of the cytochrome chain system or be generated pathologically elsewhere in the cell. Superoxide dismutase (SOD) converts superoxide to hydrogen peroxide (with the addition of $2H^+$), which allows catalase to convert hydrogen peroxide to be decomposed to water (with the addition of O_2). Catalase is relatively rare in the brain, where its role is played instead by intraneuronal glutathione peroxidase (Halliwell and Gutteridge 1985). In addition, a variety of antioxidants exist that can scavenge free radicals in order to inactivate them. These can be either endogenous or exogenous, and include vitamin E, reduced glutathione, and ascorbic acid. Therefore, oxygen radicals are a normal part of cellular biology. They are even intentionally generated by neutrophils as an antimicrobial defense (reviewed in Weiss 1989).

However, should oxygen radicals be produced at an abnormally high rate and/or the means to contain them be compromised, there are numerous ways by which the free radicals could damage a cell. Some routes are likely to be rather rapid, and of possible relevance to the neurological insults considered. These include damage to membranes and dysfunction of membrane-associated proteins via lipid peroxidation; breakdown of mucopolysaccharides through oxidative degradation, DNA damage, and inhibition of Na-K-ATPase (Goldberg et al. 1984; Palmer et al. 1985, 1988). Lipid peroxidation and membrane damage have attracted the most attention, as they can cause cross-linking between and among lipids and proteins, all with highly disruptive effects. A number of additional routes leading to damage can occur but are much slower and probably not relevant to the various insults discussed. These include accumulation of inert material in cells (such as age pigments, a point heavily emphasized by the free radical adherents in gerontology) due to oxidative polymerization of lipids and proteins, and oxidative alterations in long-lived molecules (Ames, 1983; Harman, 1984; Floyd 1991).

The Evidence for Oxygen Radicals as Sources of Neuronal Damage
Oxidative damage appears to occur quite readily in peripheral tissue after hypoxia (for example, in cardiac tissue). In such cases, the oxygen radicals are not generated during the period of hypoxia itself, but during the reperfusion period, when oxidative phosphorylation resumes and the cellular checks and balances for handling oxygen radicals safely may have been compromised by the recent hypoxic crisis. When the system of containment fails, uncontrolled free radicals are formed. Free radical production is also likely to mediate the damaging effects of various chemical toxins, oxygen toxicity, and irradiation injury. The body also appears to have evolved a way to opportunize oxygen radical generation and its dangerous effects, as leukocytes can produce them as a means to kill bacteria. Finally, some gerontologists have long promulgated the free radical theory of aging, proposing that cumulative oxidative damage is a major pacemaker of cellular aging (Harmon 1984).

There is some evidence to support a role for free radicals in mediating the neuronal damage induced by the insults under discussion (Schmidley 1990). First, catecholamine overexposure can damage neurons via oxygen radical generation (Rosenberg 1988). Second, all of the neurological insults discussed can potentially promote free radical formation (Hall and Braughler 1989); in a detailed examination of this, it was shown that the longer the ischemic period during hypoxia-ischemia, the more free radical production and lipid peroxidation in the reperfusion aftermath (Sakamoto et al. 1991). One route is via the accumulation of free fatty acids, mainly in the form of arachidonic acid and stearic acids (Westerberg et al. 1987; Bazan 1970; Yoshida et al. 1980; Fishman and Chan 1981; Huang and Sun 1986). The stearic acids are probably derived from polyphosphoinositides, released by calcium (Ikeda et al. 1986). The arachidonic acid is also released due to calcium mobilization. Calcium activates phospholipase A2 (Dumuis et al. 1988), which degrades phospholipids to release arachidonic acid. Arachidonic acid, in turn, is a precursor for thromboxanes and prostaglandins, whose syntheses involve oxygen radical formation. The high free cytosolic calcium concentrations during these insults can also generate oxygen radicals through the calcium-dependent proteolysis of xanthine dehydrogenase to xanthine oxidase (McCord 1985), a potent radical generator. While xanthine oxidase is present in tissues under all conditions, such proteolysis is markedly enhanced in the brain after ischemia, most probably during the reperfusion priod than during the ischemic period itself (Kinuta et al. 1989; Mink et al. 1990; Betz et al. 1991). As will be discussed in the next chapter, the energy deprivation typical of these neurological insults provides substrates for xanthine oxidase to generate free radicals. The result of these separate possible steps is that anoxia or ischemia cause free radical formation during the reperfusion period (Taylor et al. 1985; Cao et al. 1988; Schmidley 1990).

Not only do these insults generate free radicals, but they also compromise the means to scavenge and contain the free radicals. Tissue concentrations of scavengers such as ubiquinone, vitamin E, ascorbic acid, SOD, and reduced glutathione decline during partial ischemia or during reperfusion after total ischemia (Chan et al. 1988). As a possible explanation for this, glutamate reduces neuronal cystine uptake, which will secondarily decrease glutathione synthesis (Murphy et al. 1989). The reasons why levels of the other scavengers decline is not known.

The critical question, of course, is whether the oxygen radicals generated can cause damage. In support of this, postischemic reperfusion causes lipid peroxidation, as would be expected if oxygen radicals are damaging at such times. As more direct evidence, scavenging of oxygen radicals protects neurons following various neurological insults. This has been shown in various in vitro models. For example, superior cervical ganglion neurons that are being starved of glucose generate oxidants, and starvation-induced neuron death can be decreased by SOD (Saez et al. 1987). Similarly, vitamin E reduces anoxic damage in hippocampal slices (Acosta et al. 1987; Amagasa et al. 1989); in these studies, the endpoint was postanoxic recovery of electrical spike amplitude, rather than a more direct measure of neuronal survivorship. In the study by Acosta and colleagues, lipid peroxidation was shown not to be occurring postanoxia; the authors interpreted this as meaning that the damage induced by oxygen radicals (and prevented by the vitamin E) was presumably via some other route than membrane damage. As further support for a damaging role for oxygen radicals, inhibition of glutathione concentrations in cortical cultures enhances EAA toxicity (Bridges et al. 1991) (although the selective of this inhibition is not clear). Furthermore, antioxidants protect cerebellar granule cells against kainic acid toxicity (Lyons et al. 1991). Finally, 21-aminosteroids, which are novel antioxidents that both scavenge radicals and block arachidonic acid release, protect cortical cultures from EAA toxicity (Monyer et al. 1990).

The potential protectiveness of scavengers has been shown in vivo as well. For example, experimental ischemic neuronal damage is decreased by α-tocopherol (Yamamoto et al. 1983; Hara et al. 1990) and by oxypurinol (Lin and Phillis 1991). Moreover, kainic acid or ischemic toxicity is prevented with radical scavengers (Baran et al. 1987; Dykens et al. 1987; Kitagawa et al. 1990). Finally, 21-aminosteroids protect against ischemia (Hall et al. 1988). (In a finding similar to that of Acosta et al., the oxygen radical route of damage post ischemia in the rat forebrain was shown not to involve membrane peroxidation [Beck and Bielenberg 1990]). As one of the most powerful pieces of evidence supporting a role for oxygen radicals, infarct damage is reduced in transgenic mice, which overexpress superoxide dismutase (Chan et al. 1991).

In summary, these studies suggest that oxygen radicals can mediate neuronal damage following these insults. As a possible confound, many investigators feel that free radical damage, should it be occurring, is likely to take place in endothelial cells, rather than neurons. This is because xanthine oxidase is most probably concentrated in microvessels, rather than in neurons (Betz 1985). However, some of the studies cited above (Saez et al. 1987; Dykens et al. 1987; Monyer et al. 1990) showed protective effects of antioxidants in cultured neurons.

In contrast to these studies, some findings argue against a major role for oxygen radicals in neuron damage. In one study of bicuculline-induced seizures (Soderfeldt et al. 1983), levels of tissue oxygenation were manipulated during the insult, and animals were in some cases treated with vitamin E. Vitamin E did not protect the brain from seizure-induced damage. Moreover, conditions of low oxygen not only were not protective (as they should have been, should damage be generated predominately via an oxygen radical route), but worsened neurological outcome (probably reflecting the decreased ATP concentrations due to the low oxygen conditions). In another study, no evidence of oxygen radical generation was found following acidotic ischemia (Lundgren et al. 1991b). As evidence against one putative route of oxygen radical damage, some investigators have failed to observe lipid peroxidation after hypoxia-ischemia (Acosta et al. 1987; Koide et al. 1986).

Therefore, while oxygen radicals are probably generated during many or all of these insults and they can potentially damage through a variety of routes, I do not feel that this is as broadly credible a mechanism of damage as the EAA or calcium story. (I should note that the issue of oxygen radical involvement is not only not settled, but appears to be the most controversial of the mechanisms discussed in this chapter. In that regard, the excellent reviewers of this manuscript have uniformly been quite forceful in their, collectively, contradictory opinions regarding the subject.)

Magnesium

A growing area of interest has been in the possibility that injury-induced loss of magnesium could play a role in neuronal damage. There is a decrease in the total and free magnesium concentrations in brain regions destined to die following traumatic percussion injury (Vink et al. 1987), and the severity of neurological injury and of magnesium depletion are correlated. Furthermore, treatment with a thyrotropin-releasing hormone analog, which protects neurons from traumatic damage, also reverses the decline in free magnesium concentrations (Vink et al. 1988a). While the decline could be merely a consequence of the neuronal damage, some evidence for a causal effect has emerged with the demonstration that prophylactic treatment of rats subjected to traumatic injury with magnesium salts prevents the decline in free magnesium concentrations and improves neurological outcome (Vink et al. 1988b; McIntosh et al. 1989). Moreover, magnesium reduces the vulnerability of hippocampal neurons to anoxic injury in vitro (Kass and Lipton 1982; Rothman 1983). Finally, magnesium administration following ischemic injury in the rat decreases CA_1 damage (Tsuda et al. 1991).

Magnesium depletion may cause damage in a number of ways. Magnesium is required for all reactions involving ATP phosphate exchange, including glycolysis and the activity of all ATPase-coupled pumps, to name but a few critical areas. In addition, magnesium is critical for proper membrane fluidity. Moreover, as noted, the NMDA-coupled calcium channel is normally blocked by magnesium in a voltage-dependent manner, and a shortage of magnesium should bias the channel toward opening.

In summary, magnesium depletion is likely to be deleterious to a neuron. However, it is not clear to me where the magnesium goes following a traumatic injury. While this literature emphasizes the loss of free magnesium, a loss of total magnesium is also reported. This makes it difficult to assume that the loss of the free component is due merely to precipitation or sequestering within the cell. However, the protective effects of magnesium salts and the numerous ways in which magnesium depletion could damage neurons suggests that more research be done in this area.

The Chloride/Sodium Hypothesis

This mechanism involves a pathologic influx of chloride and sodium during varied neurological insults. In this scenario, this triggers a secondary influx of water, which causes damaging swelling of neurons. This hypothesis was based on three supporting observations. First, one of the earliest signs of hippocampal injury following various insults in vivo is acute dendrosomatic swelling (Olney 1978). Next, cultured hippocampal neurons undergoing degeneration following an insult such as anoxia often swell and burst (Rothman 1985).

Finally, and most importantly, removal of chloride from the culture media can protect neurons from exposure to EAAs (Rothman 1985); moreover, in those same studies, damage was shown to be calcium independent.

These observations, especially the final one, gave strong support to this hypothesis, which was quite dominant a few years ago. It has not held up in a general manner, however. Three problems have emerged:

1. The swelling and the neuron death are not inextricably interrelated events. For example, in vivo, the dendrosomatic swelling appears to be merely an acute response to neurological insults, which usually resolves shortly afterward and is not necessarily a marker for neurons that are going to die eventually. In vitro, the early swelling and the delayed degeneration can be dissociated. The early phase is chloride and sodium dependent, whereas the latter phase is calcium dependent (Choi 1987b; Berdichevsky et al. 1987)

2. Neuronal swelling, occurring to the point of bursting the neuron, is probably unique to in vitro cultures. This probably reflects the two-dimensional architecture of neuronal monolayers in culture, in contrast to the three-dimensional world in vivo or in slice preparations. In the monolayers, the relative size of the extracellular fluid compartment is enormous; thus, more fluid can enter neurons, and there are fewer mechanical three-dimensional constraints on a neuron by its neighbors to prevent swelling to the point of bursting. In contrast, neurons never swell that way in vivo. The neuropathology is just the opposite, namely, pyknotic collapse. Even in the simpler three-dimensional world of the tissue slice, EAAs do not cause neuronal bursting, and EAA toxicity is not chloride dependent (Garthwaite et al. 1986).

3. The phenomenon of neurons swelling to the point of bursting is probably atypical, even in the in vitro studies. The studies showing chloride dependency of excitotoxin damage (Rothman 1985) also showed a calcium independence. This both strengthened the chloride hypothesis and cast serious doubt on the calcium story. A subsequent study (Garthwaite and Garthwaite 1986), however, explains this finding quite satisfactorily. The authors studied excitotoxic damage to cerebellar slices, altering calcium concentrations in the medium. At concentrations above 1 mM, calcium exacerbated excitotoxic damage. At 1 mM calcium concentrations, the toxicity of the excitotoxins began to decline until by 0.3 mM calcium, the slices were resistant to NMDA damage. In the 1985 Rothman study just discussed, the calcium-treated cultures were only exposed to 0.5 mM calcium; thus, the system was already at a level where the calcium component was minimal, and comparison with the calcium-free condition made little difference. With the calcium component eliminated (in either the 0 or 0.5 mM calcium conditions), more toxin was needed to be toxic (1 mM of glutamate in Rothman's studies, versus 0.5 mM in Choi's studies [1987a,b,c] with more calcium present), which was sufficient to drive the chloride component to the point of fatal swelling.

Therefore, while initially attractive, the sense in the field at this stage is that while chloride/sodium influx may occur, and may even explain the acute dendrosomatic swelling seen in vivo, it is unlikely to be a broadly general route by which the neurons die in vivo (Berdichevsky et al. 1987; Choi 1988).

(However, it should be noted that some investigators feel that this mechanism explains why glial cells swell transiently after neurological insults [Kimelberg and Norenberg 1989].) This resolution of the chloride/sodium hypothesis also helps put in perspective some of the earlier thinking about EAAs. In an early formulation on the subject (Olney et al. 1971), the neurotoxicity of EAAs was thought to arise strictly and linearly from their excitatory properties. From an ionic perspective, the main consequence of excitation is sodium influx, which suggested that such influx should be intrinsic to the process of damage. This sort of thinking predicted that among the various EAA analogs, there would be a strict correlation between the extent of excitation and of toxicity. This has not been the case (reviewed in Choi 1988). Moreover, this idea predicts that other causes of neuronal excitation should be just as damaging; this has not been the case either. For example, sustained depolarization with potassium in neurons treated with NMDA antagonists is not damaging (Rothman et al. 1987). Therefore, among the EAAs, excitation means sodium influx in a fairly linear manner, but it does not necessarily mean toxicity. In contrast, a subset of EAA actions involve NMDA receptor activation, nonlinear calcium influx, and toxicity.

CHAPTER SUMMARY

This chapter reviews the ways in which neurological insults damage neurons. The hallmarks of the necrotic cell death following neurological insults typify the mystery of the process: Despite metabolic perturbation occurring throughout entire brain regions, it is characteristic subsets of neurons that show *selective vulnerability* to the particular insult (i.e., the entire brain can be equally ATP deprived after global ischemia, yet only some neurons die). Furthermore, despite the metabolic perturbations being evident almost immediately with the onset of the insult, damage is *delayed*, emerging gradually over the course of days.

Three neurological insults are considered. They are all among the most common of necrotic insults and illustrate the principles of mechanism well; all primarily damage the hippocampus, and the toxicities of all are exacerbated by glucocorticoids.

In *hypoxia-ischemia*, delivery of oxygen and nutrients to the brain is impaired, either due to global cardiac arrest or local infarct. With its onset, energy stores plummet, anaerobic metabolism commences and lactate accumulates, pH declines, and protein synthesis halts throughout the brain. Nevertheless, damage is typically most pronounced in the CA_1 region of the hippocampus (and, to a lesser extent, to the hilus of the dentate gyrus, certain neocortical pyramidal layers, cerebellar Purkinje cells, and caudate/putamen neurons); it is only with more severe ischemia that damage becomes "pan-necrotic," damaging neurons and glia indiscriminately. Moreover, the damage is delayed—with reperfusion, the metabolic indices normalize over a number of hours, and damage emerges over days. Neuropathologically, the damage involves microvacuolization of mitochondria, dendritic swelling, and ischemic cell changes. In both clinical and experimental hypoxia-ischemia, there is a paradox that contains an important clue as to mechanism of damage: A small amount of blood flow is more damaging than none at all, and hypoxia-ischemia following a meal is more damaging than when nutrients have not been stored. In general, it is believed that nutrient preloading enhances energy stores at the time of the onset of the hypoxia-ischemia; as a result, the brain is capable of more anaerobic metabolism during the hypoxia, which produces more lactate and thus more damaging acidosis.

Seizure represents a heterogeneous grouping of disorders in which there is frequent and synchronized electrical discharge. Traditionally, the brain damage associated with severe epilepsy was thought to be the cause of the seizures. It was only with the more recent development of experimental models of epilepsy that it has been shown that seizures can cause, as well as result from brain damage. Once again, damage preferentially occurs within the hippocampus, with the pyramidal neurons of Ammon's horn (CA_3 and CA_4) being most vulnerable. Preferential damage also occurs in neocortical and cerebellar Purkinje neurons. The neuropathologic changes in moribund neurons are similar to those in hypoxia-ischemia, leading to some (now generally discredited) theories that seizure damages by causing some form of ischemia (e.g., secondary to convulsive apnea, secondary to edema-induced local compression of blood vessels).

Hypoglycemia induces brain damage when circulating glucose concentrations drop below a (species-typical) threshold. This is well correlated with the point at which spontaneous EEG activity in the brain ceases (i.e., isoelectricity). Despite the metabolic deprivation being profound throughout the brain, it is again the hippocampus that is selectively vulnerable, with damage being concentrated in the dentate granule neurons. Damage also occurs in the neocortex and caudate/putamen. Neuropathologically, the features of cell damage differ from those of hypoxia-ischemia and seizure.

The remainder of the chapter is devoted to reviewing some of the most credible (and one now discredited) theories as to the mechanisms mediating damage in these neurological disorders.

Excitatory Amino Acid (EAA) Neurotransmitters

An enormous amount of attention and excitement has focused on EAAs, amino acids that also have neurotransmitter roles. Glutamate and aspartate are the most credible example of these and are probably the most plentiful of excitatory neurotransmitters in the brain. They bind to a number of different receptor types, classified as either NMDA or non-NMDA, which are both plentiful in the hippocampus. The former has received the most attention. The NMDA receptor is a complex whose binding of EAAs can be modulated by glycine, zinc, acidity, and redox state. It is associated with a channel that is permeable to sodium and calcium, but which is blocked by magnesium in a voltage-dependent manner. This is critical to its function—because of this magnesium blockade, EAA binding to NMDA receptors is normally not sufficient to cause ion flow through the channel. It is only when the local vicinity is sufficiently depolarized (for example, by EAA binding to surrounding non-NMDA receptors) that the magnesium blockade is lifted, causing an explosive depolarizing influx of sodium and calcium. Thus, the binding/response properties of the receptor are markedly nonlinear. The NMDA receptor appears to play a major physiological role in plastic events thought to underlie learning, such as long-term potentiation, and its nonlinearity fits logically with such a role.

The explosive potential for excitatory ion flow through the NMDA channel also appears to underly the excitotoxic potential of EAAs. It has been known for many decades now that EAAs can be neurotoxic. They have also been implicated indirectly in the neurotoxicity of such disorders as olivoponto-cerebellar degeneration, Guam amyotrophic lateral sclerosis/parkinsonian dementia, and Huntington's disease. A vast amount of recent work has most directly implicated EAAs as mediators of damage following hypoxia-ischemia, seizure, and hypoglycemia.

In all three cases, the insults cause considerable release of EAAs as well as cause the electrophysiological excitation that would be expected after exposure to elevated concentrations of EAAs. Most importantly, the toxicity of all of these insults can be eliminated or reduced by antagonizing the NMDA receptor. These numerous observations have fueled the "excitotoxic" hypothesis of neurological damage, which in its broadest current form states that a pathologic excess of EAAs and overstimulation of the NMDA receptor underlie the neuron death in these insults. Chapter 10 reviews how the energy depletion caused by these insults brings about the dysregulation of EAA trafficking, and its damaging accumulation in the synapse.

Despite the tremendous credibility of the excitotoxic theory of damage, it is clearly not the sole mediator of neuronal damage during these insults. As evidence, blocking the NMDA receptor is not always completely or even partially protective (especially for global ischemia). Moreover, some recent work has shown there to be dual components to, for example, hypoxic-ischemic damage, where EAAs are implicated in only one component of damage (one form being EAA and energy dependent, occurring in the range of moderate acidosis; the other, during more severe acidosis, being EAA and energy independent). Therefore, EAAs are probably the most plausible, but not sole mediators of neuron death during these insults.

Calcium Neurotoxicity

Calcium regulates a vast number of cellular events, mostly by activating calcium-dependent enzymes, and a pathologic excess of the ion has a commensurately vast potential to cause damage. The calcium hypothesis of damage is closely linked to the EAA hypothesis, as the primary damaging consequence of excessive NMDA receptor activation is pathologic mobilization of free cytosolic calcium in the postsynaptic neuron. As evidence, both EAAs and the individual neurological insults cause a decrease in extracellular calcium concentrations and a complementary accumulation of intracellular calcium. Most directly, the toxicity of EAAs and of these insults can be prevented or blunted by removing calcium from the medium, blocking calcium channels, or chelating the ion.

Because of the complexity of calcium trafficking, it is not settled which route(s) supplies the excess calcium. Most plausibly, activation of the ion channel gated to the NMDA receptor allows calcium influx. In addition, EAA-induced depolarization will also enhance influx through voltage-gated calcium channels. Calcium is also likely to be mobilized from storage sites in organelles at such times. Moreover, there is evidence that some of the pathologic accumulation of the excess calcium derives from failure to remove calcium from the cytosolic compartment, which normally occurs through sequestration back into organelles and efflux out of the cell. As will be reviewed in chapter 10, all of these regulatory steps are dependent on energy, and the energy depletion brought about by these insults is the probable cause of the pathologic accumulation of the ion.

Once calcium levels become high enough, there are a tremendous number of potential damaging consequences, mostly resulting from indiscriminate activation of calcium-dependent proteases, lipases, and nucleases. In neurons, some of the damaging consequences include generation of arachidonic acid and conversion of xanthine dehydrogenase to xanthine oxygenase; both steps favor oxygen radical generation. Moreover, there is evidence of calcium-induced proteolysis of cytoskeletal proteins such as spectrin in neurons during these insults. Finally, sufficiently high calcium concentrations will damage mitochondria and suppress oxidative phosphorylation for a number of reasons. At present, "what happens after too much calcium" remains unclear, as to which events are most responsible for the subsequent neuron death.

Acidotic Injury

Given the pH-optima for so many enzymes, when cells become even mildly acidotic or alkalotic, function is greatly perturbed. Thus, it is not surprising that there is a complex array of pumps and exchangers in cells that transport protons and thus maintain pH homeostasis. There is reasonable evidence that such homeostasis is upset during hypoxia-ischemia, and that damaging acidosis occurs. This is thought to be due to the anaerobic nature of metabolism during ischemia, where lactate is produced to an abnormal extent and pH drops. As evidence, ischemic insults cause both tissue and intraneuronal acidosis, and experimental replication of the same degree of acidity damages brain tissue. This acidotic route of damage during hypoxia-ischemia is thought to explain one of the clinical paradoxes of the insult, specifically the fact that hypoxic-ischemic brain damage is typically worse after a meal. As an explanation, nutrient preloading is thought to enhance the substrate stores available to a neuron at the time of the hypoxia-ischemia. This leads to even greater amounts of anaerobic metabolism and thus, even worse lactic acidosis.

Implicit in this acidotic model of damage during hypoxia-ischemia is the idea that neurons die not for *lack* of energy during the insult, but due to the generation of the *wrong type* of energy (i.e., energy derived from anaerobic metabolism). This is probably a simplification, and in recent years, some of the initial enthusiasm for acidosis as the sole route of hypoxic-ischemic damage has been tempered. Instead, the more severe forms of hypoxic-ischemic damage seem most acidotic in nature (i.e., the pan-necrosis that involves broad swaths of neurons and glia); in contrast, the milder selective neuron loss during less severe hypoxia-ischemia appears to be more a result of EAA/calcium dysregulation. In agreement with this tempering of the acidotic hypothesis, some experimental models of hypoxia-ischemia have shown that energy preloading can, in fact, protect neurons.

Oxygen Radical Neurotoxicity

Oxygen radicals are atoms or groups of atoms with unpaired electrons that can form chemical bonds. Because of the unpaired electron, oxygen radicals are highly reactive and can form indiscriminant bonds with a variety of molecules, damaging their function in the process. This is thought to be most common with long-chain membrane lipids, in which oxidative damage causes lipid peroxidation, inappropriate cross-linkage to membrane proteins, and so on. Normally, oxygen radicals are generated in cells during oxidative phosphorylation as a result of the electron transport chain, and normally any such radicals that escape the process (and thus become free radicals) are contained by oxygen radical scavengers and quenchers (such as superoxide dismutase or vitamin E). There is some evidence that during these neurological insults, this delicate balance between radical generation and containment is upset, producing damaging amounts of free radicals.

This case is most plausible for hypoxia-ischemia. As conceptualized, during the burst of oxidative metabolism that follows postischemic reperfusion, abnormally large amounts of oxygen radicals are generated and the containment system is functioning at less than its optimal. As evidence for this model, there is accumulation of oxygen radicals during the reperfusion period. This is probably due to more generation of them—for example, the mobilization of calcium during and after hypoxia-ischemia will cause oxygen radical generation through arachidonic acid release and xanthine oxidase generation. Moreover, hypoxia-ischemia probably compromises the ability of neurons to contain free radicals; as evidence, levels of various radical scavengers decline during the reperfusion period. As the most direct evidence for an oxygen radical role in this insult, exogenous application of radical scavengers has been reported to be neuroprotective in most reports examining the issue. Therefore, oxygen radicals appear to mediate some features of hypoxic-ischemic damage.

Depletion of Magnesium

Concentrations of total and free magnesium decline in brain tissue after insults such as trauma, and some researchers have suggested that this contributes to damage. As evidence, magnesium will decrease traumatic brain injury and EAA-induced injury. As a mediating mechanism, magnesium is critical to numerous cellular processes. It is essential for all reactions involving ATP/phosphate exchange, meaning that magnesium depletion should greatly disrupt glycolysis and ATP-coupled pumps. Moreover, as noted, an absence of magnesium will cause the NMDA-gated channel to be far more conductive of damaging calcium.

Therefore, magnesium depletion may play some role in these instances of neuron death. However, it is not clear whether its concentrations decline in all of these insults or, more importantly, why they decline.

The Chloride/Sodium Hypothesis

About a decade ago, there was considerable excitement about the possibility that an excessive influx of chloride and sodium caused neuron death during these various insults. In this scenario, the initial depolarization due to EAAs caused the influx of these ions which, secondarily, pulled in large amounts of water. Carried to a pathologic extent, the cells would then swell and burst. As evidence for this hypothesis, one of the earliest neuropathological signs in vivo following these insults is dendrosomatic swelling. Moreover, in vitro, neurons exposed to anoxia were observed to swell and burst. Finally, elimination of chloride from the medium protected the neurons from such pathology.

The enthusiasm for this hypothesis has waned for a number of reasons. First, the dendrosomatic swelling in vivo is transient and does not predict eventual neuron death. Second, the bursting of neurons appears not to ever occur in vivo but instead to be a by-product of the unique features of the in vitro environment. Finally, careful studies have shown that neuron death in vitro is chloride dependent only under the rather specialized condition in which the calcium-dependent components of damage have been eliminated.

This review of the neurological insults that damage the hippocampus, and the possible mediators of such damage, is by no means exhaustive; instead, only the major players have been considered. My guess is that, by now, the reader is quite sufficiently overwhelmed by merely this number. For the superficial reader, there is no doubt the impression that one must choose among all these different possible mediators—EAAs, calcium, acidity, oxygen radicals, etc.—and each seems quite convincing. For the reader following the interactions among them carefully, there is the equally distressing impression that each mediator has a good chance of activating one of the other mediators (for example, lack of magnesium exaggerates NMDA action; calcium can lead to oxygen radical generation, and so on). For that reader, the impression must be building that all the mediators trigger each other.

The next chapter begins to wrestle with these issues. (1) How do these various mediators of damage interact? (2) How does energy availability influence the damaging nature of each mediator alone, and their interactions? (3) How might this knowledge begin to explain individual differences in neuronal vulnerability to these insults?

Note: I would like to acknowledge two of my graduate students, Geoffrey Tombaugh and Elicia Elliott, who have shaped my thinking about this and the next chapter through their superb research and reading of the literature.

10 Metabolic Chaos II: The Role of Energy Failure in Necrotic Neuronal Injury

SUMMARY OF THE BOOK SO FAR

Various stressors trigger the endocrine and neural adaptations known as the stress-response. The adrenal secretion of glucocorticoids is central to the stress-response and typifies its two-edged quality: While glucocorticoids are essential for surviving short-term physical stressors, excessive exposure to glucocorticoids (during exogenous administration of the hormone or some instances of chronic or repeated stressors) causes numerous stress-related diseases.

Part I of this book examined how glucocorticoid secretion is regulated during aging, as well as whether excessive exposure to glucocorticoids over the lifetime can accelerate aspects of brain aging. The data reviewed in that part of the book are combined to form a model, termed the *glucocorticoid cascade*. It attempts to explain two features of aging rats—hypersecretion of glucocorticoids (including impaired negative feedback inhibition of glucocorticoid release) and degeneration of neurons in the hippocampal region of the brain. The hippocampus is shown to be an important mediator of glucocorticoid feedback inhibition, such that its senescent degeneration causes glucocorticoid hypersecretion. Glucocorticoids, in turn, are shown to be capable of killing hippocampal neurons. Therefore, these two regulatory features combine to form a feedforward cascade of senescent degeneration—glucocorticoids damage the hippocampus, which causes further glucocorticoid secretion (and numerous deleterious consequences for the aged rat).

Part II explores the mechanisms by which glucocorticoids are neurotoxic in the hippocampus. Chapter 7 demonstrated that these hormones need not be toxic. Instead, they endanger hippocampal neurons, impairing their capacity to survive coincident neurological insults, such as hypoxia-ischemia, seizure, hypoglycemia, antimetabolites, and oxygen radical generators. Therefore, glucocorticoids may not only play an important role in accelerating hippocampal aging, but might also exacerbate the toxicity of some of the most common neurological insults to the hippocampus.

This leads the way for examining the known mechanisms of neuron death, to understand which features are exacerbated by glucocorticoids. Chapter 8 examined cases of apoptotic, or programmed, cell death (such as during neuronal development) and concluded that apoptotic mechanisms are probably not relevant to understanding glucocorticoid endangerment. Therefore, the emphasis has shifted toward the mechanisms of neuron death during pathologic insults to the brain. Chapter 9 reviewed the features of the most common neuropathologic insults to the hippocampus—hypoxia-ischemia, seizure, and hypoglycemia. It also introduced the most plausible mediators of neuron death during these disorders. These are overexposure to excitatory amino acid neurotransmitters such as glutamate and aspartate, excessive mobilization of free cytosolic calcium, excessive acidosis, and generation of oxygen radicals. The present chapter reviews how neuronal energetics can modulate the toxicity of these diseases and of these putative mediators of neuron death. This lays the groundwork for appreciating how glucocorticoids disrupt hippocampal neuronal energetics, to be explored in chapter 11.

SOME IDEAS REGARDING CELLULAR ENERGY CRISES

Chapter 9 outlined the major neurological disorders that damage the hippocampus and the leading suspected mediators of their action. Much of the excitement about these mechanisms concerns their interactions and how they form a convergent cascade of damage. To understand these interactions, one needs to consider the role of energy failure in these disorders. I will suggest that all of these insults involve either an immediate or slowly emerging energy crisis, and that many of the mediating mechanisms and their interactions are exacerbated by a paucity of energy. It is in that context that the role of glucocorticoids might best be understood, to be discussed in the next chapter.

Before considering the role of energetics in the individual insults and proposed mediators of damage, I will discuss a few ideas regarding energy crises and their likely consequences. These have rarely been considered explicitly in this literature, and I feel that they can clarify some confusions that will emerge over the next two chapters.

1. *The severity of energy depletion need not be correlated with the extent of damage produced.* Put more directly, during a neurological insult two cells may have become equally depleted of energy (as assessed by some endpoint) and at equal speeds, yet only one may die. This has occasionally been used as an argument against energy failure as a route of death. I feel this is not the case, and much of the final discussion in this chapter regarding the mechanisms for selective neuronal vulnerability to insults revolves around this idea. Certainly, half the story is how *severe* an energy failure occurs; however, the second half has to be what the *consequences* are of that severe an energy crisis for a cell. Two cells may be equally strapped for energy, but the consequences may differ. I find an analogy to be quite helpful. If two individuals have gone long enough without eating, have become equally hypoglycemic, they may both ultimately pass out. From the standpoint of energy deprivation (in this case, perhaps most conveniently measured by circulating glucose levels), these individuals may be undergoing identical crises. Yet, the functional consequences and likelihood of survival may differ dramatically. If a person passes out while sitting in an armchair watching television, the pathologic consequences are likely to be far less than passing out for the same length of time while working on a girder high up on a construction site. The "selective vulnerability" in this case is not a function of the severity of the hypoglycemia or the most proximal response of passing out, but of the circumstances under which it occurs, and the damage that will likely ensue in the construction site

scenario is certainly the result of an "energy crisis." I will argue at the end of the chapter that part of the explanation for selective neuronal vulnerability must lie in the neurobiological equivalent of some neurons spending their time in armchairs and others on narrow girders high above the ground.

2. *An energy problem may not limit the rate of activity of a neuron, but rather may limit the ability of the neuron to contain the consequences of the activity.* Again, to resort to analogy, there may be the energy to throw a hell of a large party, but not to clean up the mess afterward. In neurobiological terms, this may be equivalent to having the energy to sustain high rates of excitation, oxygen and glucose consumption, and so on, yet to lack the energy to contain the neurochemical, ionic, or free radical consequences of the hyperactivity. As will be discussed, seizures seem particularly relevant to this sort of analysis, as they are characterized by enormously high levels of activity with only moderate indications of energy depletion *during* seizures. Yet, seizure-induced hippocampal damage is sensitive to energy availability, and I will argue that the energy problem does not occur during the seizures, but afterward, when the consequences of excessive EAAs, calcium, and oxygen radicals must be contained.

As a corollary of this, indices of cellular function may be normal, yet there may be an energy crisis occurring. A cell may be maintaining some aspect(s) of cellular function within a normal range, yet may be fatally overexpending energy in the process. An example of this is found in the recent report (Ben-Yoseph et al. 1990) in which a dosage of NMDA sufficient to impair energy state in cortical slices did not lead to uncontrolled mobilization of cytosolic calcium. Presumably, the energy stores were being depleted in that circumstance in order to maintain calcium homeostasis in the face of EAA challenge.

3. *A cellular energy crisis can occur even when circulating substrate concentrations are high.* In other words, high circulating glucose concentrations do not guarantee sufficient energy for neurons. This seems illogical, and usually is, but is extremely relevant to the special case of glucocorticoids. A central feature of glucocorticoid action, as noted many pages ago, is their elevation of circulating glucose concentrations. This is brought about, in part, by an inhibition of the activity of the glucose transporter in many tissues (to be discussed in chapter 11; in addition, a large part of the increase in circulating glucose concentrations is due to glucocorticoid stimulation of hepatic gluconeogenesis). Therefore, there is plentiful circulating glucose in part *because* cells cannot remove it from the bloodstream. This clarifies the observation that glucocorticoids (which increase circulating glucose) may exacerbate neuronal damage, while exogenous glucose treatment (which also increases circulating glucose) can protect neurons against neurological insults. A critical issue is whether target cells can access the glucose, and in the case of glucocorticoids, many cells cannot as readily. As will be discussed in the next chapter, glucocorticoids inhibit glucose transport in the hippocampus.

4. *Metabolic rate need not tell anything about energy state.* This can be explained most simply by pointing out that a cell may have a low rate of, for example,

glucose consumption because there is no glucose available to consume, or because it has little demand for glucose. The former case certainly occurs with hypoxia-ischemia and represents a profound energy crisis; the latter can occur with anesthetization and represents the very opposite of a crisis. In much the same way, a starving refugee and a hibernating animal both eat very rarely, yet only the former is in a state of energy crisis.

DISRUPTIONS OF ENERGY BY THE THREE NEUROLOGICAL INSULTS

With this orientation toward issues of cerebral energetics, I will review how each of the neurological insults discussed in the last chapter are crises of energy.

Hypoxia-Ischemia

Hypoxia-ischemia is the archetypal case of an energy crisis. The oxygen deprivation alone is highly disruptive, since oxidative phosphorylation yields 17 to 18 times more ATP than does glycolysis alone, and more than 95% of neuronal ATP is derived from oxidative phosphorylation (a figure much higher than in peripheral organs) (reviewed in Erecinska and Silver 1989). When coupled with glucose deprivation, a profound energy crisis ensues. Within seconds of hypoxia-ischemia, phosphocreatine and then ATP pools decline and, within minutes, disappear. ATP is broken down to ADP, then AMP, deaminated and dephosphorylated to eventually yield inosine and hypoxanthine, which can diffuse out of the cell; thus, the total adenine nucleotide pool can decrease (Kleihues et al. 1974; Kass and Lipton 1982; Yoneda and Okada, 1989; Raley and Lipton, unpublished). Moreover, the extent of ATP decline predicts the extent of subsequent damage in tissue slices (Kass and Lipton, 1982 1986).

Is this energy depletion a cause of the neuronal damage? In principle, this could be tested by seeing if preloading a neuron with glucose prior to hypoxia-ischemia is protective. The problem with hypoxia-ischemia, of course, is the paradox that glucose preloading worsens damage. This is because the elevated glucose and perhaps enhanced glycogen stores are then used anaerobically, yielding damaging lactic acid. This argues against hypoxic-ischemic damage emerging exclusively because of energy failure—these data suggest that the dangerous manner in which the energy is produced also contributes to damage.

However, as discussed, this is a simplification. As noted, Auer and Siesjo (1988) dichotomize in hypoxia-ischemia between EAA-related selective neuronal damage and acidotic pan-necrotic damage. Numerous studies of the hippocampus and basal ganglia support this dichotomy and show that energy supplementation prehypoxia in vitro can be protective (Lipton and Whittingham 1979, 1982; Kass and Lipton 1982; Goldberg et al. 1986; Raley and Lipton 1988; Tombaugh and Sapolsky, 1990a; Schurr et al. 1987). Similarly, posthypoxic glucose or fructose-1,6-diphosphate supplementation will reduce hypoxic-ischemic damage in the neonatal rat (Hattori and Wasterlain 1989) and in rabbits (Farias et al. 1990). Therefore, the massive depletion of energy that occurs during hypoxia-ischemia carries a price for the neuron.

Hypoglycemia

By definition, hypoglycemia is an energetic insult, and neuronal ATP concentrations decline to approximately 25% of control values (Siesjo, 1981. Obviously, supplementing neurons with excess energy during the hypoglycemia is protective, since it eliminates the insult. Moreover, supplementing cells with glucose prior to a hypoglycemic insult is also protective (Tombaugh et al. 1992).

Seizures

This insult is often viewed as not involving energy failure (cf. Siesjo and Wieloch 1986), because initially there is little evidence of energy depletion, and even with sustained seizures, the magnitude of depletion is less dramatic than for hypoxia-ischemia or hypoglycemia. Nevertheless, there must be a component of energy failure.

With the onset of seizure, there is a one- to three-fold increase in oxygen and glucose consumption in the brain. This is not surprising, given the metabolic demands of repeated action potentials. Cerebrovascular compensations (e.g., increased cerebral blood flow and vasodilation) successfully meet these increased demands. As a result, there is no energy mismatch early on in seizure, as measured by tissue oxygen tension, cellular redox state, or levels of high-energy phosphates (reviewed in Siesjo and Wieloch 1986). Importantly, most of these studies were carried out in anesthetized and ventilated rats or cats, such that there could be no additional confound of convulsive hypoxia.

Thus, during the initial period of seizure there seems to be no energy problem. However, even at this time, the brain is metabolically vulnerable. For example, bicuculline-induced seizures exacerbate the disruptive effects of hypoxia on phosphorylation potential, acidosis, and ammonia accumulation (Blennow et al. 1985). The authors interpreted this as showing that even if energy profiles are maintained early in seizure, this is a vulnerable, fragile state of energetic equilibrium.

With sustained seizures (generally, more than an hour), however, the compensations fail and energy mismatch becomes overt. The vasodilatory compensations fail, tissue hypoxia develops, glucose concentrations decline, redox systems are reduced, lactate accumulates, and ATP and energy charge decline (to about 75% and 90% of normal values, respectively) (Evans and Meldrum 1984; Siesjo and Wieloch 1986). As the cerebrovascular compensations fail, the brain extracts more glucose from the blood and circulating glucose concentrations decline to below the K_m for glucose transport across the blood-brain barrier, suggesting that transport becomes a rate-limiting factor at that point (Evans and Meldrum 1984).

This extent of energy disruption is not as dramatic as that seen in other types of insults. Is the disruption sufficient to cause damage? Correlative evidence supports this. For example, vulnerable brain regions (i.e., those destined for seizure-induced damage) have greater energy demands during the seizure than do resistant regions. This has been shown with 2-deoxyglucose mapping of the brain during seizure, in which vulnerable regions show a three-fold increase in glucose utilization, whereas resistant areas show essentially no rise. This is particularly well demonstrated with kainic acid–induced seizures, where damage emerges only in hypermetabolic regions, and the extent of enhanced glucose and oxygen consumption covaries with enhanced neuronal excitation (Ben-Ari et al. 1981; Lothman and Collins 1981). Moreover, vulnerable regions (such as substantia nigra) show more disruption of energy charge and far greater lactate accumulation than resistant regions (such as periaqueductal gray) (Siesjo and Wieloch 1986).

As the most direct evidence that the mild energy depletion of seizure contributes to the neurotoxicity, seizure damage is worsened by hypoglycemia (Meldrum 1983; Johansen and Diemer 1986) and decreased by energy supplementation (Sapolsky and Stein, 1988, figure 10.1).

Therefore, while sustained seizure in certain respects represents the mildest of these insults, the extent of energy disruption produced still seems sufficient to contribute to the neurotoxicity.

Protective Effects of Energy Conservation

In summary, all three insults produce some degree of energy depletion in neurons, and this appears to be central to their toxicity. Another way of demonstrating that such energetic depletion can be endangering is to show that some interventions which reduce neuronal energy utilization can protect these neurons following these insults. One such intervention is hypothermia, in which the cold is thought to decrease energy consumption. Hypothermia is at least partially protective against hypoxic-ischemic damage in vivo (Michenfelder et al. 1970; Bering 1974; Carlsson et al. 1976; Berntman et al. 1981; Welsh et al. 1990; Freund et al. 1990a; Lundgren et al. 1991a; however, see failure of protection reported by Kato et al. 1991 and Welsh and Harris 1991) and in vitro (Tanimoto and Okada 1987; Okada et al. 1988; Chopp et al. 1989, 1991; Nedergaard et al. 1991), while *hyper*thermia is detrimental (Chopp et al. 1988; Kuroiwa et al. 1990). (Note that in all of these studies, the temperature manipulations followed the insult. Periods of hyperthermia somewhat in advance of an ischemic insult can protect the hippocampus, the speculated mechanism being via induction of heat-shock proteins [Kitagawa et al. 1991]). Similarly, anesthestics decrease energy consumption in neurons and can protect them following these insults. This has most frequently been studied with barbituates or benzodiazepines, which potentiate inhibitory GABA sites (Goldstein et al. l966; Michenfelder et al. 1976; Steen and Michenfelder 1978;

Safar 1980; Yatsu 1983; Piatt and Schiff 1984; Nussmeier et al. 1986; Arako et al. 1990; Kato et al. 1990; Voll and Auer 1991. But also see Todd et al. 1982; Ward et al. 1985 for opposing conclusions). While each intervention may have effects in addition to the energetic ones, they bolster the argument that, in effect, a neuron is more likely to survive these insults if it does not have to work hard in its aftermath.

EXACERBATION OF MEDIATORS OF DAMAGE BY ENERGY FAILURE

If the three neurological insults under discussion all have their toxicities enhanced by energy depletion, the cellular mechanisms that mediate damage must also be exacerbated in some manner by energy failure. There are numerous routes by which this can occur.

EAAs

EAA signaling in the synapse is exacerbated by energy depletion. Hypoglycemic damage (induced by insulin administration), chemical hypoxia (induced by cyanide), and damage induced by uncoupling of electron transport are all prevented with NMDA receptor antagonists (Wieloch 1985; Monyer et al. 1989; Armanini et al. 1990; Dubinsky and Rothman 1991). This implies that the energy failure induces either more EAAs reaching the postsynaptic NMDA receptors, an impaired ability to withstand the EAAs, or both. The enhanced EAA signal has been shown in a number of cases. For example, hypoglycemia enhances EAA outflow and impairs high-affinity EAA reuptake in the hippocampus (Szerb and O'Regan 1988; Sandberg et al. 1986; Schaeffer and Lazdunski 1991). Neurons are also less capable of withstanding the EAAs when they are deprived of energy. For example, in vitro, glutamate causes more calcium influx and is more toxic in the presence of low glucose concentrations or sublethal cyanide concentrations (Novelli et al. 1988; Cox et al. 1989; Lysko et al. 1989; Patel et al. 1991).

How might EAA trafficking be altered by energy failure? Initial release from the axon terminal is, of course, contingent upon an action potential causing an influx of calcium, which triggers presynaptic vesicular release of EAAs (Nicholls and Sihra 1986; Sanchez-Prieto and Gonzalez 1988; Szerb 1988). After EAA interaction with the postsynaptic receptor, there can be reuptake into the presynaptic terminal via a bidirectional EAA/sodium cotransporter. So long as the Na^+-K^+-ATPase is working optimally, intracellular sodium concentrations will be quite low, and the concentration gradient will favor the inflow of EAAs along with the sodium (Sanchez-Prieto and Gonzalez 1988). A second route of removing of the EAAs out of the synapse is via uptake into glia, primarily astrocytes. A potent uptake system exists there (Szerb and O'Regan 1988), and EAAs taken up via that route (specifically, glutamate) are then eventually recycled (as glutamine) from the glia back to neurons for utilization as neurotransmitters and for metabolic purposes. Because the V_{max}

for EAA uptake is higher in glia than in neurons (Schousboe et al. 1983), a large percentage of glutamate in the synapse probably travels via the glial route (Hertz et al. 1983a) (this glial component of EAA communication will be considered below in more detail).

A paucity of energy will disrupt all of the steps just outlined.

Enhanced Neuronal Release of EAAs   With energy failure, efficacy of the Na^+-K^+-ATPase declines causing efflux of potassium and membrane depolarization (Hansen 1985). Such depolarization will sensitize neurons to EAA toxicity (Vornov and Coyle 1991). This is a particular point of vulnerability, since approximately 50% of neuronal energy is consumed by Na^+-K^+-ATPase (Erecinska and Silver 1989). This should lead to enhanced voltage-gated calcium influx at the presynaptic terminals and, in theory, increase calcium-dependent release of EAAs. However, calcium-dependent release is also ATP dependent and, at least in the instance of collapsing neuronal metabolism by poisoning glycolysis and oxidative metabolism, the absence of ATP occurs prior to the influx of calcium. Under those circumstances, calcium-dependent release of EAA is rapidly blocked and is not a source of the EAA overflow that occurs (Kauppinen et al. 1988a; Sanchez-Prieto and Gonzalez 1988; Ikeda et al. 1989; Nicholls 1989; Lobner and Lipton 1990). However, with energy failure and increased intraterminal sodium concentrations, the calcium-independent EAA/sodium cotransporter will reverse direction and release EAAs from the metabolic pool. This is the most likely source of EAA overflow during these insults (Kauppinen et al. 1988a; Sanchez-Prieto and Gonzalez 1988; Ikeda et al. 1989). This has been found to occur at a consistent point of ATP depletion (Sanchez-Prieto and Gonzalez 1988; Dagani and Erecinska 1987). Quantitatively, this is an enormous potential source of EAAs, since only 3% to 10% of EAAs are releasable via the calcium-dependent route (reviewed in Nicholls 1989). Therefore, regardless of route, energy deprivation enhances EAA outflow. As another demonstration of this, poisoning of the Na^+-K^+-ATPase with ouabain causes EAA-dependent neurotoxicity (Lees et al. 1990).

Failure of Neuronal Reuptake   The failure of neuronal reuptake is intrinsic in the reversal of the calcium-independent EAA/sodium cotransporter and the net efflux of EAAs described immediately above. With the loss of this neuronal reuptake compartment, EAAs accumulate in the extracellular space (Bradford et al. 1987). The toxicity of EAAs is greatly enhanced when reuptake is blocked (either by poisoning the pump or destruction of presynaptic neurons) (Kohler and Schwarcz 1981; McBeen and Roberts, 1985; Choi 1987a). Moreover, this seems to be a fairly vulnerable component of the system; for example, during ischemia, it is failure of reuptake that initially causes accumulation of synaptic EAAs (Drejer et al. 1985)

Enhanced Glial Release of EAAs   Astrocytic release of glutamate and aspartate is markedly enhanced by swelling (Kimelberg et al. 1990). Such cytotoxic edema occurs in glia during these neurological insults due to potassium accumulation in the extracellular space and subsequent uptake into glia. In addition, the EAA uptake pumps in glia can reverse under conditions of depolarization and export EAAs (Szatkowsski et al. 1990). Therefore, when energy deprivation causes depolarization and astrocytic edema, EAA outflow should be increased. It is not known how much this astrocytic source contributes to the extracellular EAA accumulation during neurological insults.

Failure of Glial Uptake of EAAs The glial component of this system is particularly vulnerable to energy failure for a number of reasons (Szerb and O'Regan 1988; Kauppinen et al. 1988a). First, disruption of either glycolysis or electron transport alone inhibits glutamate uptake (Kauppinen et al. 1988a). Second, the uptake of glutamate into glia depends not only upon cotransport of sodium with the EAA but with antiport movement of potassium out from the glia; thus, a large rise in extracellular potassium concentrations inhibits uptake (Barbour et al. 1988. This is seen only with high extracellular potassium concentrations; more moderate ones stimulate uptake [Schousboe et al. 1977]). Therefore, hyperexcitation or energy failure in neurons (increasing extracellular potassium concentrations) will impair neighboring glia. It should be noted that this pump cannot reverse direction of EAA movement, even with severe energy failure (Kimelberg et al. 1990).

Given the importance of the glial component of uptake, its removal should have a large and deleterious impact on the system. Supporting this, the toxicity of EAAs or of hypoxia upon cultured neurons decreases when they are cocultured with astrocytes or cultured under conditions that promote glial proliferation—the authors speculate that the astrocytic reuptake of EAAs serves as a protective sponge (Vibulsreth et al. 1987; Pauwels et al. 1989; Rosenberg 1991, 1992).

Calcium

Once the EAAs interact with the postsynaptic NMDA receptor, the calcium component of the story is also likely to have many points of metabolic vulnerability. As discussed, the initial elevation of free cytosolic calcium can come from extracellular influx or release from intracellular sequestration sites. Once calcium generates its biological signal, neurons must rapidly remove the cation from the cytosol. This is typically accomplished through the hierarchy of binding to calcium-binding proteins, sequestration into intracellular sites, and efflux.

This efficient, yet energetically costly system of control is vulnerable to energetic depletion at a number of points: First, the initial influx of calcium should be enhanced in neurons starved of energy. Because the Na^+-K^+-ATPase pump will be failing, there will be less intracellular potassium, depolarizing the cell. This will release the NMDA channel from its magnesium blockade, allowing greater calcium influx with each activation by EAAs. As evidence of the importance of the magnesium, toxicity in vitro increases with decreasing concentrations of magnesium in media (even in the presence of large amounts of glucose (Novelli et al. 1988; Garthwaite and Garthwaite 1986, 1988). In addition, the increasing intracellular sodium concentrations that will result from the depolarization will tend to open voltage-gated calcium channels, as well as release greater amounts of calcium from intracellular organelles. In agreement with this prediction, glutamate is more toxic in cultures when ouabain is used to poison Na^+-K^+-ATPase, even in the presence of large amounts of glucose and magnesium (Novelli et al. 1988).

Second, once the free cytosolic calcium level has risen, it will be more difficult to buffer. Most obviously, the efficacy of any pumps that depend upon ATP or sodium gradients will decline, and that route of removal or sequestering will be limited; this should occur at the mitochondria, the endoplasmic reticulum, and the plasma membrane. Support for this is shown in the demonstration that specific inhibition of sodium/calcium exchange in cultured cerebellar neurons enhances EAA-induced death (Andreeva et al. 1991). Even if the neuron can continue to buffer the calcium, if it is doing so to a large extent, there will be deleterious consequences. This is particularly the case with the sodium/calcium exchanger on the cell surface. The exchanger is electrogenic, with three sodium ions entering for every calcium ion extruded. Therefore, heavy use of this final (desperate?) route of efflux is counterproductive, as the neuron will become even more depolarized by the enhanced electrogenicity, elevating cytosolic calcium even further. Finally, if intracellular sodium concentrations rise high enough, not only should the sodium/calcium exchanger fail to extrude calcium, it should even reverse direction, importing more calcium into the neuron (a development, it should be noted, which should at least tend to help the neuron repolarize again).

Acidity

Even under conditions of pronounced extracellular acidosis, healthy neurons are able to maintain intracellular pH within a narrow range (Vorstrup et al. 1989), implying a highly efficient system of regulation; the emerging understanding of the cellular mechansim by which hydrogen protons and lactate are buffered suggests that this is a costly system as well. Profound energy failure can disrupt pH regulation and cause acidosis in two obvious ways— more acid would be produced and less buffered. The enhanced production would derive from the hydrolysis of ATP. Under normal conditions, such ATP hydrolysis is the greatest source of hydrogen ions in a cell (Krebs et al. 1975). These are normally consumed in the regeneration of new ATP by oxidative phosphorylation. When, during an energy crisis, ATP hydrolysis outstrips ATP production, a significant amount of acidity could be produced. As noted, however, this is probably not a major cause of acidosis in any of these insults. In addition, acid production will be enhanced by the anaerobic nature of metabolism during ischemic insults.

Along with energy failure leading to the generation of excessive amounts of hydrogen ions, the neuron is probably also impaired in removing the protons. A likely point of energetic vulnerability is in having the means to pump hydrogen ions out of the neuron. Such pumps are either directly ATP dependent or indirectly so, via their dependence on ionic gradients (Roos and Boron 1981; Kraig et al. 1985a). For example, we have shown recently that the major regulator of neuronal pH in cultured hippocampal neurons is the sodium/proton exchanger (Raley-Susman et al. 1991); obviously, a decline in the sodium gradient during energy problems will impair the ability to pump protons out of the neuron. Thus, during the early phases of hypoxia-ischemia, there is increased proton efflux out of neurons; with sustained hypoxia-ischemia and its resultant energy failure, efflux fails and intracellular hydrogen ion concentrations rise (Kuhr et al. 1988; Kraig et al. 1985b).

Does the accumulation of hydrogen ions via this route mediate damage? While this seems reasonable, this has not been tested because it has not been possible to selectively alter the activity of the sodium/proton exchanger during a neurological insult.

Oxygen Radicals

Energy depletion in neurons can cause damaging levels of oxygen radicals. For example, the oxygen radical scavenger SOD can protect cultured neurons from the damaging effects of glucose starvation (Saez et al. 1987). Energy depletion could enhance free radical-induced neuronal damage in at least three ways:

1. More oxygen radicals should be generated. Because calcium concentrations will be elevated by energy depletion, there should be more arachidonic acid release and xanthine oxidase generation. As a more direct route, energy depletion should lead to generation of more substrates for xanthine oxidase to generate oxygen radicals. This occurs via ATP hydrolysis to AMP. The latter can be dephosphorylated or deaminated to adenosine or IMP, respectively; further dephosphorylation or deamination yields inosine, which can be converted to hypoxanthine, a substrate for the enzyme.

2. Fewer scavengers may be available to contain the oxygen radicals. As noted, tissue concentrations of various scavengers decline during ischemia.

3. Less repair of free radical-induced damage is likely to occur. This invokes the obvious idea that cellular repair is costly, and energy depletion may compromise the capacity of a cell to correct oxidative damage. Few studies have explicitly addressed this, however.

Thus, these various postulated mediators of neuronal damage are exacerbated by energy depletion; EAA concentrations in the synapse, free cytosolic calcium concentrations, hydrogen ion accumulation, and free radical production can all become greater and more prolonged. Furthermore, the evidence suggests that these exacerbations are sufficient to increase toxicity. Therefore, energy depletion is clearly endangering to neurons. With this point made, a compartmentalization that has run through these last two chapters can be abandoned. Up until now, I have intentionally considered each mediator separately, to establish its credibility in playing a role in neuron death and its sensitivity to energy availability. Obviously, this compartmentalization is artificial, as the various mechanisms can interact. It is now time to review these interactions.

INTERACTIONS AMONG THE VARIOUS MECHANISMS OF DAMAGE

In this section, I will review how each mediator of damage can influence the others.

EAAs and Their Consequences

The most obvious example of interactions among the different mechanisms of damage is the mobilization of free cytosolic *calcium* by EAAs, as discussed above at length. EAAs are also likely to increase *oxygen radical* levels. EAAs mobilize free fatty acids and activate the arachidonic acid cascade system in neurons (Rordorf et al. 1991). The latter has been postulated to play some role in the EAA induction of long-term potentiation (Dumuis et al. 1988); either free fatty acids or arachidonic acid can be a source of free radicals. EAA enhancement of oxygen radical levels might be critical to EAA-induced neurotoxicity. As evidence, the EAA toxicity can be reversed by a number of scavengers (Dykens et al. 1987; Baran et al. 1987; Miyamoto et al. 1988; W. Lyons et al. 1991). A recent report also demonstrates that EAAs can cause lactate accumulation and metabolic *acidosis* in brain slices, as assessed by magnetic resonance spectroscopy (Jacquin et al. 1988).

Calcium Mobilization and Its Consequences

Such mobilization is the most likely proximal mechanism by which EAAs generate *oxygen radicals*. Specifically, calcium will activate calcium-dependent phospholipase A2, leading to arachidonic acid release (Dumuis et al. 1988; Sanfeliu et al. 1990), as well as activate a calcium-dependent protease that irreversibly converts xanthine dehydrogenase to xanthine oxidase (McCord 1985). During the neurological crises likely to have generated the high calcium signal, there will also be plentiful amounts of purine substrates available (such as inosine, hypoxanthine, and xanthine) due to depletion of the adenylate energy pool. These can then serve as substrates for oxygen radical generation. As noted briefly in the previous chapter, EAAs will trigger the synthesis of nitric oxide, and the generation of this oxygen radical is calcium dependent (Garthwaite 1991). Excessive postsynaptic calcium will also *enhance EAA release* presynaptically. This is because arachidonic acid (released by calcium [Lazarewicz et al. 1990]) can diffuse across the synapse from the post- to presynaptic neuron and enhance glutamate release (which is thought to be a possible mechanism mediating LTP) (Williams et al. 1989) (this may not in fact be a route for enhanced EAA release during ischemia, given that such release is typically calcium independent, as discussed). Finally, calcium is likely to lead to *acidosis* for a number of reasons. First, calcium accumulation will present the neuron with a choice built around the Na^+/Ca^+ exchanger and the Na^+/H^+ exchanger—does it take advantage of the costly N^+ gradiant in order to export Ca^+ or H^+? The choice is apparently to solve the calcium problem at the cost of generating intracellular acidosis (Ahmed and Conner 1980), at least in invertebrate neurons. In addition, sufficiently high calcium will damage mitochondria, or at least force the mitochondria to consume all their ATP sequestering the calcium. This could shunt the cell toward anaerobic metabolism and cause acidosis. This could be the cause of the observation (immediately above) that EAAs cause acidosis in brain slices (Jacquin et al. 1988).

Acidity and Its Consequences

This is an extremely global perturbation to a cell. To the extent that almost no proteins will be operating at their pH optima, the various pumps and exchangers needed for EAA reuptake, calcium efflux and sequestration, and so on, will probably be impaired, thus exacerbating the force of *EAA* and *calcium* signals. As a more specific interaction, calcium and hydrogen ions can compete for the same intracellular binding sites (Meech 1974); furthermore, both are exported via pumps that exchange them for sodium. Therefore, potentially, acidosis could enhance free cytosolic calcium concentrations if a neuron uses the sodium gradient to export protons rather than calcium; however, (invertebrate) neurons appear to choose to export calcium when faced with that quandary (Ahmed and Conner 1980). Furthermore, acidity causes inositol polyphosphate formation (at least in fibroblasts) which, as discussed, mobilize calcium (Smith et al. 1989).

Of some potential importance, acidity may also be a route by which one of the other putative routes is diminished. This is the situation in which the NMDA receptor-gated channel function is pH dependent, such that extracellular acidity will shut down that route of calcium entry (Morad et al. 1988; Traynelis and Cull-Candy 1990). In fact, moderate acidity can attenuate hypoxic neuronal injury, suggesting a reduction in NMDA-receptor activity (Tombaugh and Sapolsky 1990a; Giffard et al. 1990a).

Oxygen Radicals and Their Consequences

Overproduction of free radicals can potentially lead to neuronal depolarization. This is thought to be due to their decreasing the activity of Na-K-ATPase. As evidence, Na-K-ATPase activity declines after ischemia (Palmer et al. 1985; Goldberg et al. 1984; MacMillan 1982), and the extent of lipid peroxidation correlates with the extent of decline in activity (Gilbert and Sawas 1983; Sun 1972). Moreover, the decline in activity does not occur until the reperfusion period, a time when radicals are first being generated (Schwartz et al. 1976). As more direct evidence, Na-K-ATPase activity is inhibited in cortical cultures when they are incubated under conditions that generate free radicals (Kovachich and Mishra 1981; Hexum and Fried 1979) and the decline in activity in vivo can be prevented by treatment with antioxidants (Palmer et al. 1985; Hexum and Fried 1979). (It should be noted that not all investigators have found evidence for a free radical cause of this decline [Goldberg et al. 1984]). If Na-K-ATPase activity is impaired to a considerable extent, depolarization will ensue, causing a considerable potassium efflux from neurons. This may be a mechanism by which oxygen radicals promote edema (Ando et al 1989).

This may explain why free radicals can promote *EAA release* from hippocampal slices (Pellegrini-Giampietro et al. 1988, 1990). This was shown by incubating slices with xanthine oxidase plus xanthine, and could be prevented by allopurinol, mannitol, or SOD plus catalase (Pellegrini-Giampietro et al. 1988, 1990). In addition, there is the suggestion that arachidonic acid will impair glial uptake of EAAs (Yu and Chan 1988; Barbour et al. 1989). (To confuse things further, the capacity of oxygen radicals to decrease NMDA conductance via modulation of a redox site has been demonstrated as well [Aizenman et al. 1990].)

Oxygen radicals might also alter calcium trafficking directly. Free radicals impair ATP-dependent sequestration of calcium into the SER in coronary arteries (Grover and Samson 1988) and can release calcium from intact mitochondria in the liver (Richter and Frei 1988). Should either occur in neurons, this would increase *free cytosolic calcium concentrations*. Finally, by damaging membranes, oxygen radicals may promote the nonspecific leakage of extracellular calcium and calcium within organelles into the cytoplasm.

Magnesium Depletion and Its Consequences

To the extent that magnesium is a cofactor in ATP phosphate transfer, cellular energetics will be compromised, with the broad consequences discussed above. Furthermore, magnesium is also a necessary cofactor for Na-K-ATPase. With a magnesium shortage, neuronal depolarization is likely to be favored, exacerbating the other mechanisms in ways already discussed. The calcium-ATPase also uses magnesium as a cofactor, and a shortage will compromise calcium sequestration and efflux. Finally, the normal functioning of the NMDA receptor is contingent on the voltage-dependent blockade of its channel by extracellular magnesium, and a major depletion of magnesium favors enhanced sodium and calcium influx and toxicity.

Collectively, these connections form an exasperating mess. EAA overexposure leads to calcium overload, which leads to free radical generation, which can lead to EAA overexposure. Calcium overload can cause EAA release, which mobilizes more calcium. Calcium overload can lead to acidosis, which will impair the functioning of proteins needed for calcium sequestration. Magnesium depletion will exacerbate EAA signals at the NMDA receptor and compromise the energetics needed to contain all the other mechanisms. One is left with the impression that essentially every potential mediator of neuron death will exacerbate every other mediator. If everything makes everything else worse, and it all degenerates into chaos, does it really make any sense to ask how a neuron dies? One might perhaps consider it analogous to tossing a television off a tall building. After surveying the shards and fragments on the sidewalk afterward, is it interesting and useful to try to figure out just why the television no longer works, or what was the sequence of degenerative events that occurred upon encountering the insult of the concrete sidewalk? There may have been a discernable sequence of damage in the first milliseconds after hitting the ground, but the mechanisms of damage rapidly converged into a very generalized and not very interesting form of irreversible trauma for the television. After a certain point in the degenerative process, when all the potential mechanisms of damage are activated and synergizing, do hypoxia-ischemia, hypoglycemia, and seizure all converge into the same general insult? Do all the putative mediators of damage always wind up occurring as a package deal?

This cannot be the case. First, on a *qualitative* level, the pathophysiology of all the insults is not the same. In hypoxia-ischemia and seizure, there is a loss of oxygen and glucose. This causes both cytosolic and mitochondrial redox systems to be in a reduced state. In hypoglycemia, however, there is loss of glucose but not oxygen. Therefore, the redox system is very markedly in the oxidized state, as the cell struggles to carry on oxidative metabolism with substrates to replace glucose (Siesjo and Agardh 1983). Given that current flow through the NMDA receptor complex is altered by redox state (Aizenman et al. 1989), the same degree of EAA exposure should have different consequences in hypoxia-ischemia and seizure, versus hypoglycemia.

As a second qualitative difference among these insults, both hypoxia-ischemia and seizure produce an acidosis in neurons, while hypoglycemia produces an alkalosis (Pellegrino et al. 1981). This is because in hypoglycemia, the cell tries to oxidize anything it can lay its proverbial hands on, predominately the anions of numerous metabolic acids.

The pathophysiological consequences of the insults also differ *quantitatively*. For example, they do not produce equivalent extents of energy depletion. In general, hypoxia-ischemia is the most profoundly disruptive, depleting neurons of essentially all ATP and phosphocreatine. Next most disruptive is hypoglycemia, and then status epilepticus. Similarly, the minimum duration of insult needed to trigger brain damage is shortest for hypoxia-ischemia (2 to 10 minutes), followed by hypoglycemia (10 to 20 minutes), and then status epilepticus (excess of an hour) (emphasized by Auer and Siesjo 1988).

Most importantly, the *neuropathological pattern* of damage differs among these insults. This is most obvious when considering which neurons are vulnerable. Within the hippocamus, hypoxia-ischemia preferentially damages CA_1 neurons, status epilepticus CA_3 and (with more severe seizures) CA_1 neurons, and hypoglycemia neurons of the dentate gyrus. In the same way, the patterns of damage within the cortex differ by insult, as with other brain regions (thalamus, caudoputamen). Moreover, the neuropathological responses differ on a cellular level, depending on the insult. Many decades ago, *ischemic cell change* was used to describe the degenerative response to all three

The Role of Energy Failure in Necrotic Neuronal Injury

insults. More recent work has shown that this grouping is not justified. Hypoxia-ischemia and seizure are similar, in that both cause massive accumulation of calcium in mitochondria, mitochondrial swelling and eventual micro-vacuolization. Hypoglycemia, in contrast, while causing calcium influx into neurons, does not seem to have these cellular sequelae. Instead, its typical features are dark cell changes, swollen Golgi bodies, and dilated smooth endoplasmic reticulum (Simon et al. 1986).

Thus, one must back away from the simplistic notion that all three insults ultimately converge into the same cellular event. But hypoxia-ischemia and seizure seem to go hand in hand in terms of their redox state, cellular neuropathology, and to a certain extent, the anatomical pattern of vulnerability within the hippocampus. Is it at least the case that these two insults are highly interrelated? This is not a new idea. The vulnerability of CA1 to hypoxic-ischemic damage and to seizure damage suggested to some that when seizure is severe enough to involve CA_1 neurons, the insult is essentially hypoxic-ischemic in nature (cf. Ben-Ari 1985; Lassmann et al. 1984; Sperk et al. 1983). This idea has gone through some transformations over the years. The earliest formulations were that seizure-induced convulsions produced apnea and thus hypoxia. This possibility was ruled out by the demonstration that similar damage could be induced in ventilated animals (who were, thus, not apneic) undergoing seizure (Meldrum 1983; Nevander et al. 1985). Another early idea was that seizure induced hypoxia via cerebral vasoconstriction; this was undermined by the demonstration that seizure, in fact, produced vasodilation. A more recent version of this idea is that seizure induces a local hypoxia-ischemia in the brain through edema-induced compression of local vessels (Lassmann et al. 1984). As an even more subtle idea, the hypoxia induced by seizure could be intracellular—with sufficient seizure intensity and influx of calcium, mitochondria become inoperable. This could be because the mitochondria are damaged in the process of sequestering so much calcium (from swelling due to osmotic pressure), or they may be able to sequester the calcium without damaging themselves but may wind up producing no energy for the rest of the cell, consuming all their own ATP in their introverted task of sequestering the calcium. In either scenario, while there would not be a true hypoxia-ischemia occurring (i.e., glucose and oxygen would still be available to the cell), the oxygen would be superfluous with the mitochondria out of business, and all cellular metabolism would have to be anaerobic, producing damaging lactate, much as with hypoxia-ischemia (Ingvar et al. 1987).

In any of these scenarios, if seizure damages CA_1 neurons via a hypoxic-ischemic route, a prediction is generated: Seizure damage to CA_1 should be worsened by glucose preloading, much as is hypoxic-ischemic damage. This is not the case.

We have shown this by manipulating glucose concentrations over a broad range (70 to 350 mg/dl) in rats prior to kainic acid–induced status epilepticus. Under these conditions, glucose preloading *reduced* damage in CA1 (and CA_3; Sapolsky and Stein 1988; see figure 10.1). Other studies have shown this as well. For example, loss of CA1 pyramidal neurons, as well as of two of three

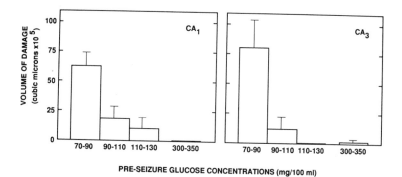

Figure 10.1. Relationship between circulating glucose concentrations at the time of kainic acid–induced seizures and resultant volume of CA_3 (*top*) or CA_1 (*bottom*) damage. (From Sapolsky and Stein, 1988, Neurosci Lett 97, 157. Reproduced by permission of Elsevier Scientific Publishers Ireland Ltd.)

types of CA_1 interneurons is worsened by hypoglycemia prior to kainic acid administration (Johansen and Diemer 1986; oddly, in the discussion in that study, the emphasis was put on the one type of interneuron in which the opposite occurred, and the conclusion was reached that hypoglycemia protected the hippocampus from kainic acid, ostensibly supporting a hypoxic-ischemic route of damage). As further evidence, hypoglycemia enhances hippocampal damage following bicuculline-induced seizures (Meldrum 1983). Furthermore, while hyperglycemia prior to status epilepticus does indeed elevate hippocampal lactate content, in agreement with the "hypoxic-ischemic" view of seizure damage, the concentrations of lactate achieved are below that needed to produce acidotic damage (Swan et al. 1988). Collectively, these observations argue against a hypoxic-ischemic route of injury to CA_1 neurons during status epilepticus. Even if hypoxia-ischemia and seizure share many features, they ultimately appear to represent different routes of damage to neurons.

Even within the context of any single neurological insult, there seem to be multiple routes by which damage occurs, and hierarchies of induction of the different mechanisms. For example, we have found, in vivo, that at low concentrations, the antimetabolite 3-acetylpyridine damages the hippocampus in an NMDA-independent manner, whereas at higher concentrations, an NMDA-sensitive component is recruited as well (Armanini et al. 1990). Furthermore, as noted, one component of hypoxic damage to hippocampal cultures is NMDA and energy dependent, while another type of damage (acidotic), at a lower pH, is not (Tombaugh and Sapolsky 1990b). Similarly, Monyer and colleagues (1990) found that in primary neuronal cultures, a moderate hypoglycemic insult is NMDA mediated, whereas more severe hypoglycemic insults recruits non-NMDA mechanisms as well.

Two conclusions emerge from the study of the interaction of the various mediators of damage. First, even the most credible of mechanisms may be necessary but rarely sufficient to explain toxicity. When thinking about the causes of neuron death, there seems diminishing support for a lone gunman

The Role of Energy Failure in Necrotic Neuronal Injury

hypothesis. Instead, conspiracies among multiple mediators seem more the rule. The second conclusion is that even though there are vast interactions among the conspiring mediators, all insults that activate these mediators do not converge into a single route of degeneration.

INDIVIDUAL DIFFERENCES IN VULNERABILITY: THE ROLE OF NEURONAL PERSONALITY

How then to make any sense of the three persisting mysteries raised in the last two chapters? As was just shown, essentially every putative mediator of damage can give rise to or enhance one of the other mediators; despite this, why does there appear to be selective activation of only some of the cellular mechanisms of damage in different neurological insults? Why is there selective neuronal vulnerability—given the same insult, why do only some neurons die? Moreover, why does it occur in a delayed manner? A beautiful example of this was shown recently (Mattson et al. 1989). Cultured hippocampal neurons differed dramatically from one another in their vulnerability to EAA toxicity and in the extent of calcium mobilization triggered by the EAAs. As an interesting addition, two neurons were shown to have identical vulnerabilities if they descended from a common progenitor cell in the culture—what the authors referred to as "sister neurons." As an important control, "non-sister" cells that just happened to be in contact did not have the similar sharing of traits. Therefore, intrinsic differences arising from mitotic history have something to do with the selective vulnerability.

At this stage, there is little means of answering why only some mechanisms of damage are triggered in a particular insult, or why only some neurons die. Yet on one level, the answers are simple—the individual differences have to be a function of, for want of a better term, the individual "personalities" of the neurons.

What do I mean by this unlikely term? First, there must be differences in the sort of tasks and levels of activity that different neurons maintain. These can be long-term differences or can reflect what different neurons were busy with at the time the neurological disaster struck. To return to the anthropomorphisms of the beginning of this chapter, when discussing the nature of energy problems, passing out in your armchair carries a different risk than passing out while walking a girder high up on a construction site. Similarly, surviving a life-threatening physical challenge is easier when you are well fed than when you haven't eaten for days. Some of the differences in selective vulnerability must reflect a neurological equivalent of luck—some neurons just happen to have the day off and be sitting in armchairs when the disaster strikes, some neurons just happen to have finished their metaphorical breakfast. This sort of factor accounts for short-term individual differences. The consistency of the differences—CA_1 neurons are the most vulnerable to hypoxia-ischemia in most everyone's brains, for example—must reflect habit that transcends short-term luck; in effect, some neurons must pass their days working high up on girders, while others have desk jobs.

The armchair metaphor might be translated most readily into both extrinsic and intrinsic variables. A neuron that receives numerous inhibitory GABAergic projections would probably constitute a cell that is habitually sitting in an armchair. Thus, for the same unit of exposure to an excitatory EAA signal, such a neuron would undergo less excitation than a neuron lacking such inhibitory inputs (and this idea has been made explicit by Globus and colleagues [1991] in discussing the ratio of glutamatergic-GABAergic inputs to a neuron as contributing to the "excitotoxic index.") The intrinsic variables most relevant to the armchair metaphor probably revolve around differences in energy stores at the time of the insult. This is a first pass, however. It is clear that an increased availability of glucose prior to hypoxia-ischemia is not necessarily a good thing. Even excluding that insult, mere energy availability is not all there is to it. As discussed at the beginning of the chapter, two neurons can be equally depleted of ATP or phosphocreatine during the course of an insult, yet only one dies. There must be additional factors.

If neurons differ as to how hard they work in general and how hard they were working and how hungry they were at the time of the insult, they must also differ in their basic constitutions. By this personification, I mean that neurons must differ in their numbers and workings of molecules relevant to dealing with the crises. One can generate an enormous list of sources of potential variability—neurons differing from one another in their numbers of NMDA receptors, in their second messenger coupling systems, in their amounts of cytosolic calcium binding proteins, in their numbers and efficiency of proton pumps, in their levels of antioxidants, and so on.

Some first hints at this variability are emerging from the literature. For example, cortical neurons appear to differ dramatically in their vulnerability to EAAs. One subset of neurons is relatively resistant to NMDA, aspartate, and quinolinate but quite sensitive to AMPA and kainic acid. These cells contain particularly high concentrations of the enzyme reduced nicotinamide adenine dinucleotide phosphate diaphorase (NADPH-d) (Koh et al. 1986; Beal et al. 1986; Koh and Choi 1988). As support for the NMDA receptor playing a role in the selective brain damage in Huntington's disease, such patients have selective sparing of NADPH-d–positive neurons (Ferrante et al. 1985). It is not clear if the NADPH-d itself is instrumental in the protection or if it is merely a correlative marker. Some recent evidence links the NADPH-d to nitric oxide synthetase, the enzyme that generates nitric oxide, a gas recently recognized to have neurotransmitter function (Snyder and Bredt 1991; this subject will be reviewed in chapter 11). Koh and Choi (1988) speculate that the pattern of vulnerability derives from relatively fewer NMDA receptors and more quisqualate/kainic acid receptors in NADPH-d–positive neurons. Therefore, the selective vulnerability might derive from a very basic difference—whether or not the cell is particularly sensitive to NMDA receptor ligands.

Selective vulnerability could also arise from differences distal to this step. For example, levels of all of the cytosolic calcium-binding proteins disovered to date differ considerably from one hippocampal cell field to another (McBurney and Neering 1987). This may have important implications. A great deal of attention has focused on calbindin D-28K as being a critical player determining individual differences in neuronal vulnerability. For example, the adult pattern of CA_1 vulnerability to hypoxia-ischemia is not seen in the perinatal brain. There, instead, the dentate gyrus neurons are most vulnerable. At both ages, the vulnerable hippocampal region has particularly low levels of calbindin D-28K, and it is speculated that this may play a role in the vulnerability (Wasterlain et al. 1988). Supporting this idea, cultured hippocampal neurons destined to die when exposed to glutamate, excessive stimulation, or high calcium concentrations are those with low calbindin D-28K and parvalbumin concentrations (Baimbridge and Kao 1988; Scharfman and Schwartzkroin 1989; Mattson et al. 1991b), while dopaminergic substantia nigra neurons spared in Parkinson's disease are those containing calbindin D-28K (Yamada et al. 1990). (One recent study should be noted in which high calbindin concentrations were not associated with resistance to ischemic injury in all neuronal populations in the brain [Freund et al. 1990b]).

Sometimes the features of individual vulnerability are less readily associated with a molecular marker but nevertheless still make a great deal of sense, physiologically. For example, in hippocampal slices, when glucose concentrations are decreased to 0.5 mM, field potentials in the dentate gyrus begin to be lost. As a predictor of this vulnerability, neurons that were the least excitable in the normoglycemic media were most resistant to the disruptive effects of the low glucose media (Cos and Bachelard 1988). Although one should be careful not to overgeneralize from a single study, these may be the neurons that habitually are sitting in armchairs. Some of the markers are less clear in their meaning at this point. For example, following hypoxia-ischemia, hippocampal neurons destined to die (i.e., CA_1 neurons) induce less hsp70 and c-fos than those that will survive (CA_3 neurons) (Vass et al. 1988; Uemura et al. 1991).

These putative mechanisms mediating individual differences are all intracellular—neurons simply differ from each other. This must account for some of the variations in the hippocampus, as neurons from separate hippocampal regions still retain dramatic differences in vulnerability to insults even when in cell cultures (Mattson and Kater 1989). But some of the individuality might come from a level greater than that of the single cell. For example, hippocampal cell fields differ in their extracellular volume fraction, and this has been suggested to explain variability in the postischemic neuronal hyperexcitability—different fractions would concentrate potassium to differing extents during periods of repeated action potentials (McBain et al. 1990). In effect, individual vulnerability might arise from differences in the sort of ionic "neighborhood" in which a neuron resides.

This all seems very logical—individual differences in vulnerability to damage must be derived from individual differences in the molecules, energy substrates, and physiological processes relevant to coping with insults. There is the temptation at this stage to attribute great significance to these sorts of individual differences as they are detected; for example, one could imagine a global theory about levels of calbindin D-28K as the predictor of neuronal vulnerability. This has not been done, as such conclusions are obviously premature. Most likely, one must keep track of the levels of all the different calcium binding proteins, antioxidants, regulators of the NMDA receptor, and so on, including the many that, no doubt, have not yet been discovered. This leads to the not very surprising conclusion that there are multiple levels of potential defenses in neurons, and individual differences in vulnerability must reflect all these levels. I do not think the field is anywhere near the point of being able to make any conclusions regarding the critical points of vulnerability. This is still the stage of collecting large numbers of individual facts, and a vast amount of work still needs to be done.

CHAPTER SUMMARY

Chapter 9 reviewed the features of neuron death during hypoxia-ischemia, seizure, and hypoglycemia, and examined the considerable evidence that these instances of neurotoxicity are mediated by excessive EAAs, cytosolic calcium, acidosis, and oxygen radicals. The present chapter shows how these insults, and their mediators, are influenced by neuronal energetics.

Initially, it is important to consider a few ideas regarding energy crises in the brain and their likely consequences. (1) The severity of energy depletion need not correlate with the extent of damage produced. Two neurons may be equally deprived of energy after an insult, yet only one dies. However, this does not prove that energetics are irrelevent to that instance of neuron death. Instead, while half the story depends on the *severity* of the energy crisis, the other half depends on the *consequences* of that crisis; some neurons handle crises better than others. (2) An energy problem may not limit the rate of activity of a neuron, but rather may limit the ability of the neuron to contain the consequences of the activity. This is particularly the case for seizure, where there is little evidence of a major energy crisis *during* the insult. Instead, the energetic constraint may be felt in the *aftermath*, when the neuron is trying to cope with the ionic and neurotransmitter consequences of the seizure. (3) A cellular energy crisis can occur even when circulating substrate concentrations are high. This is seemingly paradoxical, except in the case where circulating concentrations are high *because* the many target tissues cannot extract them from the circulation. This is extremely relevant to glucocorticoid effects on neuronal energetics. (4) Metabolic rate need not tell anything about energy state. Neurons may have low metabolic rates because they are *deprived* of energy, or because their *demands* are low. Only the former represents a pathologic state.

With this orientation, the neurological insults can be examined. Hypoxia-ischemia, seizure, and hypoglycemia all are energetic insults, in that all cause declines in ATP and phosphocreatine (although to differing extents). Even more importantly, the toxicity of each insult can be lessened by energy supplementation.

This suggests that the putative mediators of damage during these insults can have their actions exacerbated by energy failure. This is the case. (1) The release of EAAs by neurons and glia increases during energy failure, while uptake by neurons and glia declines. The result is a larger and more prolonged EAA signal in the synapse. (2) Similarly, energy failure produces a larger and longer cytosolic calcium signal. This is because more calcium will enter the neuron and be mobilized from intracellular stores, and less will be sequestered or exported. (3) Acidosis should be exacerbated during energy failure, mainly because the pumps that remove protons from the neurons are all either directly ATP dependent or dependent on costly ionic gradients. (4) Oxygen radical damage is enhanced with energy failure. More radicals are generated, mainly due to more substrate availability. Moreover, less scavengers are likely to be available to prevent cell damage, and less energy will be available for repairing the damage.

The various mediators of damage (EAAs, calcium, acidosis, etc.) can interact, each typically being able to exacerbate the other. Thus, there is rarely a "lone gunman" causing neuron death. Instead, the mediators converge in a web of dysregulation. However, the identical web is not triggered for all insults, and certain mediators in the web predominate for different neurological disorders.

This knowledge about the mediators of neuron death and their interactions allows one to return to the mystery posed at the beginning of chapter 9—What is the basis for selective neuronal vulnerability? Personifying, I suggest that individual neurons must differ in many features of "personality"—their "work habits" (determining, for example, their energetic profile at the time of a metabolic disaster), their "constitution" (levels of EAA receptors, calcium binding proteins, antioxidants, and so on), and the sort of "neighborhood" in which they reside (for example, differences in extracellular volume fraction determining the degree of dilution of potassium released during hyperexcitation). While these ideas begin to hint at the bases of individual differences in neuronal vulnerability, knowledge is still far too scanty to attempt an explanatory synthesis.

11   How Do Glucocorticoids Endanger the Hippocampal Neuron?

SUMMARY OF THE BOOK SO FAR

A variety of stressors trigger the endocrine and neural adaptations that constitute the stress-response. The adrenal secretion of glucocorticoids dominates this stress-response, and typifies its two-edged quality: While glucocorticoids are vital for surviving short-term physical stressors, an excess of glucocorticoids causes a variety of stress-related disorders.

Part I examined how the regulation of glucocorticoid secretion is impaired during aging and how excessive exposure to glucocorticoids over the lifetime can accelerate aspects of brain aging. The data reviewed are combined to form a model, termed the *glucocorticoid cascade*. It attempts to explain two features of aging rats—hypersecretion of glucocorticoids (including impaired negative feedback inhibition of glucocorticoid secretion) and degeneration of neurons in the hippocampal region of the brain. The hippocampus is shown to contribute to glucocorticoid feedback inhibition, such that its senescent degeneration causes glucocorticoid hypersecretion. Glucocorticoids, in turn, were shown in chapter 6 to be capable of damaging hippocampal neurons. These two regulatory features combine to form a feedforward cascade of senescent degeneration—glucocorticoids damage the hippocampus, which causes further glucocorticoid secretion (as well as numerous deleterious consequences for the aged rat, including further hippocampal damage). Chapter 6 explored some of the features and limitations of this model.

Part II explores the mechanisms by which glucocorticoids are neurotoxic in the hippocampus. Chapter 7 demonstrated that these hormones need not actually be toxic. Instead, they endanger hippocampal neurons, impairing their capacity to survive coincident neurological insults, such as hypoxia-ischemia, seizure, hypoglycemia, antimetabolites, and oxygen radical generators. Therefore, glucocorticoids may not only play an important role in accelerating hippocampal aging, but might also exacerbate some of the most common neurological insults to the hippocampus.

This leads one to examine the mechanisms of neuron death, in order to understand which features are worsened by glucocorticoids. Chapter 8 reviewed the mechanisms of apoptotic (programmed) cell death and concluded that glucocorticoids probably do not endanger hippocampal neurons through apoptotic means. Chapters 9 and 10 examined necrotic neuron death. The features of the most common of neurological insults to the hippocampus (which are all exacerbated by glucocorticoids)—hypoxia-ischemia, seizure, and hypoglycemia—were reviewed. The likely mediators of damage in these insults, including excitatory amino acids, excessive calcium, oxygen radicals, and acidosis are also considered. Finally, Chapter 10 emphasized that these insults are all metabolic ones, causing energy crises that are central to the toxicity of these insults. This lays the groundwork for the present chapter, which reviews how glucocorticoids disrupt hippocampal neuronal energetics and, thus, exacerbate the ionic and neurotransmitter perturbations that occur during these insults.

It is now time to attempt a synthesis as to how glucocortiocids endanger neurons. This is the most speculative chapter in the book, based on the most recent data, and thus it should be read keeping in mind how quickly a scientific story can change. Despite this caveat, very recent data are emerging that suggest how glucocorticoids might endanger the hippocampus. The punchline of this chapter is that glucocorticoids appear to exacerbate the EAA/NMDA/ calcium cascade, and this is due, at least in part, to a problem of energy. This chapter will examine some effects of glucocorticoids on cell biology that are relevant to the endangerment of neurons, as well as some which appear to be of less relevance than one might initially expect. Out of this, I will attempt a synthesis as to the most likely route by which glucocorticoids exert their endangering actions in the hippocampus.

GLUCOCORTICOIDS ACTIONS NOT LIKELY TO CAUSE NEURONAL ENDANGERMENT

Glucocorticoids and Regulation of Glutamine Synthetase

A puzzling, circuitous aspect of EAA trafficking involves glia. As discussed at length in chapter 9, following its interaction with receptors, glutamate can be taken up into the neuron from which they were released (i.e., reuptake) or taken up into neighboring astrocytic glia through a high-affinity uptake system. Such astrocytes use glutamate for energy and may even metabolize glutamate preferentially over glucose (Hertz et al. 1988; Swanson et al. 1990). Astrocytes also convert the glutamate into glutamine, which is used in various aspects of glial metabolism. But in addition, glutamine is transferred back to neurons for reconversion to glutamate (Hertz et al. 1983b).

This last step seems a particularly roundabout way of recycling a neurotransmitter. This "glutamate/glutamine" shuttle might make sense from the standpoint of providing an additional means of removing glutamate from the synapse before it becomes excitotoxic. The high-affinity nature of glutamate uptake by glia supports this view. Once the glutamate is in the glia, it must be returned to the presynaptic neuron, and repatriation in the form of glutamine probably represents a safety precaution—shuttling the glutamate around in the extracellular space in an unexcitatory, inactive form (Norenberg and Martinez-Hernandez 1979; Hertz et al. 1983a). The process is probably best viewed as a protective shuttle to remove the glutamate from the synapse quickly and return it back to neurons as safely as possible. This shuttle is but one of a number of ways in which astrocytes can aid neurons, especially during metabolic insults. Other possible routes include uptake of potassium and of protons or detoxification of ammonia, and support the growing emphasis on the critical role of these cells in local glia/neuron communities (Kimelberg and Norenberg 1989).

The rate-limiting step in this shuttle is the astrocytic conversion of glutamate to glutamine by glutamine synthetase. The V_{max} for EAA uptake into astrocytes is even higher than in neurons (Schousboe et al. 1983), and as much as 80% of the glutamate used as a neurotransmitter in the brain is thought to shuttle through this astrocytic cycle, rather than being returned to the presynaptic neuron via direct reuptake (Hertz et al. 1983a). In support of this, during hypoxia-ischemia, there is a net transfer of glutamate from neurons to astrocytes in the hippocampus (Torp et al. 1991).

Therefore, anything that changes the workings of this shuttle could dramatically influence the availability of the glutamate as a neurotransmitter and as a neurotoxin. In hypoglycemia, for example, large amounts of glutamate are released into the synapse (in the hippocampal slice). This outpouring eventually is exhausted as the presynaptic neuron is depleted of glutamate. However, if glutamine is made available to the slice during this time, glutamate outflow is enhanced, as is toxicity (Szerb 1988). Further evidence for the importance of this shuttle system is that selective poisoning of glutamine synthetase (with sulfoximine methionate) decreases the toxicity of insults that involve endogenous glutamate release (Rothstein and Tabakoff 1985).

Critically, glucocorticoids induce glutamine synthetase. This is well documented in muscle and in the developing brain (Max et al. 1988; Patel et al. 1983). This immediately suggests that glucocorticoids, by inducing this enzyme, might increase the amount of glutamate delivered to neurons for use as EAA neurotransmitters. Therefore, the steroids might enhance the strength of a glutamatergic signal (and thus exacerbate EAA-related neurological insults). What was not clear was whether glucocorticoids regulate the enzyme in the adult hippocampus, and whether the regulation occurs physiologically. We pursued this possibility and, disappointingly, did not find support for this idea. Neither physiological elevations of glucocorticoids nor the stressor kainic acid infusions induce glutamine synthetase activity in the adult hippocampus under conditions where we observe a robust induction of muscle glutamine synthetase; moreover, adrenalectomy, which decreases muscle enzyme activity, does not influence hippocampal activity, showing that basal glucocorticoid levels in the adult do not regulate hippocampal activity of the enzyme (Tombaugh and Sapolsky 1990c). As one other possible route by which glucocorticoids might be endangering by priming neurons with glutamate, a specific glutamine efflux pump appears to occur in rat skeletal muscle whose activity is stimulated by glucocorticoids (Babij et al. 1986). Should the same occur in hippocampal astrocytes, glucocorticoids might enhance glutamine efflux into the extracellular space. No evidence exists for this, however. Therefore, at present, there is little reason to believe that the glucocorticoids are endangering by augmenting some feature(s) of the glutamate/glutamine shuttle.

(It should be mentioned that some investigators are becoming less impressed with the importance of this glutamate/glutamine shuttle as a source of neurotransmitter glutamate [Cohen et al. 1988; McMahon and Nicholls 1990]. For example, many studies have shown that in tissue slices, glutamine is preferentially shunted toward forming glutamate destined for neurotransmitter use and that glutamine preloading leads to vast spontaneous release of glutamate. However, McMahon and Nicholls [1990] examined this in synaptosomes and showed that most of the "spontaneous release" of neurotransmitter glutamate was actually glutamate released by mitochondria that have ruptured into the extracellular space as an artifact of synaptosome formation. They also note that few investigators [including themselves] have shown that glutamine preloading leads to enhancement of *calcium-dependent* glutamate release. Such calcium dependency is a hallmark of traditional neurotransmitter release. Therefore, that argues further that the supposed priming of neurotransmitter glutamate release by glutamine preloading is mostly an artifact.)

Glucocorticoids and Edema

Brain swelling (edema) is a frequent consequence of neurological insult, particularly tumor, stroke and trauma. In a broad and simplified way, one type of edema is *vasogenic* (also known as *vascular*) in nature, with an inappropriate amount of water and large molecules (including proteins) leaving the vascular space and moving into the extracellular compartment in the brain. This is due to the integrity of the blood-brain barrier being compromised. Originally, such edema was thought to be due entirely to a defect in tight endothelial cell junctions, but there is also aberrant and enhanced vesicular transport across endothelial cells. Vasogenic edema is triggered by prostaglandins, leukotrienes, and free fatty acids, which cause vasodilation and plasma exudation (Chan and Fishman 1978; Iannotti et al. 1981; Chan et al. 1983). As discussed in the previous chapters, these compounds can be produced during neurological insults (Gaudet and Levine 1979; Shohami et al. 1982, 1987; Moskowitz et al. 1984). This is most probably due to oxygen radical attacks on cell membranes, triggering arachidonic acid release from membrane phospholipids (arachidonic acid, as a reminder, being the precursor of the prostaglandins and leukotrienes) (Schmidley 1990).

Alternatively, edema can be *cellular* (also known as *cytotoxic*), in which an inappropriate amount of extracellular water enters the brain cells, resulting in swelling. Cytotoxic edema is mostly driven by ionic dysregulation—in effect, various ions wind up in the wrong place, and water follows. Most commonly, such edema occurs in the glia (although it also occurs in neurons); massive amounts of potassium, released by repeated depolarizations in neurons, are removed from the synapse by the glia, and the potassium uptake pulls in water as well. As another route, during neurological insults, the failing sodium gradient in neurons will produce an aberrant influx of sodium, which will pull water in with it. As a third route, during neuronal intracellular acidification (e.g., following hypoxia-ischemia), protons are most readily pumped out via a sodium exchanger (Gaillard and Dupont 1990; Raley-Susman et al. 1991), and theoretically, the massive sodium influx can cause swelling. In glia, acidification causes swelling (Jakubovicz and Klip 1989), although it is not yet known whether a sodium/proton exchanger is involved in this. (As discussed in chapter 9, microvacuolization bears some similarities to cytotoxic edema. Recall that the former occurs in mitochondria during hypoxia-ischemia and seizure, perhaps as a result of the organelle taking up calcium to buffer the huge mobilization of free cytosolic calcium. Under some conditions, water will follow, causing mitochondrial swelling [or even bursting] and dysfunction.) Under some conditions, both vascular and cytotoxic edema can occur simultaneously.

Clearly, neither is a particularly pleasing state to be in for the brain. In cytotoxic edema, cellular functioning is likely to be compromised by the swelling, causing cytoskeletal damage, disruption of subcellular compartmentalization, and so on. At the extreme, the cell may even burst. Despite this, the pathologic consequences of such edema have not received much attention. The swelling occurs acutely after injury and is transient. Moreover, there is not a good correlation between sites of marked cytotoxic edema and eventual selective neuronal loss. Finally, while the edema can theoretically lead to cells bursting, that seems rather rare; the best-documented case is in the chloride-mediated acute cell bursting following insults in vitro. As discussed in chapter 9, it seems plausible that this bursting is an artifact of neurons in tissue culture monolayers, where there is not the three-dimensional constraint on soma swelling that occurs in vivo.

The pathologic consequences of the vascular edema have received far more attention, principally because of the potential for compression injury, where the fluid occludes capillaries or presses on cells. Recall that in earlier periods, this was speculated to be a mechanism for seizure-induced neuron damage—the postseizure edema caused compression and local hypoxia-ischemia (which, as reviewed in chapter 9, was a basis for emphasizing the similarities between seizure and global ischemia).

Where glucocorticoids fit in is with their long-recognized capacity to block or reverse vascular edema (as part of their general anti-inflammatory effects). These qualities were inferred even prior to the isolation of corticosteroids, in that as early as 1945, ACTH and adrenal extracts were reported to decrease experimental edema in the cat brain (Prados et al. 1945). Over the subsequent decades, glucocorticoids were shown to decrease potently the edema arising from brain tumors (Ingraham et al. 1952; Galicich et al. 1961; Galicich and French 1961), and the use of glucocorticoids in this situation has become standard clinical practice. The glucocorticoid effect arises because the steroids inhibit prostaglandin synthesis (Flower 1974; Hirata 1981), including in the brain (Weidenfeld et al. 1987). The molecular biology of this effect is well understood. Glucocorticoids induce the synthesis of lipocortin (also known as lipomodulin or macrocortin). Lipocortin, in turn, is a potent inhibitor of phospholipase A2, which is the rate-limiting enzyme for prostaglandin synthesis. In addition, glucocorticoids also block the activity of cyclo-oxygenase, which is necessary for a later step in the synthesis of prostaglandins (reviewed in Blackwell et al. 1980; Hirata et al. 1980; Flower 1986; Wallner et al. 1986).

These findings predicted that glucocorticoids should also reduce the edema arising from hypoxia-ischemia, hemorrhage and infection, and should thus *help*, rather than *endanger* the hippocampus in such circumstances. This has turned out not to be the case for the simple reason that the edema arising in these circumstances is predominately cytotoxic, rather than vasogenic (Fishman 1982). Vascular edema is more a phenomenon of white matter than of gray matter, and the antiedemic effects of glucocorticoids are via the steroids working on endothelium, rather than on neurons or glia. In contrast, glucocorticoids do not particularly inhibit cytotoxic edema (Sztriha et al. 1986).

This lack of effectiveness has been shown in a large number of studies examining the antiedemic quality of glucocorticoids following various insults that induce cytotoxic edema. Typically, efficacy is measured by the extent of edema, of intracranial pressure, blood-brain barrier permeability, or neurological outcome. There is conflict whether the steroids show protective effects against seizure-induced edema, against edema following global ischemia and stroke, and whether glucocorticoids reduce blood-brain barrier permeability in rats without a coincident neurological insult (table 11.1). Moreover, there are also reports that glucocorticoids do not induce lipocortin in the brain (Strijbos

Table 11.1. Conflicting findings as to whether glucocorticoids inhibit cytotoxic edema

	Yes	No
Do glucocorticoids protect against seizure-induced edema?	Eisenberg et al. 1970; Sztriha et at. 1986 (in the thalamus)	Sztriha et al. 1986 (in the hippocampus)
Do glucocorticoids decrease edema following global ischemia or stroke?	Fenske et al. 1979; Harrison et al. 1973; Jarrott and Domer 1980; Bremer et al. 1980; Taylor et al. 1984; Temesvari et al. 1984; Barbrosa-Coutinho et al. 1985	Jane et al. 1984; Giannotta et al. 1984; Gudeman et al. 1979; Deardeu et al. 1986; Plum et al. 1963; Lee et al. 1974; DeLaTorre and Surgeon 1976; Goldstein et al. 1989; Grafton and Longstretch 1988; Jastremski et al. 1989; Norris and Hacinski 1986; Altman et al. 1984; Anderson and Cranford 1979; Donley and Sundt 1973
Do glucocorticoids reduce blood-brain barrier permeability in rats who are not undergoing a coincident neurological insult?	Hedley-Whyte and Hsu 1986; Reid et al. 1983a, b; Ziylan et al. 1989	Chan et al. 1983

et al. 1991—although it should be noted that in this latter study, glucocorticoids were administered only 2 hours before) and do not inhibit prostaglandin synthesis in the brain after all (Shapira et al. 1988; Jane et al. 1984; Giannotta et al. 1984).

In viewing these results, Fishman (1982), in an influential review, concluded that with respect to these forms of edema, "Steroid therapy has been found wanting, even deleterious," while a World Health Organization task force on the subject (Goldstein et al. 1989) concluded that "Steroids are of no value. There is good experimental and clinical evidence that steroids could be more harmful than helpful."

In conclusion, glucocorticoids do not appear to decrease the edema that can arise after the neurological insults discussed in this book. There is even the possibility that they exacerbate cytotoxic edema. As discussed later in this chapter, glucocorticoids increase calcium-dependent potassium efflux in the hippocampus. Importantly, this is a major source of the potassium that drives the cellular edema (Tominaga et al. 1988). Therefore, this arena of glucocorticoid actions does not contradict the general observation that glucocorticoids endanger hippocampal neurons and exacerbate the toxicity of these insults in the hippocampus.

Glucocorticoids and Oxygen Radicals

There are a number of routes by which glucocorticoids might modulate either oxygen radical generation or the severity of oxidative damage—some of these effects predict that the steroids should worsen oxidative damage, while others predict protective actions. As will be discussed later in this chapter, glucocorticoids enhance the mobilization of calcium following EAA exposure. Because of the role of calcium in oxygen radical formation (see chapter 10), glucocorticoids are thus likely to enhance the generation of such radicals. As will also be discussed, glucocorticoids disrupt neuronal energetics in the hippocampus, and this should worsen oxidative damage by impairing the ability of the neuron to repair such damage. Thus, these two steps predict that glucocorticoids should worsen oxygen radical toxicity in the hippocampus.

The inhibition of prostaglandin synthesis by glucocorticoids generates the opposing prediction. Since such synthesis is a potent source of oxygen radicals, the glucocorticoids should protect against oxidative toxicity in hippocampal neurons. This was the stated rationale for the use of dexamethasone in one experimental model of hypoxia-ischemia where instead, "unexpectedly," the glucocorticoids were found to increase the hippocampal damage (Koide et al. 1986). However, the glucocorticoid inhibition of prostaglandins is predominately a phenomenon of peripheral tissue or brain endothelium. To date, there are no reports of glucocorticoids inducing lipocortin within neurons, and as mentioned, the majority of studies show that glucocorticoids do not inhibit prostaglandin synthesis in the brain. Furthermore, glucocorticoid treatment does not alter levels of lipid peroxidation (one marker of oxygen radical damage) in the brain (Koide et al. 1986).

Another, rather unorthodox, feature of glucocorticoid action also should *protect* the nervous system from oxidative damage. Because of their lipophilic, steroidal nature, glucocorticoids in sufficiently high concentrations can potentially intercalate into cell membranes and stabilize them, protecting them against peroxidative attack. This is probably the basis of the highly publicized ability of glucocorticoids to reduce spinal cord injury (reviewed in Bracken et al. 1990). A number of pieces of evidence support the view that glucocorticoids are exerting these protective effects independent of their more tradiational, receptor-mediated actions: (1) The hormones are most efficacious against spinal cord injury when administered in megadoses that are vastly supersaturating of even the high-capacity type II receptor (Bracken et al. 1984, 1985, 1990; Braughler et al. 1987). (2) The glucocorticoids can be protective more rapidly than can be explained by their classic receptor-mediated, genomic effects (Hall 1985). (3) The spinal cord does not have a particularly large number of corticosteroid receptors, and is thus not likely to be particularly sensitive to receptor-mediated glucocorticoid effects. (4) Glucocorticoids protect against trauma only so long as the steroid molecules are physical present (Braughler and Hall 1984, 1985). This fits a model of the steroids physically intercalating in the membrane and contradicts the classic receptor model where, by altering genomic events, the steroids influence events long after they have disappeared from the scene. (5) The lazaroid steroids, which lack glucocorticoid action, also protect against spinal cord injury (Hall et al. 1987). (6) Of the various beneficial cellular and biochemical consequences of administration of glucocorticoids or lazaroids following spinal cord injury, the extent of lipid solubility of the steroid and the extent to which it inhibits lipid peroxidation are the best predictors of neuroprotection (Hall et al. 1987).

In summary, these various findings generate opposing predictions—glucocorticoids should exacerbate oxidative damage through their effects on metabolism and calcium mobilization; they should protect via their nonspecific effects on membranes. How do these opposing trends balance out? Tentatively, it appears that when glucocorticoids are administered in the high but physiologic range (as opposed to the supraphysiologic megadoses required in the spinal cord studies), their deleterious effects predominate. Thus, glucocorticoids exacerbate hypoxic-ischemic injury (Sapolsky and Pulsinelli 1985; Koide et al. 1986; Morse and Davis 1990b) and exacerbate the toxicity of oxygen radical generators (Sapolsky et al. 1988). When megadoses of glucocorticoids are used to protect against trauma that does not involve the hippocampus (e.g., spinal cord injury), the steroids are highly protective, as noted. When megadoses of glucocorticoids are used to protect against trauma in which the hippocampus is endangered (i.e., brain trauma), the protective and deleterious effects appear to cancel each other out. Thus, while some studies have observed protective effects of glucocorticoids against brain trauma in humans, the majority have not (discussed in chapter 14).

Therefore, while glucocorticoids can potentially protect neurons against oxidative damage, they do not do so within the concentration range of the studies discussed in this section of the book. The clinical implications of these ideas will be the subject of speculation in the final chapter.

Glucocorticoid Induction of Synapsin I

Synapsin I, along with synapsin II, form a family of proteins located in axon terminals of essentially all central nervous system neurons. Synapsin I is found on the surface of vesicles, and it can regulate the release of vesicular neurotransmitters. The number of synapsin I molecules per vesicle is quite high, allowing the formation of a "cage" around the vesicle. Originally, it was thought that the protein might stabilize vesicles, regulate their size, or preserve the integrity of their membranes during vesicular fusion with the plasma membrane, so as to facilitate the reformation of vesicles.

More recent studies suggest instead that synapsin I regulates neurotransmitter release via interaction with cytoskeletal proteins. In its dephosphorylated form, synapsin I binds to a variety of such proteins, including actin, fodrin, microtubules, and neurofilaments. This is thought to form a constraining anchor which keeps vesicles from migrating toward and fusing with the plasma membrane. With the influx of calcium following an action potential, the protein is phosphorylated, which releases it from the cytoskeletal matrix, facilitating vesicular fusion and neurotransmitter release (reviewed in Bahler et al. 1990).

Of significance, glucocorticoids induce synapsin I in the hippocampus via the Type I receptor (Nestler et al. 1981). This immediately suggests that glucocorticoid induction of the protein might somehow enhance the vesicular release of EAAs and that this might explain the endangerment. There is not yet direct evidence for this attractive idea. First, it is not clear what effects more synapsin I would have, since it is not known if the result would be more phosphorylated or dephosphorylated synapsin I. Moreover, there is no reason to believe that glucocorticoids are preferentially inducing synapsin I in some neuron types (for example, those containing EAAs) as opposed to those containing, for example, inhibitory neurotransmitters such as GABA. Finally, as reviewed in chapter 7, the glucocorticoid endangerment appears to be mediated by Type II corticosteroid receptors, rather than the Type I receptor which is involved in the synapsin effect. Therefore, there is little reason at present to believe that the glucocorticoid endangerment is mediated by induction of synapsin.

Glucocorticoid Induction of Calbindin D-28K

As an additional feature of glucocorticoid action in the brain, the steroids induce calbindin D-28K in the hippocampus (Iacopino and Christakos 1991). This is one of the more important of the calcium-binding proteins in terms of potentially serving as a buffer against damaging excesses of free cytosolic calcium. As was reviewed in the previous chapter, a number of studies have presented correlative evidence in support of this, in that neurons most resistant to EAA toxicity tend to be those with the highest concentrations of calbindin D-28K (reviewed in Mattson et al. 1991b).

Therefore, if glucocorticoids induce this protein, the steroids should be neuroprotective. However, a few features of this induction appear to make this phenomenon of limited relevance. First, the induction is a rather slow one; in the published report of the induction, glucocorticoid concentrations were manipulated for 2 weeks (Iacopino and Christakos 1991), and in the shortest time course tested to date, 5 days of glucocorticoid manipulation was insufficient to alter calbindin D-28K levels (S. Christakos, personal communication). Moreover, we have found that 2 days of glucocorticoid manipulation fails to induce the protein in hippocampal cultures (Packan, Sapolsky, and Christakos, unpublished observation). Therefore, glucocorticoids are not inducing calbindin D-28K within the time frame in which the steroids are endangering.

The induction might have some relevance to the gradual glucocorticoid toxicity in the hippocampus that occurs during aging (i.e., the ability of glucocorticoids to directly damage the hippocampus over the course of weeks to months, in contrast to their ability to exacerbate neurological insults to the hippocampus over the course of hours to days). As will be recalled from chapter 6, the studies showing the toxic effect of long-term glucocorticoid exposure and the protective effect of long-term diminution of glucocorticoid exposure all focused on Ammon's horn neurons (i.e., those of CA_2, CA_3, and CA_4). Consistently, CA_1 and dentate gyrus neurons were reported to be resistant to glucocorticoid toxicity. Moreover, during normal aging, neuron loss was nil or minimal in CA_1 and dentate, and was most dramatic in the CA_3 region. Intriguingly, the induction of calbindin D-28K by glucocorticoids occurs only in CA_1 and dentate gyrus (Iacopino and Christakos, 1991). One might hypothesize that while sustained glucocorticoid exposure is predominantly catabolic in the CA_3 region, resulting in eventual neuron death, the delayed induction of calbindin D-28K in CA_1 and dentate gyrus offsets the glucocorticoid toxicity in those cell regions. This idea has yet to be tested. However, as interesting correlative evidence, in the aged hippocampus, there are substantial amounts of calbindin D-28K in the CA_1 region, lesser amounts in dentate gyrus, and no detectable amounts in CA_3 (Smith and Booze 1991).

Glucocorticoids and Nitric Oxide

Nitric oxide (NO) is known to play a role in macrophage-mediated cytotoxicity, as well as in vasodilatation of smooth muscle (and NO, in fact, is endothelium-derived relaxing factor). Recently, NO has been shown to play a neuromodulatory and/or neurotransmitter role in the brain. Despite the awareness for centuries that nitrous oxide ("laughing gas," N_2O) is neuroactive, this finding regarding NO still runs counter to a lot of the current dogma of neurochemistry—gases are simply not likely candidates for neurotransmitters. Nevertheless, there has been a veritable avalanche of data regarding NO in the last year (for reviews, see Garthwaite 1991; Snyder and Bredt 1991; Bredt et al. 1991). One facet of the NO story may be of relevance to the glucocorticoid endangerment.

Nitric oxide is enzymatically produced in neurons in an NADPH-requiring reaction by the calcium-calmodulin–dependent enyzme nitric oxide synthase (NOS). The primary consequence of NO generation is the activation of guanylate cyclase which, in turn, generates cGMP. The understanding of cGMP actions is limited (as compared to, say, information regarding cAMP). Nevertheless, it is known that cGMP can interact directly with ion channels, can trigger phosphorylation cascades via a cGMP-dependent protein kinase, or can regulate cAMP levels (Garthwaite 1991).

There appear to be two general scenarios by which NO serves as a neural messenger. In its neurotransmitter role, the gas can be released by axon terminals in response to action potentials and calcium influx. In this case, the trafficking of NO differs from that of more traditional neurotransmitters in that the gas, obviously, cannot be stored in vesicles. Instead, the calcium influx is thought to trigger the immediate synthesis and release of NO. The gas can then diffuse across the synapse and trigger cGMP accumulation post-synaptically. In general, this model is thought only to apply to the release of NO by peripheral nerves, with the postsynaptic target being smooth muscle.

In the scenario that probably accounts for most NO activity within the brain, the gas is generated postsynaptically. It can then diffuse out of the dendrite and generate cGMP in the presynaptic axon terminal and/or in neighboring neurons and glia. There is some speculation in the literature that NO can also generate cGMP in the postsynaptic neuron while in the process of diffusing out. Critically, NO is best implicated in this neuromodulatory role in the brain in glutamatergic synapses.

It is this EAA-NO link which is of interest, particularly since EAAs stimulate cGMP accumulation in the adult and perinatal hippocampal slice (Garthwaite 1991). This suggests that NO might play some role in the toxicity of the EAA/NMDA/calcium cascade. Potentially, this could be either a damaging or protective role—the mere generation of NO by EAAs does not guarantee that the gas mediates glutamatergic toxicity (for example, as discussed in the previous chapter, EAA exposure can cause release of adenosine, which is neuroprotective). Unfortunately, at present, the issue is completely confused as to whether NO is damaging or protective.

The evidence for a damaging role is as follows:

• It has been shown recently that NO mediates glutamatergic toxicity in primary rat cortical cultures (V. Dawson et al. 1991). This was accomplished by blocking the generation of NO with a number of NOS inhibitors and thus decreasing glutamatergic toxicity.

• Nitroprusside, a drug which generates NO, is also toxic in a dose-dependent manner to cortical cultures. Furthermore, nitroprusside generates cGMP in parallel with its toxicity (V. Dawson et al. 1991).

• Separate of the NO/cGMP link, NO can be a potent oxygen radical on its own and can interact synergistically with a number of other radicals (Snyder and Bredt 1991).

This seems rather convincing for a damaging role for NO. However, some evidence suggests that the gas can be neuroprotective:

• Within the brain, NOS is colocalized with the enzyme NADPH-d, and NOS appears to account for all of the activity of the latter (T. Dawson et al. 1991). As reviewed at the end of the previous chapter, the subpopulation of neurons that contain NADPH-d are remarkably resistant to NMDA and hypoxia-ischemia and in the human brain to degeneration in Huntington's disease and in Alzheimer's disease (Ferrante et al. 1985; Koh et al. 1986; Beal et al. 1986; Koh and Choi 1988). This suggests that NOS is associated with neuroprotection.

• Despite the finding of nitroprusside-induced toxicity in cortical cultures, the same compound *protects* rat cerebellar slices from EAA-induced damage (Garthwaite and Garthwaite 1988) and inhibits the calcium response to kainic acid (Kaiser et al. 1991) and to NMDA (Manzoni et al. 1991) in cultured neurons.

• NO has been reported to inhibit glutamate binding to synaptic membranes in the rat brain (Fujimori and Pan-Hou 1991).

• Finally, one recent abstract suggests that NO production is independent of kainic acid neurotoxicity in cultured granule cells (Puttfarcken et al. 1991).

Therefore, at present, the issue is quite confused. Some of this confusion might arise over the uncertainty as to whether NO acts primarily in the neuron in which it is generated (i.e., in the postsynaptic neuron, in the model by which NO most likely works in the CNS), or in some neighboring neuron and/or glia to which it diffuses. This more complex latter scenario is offered to explain some puzzling observations. It is known that neurons which contain NADPH-d, while being resistant to NMDA-induced toxicity, are quite vulnerable to quisqualate-induced toxicity (Koh and Choi 1988), perhaps arising from a preponderance of receptors for the latter. In one tissue culture study in which NADPH-d—containing neurons were first killed with quisqualate, the subsequent toxicity of NMDA was reduced. The interpretation given was that part of the normal degree of NMDA toxicity was mediated by NOS/NADPH-d—positive neurons releasing NO which would diffuse to neighboring neurons, damaging them. In the absence of those NOS/NADPH-d—positive neurons, the NO component of NMDA toxicity was removed (unpublished data cited by V. Dawson et al. 1991).

Not surprisingly, given the recency of these data, the role of NO in neuron death has not been settled. Of considerable interest, glucocorticoids have been shown to inhibit the induction of NOS in a variety of peripheral tissues (Moncada and Palmer 1991). This has been offered as a possible new mechanism by which glucocorticoids are anti-inflammatory (by blocking vascular dilatation), as well as an explanation for why glucocorticoids can facilitate the spread of infection (by disrupting NOS-mediated cytotoxicity by activated macrophages). At present, there is no information available as to whether glucocorticoids have any effect on NOS expression or activity in the brain. Were that to be the case, it might have some striking implications for the glucocorticoid endangerment and/or toxicity.

GLUCOCORTICOID ACTIONS LIKELY TO CAUSE NEURONAL ENDANGERMENT

The previous sections of this chapter have reviewed various glucocorticoid actions in the brain that do not seem to explain the features of glucocorticoid endangerment of the hippocampus or whose relevance is not clear (induction of glutamine synthetase, synapsin I, calbindin D-28K, or nitric oxide synthase, inhibition of vasogenic edema, protection from peroxidative damage). The remainder of the chapter is devoted to the glucocorticoid actions in the brain that, I feel, are most relevant to explaining the endangerment. To summarize, they are as follows:

1. The glucocorticoid endangerment appears to be energetic in nature. As evidence, the steroids exacerbate some of the indices of energy depletion that accompany the various neurological insults in the hippocampus. Moreover, supplementation of neurons with excess energy protects them from the glucocorticoid endangerment.

2. The best-documented route by which glucocorticoids cause an energetic endangerment in the hippocampus is through their inhibition of glucose transport. A number of other mechanisms have also been suggested.

3. By exacerbating the energy depletion during these neurological insults, glucocorticoids impair the capacity of hippocampal neurons to contain the EAA/NMDA/calcium cascade, exaggerating its damaging features. As evidence:

• Glucocorticoids augment the accumulation of extracellular EAAs in the hippocampus during seizures, and this augmentation can be reversed by energy supplementation.

• As a possible explanation for that effect, glucocorticoids inhibit hippocampal glial uptake of EAAs, and this inhibition can be reversed by energy supplementation.

• The glucocorticoid endangerment of the hippocampus can be prevented by blockade of NMDA receptors.

• Glucocorticoids raise basal free cytosolic calcium concentrations in hippocampal neurons and increase the mobilization of calcium during EAA exposure. This latter effect can be reversed by energy supplementation.

• Glucocorticoids will augment EAA-induced, calcium-dependent proteolysis of cytoskeletal proteins in the hippocampus in a manner that can be reversed by energy supplementation.

Energetic Endangerment of the Hippocampus by Glucocorticoids

Effect of Energy Supplementation   In considering seizure, hypoxia-ischemia, and hypoglycemia, one can concentrate on their similarities or on their differences. Chapter 7 focused on the differences—it is quite a different thing for a neuron to be deprived of oxygen than to be hyperexcited. The fact that glucocorticoids exacerbate all of those insults suggested that, whatever the steroids are doing, it is a very broad and general endangerment that they produce. Chapters 9 and 10, in contrast, focused on the similarities of these insults—the similarity of the EAA cascade, and the common property of the energy crisis. Could the endangerment produced by the glucocorticoids be an energetic one?

If glucocorticoids were causing such a crisis, this should be confirmed in a fairly simple test: Under conditions where glucocorticoids exacerbate one of these neurological insults, treatment with glucocorticoids plus some additional source of energy should be able to protect the neurons from the steroid endangerment. This is the case.

In one demonstration, adrenalectomized rats were microinfused in the hippocampus with 3-acetylpyridine (3AP), the antimetabolite that produces dentate gyrus damage very similar to that seen in hypoglycemia. A dose was chosen that produced only minimal damage (figure 11.1A, column 1, from Sapolsky, 1986b). As discussed in chapter 7, when rats were exposed to high physiological concentrations of glucocorticoids for a few days before and after the 3AP insult, the damage was greatly increased (column 3). Additional groups of rats were infused with additional energy substrates every 3 hours during the period of glucocorticoid treatment. Some rats were made hyperglycemic with glucose infusions, and this produced a trend toward protection of the hippocampus (column 4). A much more protective strategy was to use mannose, a monosaccharide that penetrates the blood-brain barrier, is metabolized by the brain, and whose uptake is probably unaffected by glucocorticoids (Siesjo 1978). Treatment of rats with mannose (which did not change circulating glucose concentrations) decreased the hippocampal damage dramatically (column 5). In contrast, treatment with as much as twice the dose of fructose was not particularly protective (columns 6 and 7)—fructose does not pass the blood-brain barrier. Finally, infusion of rats with the one other class of energy substrates that are normally used by the brain—ketone bodies such as β-hydroxybutyrate—was also protective (figure 11.1B).

This turned out to be a general phenomenon. Excess energy substrates (in this case, mannose) decreased the in vivo synergy between glucocorticoids and kainic acid (Sapolsky 1986b). These data suggested that glucocorticoids exacerbate the toxicity of these insults through some energetic means. The problem, however, was that substrates such as mannose could be protective by decreasing the endangering effects of the steroids, and/or by decreasing the toxicity of the toxins themselves. The latter is certainly a possibility, given the emphasis in chapter 10 on the energetics of these insults. Initially, this latter interpretation appears not to be valid, since the toxicity of 3AP alone and 3AP

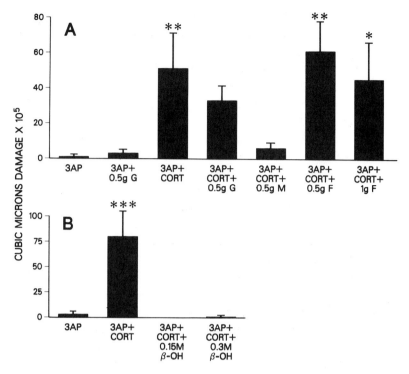

Figure 11.1. Potentiation of 3-acetylpyridine-induced hippocampal damage by corticosterone and reversal of this potentiation with brain energy substrates. Volumes of damage from entire unilateral hippocampi are presented. (A, bars left to right) Damage due to 3-acetylpyridine (3AP); 3AP plus 0.5 g glucose i.p. every 3 hours for 1 day before and after 3AP microinfusion; 3AP plus high physiologic concentrations of corticosterone; 3AP plus corticosterone plus glucose; 3AP plus corticosterone plus mannose; 3AP plus corticosterone plus fructose (same dose and schedule as for glucose and mannose); 3AP plus corticosterone plus 1 g fructose per injection. (B, bars left to right) 3AP alone; 3AP plus corticosterone; 3AP plus corticosterone plus 0.15 M β-hydroxybutyrate; 3AP plus corticosterone plus 0.3 M β-hydroxybutyrate. (From Sapolsky, 1986, J Neurosci 6, 2240. Reprinted with permission of Oxford University Press.)

plus glucose were no different (figure 11.1, columns 1 versus 2). However, because there was so little damage due to 3AP alone, it would not be possible to decrease damage further with glucose.

In a subsequent attempt to answer this, we sought an insult that did not appear to damage the hippocampus via energetic means, yet which was made worse by glucocorticoids. One example of this is paraquat, the oxygen radical generator. We studied this in vitro, in primary hippocampal cultures. Under these conditions and at this concentration, paraquat was toxic to the cultures, but supplementing the neurons with as much as 0.4% glucose did not alter the toxicity of paraquat. As discussed previously, addition of the glucocorticoid corticosterone exacerbated paraquat-induced damage. Critically, addition of from 0.2 to 0.4% glucose removed the glucocorticoid component of the endangerment (Sapolsky et al. 1988). More recently, we have shown that the glucocorticoid component of the synergy with hypoxia in vitro could also be reduced by glucose supplementation (Tombaugh et al. 1992).

Finally, a similar story appears to hold regarding glucocorticoid endangerment of hippocampal astrocytes. As reviewed in chapter 7, glucocorticoids can exacerbate damage to such cells, and we observe that glucose supplementation, either at the time of or prior to hypoxia, will decrease the glucocorticoid exacerbation of damage. This occurs under circumstances where the glucose manipulation fails to alter the toxicity of the hypoxia itself (Tombaugh and Sapolsky 1992).

In summary, it appears that it is a metabolic cliff upon whose edge glucocorticoids place neurons. Naturally, at this point, the question becomes how glucocorticoids disrupt hippocampal energetics. We believe we have an answer, one that constitutes relatively new information for neurobiologists, but that is old news for endocrinologists.

Glucocorticoid Inhibition of Glucose Transport in the Hippocampus
As discussed many chapters ago, one of the hallmarks of the metabolic stress-response is the capacity of glucocorticoids to mobilize circulating glucose in order to divert energy to voluntary muscles. This makes sense, as most stressors are physical, demanding some sort of muscular response. It has been known for decades that glucocorticoids accomplish this, in part, by inhibiting the uptake of glucose into a variety of peripheral tissues (reviewed in Munck 1971; Munck et al. 1984). The molecular biology of this inhibition is fairly well understood. Glucose enters target cells through facilitated diffusion via a glucose transporter. The transporter actually exists as a family of different but highly conserved molecules that transport glucose in different tissues; they vary as to their affinity for glucose, membrane concentration, insulin sensitivity, and ability to transport bidirectionality (Baly and Horuk 1988). Glucocorticoids inhibit glucose entry into the affected target cells by decreasing the number of glucose transporters. This is accomplished in two ways (figure 11.2). During the first 8 to 12 hours of steroid exposure, glucocorticoids cause transporters to be removed from the cell membrane and sequestered in inactive forms into intracellular storage sites (Carter-Su and Okamoto 1985; Horner et al. 1987; Garvey et al. 1989a). This is the opposite of the mechanism by which insulin promotes glucose uptake (Suzuki and Kono 1980; Cushman and Wardzala 1980). Glucocorticoids translocate the receptor by inducing a "sequestering" protein; this has not yet been identified, although it is known not to be lipocortin (Horner, personal communication). With more prolonged glucocorticoid exposure, there are decreased levels of mRNA for the transporter and less total cellular transporter (Garvey et al. 1989b). The final result of these actions is that glucocorticoids inhibit glucose uptake into some peripheral tissues by as much as 70%.

This suggested that glucocorticoids might metabolically endanger the hippocampus through a similar inhibition of glucose transport. This appears to be the case.

In the first demonstrations of this, local cerebral glucose utilization (LCGU) was studied in vivo using the classic Sokoloff technique for measuring radioactive 2-deoxyglucose uptake autoradiographically. Adrenalectomy increased,

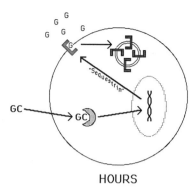

HOURS

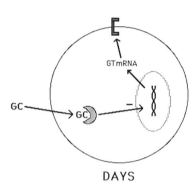

DAYS

Figure 11.2. Schematic representation of the two documented routes by which glucocorticoids (GC) decrease glucose transport. *Top*, Over the course of hours, glucocorticoids induce the expression of an as yet uncharacterized "sequestering" protein, which translocates glucose transporters from the cell membrane to intracellular storage sites. *Bottom*, Over the course of days, glucocorticoids can directly inhibit transcription of the glucose transporter gene.

while glucocorticoids decreased LCGU throughout the brain, with the modulation in the hippocampus being one of the most dramatic sites (25% to 30% change) (Kadekaro et al. 1988; Bryan and King 1988). (In an apparent contradiction, Domer et al. [1988] failed to show an effect of dexamethasone on LCGU. However, they applied the glucocorticoid only 15 minutes before the start of the experiment, a time insufficient for the steroid to exert its known genomic inhibition of glucose transport [Munck 1971].) These reports showed that even basal glucocorticoid concentrations could inhibit glucose utilization in the brain. However, because of the limits of resolution with the technique, it was not possible to tell where the inhibition occurred—was there less movement of glucose from the bloodstream into the extracellular space via the endothelial glucose transporter, was there less transport directly into neurons and glia, or both?

We examined this by measuring glucose uptake directly into cultured hippocampal neurons and glia and found that high nanomolar concentrations of glucocorticoids inhibit uptake into both cell types. The magnitude of inhibition is approximately 25% to 30% in neurons and approximately 15% to

How Do Glucocorticoids Endanger the Hippocampal Neuron?

20% in glia. In agreement with the known mechanisms of glucocorticoid action, the effect takes a few hours to develop, is not induced by nonglucocorticoid steroids (estadiol, testosterone, and progesterone), and is mediated by the Type II glucocorticoid receptor (Horner et al. 1990; Virgin et al. 1991).

Interestingly, glucocorticoids do not inhibit glucose uptake in cerebellar, cortical, or hypothalamic cultures, despite their containing Type II receptors (Horner et al. 1990). This restriction of the inhibition to the hippocampal cultures appears to contradict the in vivo studies, in which the glucocorticoid inhibition of LCGU was most pronounced in, but certainly not exclusive to, the hippocampus. We interpret this as showing that glucocorticoids probably inhibit neuronal and glial glucose transporters only in the hippocampus, whereas inhibition of endothelial transporters occurs additionally throughout the brain. Of relevance, glucocorticoids inhibit glucose transport in peripheral endothelium (Olgemoller et al. 1985).

Thus, in agreement with their classic peripheral action, glucocorticoids inhibit glucose transport into hippocampal neurons and glia. It is important here to reiterate an idea discussed at the beginning of chapter 10. In that section, I reviewed a few ideas about the nature of neuronal energy crises that appear to have been underemphasized or unappreciated in the literature. One was the idea that high concentrations of an energy substrate in the circulation do not necessarily translate into high concentrations of energy for target tissues. This was seemingly paradoxical, but is the case just discussed—in the instance of glucocorticoids, circulating glucose concentrations rise in part *because* of the inhibition of glucose entry into many target tissues (including, perhaps, the hippocampus) (although it should be noted that most of postglucocorticoid hyperglycemia is due to effects of the hormone on hepatic gluconeogenesis).

Additional Disruptions of Hippocampal Energetics by Glucocorticoids

Glucocorticoids may disrupt neuronal energetics in a second way. During starvation, protein synthesis in most cells declines sharply, with the exception of the induction of a class of *glucose-regulated proteins* (GRPs). This pattern of selective induction during an energetic stressor is reminiscent of the heat-shock proteins (with which the GRPs share considerable homology). Presumably, GRPs serve some adaptive role during this emergency. One might predict that the GRPs are glucose transporters; teleologically, it makes sense to increase transporter number at such times, and starvation does indeed induce an increase (reviewed in Baly and Horuk 1988). However, the GRPs appear not to be glucose transport proteins (Wertheimer et al. 1991). Perhaps they are the putative proteins that translocate glucose transporters to the cell surface. Of considerable interest, glucocorticoids block their induction by glucose starvation in cultured L929 cells (Kasambalides and Lanks 1983). If the GRPs do translocate the glucose transporter, this explains why glucocorticoids can antagonize insulin action and decrease glucose transport. Regardless of what these GRPs do, to the extent that they represent a cellular response to an energetic emergency, it is bad news for the cell that they are inhibited by glucocorticoids. We are currently examining whether glucocorticoids inhibit GRP expression in the hippocampus as well.

Glucocorticoid Alteration of Energetic Profiles in Hippocampal Cells If the glucocorticoid effects on glucose transport (and perhaps on GRPs and oxidative metabolism) are physiologically relevant, they should be reflected in decreased levels of energy substrates in the hippocampus and/or impaired metabolism.

As a test of this idea, do glucocorticoids decrease concentrations of ATP and/or phosphocreatine in hippocampal neurons? As a biochemical correlate of the glucocorticoid "synergy" with insults, one might predict that glucocorticoids will not neccesarily depress *basal* concentrations of either of those compounds, but might accelerate their decline during a neurologic insult. This is because under basal conditions, glucose transport across the blood-brain barrier into neurons is in no way rate limiting. Therefore, the normal rate of glucose influx exceeds the rate of phosphorylation (discussed in van der Kuil and Korf 1991) and is likely to be able to withstand an approximately 30% inhibition of glucose transport induced by the hormone. In contrast, glucose transport becomes rate limiting during times of enhanced energy demand during neurological crises such as hypoxia-ischemia (Lewis et al. 1974; Betz et al. 1974) or seizure (Chapman et al. 1977); at such times, a 30% decrease in transport may be critically endangering.

No study, to my knowledge, has examined glucocorticoid effects on ATP or phosphocreatine concentrations in hippocampal neurons during energetic crises. However, we have obtained indirect evidence that glucocorticoids hasten the metabolic crash in the hippocampus during such an insult. We have used a silicon-based microphysiometer, a novel instrument that allows the measurement of real-time metabolism in a small number of plated cells by measuring the slight extracellular bursts of acidity due to proton extrusion following ATP hydrolysis (Parce et al. 1989; Raley-Susman et al., in press). We have observed that a variety of EAAs cause an immediate increase in metabolic rate in hippocampal cultures; over the subsequent day, metabolism declines precipitously in a manner preceding cell death (Raley-Susman et al., in preparation). This fits in quite neatly with the delayed and excitatory nature of EAA toxicity. Critically, glucocorticoids appear not to alter basal metabolic rate nor the slope and magnitude of the EAA induced metabolic enhancement, but instead accelerate the delayed metabolic crash.

The inhibition of glucose transport into hippocampal glia predicts that energy profiles should be disrupted there as well. In support of this, we observe that glucocorticoids decrease glycogen stores in hippocampal astrocytes in vitro (Virgin et al. 1991). Moreover, glucocorticoids decrease the tissue glucose: glycogen ratio in the hippocampus in vivo (with no change in the cortex) (Tombaugh et al., in preparation). Because glycogen in the brain is stored far more readily in glia than in neurons, this implies that glucocorticoids inhibit glycogen storage in hippocampal glia in vivo. Thus, glucocorticoids disrupt energetic stores in glia under basal conditions. The notion of glucocorticoid synergy with insults again predicts that the hormones will exacerbate the decline in energy stores occurring during an energetic insult. We have observed this pattern in cultured astrocytes, monitoring the decline in ATP concentrations during excitotoxic insults (Tombaugh et al., in preparation).

The disruption of glucose transport and depletion of energy stores in hippocampal glia by glucocorticoids taps into a theme that is receiving more attention in neurology. Glia are coming to be recognized increasingly for the varied and dynamic roles that they play and their potential for altering the severity of neurotoxic evens in the brain. In general, glia are viewed as playing a salutary role. For example, cultured neurons are less vulnerable to hypoxia or EAA exposure when cocultured with glia (Vibulsreth et al. 1987; Rosenberg and Aizenman 1989; Mattson and Rychlik 1990). Glia can be "good neighbors" in a number of ways. As reviewed earlier in this chapter, they can remove EAAs from the synapse, playing a critical role in terminating an excitatory signal. They can act as a sink for protons or potassium, regulating the severity of neuronal or extracellular acidosis or the extent of edema. Moreover, they can take up ammonia. They can also release a wide variety of neuroactive substances. The importance of these roles has been shown in a number of studies. For example, pharmacological disruption of EAA removal by glia from the synapse potentiates EAA neurotoxicity (Sugiyama et al. 1989; Harris et al. 1990; Saito 1990; Swanson and Choi 1990).

Not surprisingly, essentially all of these "neighborly" activities on the part of glia are energetically costly, typically depending directly on ATP-consuming processes or indirectly on costly ionic gradients. Therefore, the extent of glycogen storage in glia (and thus, the glial potential for carrying out some of these costly acts of Samaritanism) is a powerful predictor of the extent of neuronal vulnerability during in vitro hypoxia (Swanson and Choi 1990).

This digression is meant to emphasize the importance and costliness of glial function in modulating neuronal survivorship and, therefore, the potential importance of the glucocorticoid disruption of glial energetics in the hippocampus. As will be seen shortly, this glucocorticoid effect in glia appears to have at least one important consequence for the phenomenon of neuronal endangerment, namely disruption of glutamate uptake.

In summary, a variety of studies suggest that glucocorticoids endanger the hippocampus by inducing some form of metabolic vulnerability. As the most plausible explanation, glucocorticoids induce the vulnerability by inhibiting the entry of glucose into these cells. Neurons are notorious for their fragile energetic state—they consume almost nothing but glucose and store it poorly. Furthermore, their health depends, to some extent, on energy-dependent processes carried out by neighboring glia. Despite these features of neuronal and glial energetics, there is little reason to believe a priori (and very little experimental evidence to support the view) that the small inhibition of glucose transport demonstrated is enough to *kill* a hippocampal neuron. However, it seems quite plausible that it may *endanger* a neuron, impairing its ability of the neuron to deal with an energetic crisis. The interminable chapters 9 and 10 will have served their purpose if the reader now is wondering whether glucocorticoids, by disrupting neuronal energetics, exacerbate the EAA/NMDA/calcium cascade.

Glucocorticoids and the Glutamatergic Synapse: NMDA Receptor Dependency

If glucocorticoids exacerbate the EAA/NMDA/calcium cascade, one prediction must be true: Regardless of which particular steps in EAA or calcium trafficking are affected by glucocorticoids, the endangerment should be NMDA receptor dependent.

In theory, this should be easy to demonstrate. Under conditions where glucocorticoids exacerbate the toxicity of an insult, blockade of the NMDA receptor should subtract out that glucocorticoid endangerment. The trouble with this approach, however, is that blocking the NMDA receptor should decrease the toxicity of the primary insult itself. Thus, it is difficult to determine whether a demonstrated protection is due to less of an insult or less glucocorticoid augmentation of that insult. Our strategy became to find an insult that was exacerbated by glucocorticoids, but which itself did not damage via the NMDA cascade.

We found a dose of 3AP that damaged the dentate gyrus but which was insensitive to blockade of the NMDA receptor with the competitive antagonist APV. Therefore, in adrenalectomized rats, APV did not alter 3AP-induced damage (figure 11.3, column 1 versus column 3; Armanini et al. 1990). As

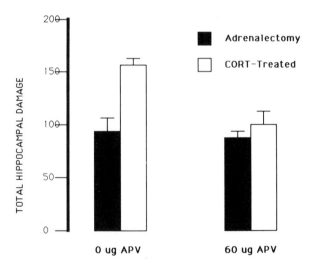

Figure 11.3. Glucocorticoid endangerment of the hippocampus is NMDA receptor dependent. Rats were either adrenalectomized or treated with exogenous glucocorticoids (GC), generating constant concentrations in the upper physiologic range. Rats were either treated with 0 or 60 μg of the NMDA receptor antagonist APV at the time of the 3-acetylpyridine infusion. (From Armanini et al., 1990, Brain Research 532, 7. Reprinted with permission from Elsevier Science Publishers.)

shown previously, glucocorticoid treatment increased 3AP-induced damage (column 1 versus column 2). However, when the NMDA receptor was blocked with APV, the exacerbating effects of glucocorticoids were subtracted out (column 4).

Glucocorticoids and the Glutamatergic Synapse: Increased Synaptic Concentrations of EAAs

In summary, at least in this particular model, the glucocorticoid endangerment of the neurons is NMDA receptor mediated. One must then begin to explore which particular steps in EAA and calcium trafficking are being exacerbated by the steroids (figure 11.4). At each point in such a tree diagram, there are three types of questions to be asked: (1) Do glucocorticoids disrupt that particular point of EAA or calcium trafficking? (2) If so, is it because of the energetic effects of the glucocorticoids? Specifically, can the glucocorticoid effect be overridden by supplementing the neurons with more energy substrates? (3) As a further means of testing the energetic nature of the glucocorticoid action, can it be replicated by depriving the neurons of 25% to 30% of their glucose (i.e., the magnitude of the glucocorticoid inhibition of glucose transport into hippocampal neurons)?

The first step in exploring that tree diagram of possibilities is to determine whether glucocorticoids increase the amount of synaptic EAAs in the synapse and/or increase the postsynaptic calcium response to EAAs. We have recently observed that there is an increase in the EAA signal. Specifically, we micro-dialyzed the hippocampi of rats before and after kainic acid–induced seizures, and measured the concentrations of various amino acids in the extracellular space. In adrenalectomized rats, we observed the kainic acid–induced rise in

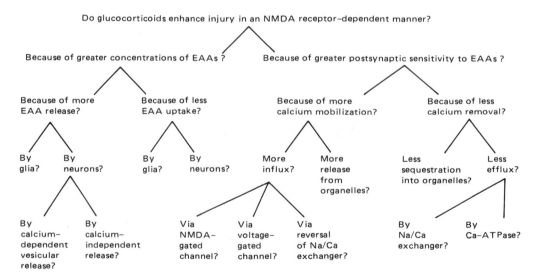

Figure 11.4. Schematic tree diagram demonstrating the possible mechanisms underlying the NMDA receptor dependency of the glucocorticoid endangerment.

How Does a Neuron Die?

EAA concentrations reported in numerous previous publications (reviewed in chapter 9) (in this paradigm, kainic acid was perfused directly in the dialysate buffer, affording a fair confidence as to when, precisely, it reached the hippocampus). Glucocorticoid pretreatment elevated the extracellular concentrations of glutamate (figure 11.5) and aspartate. In the former case, the hormone treatment elevated pre-kainic acid concentrations, while the magnitude of the kainic acid response was unchanged. With aspartate, glucocorticoids elevated the response to kainic acid. Furthermore, the glucocorticoid effect was prevented by administering the rats additional mannose. Glucocorticoids did not increase the extracellular concentrations of taurine or alanine (figure 11.5 also shows the data regarding alanine as a demonstration of a lack of effect) (Stein-Behrens et al., in press). (As discussed already, the glucocorticoid-induced increase in the glutamate concentration in the extracellular volume is not likely to be due to the glucocorticoids preventing seizure or trauma edema [i.e., causing a smaller extracellular volume and thus artifactually concentrating the glutamate]. Furthermore, were that the case, glucocorticoids should have artifactually increased the concentration of other amino acids as well.)

(Interestingly, we also observed that while kainic acid infusion failed to change glutamine levels, overall extracellular glutamine concentrations were significantly higher in the glucocorticoid-treated rats. Moreover, this hormone effect was not reversible with mannose, unlike the increased levels of aspartate and glutamate. This suggests that glucocorticoids are increasing the trafficking of glutamine in the extracellular space in a way that is independent of the energetic effects of the hormones as well as of glutamate concentrations. As a possible explanation, the small but not significant increase in glutamine synthetase activity in the adult hippocampus which I dismissed earlier in this chapter may actually be sufficient to cause the synthesis of more glutamine. This strikes me as rather unlikely, however.)

GLUCOCORTICOIDS AND THE GLUTAMATERGIC SYNAPSE: DISRUPTION OF EAA UPTAKE

In summary, glucocorticoids appear to exacerbate an EAA signal during a neurological insult. Is this because of enhanced EAA release, or less removal from the synapse? We do not have any information on release, nor on neuronal reuptake of EAA, but our data indicate that glucocorticoids disrupt EAA uptake into astrocytes. This is energetic in nature. As noted, glucocorticoids inhibit glucose transport into hippocampal glia as well as neurons (Horner et al. 1990). As a probable consequence of this, the high affinity uptake of ^{3}H-glutamate is impaired. Specifically, we find that both decreased glucose availability and glucocorticoid exposure cause an approximate doubling in the K_m of glutamate uptake into astrocytes, without affecting the V_{max} (Virgin et al. 1991). This makes considerable sense. As outlined in chapter 10, EAA uptake into astrocytes depends on low intracellular sodium concentrations and low extracellular potassium concentrations. Both of these conditions favoring uptake are disrupted by a paucity of energy.

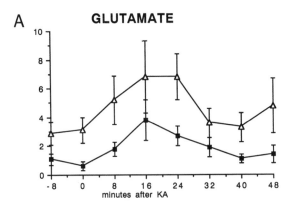

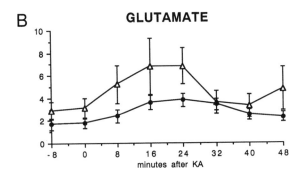

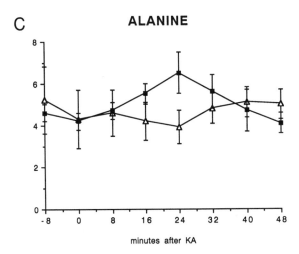

Figure 11.5. Glucocorticoid administration increases extracellular concentrations of glutamate in the hippocampus, as measured by microdialysis. (*A*) Concentrations of glutamate (in μM) before and after exposure to kainic acid in the dialysate in adrenalectomized rats replaced with doses of corticosterone generating either low basal concentrations (square) or concentrations in the upper stress range (triangles). (*B*) Concentrations of glutamate before and after exposure to kainic acid in the dialysate in adrenalectomized rats replaced with a dose of corticosterone generating concentrations in the upper stress range (triangles—these are the same data as in part *A*), and in rats treated the same way but supplemented with mannose (circles). (*C*) Concentrations of alanine (in μM) before and after exposure to kainic acid in the dialysate in

These findings replicate the indirect finding of two previous studies. In the first, glucocorticoids were shown to decrease a combination of EAA receptor binding and EAA uptake in the hippocampus (Halpain and McEwen 1989). Subsequently, glucocorticoids were shown not to have an effect on receptor binding alone (Clark and Cotman 1990), implying that the effect in the former study was on uptake (by neurons and/or glia).

(It should be noted that, theoretically, there is a mechanism by which glucocorticoids might *increase* astrocyte glutamate uptake. Such uptake is inhibited by arachidonic acid [Barbour et al. 1989] and, as discussed, glucocorticoids in general inhibit arachidonic acid synthesis. However, there is little evidence that this glucocorticoid effect occurs within neurons or astrocytes.)

Glucocorticoids and the Glutamatergic Synapse: Increased Basal and EAA-induced Calcium Mobilization

In summary, glucocorticoids appear to increase EAA accumulation in the synapse during a neurological crisis, and as one mediating mechanism, they inhibit the removal of EAAs from the synapse by astrocytes. We are at present examining whether glucocorticoids enhance the EAA signal by also disrupting neuronal EAA reuptake, by enhancing the initial EAA release, or both. Regardless of the mechanism, the enhanced extracellular EAA concentration predicts that glucocorticoids should exacerbate calcium mobilization as well. We have observed this.

Working with primary hippocampal cultures, we have measured free cytosolic calcium with the calcium-sensitive dyes fura-2 and fluo-3. Under such conditions, the excitotoxin kainic acid produces a prompt and transient increase in free calcium in a dose-related manner (see figure 9.2). Working with a dose of kainic acid that produce approximately 50% of the maximal calcium mobilization (100 μM kainic acid), we observed that pretreatment with concentrations of glucocorticoids typically generated during stress exacerbated this mobilization. The amount of calcium mobilized was increased, as was the length of time it took for calcium concentrations to return to baseline (Elliott and Sapolsky, in press). Moreover, this glucocorticoid effect could be blunted by glucose supplementation and mimicked by energy deprivation (30% decrease in glucose concentrations, to roughly approximate the 30% decrease in glucose transport induced by glucocorticoids). Glucocorticoids appear to exacerbate the calcium mobilization induced by other EAAs as well (M. Mattson, personal communication). Furthermore, we observed that glucocorticoids cause a 30% increase in the basal free cytosolic concentrations of kainic acid–responsive neurons (Elliott et al., in preparation).

adrenalectomized rats replaced with doses of corticosterone generating either low basal concentrations (squares) or concentrations in the upper stress range (triangles). (From Stein-Behrens et al., Glucocortiocids exacerbate kainic acid-induced extracellular accumulation of excitatory amino acids in the rat hippocampus. J Neurochem, in press. Reprinted with permission of Raven Press, Ltd.)

This glucocorticoid-induced increase in free cytosolic calcium in the hippocampus was implied in a number of recent studies. Concentrations of free cytosolic calcium are increased in the aged brain, as assessed by direct synaptosomal measurement or via indirect electrophysiological measures (Martinez et al. 1987; Reynolds and Carlen 1989). In at least one instance, this enhanced calcium tone is due to the elevated glucocorticoid concentrations observed in aged rats. In aged rats, there is augmentation of a calcium-dependent electrophysiological phenomenon in the hippocampus (the calcium-dependent, potassium-mediated slow afterhyperpolarization) (Landfield and Pitler 1984) as well as a prolonged calcium spike duration in hippocampal slices from aged rats (Pitler and Landfield 1990) and increased calcium influx during repetitive activation of the aged hippocampus (Landfield et al. 1986). Critically, the enhanced calcium mobilization was reversed by adrenalectomy of aged rats and enhanced by glucocorticoid administration in young rats (figure 11.6; Joels and de Kloet 1989a,b; Kerr et al. 1989). (Note: Kerr and colleagues interpret their findings much as I do here, namely that the glucocorticoid enhancement of calcium levels in the aged hippocampus may bear some relevance to the glucocorticoid neurotoxicity evident during aging. In contrast, de Kloet places a different emphasis on his findings with Joels, namely that this electrophysiological effect of glucocorticoids is not likely to be endangering, insofar as it enhances the inhibitory phenomenon of afterhyperpolarization [personal communication]. This inhibitory effect is consonant with an existing literature on the subject [reviewed in McEwen et al. 1986]. As a possible response, the enhanced afterhyperpolarizations may be a very different phenomenon from the glucocorticoid endangerment—the former concerns the effect of glucocorticoids on hippocampal neurons, while the latter concerns the modulation by glucocorticoids of the effects of other agents on such neurons.)

Do glucocorticoids increase free cytosolic calcium concentrations by enhancing influx, by enhancing mobilization from organelles, by inhibiting efflux, or by inhibiting sequestration back into organelles? This is a daunting set of questions to answer. At present, we have determined that glucocorticoids inhibit calcium efflux from the neuron. Cultured neurons were depolarized with potassium and, at the end of the potassium stimulus, the rate of decline of the intracellular free cytosolic calcium signal was monitored. Under those conditions, the decline is predominantly a function of sequestration of calcium into organelles and pumping of calcium out of the neuron (Blaustein 1988). Typically, the greater the free cytosolic calcium concentrations provoked by the potassium stimulus, the greater the subsequent efflux rate (i.e., the neuron works harder at efflux when the calcium load is greater).

Using this protocol, we observed that glucocorticoids decreased the efflux rate. Importantly, the steroids did not have this effect at all rates of efflux. Instead, the inhibition only occurred at the higher efflux rates (triggered by the heavier potassium-induced calcium load). In other words, glucocorticoids disrupted calcium efflux only when it was at its most expensive. This suggests

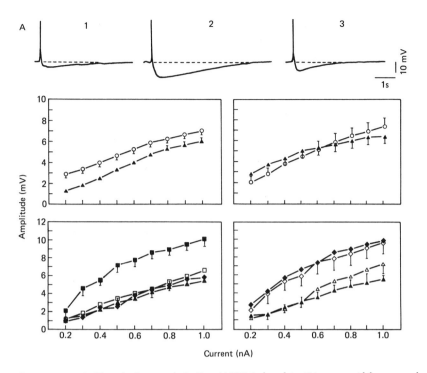

Figure 11.6. *A*, The afterhyperpolarization (AHP) induced in CA_1 pyramidal neurons by a 0.5-nA depolarizing pulse of 50-ms duration. The relatively small AHP in (A_1) is a typical example of the AHP obtained for neurons in slices from rats 7 days after adrenalectomy (ADX). (A_2) Treatment of a slice with 10^{-7} M of the selective glucocorticoid agonist RU 28362 results in a marked increase in the amplitude and duration of the slow AHP. (A_3) Recording of AHP in a slice from a sham-operated rat. In all three records, action potentials are truncated. *B*, Amplitude of the slow AHP evoked in CA_1 pyramidal cells by 50-ms current pulses of increasing intensity. (*Left*) Neurons recorded in slices from rats 7 days after ADX (triangles, $n = 62$) displayed a smaller AHP amplitude when compared with their sham controls (circles, $n = 38$). (*Right*) When the slices were prepared within 1 hour after ADX, no differences were observed between the CA_1 neurons from ADX rats (triangles, $n = 14$) and their time-matched sham controls (circles, $n = 11$). *C* (*left*) A 20-minute exposure of slices from ADX rats to 10^{-6} M corticosterone (solid squares, $n = 6$) 30 to 90 minutes before recording resulted in a marked increase in the AHP amplitude when compared to the neurons recorded before the slices were exposed to corticosterone (triangles, $n = 18$). If the glucococorticoid antagonist RU 38486 (10^{-6} M) was present during the whole experiment, no differences were observed between neurons before (circles, $n = 6$) and after (open squares, $n = 9$) corticosterone treatment. (*Right*) Perfusion of the slices from ADX rats with 10^{-6} M (solid diamonds, $n = 9$) or 10^{-8} M (open diamonds, $n = 7$) of the selective glucocorticoid agonist RU 28362 (30 to 90 minutes before recording) increased the amplitude of the AHP significantly when compared with the AHP obtained in CA_1 neurons before exposure to the agonist (solid triangles, $n = 18$). The amplitude of the AHPs recorded after slices were exposed to 10^{-9} M RU 28362 ($n = 8$) was somewhat smaller but still significantly different from the controls ($p < 0.05$). With 10^{-10} M RU 28362 (open triangles, $n = 4$) the increases were not significant. Statistics were done with a multivariate analysis of variance test for repeated measurements. (From Joels and de Kloet, 1989, Effects of glucocorticoids and norepinephrine on the excitability in the hippocampus. Science 235, 1502. Copyright AAAS.)

that glucocorticoids do not directly disrupt the mechanics of calcium efflux, but rather disrupt the energetic fueling of efflux. This is consonant with the energetic flavor to the glucocorticoid endangerment (Elliott and Sapolsky, in preparation).

Thus, glucocorticoids appear to enhance a variety of indices of calcium activity in the hippocampus and, most relevant to the present discussion, enhance the calcium mobilization during at least one neurological insult. At present, we do not yet know whether the same occurs after other neurological insults. Moreover, we do not know whether other components of calcium trafficking are disrupted by glucocorticoids (i.e., calcium influx and mobilization from organelles) or which component(s) of efflux is inhibited (e.g., sodium/calcium exchange, activity of the calcium-ATPase). The critical point, however, is that glucocorticoids augment the levels of this damaging ion under both basal conditions and following at least one neurological insult.

Glucocorticoids and the Glutamatergic Synapse: Enhanced Calcium-induced Proteolysis

Regardless of which mechanisms contribute to the enhanced calcium signal, these findings predict that glucocorticoids should enhance some of the calcium-mediated degenerative events in the hippocampus during neurological insults. Our data support this prediction. As discussed in chapter 10, excessive calcium following EAA exposure in the hippocampus leads to proteolysis of spectrin, MAP2, and the amyloid precursor protein, as well as accumulation of tau- and ubiquitin-like immunoreactivity. (The similarity between these degenerative changes and the neuropathology of Alzheimer's disease is striking and will be discussed in chapter 14.) We are presently exploring whether glucocorticoids exacerbate the emergence of these degenerative markers following EAA exposure. We have observed that glucocorticoids enhance the breakdown of spectrin and augment the accumulation of tau-immunoactivity in the rat hippocampus following kainic acid exposure. Additionally, we observed that the glucocorticoid effect on spectrin proteolysis could be reversed by energy supplementation; the equivalent experiment has not been carried out examining tau immunoactivity (Elliott et al., submitted). Therefore, these data suggest that glucocorticoids, by exacerbating the EAA/calcium cascade, augment the most proximal known markers of neurodegeneration.

CONCLUSIONS

The preceding sections of this chapter suggest that by disrupting energetics within the hippocampus (in both neurons and glia), glucococorticoids exacerbate some of the features of the EAA/NMDA/calcium cascade, making neurons more likely to be killed. These are among the most speculative ideas presented in this book, and are based on the most recent and least replicated data. Therefore, they should be evaluated in that context.

In considering this model of glucocorticoid interaction with this degenerative cascade, a number of caveats and disclaimers should immediately be voiced:

1. While I believe that the data suggest that glucocorticoids exacerbate the EAA/NMDA/calcium cascade, none of the data suggests that this is the *sole* way that glucocorticoids exacerbate damage. The non-NMDA glutamatergic receptors are coming to be viewed as playing an increasingly important role in neuron death, and these may well also be sensitive to glucocorticoid actions (as might be mechanisms completely independent of EAAs). For example, glucocorticoids might, by enhancing the EAA signal in the synapse, very well increase the strength of an NMDA receptor-mediated signal in the post-synaptic neuron. However, the proximal mechanism by which this might be endangering could be via subsequent modification of non-NMDA receptor responsiveness to ligands (for which there is precedent in the long-term potentiation literature). In such a scenario, the glucocorticoid endangerment would indeed be NMDA receptor dependent (as we have reported; Armanini et al. 1990), while still involving other routes of damage.

2. While the data suggest that glucocorticoids endanger the neurons energetically, this need not be the *sole* route of endangerment. The strongest evidence in favor of an energetic role was that supplementing neurons with additional energy around the time of insults buffered them from the glucocorticoid synergy. Essentially, those experiments could have been carried out in one of two ways. First, if the hippocampus were given a great deal of excess energy substrates and the glucocorticoid endangerment lessened (without the toxicity of the insult itself changing), this implies that glucocorticoids are endangering through some energetic means. Second, if the *precise* amount of energy depleted by glucocorticoid exposure were replaced in the hippocampus and had no additional effect on the hippocampus, and the glucocorticoid endangerment were completely eliminated, this implies that glucocorticoids are endangering exclusively through some energetic means. The experiments carried out were of the relatively nonquantitative first scenario. They implied an energetic involvement, but did not eliminate nonenergetic mechanisms.

3. The glucocorticoid inhibition of glucose transport into hippocampal neurons and glia strikes me as the most plausible and best implicated mechanism by which the steroids might be energetically disruptive. However, nothing in the data implies that this is the *sole* route by which energetics are disrupted. Some of the (more speculative) additional routes were discussed earlier in this chapter.

Thus, while this chapter reviews the (very thin thread of) data linking glucocorticoid inhibition of glucose transport, disruption of hippocampal energetics and augmentation of the EAA/NMDA/calcium cascade, these links are not meant to exclude other routes of endangerment.

Some data have already emerged indicating that it is probably naive to overemphasize the glucose transport step of the story. I have already discussed the confusion that has arisen in the literature over the fact that glucocorticoids increase circulating glucose concentrations yet are catabolic for target tissues.

The idea I tried to emphasize is that just because there is a lot of potential energy in the circulation does not necessarily mean it will reach target tissues—if circulating glucose concentrations have risen (in part) because glucocorticoids are inhibiting their entry into target tissues, energy in the bloodstream does not translate into energy for cells. However, it is possible that I have taken that idea too far; a converse must be considered as well: Just because glucocorticoids inhibit glucose transport in the hippocampus, that does not necessarily mean that glucocorticoids must decrease glucose availability to those neurons. This is due to the magnitude of the inhibition of transport in peripheral tissues. In a rough way, the increase in circulating glucose concentrations should reflect the magnitude of the decrease in transport into target tissues plus the extent of hepatic gluconeogenesis. Such gluconeogenesis can be considerable, and the scale of inhibition of glucose transport in peripheral tissues by glucocorticoids can be quite large (for example, 60% to 70% inhibition in thymocytes [Munck 1971]). Thus, prolonged glucocorticoid exposure in rats can elevate circulating glucose concentrations as much as 60% (cf. Koide et al. 1986). In contrast, the steroids inhibit glucose transport only approximately 25% in the hippocampus. Therefore, conceivably, glucocorticoid actions in the periphery might bring about a sufficiently large increase in circulating glucose concentrations to override the milder inhibition of transport in the hippocampus.

This possibility was implied in the careful study of Koide and colleagues (1986), who reported that glucocorticoids exacerbate hypoxic-ischemic injury in the rat hippocampus. They also observed that under those circumstances, glucocorticoids partially *buffered* the hippocampus from the disruptive effects of hypoxia-ischemia upon total energy charge and concentrations of ATP, phosphocreatine, glucose, and glycogen (while greatly exacerbating lactate accumulation). Yet, the glucocorticoids still made damage worse. Moreover, infusing glucose (in an amount that matched the glucocorticoid-induced increase in circulating glucose concentrations) also protected the energy profile of the hippocampus, yet did not exacerbate lactate concentrations anywhere near as much as did glucocorticoids. These findings at least conflict with the spirit of our recent observation that glucocorticoids exacerbate the declines in ATP and glycogen concentrations in hippocampal astrocytic cultures subjected to anoxia and/or glucose reduction stores (Tombaugh et al., submitted). It is not yet clear how to resolve these somewhat conflicting sets of data. However, amid this confusion, probably the safest interpretation is that the inhibition of glucose transport by glucocorticoids cannot be the sole bottleneck accounting for the endangerment. There must be some rather powerful and catabolic effects of glucocorticoids far downstream from this point.

Leaving aside the intricacies of glucocorticoid effects on neuronal energetics, a number of recent studies reviewed in this chapter suggest that glucocorticoids ultimately exacerbate the EAA/calcium cascade. It seems to me that this shifts the phenomenon of glucocorticoid neurotoxicity from being a fairly obscure sideshow in neurology to being in the mainstream.

One feature of these interactions with the cascade emerges repeatedly in these studies and reflects, perhaps, the central idea of part II of this book. Consistently, glucocorticoids fail to do anything particularly catabolic or pathogenic on their own. This is supported by the demonstration that a broad range of enzymes and energetic processes in the hippocampus are not altered under basal, nonchallenged conditions by glucocorticoids (Meyer et al. 1979; Meyer 1985; McEwen et al. 1986) and the fact that glucocorticoids, on their own, tend to inhibit hippocampal electrophysiology (McEwen et al. 1986). It is only when the neurons are pummeled with a simultaneous neurological insult that the subtle glucocorticoid action becomes the last straw. These chapters are laden with notions of "synergy," "enhancement," "exacerbation," "augmentation," and so on. For example, glucocorticoids were shown to enhance the effect of kainic acid on aspartate accumulation and cytosolic calcium mobilization, to augment the decline in ATP and glucose concentrations in astrocytes during hypoxia, and to exacerbate seizure-induced cytoskeletal breakdown. This is fine and represents the mechanistic underpinnings that are neccesary to explain the basic observation of part II, namely that under all sorts of circumstances in which glucocorticoids are not directly damaging, they nevertheless compromise the ability of the hippocampus to survive neurological insults.

Yet, do these findings have any relevance to the cases where glucocorticoids are, indeed, directly toxic on their own? By this, I mean the issues of gradual glucocorticoid neurotoxicity in the hippocampus over the course of aging in the rat. Without having yet introduced the cellular biology of neuron death, this question was indirectly voiced at the end of chapter 7 (see figure 7.9). Is hippocampal neuron loss during aging an incremental and intrinsic process, where the smooth slope of decline is made steeper by glucocorticoids? Alternatively, is the senescent loss due to a series of punctate declining steps due to extremely small extrinsic insults, where glucocorticoids make the magnitude of each explicit downward step larger? In the latter scenario, the extrinsic insults could be tiny versions of the neurological disasters that have dominated the last three chapters. For example, animals are fed a bit later than usual, resulting in a slight hypoglcyemia, or an animal suffers a brief cerebral vasospasm, causing a mild transient hypoxia. In a young rat, these subtle insults might kill a single hippocampal neurons, whereas in an aged rat with elevated glucocorticoid exposure, two neurons die instead; the tiny downward step has just been magnified by glucocorticoids.

If the latter is what goes on in the aging hippocampus, the glucocorticoid interaction has exactly the same flavor of "synergy" and "exacerbation" as during these major neurological insults, merely writ small. However, it is not clear how much this punctate model of decline does indeed apply to hippocampal aging. What if glucocorticoids can in some cases kill neurons directly, independent of a coincident insult of even the most subtle nature. Are any glucocorticoid actions discussed in this chapter likely to be of relevance?

The only possibilities are those glucocorticoid effects on EAA and calcium trafficking that occur even in the absence of the neurological insults. Of these, only two were uncovered: Glucocorticoids were shown to elevate basal extracellular glutamate concentrations in the hippocampal microdialysis studies (i.e., prior to the kainic acid exposure). In addition, in cultured hippocampal neurons, glucocorticoids increased basal free cytosolic calcium concentrations (in addition to exacerbating the magnitude of the rise following kainic acid exposure). Interpretive problems exist with both. In the microdialysis study, it is questionable whether it is possible to measure basal concentrations of anything after inserting the relatively enormous dialysis probe; thus, the increased "basal" glutamate concentrations may instead represent glucocorticoids exacerbating trauma-induced release. In the case of the basal calcium concentrations, the glucocorticoid-induced elevation is rather small (less than a 40% increase). Either of these effects occurring in the hippocampus in vivo under truly basal conditions could represent a mechanism by which glucocorticoids are slowly neurotoxic on their own. Obviously, this will be rather difficult to test.

A second theme of the glucocorticoid interaction with hippocampal energetics and the EAA/NMDA/calcium cascade is the magnitude of the hormone effects. In general, the EAA/NMDA/calcium cascade during hypoxia-ischemia, seizure, and hypoglycemia is anything but subtle—these are massive insults, the extent of energy depletion is often profound, the accumulation of EAAs can be enormous, and so on. In contrast, I suspect that individual steps by which glucocorticoids are endangering, when fully understood, will be extremely subtle. The pieces understood already support this view: The inhibition of glucose transport is far smaller than in peripheral tissues; the change in the affinity of astrocytic glutamate uptake is demonstrable but not dramatic; the same applies to the glucocorticoid enhancement of EAA concentrations in the synapse, the effects on basal free cytosolic calcium concentrations and on spectrin breakdown. To date, only the exacerbation of free cytosolic calcium accumulation following kainic acid exposure seems particularly dramatic. I have every expectation that any additional steps modulated by glucocorticoids (e.g., enhanced EAA release, impaired neuronal reuptake of EAAs) will be just as minimal. Once again, I suspect that many or most of these effects will not be demonstrable under basal condtiions, but only when the neurons are being challenged by a coincident insult.

This makes things immensely difficult to study, as effects will often be lost in the noise of imperfect techniques. However, it makes a great deal of sense, teleologically. The glucocorticoids are endangering, rather than being outright fatal, and the most plausible mechanism that dominates the endangerment—induction of a mild energy problem—is likely to perturb many systems only slightly. Glucocorticoids probably do not kill neurons directly; instead, they probably just kick at their proverbial ankles repeatedly during a time when the neurons already have enough problems. During a crisis, even a mild amount of kicking at ankles makes it more likely that the neuron will ultimately topple over. While perhaps a misery to study, it is still intellectually pleasing to explore something subtle within a neurological landscape that is, far too often, so tragically unsubtle. In the final part of the book, I explore what interventions this knowledge may afford us in decreasing neurodegeneration during aging and following neurological insults, and whether these findings are likely to apply to the human.

CHAPTER SUMMARY

In this chapter, I present a synthesis of how glucocorticoids endanger the hippocampus; the conclusion is that, by disrupting neuronal energetics, the glucocorticoids exacerbate the EAA/NMDA/calcium cascade of damage.

In reviewing the biochemical and physiological effects of glucocorticoids in the brain, a few that could potentially play a role in endangering the hippo-campus can be eliminated. One concerns the induction, by glucocorticoids, of the enzyme *glutamine synthetase*. As discussed previously, some of the gluta-mate released into the synapse as a neurotransmitter can be removed via the glial, rather than neuronal route. Such glutamate is rapidly converted within glial astrocytes to glutamine by glutamine synthetase. The glutamine is then repatriated to the presynaptic neuron, where it is converted back to glutamate. The conversion can be viewed as a means to "deactivate" the dangerous glutamate and transfer it back to the neuron in the more benign form of glutamine. Importantly, estimates are that the majority of glutamate is cycled through this glial route, and glutamine synthetase is the rate-limiting enzyme in this process. Therefore, enhancement of glutamine synthetase levels should enhance the supply of glutamate to the synapse. The fact that glucocorticoids induce that enzyme immediately suggests that the steroids exacerbate the EAA cascade by enhancing the delivery of precursor glutamine to neurons. However, this glucocorticoid induction appears to be a developmental phe-nomenon; under conditions where glucocorticoids exacerbate hippocampal damage in the adult in vivo, they fail to increase activity of the enzyme.

A second route by which glucocorticoids might modulate neuronal damage after these insults, is their *inhibition of edema*. Such edema can occur after global ischemia or seizure, and it can be damaging. This leads to the prediction that glucocorticoids should *decrease* neuronal damage after these insults (and this, indeed, is the basis for their use in clinical neurology). However, there are two types of edema, vascular and cellular, and while glucocorticoids are efficacious against the former, it is the latter which occasionally occurs after seizure or hypoxia-ischemia.

A variety of glucocorticoid actions might *modulate the generation and toxicity of oxygen radicals*. Because glucocorticoids can enhance calcium mobilization in neurons and disrupt them metabolically, the steroids should enhance oxidative damage. Because glucocorticoids can inhibit prostaglandin synthesis and can intercalate into membranes and stabilize them against peroxidative attack, the steroids should decrease oxidative damage. These opposing trends can be reconciled when considering the mechanisms and dose requirements for these various effects. Within the physiologic range of glucocorticoid concentrations utilized in the various studies in these preceding chapters, the deleterious effects of glucocorticoids predominate. When supraphysiologic megadoses of glucocorticoids are used in cases of oxidative neurological insults that do not endanger the hippocampus (e.g., spinal cord injury), the steroids are quite protective. In cases where the oxidative insult dose involve the hippocampus (e.g., brain trauma), the trends cancel each other out and the steroid is neither particularly protective nor endangering.

There are also biochemical effects of glucocorticoids that may bear relevance to the endangerment but which have not yet been tested for the possibility. For example, in the hippocampus, glucocorticoids induce the protein *synapsin I*, which helps regulate vesicular release of neurotransmitters, including EAAs. The relevance of this is not clear, since it is not the quantity, but the phosphorylation state of the protein that modulates vesicular release. As another example, glucocorticoids induce the expression of *calbindin D-28K*, an important calcium-binding protein. As was reviewed in an earlier chapter, this protein can bind cytosolic calcium that might otherwise contribute to neuron death, and levels of calbindin D-28K correlate with neuronal survival during various insults. Thus, an induction of this protein by glucocorticoids might be a route of neuronal protection. However, the time course of the induction is rather slow and does not occur rapidly enough to be relevant to the demonstrated glucocorticoid synergies with various insults. Finally, some very recent work suggests that *nitric oxide* may play an important neuromodulatory role in glutamatergic synapses, one with potentially a great deal of relevance of excitotoxicity. In peripheral tissues, glucocorticoids inhibit the induction of the rate-limiting enzyme for nitric oxide. If the same were to occur in the brain, glucocorticoids might modulate the workings of glutamatergic synapses by this route. At present, it is quite confused whether nitric oxide is likely to increase or decrease excitotoxicity; thus, the consequences of any putative glucocorticoids effects on nitric oxide in the brain is highly speculative.

Therefore, a variety of mediators of the glucocorticoid endangerment of the hippocampus can be eliminated or at least deemphasized. The remainder of the chapter suggests the most plausible link between the biochemistry of glucocorticoid actions in the hippocampus and the glucocorticoid endangerment. I suggest that glucocorticoids exacerbate the EAA/NMDA/calcium cascade of degeneration outlined in chapters 9 and 10. Specifically, glucocorticoids disrupt hippocampal energetics, most plausibly by inhibiting glucose transport. This produces a mild energy deficit in neurons, one that is readily survived under normal circumstances. However, when this deficit occurs at the time of an insult that invokes the EAA/NMDA/calcium cascade, various steps of the cascade are augmented because of the energy deficit.

This model is introduced by reviewing how glucocorticoids *disrupt hippocampal energetics*. This makes sense—all of the neurological insults that are exacerbated by glucocorticoids constitute energetic crises for the neuron, in that they either involve pathologic demands for energy (seizure) or disruption of energy production (hypoxia-ischemia and hypoglycemia). This suggests that glucocorticoids augment their toxicity by exacerbating the energy crisis. If true, the glucocorticoid synergy with these insults should be reduced with energy supplementation. This has been shown both in vivo and in vitro, using substrates such as excess glucose, mannose, or ketones.

Recent work has demonstrated a possible mechanism by which glucocorticoids disrupt hippocampal neuronal energetics and thus impair the ability of the neurons to survive these energetic insults. For decades, endocrinologists have known that glucocorticoids *inhibit glucose transport* in numerous peripheral tissues (an effect that makes sense in the larger context of the teleology of the stress-response). The same occurs in the brain, with the hippocampus being the region most sensitive to this effect. The inhibition occurs both in vivo and in vitro, and in both neurons and glia. Transport is inhibited about 20% to 30% and in peripheral tissues, a number of mediating molecular mechanisms have been identified.

At present, there are a number of additional routes by which glucocorticoids might disrupt hippocampal energetics, although these have just begun to be studied. Collectively, glucocorticoids cause a significant decrease in hippocampal glial glycogen stores. While it is not yet clear whether they effect neuronal energy substrates (e.g., ATP and/or phosphocreatine) as well, glucocorticoids accelerate the decline in hippocampal metabolism following EAA exposure.

When recalling the emphasis of chapter 10, this ability of glucocorticoids to disrupt hippocampal energetics immediately suggests that glucocorticoids *exacerbate the EAA/NMDA/calcium cascade*. Very recent data support this hypothesis. The glucocorticoid endangerment is NMDA receptor dependent. This is at least partially due to glucocorticoids *exacerbating the accumulation of EAAs in the synapse* after an insult such as seizure. This enhanced accumulation could be due to enhanced EAA release or to impaired EAA removal from the synapse. To date, only the latter has been examined, and glucocorticoids have been shown to *impair astrocytic glutamate uptake* in an energy-dependent manner.

To continue working through the steps of the EAA/calcium cascade, if glucocorticoids enhance EAA concentrations in the synapse during these neurological insults, they should *enhance calcium mobilization* in the postsynaptic neuron, and this has been demonstrated recently. The steroids increase the height and duration of EAA-induced calcium mobilization in vitro. This effect is energetic, as it can be reduced by glucose supplementation and mimicked by glucose deprivation. This appears to involve a glucocorticoid inhibition of calcium efflux during a depolarizing challenge. Furthermore, glucocorticoids cause a mild but significant increase in free cytosolic calcium concentrations in cultured hippocampal neurons under even basal conditions.

As a final prediction, if glucocorticoids exacerbate calcium mobilization during excitotoxic insults, then they should *exacerbate the degenerative consequences of excess calcium*. In support of this idea, glucocorticoids enhance kainic acid–induced proteolysis of the cytoskeletal protein spectrin and enhance the accumulation of tau antigenicity. Furthermore, energy supplementation will reverse the glucocorticoid effect on tau (the equivalent experiment with spectrin has not yet been carried out).

In summary, glucocorticoids disrupt hippocampal energetics and, as a result, impair the trafficking of EAAs and calcium during these neurological insults. In this manner, the steroids might exacerbate the toxicity of these insults. It should be emphasized that this model is speculative and based on very recent data. Moreover, the effects are quite small—the glucocorticoid inhibition of glucose transport is far smaller than in peripheral tissue, and the glucocorticoid effects on EAA and calcium trafficking are, for the most part, quite small. This makes a considerable amount of sense—glucocorticoids are probably not directly fatal to hippocampal neurons, but instead endanger them. This fits with the picture of the hormone causing a mild disruption of a variety of steps of EAA and calcium trafficking. To use a metaphor, glucocorticoids do not so much kill hippocampal neurons as repeatedly kick them in the ankles when they are distracted with some serious problems. During such a crisis, even a mild amount of kicking at ankles makes it more likely that the neuron will topple.

III   How Depressing Is All of This?

12

Individual Differences and Adrenocortical Function: Why Do Some Individuals Secrete More Glucocorticoids Than Others?

SUMMARY OF THE BOOK SO FAR

Various stressors trigger the endocrine and neural adaptations known as the stress-response. Glucocorticoid secretion is central to such adaptations and typifies the two-edged nature of the stress-response: While glucocorticoids are essential for surviving short-term physical stressors, prolonged glucocorticoid exposure is pathogenic in a variety of ways.

Part I examined how the regulation of glucocorticoid secretion is impaired during aging, and how excessive exposure to glucocorticoids over the lifetime can accelerate aspects of brain aging. The data reviewed combine to form a model, termed the *glucocorticoid cascade*. It attempts to link two features of aging rats—hypersecretion of glucocorticoids and degeneration of neurons in the hippocampus. The hippocampus is shown to be an important mediator of glucocorticoid feedback inhibition, such that its senescent degeneration causes glucocorticoid hypersecretion. Glucocorticoids, in turn, are shown to damage hippocampal neurons. These two regulatory features combine to form a feed-forward cascade during aging—glucocorticoids damage the hippocampus, which causes further glucocorticoid secretion (and numerous deleterious consequences for the aged rat, including further hippocampal damage).

Part II presented a model by which glucocorticoids damage the hippocampus. The hormones are shown not to necessarily be toxic as much as endangering, in that they impair the capacity of neurons to survive coincident neurological insults, such as hypoxia-ischemia, seizure, hypoglycemia, antimetabolites, and oxygen radicals. Therefore, glucocorticoids may not only play an important role in accelerating hippocampal damage during aging, but might also exacerbate some of the most common neurological insults to the hippocampus.

I reviewed how these neurological insults can become toxic by activating a cascade, in which there is excessive synaptic accumulation of excitatory amino acid (EAA) neurotransmitters. This may cause excessive postsynaptic mobilization of free cytosolic calcium which, in turn, causes various degenerative events in cells. Critically, these insults are energetic in nature, and a paucity of energy will impair the ability of the hippocampus to properly control the trafficking of EAAs and of calcium. It is shown that glucocorticoids can disrupt hippocampal neuronal energetics (most plausibly by inhibiting glucose transport in the hippocampus) and, thus, exacerbate this degenerative EAA/calcium cascade.

The model developed in chapter 11 regarding the mechanisms of glucocorticoid endangerment of the hippocampus is the most speculative section of this book, based on the most recent (and sparse) data. While this model as to how glucocorticoids cause damage may prove entirely incorrect, the evidence seems reasonably strong that endangerment and also irreversible damage can occur in the face of heavy glucocorticoid exposure. This is rather depressing and raises the question regarding the inevitability of such degeneration. This and the following chapter approach these issues. This chapter examines individual differences in glucocorticoid secretion. How do differences in genetics, behavior, and early experience change adrenocortical function, and what neuroendocrine mechanisms mediate those changes? Do organisms with less cumulative glucocorticoid secretion show less senescent hippocampal degeneration? What manipulations are available over the lifetime to alter the gradual impact of glucocorticoids on hippocampal senescence? In the following chapter, the emphasis will be different. There, the question is: What can be done immediately following a neurological insult to decrease the endangering effects of glucocorticoids?

In some ways, the present chapter bears a certain resemblance to the self-help books that have festered in the psychology sections of bookstores. By exploring the degree of and sources of variability in glucocorticoid secretion among individuals, it indirectly asks what can be done to help ourselves—can we manipulate the adrenocortical axis in order to produce less pathogenic profiles of glucocorticoid secretion? A critical place to begin is to understand how psychological variables can modulate the stress-response.

WHY IS PSYCHOLOGICAL STRESS STRESSFUL?

The most obvious reason why two organisms might differ in the amount of glucocorticoids they secrete is if they differ in the amount of stressors to which they are exposed. Superficially, that might seem straightforward or even trivial, and not the level of analysis that is likely to be of importance. It would appear that we can move to the next level of analysis—two organisms perceive a stressor and then differ in the strength and duration of the neuroendocrine mechanisms with which they respond to the stressor. This carefully worded leap to the next level of analysis was a mistake that dominated the first decades of stress physiology. Yes, organisms will differ as to how much stress they experience, and that will give rise to individual differences in endocrine responses, but that is obvious and dull. It would seem that the only interesting question is, once having perceived the same stressor, how can organisms then differ in their responses? What was just leaped over, of course, is the intervening step—two organisms rarely *perceive* the same external events to be equally stressful. My bias is that this difference accounts for the bulk of individual differences in adrenocortical activity—that is to say, it is not so much a question of why organisms respond differently to a stressor, but why organisms differ as to whether they perceive an event to be stressful in the first place.

In retrospect, it is logical why that kind of idea was not at the forefront of stress physiology's early years. If you are studying a phenomenon that is new, uncertain, of questioned importance or replicability, the scientific reflex is to study it under extreme conditions. In effect, if you can't observe it then, don't bother with more subtle cases. Therefore, the early stress physiologists tended to study the physiological and pathophysiological responses to major physical perturbations of homeostasis. The dominant view was that of Selye's, namely, that a stressor is something that throws an organism out of homeostasis, and the stress-response is the set of nonspecific bodily reactions that help to reestablish homeostasis.

Selye's first generation of intellectual descendents were physiologists at heart, and they examined the sensitivity of the stress-response to different physiological stressors—hypoglycemia, hypotension, hemorrhage, pain, surgical incision, and so on. Some of the researchers were very mechanistic, coming from a bioengineering orientation, and careful studies tested the sensitivity of the system to different magnitudes of perturbation. For example, if hemorrhage causes glucocorticoid secretion (as part of the stress-response), can the adrenocortical axis differentiate between loss of 5%, 10%, and 15% of blood volume? The answer has generally been yes (reviewed in chapter 2). Can the system differentiate between an identical magnitude of blood loss but with a difference in the speed with which it happens? The answer there also turned out to be yes, indicating the capacity of the adrenocortical axis to calculate rate of change as well as magnitude of change (Gann 1969). The work on negative feedback regulation showed that the adrenocortical axis is differentially sensitive to absolute levels of signal versus rate of change of signal, to absolute versus relative rates of change, and so on (Dallman and Yates 1969).

These were pleasing times for the bioengineer, as the adrenocortical axis turned out to be immensely more complicated than anyone had guessed but tractable, understandable, in this rational manner. Many years after that golden era, when it comes to neuroendocrine systems, the adrenocortical axis remains the sweetheart of bioengineering modelers (cf. Yates 1981). Stressors were perturbers of homeostasis, and the stress-response was turning out to be wonderfully complex, sensitive, yet rational in measuring just how much of a perturbation there was. In that framework, it would be obvious how the question of individual differences would be approached. Two organisms are stressed to an equivalent extent—identical magnitude of hemorrhage, identical pattern and severity of exposure to electric shocks—yet they differ in their glucocorticoid secretion in response. The rational response must be that those individual differences arise from some mechanistic difference in rates of steroid synthesis, clearance rates, receptor levels for hormones, and so on.

One simple experiment, of a large number that could be chosen, bursts that lucid mechanistic bubble. Two rats are exposed to identical stressors—intermittent electric shocks. They receive the same pattern and intensity of shocks. The two differ in only one way. One rat receives a signal indicating when the shock session has ended. That individual secretes far less corticosterone than its conspecific. Nothing in the mechanistic world of measuring the extent of perturbation induced by the stressor itself could have predicted that finding (Weiss 1971b,c).

To expand Selye's world, the experiment just discussed shows that the stress-response not only consists of the adaptations triggered by a perturbation, but are also those triggered by our belief that a perturbation is *about to happen*. This is a very different picture. We have some intuitive feeling for these ideas. When we have a stress-response in anticipation of a perturbation that is indeed about to happen, we often call it conditioned fear. When it is anticipating a perturbation that is, in fact, not about to occur, we call it anxiety neurosis, or irrational fear.

These experiments opened up a new world in stress physiology. The stress-response, when triggered by homeostatic perturbations, can be modulated by the psychological settings in which they occur. Soon, it became apparent that purely psychological stressors could activate the system as well. The hormones of the stress-response were shown to change in response to bereavement, difficult cognitive tasks, conditioned fear, and so on (Mason 1975a,b). In a classic series of studies that covered hundreds of pages of a single celebrated issue of *Psychosomatic Medicine*, John Mason and colleagues studied nonhuman primates given sustained cognitive tasks and methodically examined essentially all of the endocrine systems that were, at that time, recognized as being responsive to physical stressors. The verdict was clear— the system was just as responsive to psychological stressors as to physical stressors (summarized in Mason, 1968). In a particularly expansive state of mind, it was argued by some that Selye's treasured stress-response was, in fact, *only* triggered by psychological stressors (Mason 1975a,b). In this view, injury, pain, forced exercise, hypotension, and so on, are stressful because they all typically trigger the same psychological associations—senses of lack of control and of predictability.

The old guard of stress physiology was not amused, particularly Selye. A lot of that period was spent in debate between the two factions, often in single-warrior combat between Selye and Mason (cf. Mason 1975a,b; Selye 1975). The physiological school was forced to give a lot of ground and finally contented itself with holding onto the view that at least *some* stressors had no psychological component. As a prime example, they would cite that the stress-response was provoked quite robustly by a surgical incision made in an anesthetized organism. As another example, they would cite the newly developed technique for surgically isolating the hypothalamus by making a circular cut around the structure (using the Halasz knife). If glucocorticoid secretion was always a response of the brain, in effect, perceiving a psychological stressor, there should be no secretion in animals with isolated hypothalami. Yet, there would still be (at least some) adrenocortical activity triggered by stressors such as ether, tourniquet shock, or formalin injection (Selye 1975). The psychologists would return with examples where the magnitude of a stress-response to the same physiological perturbation would vary enormously as psychological variables were manipulated.

In smug retrospect, it is obvious how the system is sensitive to both physiological and psychological factors and to their rich interactions. It is also obvious why, at the time, the psychological data were so distressing to the physiologists. In its early period, the psychological school and the data base that it was generating must have seemed so, well, messy, unsystematic, ad hoc, and anecdotal. Data poured in from all sorts of odd quarters: parents of children with cancer; rats receiving electric shocks with and without warning lights; soldiers about to face battle in Vietnam urinating in Dixie cups for researchers; social primates having their ranks manipulated; people in nursing homes having their lunch schedules manipulated. No wonder the bioengineers were horrified—the nice clean carpet was being muddied by some mongol horde of psychologists.

Not surprisingly, the psychobiological components of stress have become less threatening to the purer physiological school as the former has acquired the beginnings of wrinkles and gray hair and some table manners. Essentially, there has been enough time for the data base concerning the psychobiology of stress to mature and grow, and for some clarity and systematization to emerge. These studies have made it possible to answer the question, What is stressful about psychological stress? It appears to include a lack of control, lack of predictability, lack of outlets for frustration, and a perception that circumstances are worsening. Other terms and constructs have been used in the field, but these encompass many of the important ideas.

The issue of *loss of control* is at the forefront of psychological stress. In a classic experimental style pioneered by Jay Weiss, rats were subjected to intermittent electric shocks. One rat would have control over the situation, being able to press a level in order to decrease the rate of shocks to a certain extent. The second rat was yoked to the first, receiving whatever pattern and intensity of shocks the first received, but without the control. Over a wide range of shock schedules, the lack of control was associated with higher corticosterone secretion and a greater likelihood of formation of gastric erosions (Weiss 1971a,b,c, 1984; Davis et al. 1977; Swenson and Vogel 1983). Similar studies, with glucocorticoid secretion as an endpoint, have been carried out with nonhuman primates (Hanson et al. 1976), dogs (Dess-Beech et al. 1983), and humans (Brier et al. 1987). As a subtle elaboration, if a rat has been trained to actively avoid a shock and is then prevented from making that avoidance behavior, there is adrenocortical activation, even if no shock is actually delivered (Coover et al. 1973). Here, loss of control is a trigger, even in the absence of an external physical stressor.

Similarly, *lack of predictability* is a major stimulant of the adrenocortical axis. If rats were given a signal indicating the impending delivery of a shock, the adrenocortical response was lessened, as compared to rats who could not predict the stressor (Weiss 1984). Similarly, as noted, smaller adrenocortical responses were seen in rats given a signal indicating the end of the shock period (Hennessy et al. 1977). In both of these experiments, inserting the signal allowed a rat to predict when a shock was and was not about to occur, and thus, when it could let down its vigilance. Similar studies have been shown with dogs (Dess-Beech et al. 1983). In these studies, glucocorticoid concentrations vary two- to threefold between groups.

Some have considered the components of control and predictability to combine to form any of a number of larger categories. Some have emphasized that both conditions share the trait of the outcome being *discrepant with expectations*, or in other words, *novel*. That is surely the case with a lack of predictability, when one does not know what to expect, or under conditions of loss of control, where responses that previously worked no longer do (Levine et al. 1989). This has been studied in rodents who were trained to expect water after pressing a lever. When that expectation failed to be met, corticosterone secretion increased (Levine et al. 1972; Coover 1983; Coe et al. 1983). This seems very explicable in the context of loss of both control and predictability, and numerous other studies show similar results whenever reinforcement schedules are altered.

This has also been seen in nonhuman primates. In general, infant primates, when separated from their mothers, elevate glucocorticoid secretion. Moreover, placing them in a social group will inhibit that stress-response. To some, this has suggested the important calming influence of members of one's species, regardless of who they are. Subsequent study has shown that the critical thing here is that they be familiar, and not merely members of one's own species. Therefore, placing of infant squirrel monkeys into a novel social group not only does not prevent the stress response, but adds to it (Levine et al. 1989). Identical findings emerge with studies of adult primates placed in novel social settings (reviewed in Sapolsky 1992c). In a demonstration of the importance of novelty in humans, young men going through parachuting training were studied. With their first jump, a robust stress-response was observed in almost every endocrine system examined, both at the time of the jump itself and in anticipation of the event. With subsequent jumps, however, the magnitude of the anticipatory stress-response declined until eventually there was a response only at the time of the jump. This was interpreted as showing the importance of novelty as a stimulus (Levine 1978).

Some have also emphasized that loss of control or predictability cause *arousal* or *vigilance*, and that this is the primary stimulus on both the adrenocortical axis and sympathetic catecholamines (Hennessy and Levine 1979). It is easy to understand this conceptualization. Loss of control over an aversive stimulus immediately demands vigilance and arousal, as one searches for the new rules of control, while loss of the ability to predict when an aversive event will take place commands arousal and vigilance as well. Others have emphasized that circumstances in which there is loss of control and/or predictability indicate *loss of feedback* of information (Weiss 1971a,b,c). One can see the similarity of themes in these different emphases.

A number of studies have touted the importance of *outlets for frustration*. This can be shown in studies in which rats receive electric shocks and one individual has an outlet, such as being able to chew on a stick of wood. That individual typically has a significantly smaller corticosterone stress response and less of a chance of developing ulcers than does the rat without that outlet

(Levine et al. 1989). Various outlets include being able to displace aggression by attacking a conspecific (Azrin et al. 1966), being allowed a consummatory event such as eating or drinking at the time of the stressor, or being allowed a physical outlet such as access to a running wheel (Levitsky and Collier 1968; Gray et al. 1978; Levine et al. 1979; Heybach and Vernikos-Danellis 1979). This has been shown in other mammals as well (Dantzer and Moremede 1981) and appears to be independent of the physical features of the outlet itself (Levine et al. 1989); thus, it is probably not the particular outlet or coping strategy, but its effectiveness that is critical in attenuating the stress-response (Ur 1991).

Stress psychobiology has progressed far enough to allow the asking of some of the more subtle, elegant questions of the physiological school. For example, When the stress-response is triggered by psychological stressors, is it in an all-or-none fashion, or is it sensitive to the magnitude of the psychological variable in a dose-response manner? Much as with physiological stressors, there appears to be a dose-response relationship. For example, when a rat is placed into a novel cage, the greater the difference between that cage and the home cage, the greater the adrenocortical activation (Hennessy and Levine 1979; Hennessy et al. 1979). Similar results have emerged from studies of primates as well (Levine et al. 1989).

In summary, not only can the adrenocortical axis be triggered by purely psychological stressors in a sensitive linear fashion, but the stressfulness of a physical stressor can be altered considerably by the psychological setting in which it occurs. These ideas are now generally accepted, and the concentration on control, predictability, outlets for frustration, and forming of social support is the backbone of stress management therapy. What remains surprising, perhaps, when reviewing the literature is the strength of these effects. The stress-response, and especially the adrenocortical axis, is exquisitely sensitive to psychological manipulation. It is now time to examine some individual differences in adrenocortical function that probably reflect differences in these psychological factors. I will first review how glucocorticoid levels vary as a function of the social rank of the animal within a dominance hierarchy. Next, I will examine how adrenocortical function can also vary as a function of personality (in this case, of the individual, rather than of the neuron, as in my unorthodox usage in chapter 10).

SOCIAL STATUS, PERSONALITY, AND ADRENOCORTICAL FUNCTION

The Phenomenon of Social Dominance

Regardless of how rich an ecosystem might be, its resources are finite and are typically divided unevenly. Resource competition is central to much of animal behavior, taking various forms—niche separation, optimal foraging strategies, territoriality. Among the solutions evolved by numerous social species is the phenomenon of social dominance. Pairs of individuals, in their dyadic interactions, are not equally likely to obtain a disputed resource. Critically, this asymmetry need not be reestablished by overt aggression each time something is contested. Instead, a status quo emerges with a recognition of the inequality of the two. This inequality is usually signaled with ritualized displays of dominance or subordinance. The former typically involve stylized elements of threat—displaying of dangerous canines, semilunges, chest-thumping, so on (depending, obviously, on the species), while the latter suggests submission—crouching, fear-grimacing, averting eyes, rolling onto one's back.

The power of the status quo of inequalities in these dyads is demonstrated frequently. For example, two primates approach a bush full of ripe fruits at the same time. In the absence of the recognized status quo, there would be a fight to determine primacy. Instead, the status quo typically holds sway—the higher ranking animal will give a threat gesture, the subordinate will move away without having fed. The advantages to ritualizing the inequalities, instead of having to retest them each time, are clear. Early theorizing about the evolution of social behavior focused on "group selectionist" models, asking how such patterns are for the good of the species (cf. Wynne-Edwards 1962). This style of thinking has been largely discredited by sociobiological thinking, and the current emphasis is on selection for the individual and its kin (Hamilton 1964). In this context, ritualized asymmetries are adaptive, even for the subordinate individual—if one is not going to get any of the ripe fruit anyway, better to simply walk away than to have that outcome follow a taxing, potentially injurious fight. Such a system is evolutionarily logical only if the status quo is tested intermittently—every now and then, the subordinate animal should provoke overt aggression, just in case the direction of inequality in the dyad has shifted.

In summary, within social species, individuals within the group typically "know" where they stand with respect to other individuals. Out of these dyads come dominance hierarchies, with the highest ranking individual dominating in the most dyads, the second highest in the second most, and so on. Such hierarchies can be fairly linear (A dominates B dominates C...) or can have circularities embedded in them (A dominates B dominates C dominates A), and can involve coalitions (A dominates B, only with the assistance of C...). Hierarchies can encompass both sexes or be sex specific, can be expressed only at certain times, can remain static for long periods of time, or be in frequent states of flux. These hierarchies, and their psychological implications, are richest when occurring among social primates; I will devote most of the discussion here to them.

The most striking thing about dominance hierarchies among primates is how defining one's social rank is. The quality of one's life differs tremendously depending on where one stands in the hierarchy. When it is a stable one, the daily life for subordinate animals is filled with a great deal of social stress. The stressors reflect many of the themes of psychological stress. A subordinate individual may carefully search for a tuberous root to eat, sit and dig it out of the ground, clean it off—only to have it taken away at the last second by a dominant individual. This might occur repeatedly during a day. During dry seasons, when food resources become limited, this can mean considerably more time spent each day to get one's calories, or can even mean insufficient calories. During mid-day's heat, a subordinate individual may find a spot of shade, only to be displaced from it repeatedly. When individuals are grooming socially, it is the subordinate one who is least likely to be groomed and whose grooming bouts are most likely to be disrupted. When males are in sexual consortships with sexually receptive females, it is subordinate males whose liaisons are most likely to be harassed and disrupted. Finally, as an extremely important route of social stress for the subordinate, primates excell at displaced aggression—a high-ranking individual, after losing a fight, often attacks a subordinate bystander without warning. Such attacks can cause serious injury. This implies that even a subordinate individual who attempts to remove him or herself from the most stressful social competition can still get pulled into someone else's problems (for masterly discussions of the intricacies of social dominance in apes and Old World primates, see de Waal 1982, Goodall 1986, and Smuts 1986).

Therefore, life for a subordinate animal is filled with problems that can range from petty harassment, in which one's nose is rubbed rudely in one's lack of social status, to extremely serious forms of menace—unpredictable and injurious attacks, insufficient food, inability to depend on finding a safe spot when a predator attacks. Collectively, these social stressors incorporate many features of psychological stress—lack of control, of predictability, and of outlets for frustration.

Glucocorticoid Secretion in Subordinate Individuals

This portrait of social subordinance and its stressfulness suggests that low rank should be associated with adrenocortical hyperactivity. Many studies of captive primates living in stable dominance hierarchies have shown this, with subordinate animals having elevated basal cortisol concentrations (Keverne et al. 1982, Herbert et al. 1986, for talapoin monkeys; Manogue et al. 1975, for squirrel monkeys), a sluggish secretory response to stress (Manogue et al. 1975), and enlarged adrenals (Shively and Kaplan 1984, for fascicularis macaques). As a complement to the more traditional laboratory approaches, I have studied these issues with male olive baboons living freely in the Serengeti Ecosystem of East Africa. Each year, I abandon my Stanford laboratory for the summer months and return to the same troop of individuals, studying their physiology and behavior. For such study, I must anesthetize animals, using a blowgun, under highly controlled conditions. These include that the anesthetic itself not affect the hormones under study; that all animals be darted at the same time of day to control for circadian rhythms; that no one be darted who has recently been injured, had a fight, mated, or been sick, to avoid taking samples at a time when basal values are distorted; that animals be darted unawares, so that there is no anticipatory stress prior to darting; and that the

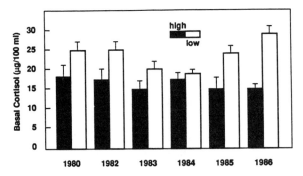

Figure 12.1. Low-ranking male baboons have elevated basal cortisol concentrations. Basal cortisol concentrations of the six highest-ranking and six lowest-ranking males in each of 6 years of study of a population of wild olive baboons. Total number of males under study per year ranged from 12 to 16. Values are derived from a single anesthetization per animal per season. (From Sapolsky, 1989, Arch Gen Psychiatry 46, 1047.)

first blood sample be taken within a few minutes of the onset of the stressful anesthetic effects, so that the sample's cortisol concentrations reflect basal values (see Sapolsky 1982, for validation of some of these controls). Among these animals, social subordinance is associated with elevated cortisol concentrations (Sapolsky, 1989; figure 12.1). Moreover, subordinate animals are also sluggish in elevating cortisol concentrations with the onset of stress (Sapolsky 1982). Elevated basal glucocorticoid concentrations have been observed among subordinate individuals in species other than primates, including mice (Davis and Christian 1957; Southwick and Bland 1959; Bronson and Eleftheriou 1964; Louch and Higginbotham 1967; Archer 1970; Schuhr 1987), rats (Barnett 1955; Popova and Naumenko 1972; Sakai et al. 1991), wolves (Fox and Andrews 1973), tree shrews (Uno et al. 1991), and even salmon (Ejike and Schreck 1980).

Mechanisms Underlying the Hypersecretion in Subordinate Animals

If the hypercortisolism of subordinate primates is due to their being exposed to more stressors, then it should originate at the level of the brain, rather than from peripheral dysfunction (for example, enhanced adrenal sensitivity to ACTH). My studies support this idea. Obviously, the easiest way to answer whether the hypercortisolism of subordinance is driven at the CNS level is to simply measure hypophysial-portal concentrations of CRF, vasopressin, oxytocin, and so on, and just as obviously, this cannot be measured in these long-term study subjects (much as it is impossible to study the hypercortisolism of depression or anorexia in humans in this manner, as will be discussed in the final chapter). Instead, one must implicate the CNS indirectly by eliminating the other possible causes of the hypercortisolism.

As a first possible alternative mechanism, there could be elevated concentrations of cortisol in the circulation of subordinate animals, not because of enhanced secretion of the hormone, but because of impaired clearance. This was eliminated as a possibility with the demonstration that the clearance rate of ^{3}H-cortisol does not differ by rank (Sapolsky 1983a). Therefore, the focus shifts to hypersecretion of cortisol in subordinate animals. This could be due to the adrenals being stimulated with excessive amounts of ACTH, to enhanced adrenal sensitivity to ACTH, or both. This could be answered most directly by measuring basal ACTH concentrations and seeing if they are elevated in subordinate individuals (as they are in many hypercortisolemic human depressives [Kalin et al. 1982; Reus et al. 1982; Herevanian et al. 1983]). This is not possible, however. While it takes perhaps 5 minutes for basal concentrations of cortisol to be changed by stress, making it possible to obtain a first "basal" sample in these baboons within a few minutes of anesthetic effects, ACTH changes more rapidly than that (within seconds). Therefore, it is not possible to determine basal concentrations of the peptide directly. Therefore, I challenged high- and low-ranking individuals with ACTH concentrations over the physiologic range. Both groups secreted cortisol in an equivalent pattern, implying that the hypercortisolism of the subordinate males was driven by excessive ACTH, rather than by excessive adrenal sensitivity to ACTH (Sapolsky 1990a). As will be discussed in the final chapter, this lack of an adrenal component differs from the data concerning the hypercortisolism in human depressives.

The possible cause of hypersecretion was thus moved to the level of ACTH secretion. The hypersecretion could be due to the pituitary being overstimulated with CRF (or one of the other secretagogs) or to pituitary sensitivity to the releasing factor being enhanced. I recently tested this with a CRF challenge, monitoring ACTH outflow. Rather than the pituitaries of subordinate males having enhanced sensitivity to CRF, their responsiveness was actually blunted (Sapolsky, 1989; figure 12.2). This same has been observed following CRF challenges in hypercortisolemic depressive humans (Gold et al. 1986; Holsboer et al. 1984a; Risch et al. 1988). In both cases, the conclusion must be the same—if the pituitary has damped sensitivity to CRF, yet it still hypersecretes ACTH, then that implies it is subject to a very strongly elevated stimulatory signal from the hypothalamus. The damped pituitary sensitivity, if anything, can be viewed as an only partially successful attempt to counteract the enhanced hypothalamic signal (which could be easily explained by CRF-induced down-regulation of CRF receptors on pituitary corticotrophs [Wynn et al. 1985]). Therefore, the brain becomes a likely site driving the hypersecretion.

This fits well with the notion that subordinate individuals are subject to more social stressors and are initiating more stress responses at the CNS level. This is, in effect, a "psychosocial" explanation for the hypercortisolism. Baboons provide a particularly appropriate population with which to make this argument. For a baboon, the Serengeti is an ideal place to live, as animals spend only a small part of each day obtaining their calories, have low rates of being preyed upon and of infant mortality. In effect, much like humans in our own

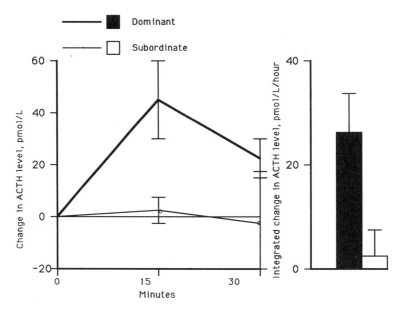

Figure 12.2. The pituitaries of low-ranking baboons are relatively insensitive to CRF. Absolute change in the circulating ACTH concentrations in response to CRF challenge among high- and low-ranking males in the absence of cortisol feedback (following metyrapone administration). (*Right*) Areas under the curve of the data from the left. (From Sapolsky, 1989, Arch Gen Psychiatry 46, 1047.)

society, they live well enough to be buffered from many ecological stressors. Instead, they have the luxury to devote their energies to generating social and psychological stressors, and it is the subordinate individual who is most frequently the victim of these energies.

In addition to the psychosocial explanation, there appears to be a "neuroendocrine" explanation for the hypercortisolism as well, in that baboons with elevated basal cortisol concentrations are relatively dexamethasone resistant (Sapolsky 1983a; figure 12.3). It was not possible to administer the standard dexamethasone suppression test (in which 5 mg dexamethasone is given at 8 PM, and responses up to 48 hours later are monitored), given the limited amounts of time that animals could be kept anesthetized. Nevertheless, even in this limited field version of the dexamethasone suppression test, the higher the basal cortisol concentrations, the slower and smaller the decline in cortisol concentrations post dexamethasone.

The psychosocial model suggested that subordinate males hypersecrete cortisol because they are exposed to frequent psychological stress; the neuroendocrine model suggests it occurs because their adrenocortical axes have lost sensitivity to negative-feedback regulation. Part I of this book suggested that these two models are not only not mutually exclusive, but are highly interconnected, in that sustained stress, via glucocorticoid hypersecretion, will lead to corticosteroid receptor down-regulation in the hippocampus and blunting of feedback efficacy. Thus, initially, subordinate animals might be hyper-

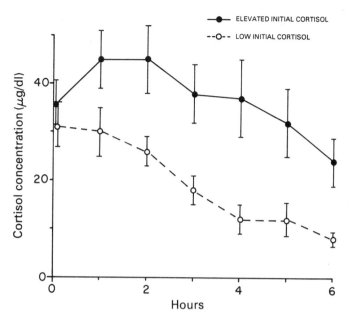

Figure 12.3. Cortisol concentrations after 5 mg dexamethasone administration. Subjects were divided into the 50% with below-average basal cortisol concentrations (solid line; this group was predominately high-ranking, with mean basal cortisol concentrations of 13 ± 2 μg/dl) and the 50% with above-average basal cortisol concentrations (broken line; this group was exclusively low- and middle-ranking, with mean basal cortisol concentrations of 36 ± 4 μg/dl). The two groups did not differ in body weight. (From Sapolsky, 1983, Individual differences in cortisol secretory patterns in the wild baboon: Role of negative-feedback sensitivity. Endocrinology 113, 2263–2268. Reprinted with permission of Williams and Wilkins Publishers.) We recently replicated the observation that dominant male baboons are more responsive to dexamethasone than are subordinates (in a study of 60 male yellow baboons [*Papio cynocephalus*]). (From Sapolsky and Altmann, unpublished.)

secretory simply because they are exposed to more frequent stressors (i.e., they have more stress-responses than do dominant animals). With time, these frequent bursts of glucocorticoid secretion will alter feedback sensitivity and cause hypersecretion basally as well (Sapolsky 1990b).

In summary, optimal adrenocortical function is associated with being socially dominant. Such individuals have lower basal cortisol concentrations, a more rapid adrenocortical stress-response, and greater sensitivity to feedback inhibition. This suggests that subordinate animals might be more at risk for the pathophysiological consequences of glucocorticoid overexposure (although it should be emphasized that these differences in basal cortisol concentrations as a function of rank are generally rather subtle). Nevertheless, subordinate primates are more likely to show some pathologies or markers of pathology that are sensitive to glucocorticoid concentrations: Subordinate primates in stable hierarchies have more atherosclerotic occlusion (Kaplan et al. 1982), lower HDL-cholesterol concentrations (Sapolsky and Mott 1987), and fewer total circulating lymphocytes (Sapolsky 1992b).

Some Limits to the Association Between Social Subordinance and Hypercortisolism

At first glance, social dominance appears to be a fairly important and straightforward variable in explaining individual differences in adrenocortical function. Among complex social primates, however, it is far from straightforward. This is the case for at least three reasons:

1. *Social ranks can change over time.* This occurs often in many primate species. Young subordinate individuals undergo a growth spurt and can reverse the direction of dominance with a rival; new males transfer into a troop and patterns of coalitions shift; high-ranking males pass their prime, sustain injuries, or occasionally "voluntarily" (to use a term that I think is valid when applied to these complex individuals) relinquish dominance and cease to compete. The complexity of these dominance hierarchies is shown by the interesting fact that if, for example, a male of rank 3 is abruptly killed, ranks 4 to 20 need not merely shift to 3 to 19, but interchanges may occur throughout the hierarchy.

This plasticity is most pronounced among males of the Old World monkey species that have large social groups; female Old World hierarchies tend to be more static, where rank is often "inherited" (i.e., transferred from the mother; Jolly 1985). The plasticity of the male hierarchies has two important implications for adrenocortical physiology. First, it is faulty to generate simple predictions about the pathophysiologic consequences of the hypercortisolism in subordinate males. The glucocorticoids may lead to hypertension, immunosuppression, or diminished fecundity. But when extrapolating these consequences into changes in lifelong patterns of disease, one must incorporate the fact that the ranks will change—this season's hypercortisolemic male at the bottom of the hierarchy may be dominant a few years later. Moreover, not only do ranks change over time, but each individual's cumulative pattern may be idiosyncratic, with some rising in rank slowly over the years and declining abruptly, others with a single high-ranking season, and others who are subordinate for their entire lives. Therefore, detailed longitudinal data over many years must be collected before predictions can be made as to the pathologic consequences of hypercortisolism. To extrapolate from a single cross-section of dominance, during a single season of the life of an animal that can live 25 years or more, is insufficient.

The changing ranks also complicate the adrenocortical picture in terms of the neuroendocrine mechanisms discussed in this book. It is easy to consider a prime-aged, high-ranking male in whom rank declines and basal cortisol concentrations rise as he subsequently senesces. This echoes the glucocorticoid cascade model of part I of this book. But what should one make of the subadult, low-ranking male, with elevated basal cortisol concentrations and dexamethasone resistance, where, with each passing year as he approaches his prime, his rank rises and his adrenocortical axis works *better*? This is the sort of problem confronting anyone doing developmental biology, watching this mysterious decrease in entropy.

2. *The physiological correlates of dominance depend on the sort of society in which the dominance occurs.* The various studies of dominance and physiology outlined above suggest a general correlation between rank and adrenocortical physiology. Numerous additional studies have shown nearly as strong associations between rank and other physiological systems. But what does this correlation mean? Does rank cause the physiology, or physiology the rank, or are they mere correlates of some other variable that is hidden? For example, high-ranking male baboons tend to be prime-aged, in good health, and well fed. Perhaps low basal cortisol concentrations are simply a marker of these traits and have nothing to do with social dominance itself.

An important body of studies show that there is causality, in that the physiology seems to arise from the rank; moreover, it is not merely the rank, but the social setting in which the rank occurs.

In my own work, I obtained evidence for this during the 1981 season in Africa. Typically, when an alpha male is nearly past his prime, there is an obvious male in the number 2 position who is, in effect, breathing down his neck. In this particular season, I arrived to find the previous year's alpha male barely holding on. Atypically, however, there was no heir apparent. Instead, a coalition of young adult, of ranks 2 to 7, were harassing him. Shortly into that season, the coalition crippled him in a fight, removing him from social competition. In the aftermath, the cooperative coalition promptly disintegrated, and a sustained period of social instability ensued for the next 3 months. Any of these six males dominated the remaining dozen males in the troop. Moreover, they were all prime-aged, in good health, and well fed, like dominant males in more stable seasons. However, among themselves, no clear hierarchy emerged. Ranks among them shifted daily. Coalitions formed and disintegrated hourly. Rates of dominance interactions and of aggression soared, feeding and mating were suppressed. Critically, during this period of sustained social instability, the psychological advantages of dominance in a stable setting had disappeared. Now, being in this top-ranking half dozen meant a life of highly charged unpredictability and lack of control. Sitting precariously at the top of a threatened, shifting hierarchy is, psychologically, a very different experience than sitting atop a stable one—just consider the likely psychological state of one of the Romanov's during the pre-Soviet winter of 1917.

During this unstable season, all of the physiological markers of dominance detected in other stable seasons had disappeared. In terms of adrenocortical function, for example, dominant males no longer had the lowest basal cortisol concentrations nor the fastest elevations in cortisol during stress (Sapolsky 1983b). This begins to show that a particular physiological profile is not a prerequisite for dominance. Instead, it is a consequence of dominance, but only of certain types of dominance.

This is shown more clearly in studies of captive primates, where social instabilities can be generated artificially by the formation of new groups. The first conclusion from these studies is that a particular physiological profile is not a *cause* of dominance. As evidence, almost no studies have shown a physiological marker in monkeys living singly in cages that predicts high or low rank when they are put in a social group. Instead, once the social groups are formed, the distinctive physiological profiles emerge. During the period immediately after formation, a picture emerges very much like during the 1981 unstable season with my baboons. High-ranking animals have their ranks shift, with high rates of interactions and of aggression. This is to be expected during the period when the directions of dominance in dyadic relations are first being tested and are not yet settled. During this time, dominant males have basal cortisol concentrations at least as high as do subordinates (Keverne et al. 1982, for talapoin monkeys; Mendoza et al. 1979 and Coe et al. 1979, for squirrel monkeys; Chamove and Bowman 1976, for rhesus monkeys) and do not have the most rapid adrenocortical responses to stress (Coe et al. 1979). They also show elevated testosterone concentrations at that time (Eberhart and Keverne 1979, for talapoin monkeys, Mendoza et al. 1979 and Coe et al. 1979, for squirrel monkeys; Rose et al. 1971, for rhesus monkeys; Sapolsky 1983a, for baboons).

With time, the picture resembles that of the wild baboons during their stable seasons. Rates of dominance interactions and of aggression by dominant males decline. The direction of dominance in dyads stabilizes (i.e., the dominant male wins perhaps 90% of his interactions with the particular opponent, instead of 51%). The endocrine picture is quite different than during the period of initial organization of the hierarchy. Dominant individuals now have the lowest basal cortisol concentrations (Manogue et al. 1975 for squirrel monkeys; Keverne et al. 1982, for talapoin monkeys) and greater cortisol secretion in response to stress (Manogue et al. 1975). (In addition, testosterone concentrations are no longer elevated in dominant males [Gordon et al. 1976, for rhesus monkeys]. Moreover, dominant males have the lowest rates of atheroslcerotic plaques, a feature not seen during periods of social instability [Kaplan et al. 1982, for fascicularis macaques].) This picture emerges in captive groups that have been together for more than 12 to 15 months (reviewed in Sapolsky 1992c). In one case, longitudinal study of the same group over time was carried out (Keverne et al. 1982). As further support for this picture, a captive population was studied in which there never was an unstable period of group formation—this was an entire troop of Japanese macaques that had become agricultural pests and were trapped in toto and transported overseas to an outdoor corral at a primate center in Oregon. They have thus been intact as a social group for decades and show most of the behavioral indices of having stable dominance hierarchies. Their dominant animals have endocrine profiles very similar to those of the dominant baboons during their stable seasons (Eaton and Resko 1974).

Collectively, these studies show that there is not a single physiological profile of dominance among social primates, particularly as it pertains to adrenocortical function. Instead, it depends on the type of society in which it occurs, and a critical variable seems to be whether it is a stable or unstable one. It is my feeling that the psychological advantages and disadvantages of dominance, varying according to social setting, are the critical variables in this stable/unstable dichotomy.

Some recent data suggest a further refinement of this idea. The studies outlined above examine endocrine differences between social groups which, collectively, can be characterized as having either stable or unstable hierarchies. Within a hierarchy that is stable overall, there can still be individuals whose own individual rankings are nevertheless unstable—they are in the process of moving up or down in the rankings. Quantitatively, such individuals have high rates of "reversals" of the direction of dominance in their interactions. One would predict then that within stable hierarchies, higher basal cortisol concentrations are observed, after correcting for rank, among individuals whose ranking is unstable.

I recently analyzed the behavioral data from my baboon population to test whether such a pattern occurred. Intriguingly, this was only partially the case. Among these males, higher basal cortisol concentrations were indeed observed when the individual experienced a high rate of dominance reversals—but only when those reversals were with males immediately *lower* ranking. In contrast, high rates of reversals with males immediately *higher* ranking were not associated with elevated cortisol concentrations. High rates of reversals with animals higher ranking mean that the male is gradually usurping their higher ranks. Conversely, high rates of reversals with animals lower ranking means that the male is in the process of being usurped himself. Thus, social instability is not automatically associated with elevation of cortisol concentrations in an individual—only if the instability means that that individual is losing, rather than gaining ground in the competition (Sapolsky 1992b).

3. *The physiological correlates of dominance may be more related to personality than to the dominance itself.* The previous two sections show that the plasticity and the stability of hierarchies are two important variables in determining what sort of adrenocortical profiles are seen in a primate. However, the picture is more complicated than this. Social primates do not merely come in two flavors—dominant or subordinate; they cannot even be simply described as, for example, "A male who is number 3 in a stable hierarchy." A critical feature of these individualistic animals is that they have different *styles* of their rank.

The notion of style is apparent to anyone who observes social primates. A high-ranking male may have a history of frequent and successful cooperative coalitions; in contrast, in the next troop or in a different year, a male of the same high rank may have attained his position without ever having had a cooperative partner. Males may differ in how much they play with infants, how much they groom, whether they have nonsexual affiliations with females. They may differ in their responses to ambiguous social situations or to losing a fight. In a stable hierarchy, do dominant males of very differing styles of dominance all have the same low basal cortisol concentrations?

We have explored this question by analyzing 10 years of behavioral data, formalizing styles of male-male competition, of male-female sexual interactions, of nonsexual interactions, and so on. We found subsets of males with certain extremes of particular behaviors, with groups of behavioral extremes tending to form clusters. Most importantly, we found that low basal cortisol concentrations not only differentiated dominant from subordinate animals; in addition, within the dominant cohort, extremely low basal cortisol concentrations were a marker of a certain stylistic subset of dominant males.

The traits themselves were quite informative, as they strongly reflected many of the themes of psychological stress and of stress management. Being at the extreme of a number of behavioral styles was associated with low basal cortisol (Sapolsky and Ray 1989; Ray and Sapolsky 1992; figure 12.4):

• Low basal cortisol concentrations were observed in males who were best at differentiating between threatening and neutral interactions with social rivals. This was determined by looking at the transitional probabilities for certain events. The rival of a male walks up to him and gives him an open-mouthed

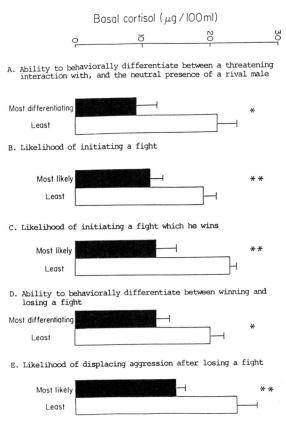

Figure 12.4. Dominant baboons with certain personality traits (solid bars) have lower basal levels of cortisol than do other dominant males (open bars), suggesting that attitude is a more important mediator of physiology than is rank alone. Dominant males who can distinguish between the threatening and neutral actions of a rival have cortisol levels that are about half as high as those of other dominant males (A). Similarly, low cortisol levels are found in males who start a fight with a threatening rival instead of waiting to be attacked (B); who know which fights to pick and so are likely to win fights they initiate (C), who distinguish between having won and lost a fight (D), and who, when they do lose, displace aggression onto a subordinate (E). (From Sapolsky and Ray, 1989, Am J Primatol 18, 1.)

threat display from a foot away. What is the probability that this will disrupt whatever he was doing previously? In contrast, the same rival shows up on the scene and falls asleep 50 feet away. What is the probability here that the male's behavior will be disrupted by this? One subset of males was very poor at differentiating between the two circumstances—the mere presence of a sleeping rival was as disruptive as an overt threat. At the other extreme, a subset was extremely discriminating between the two situations (with, invariably, little disruption of behavior when the rival was not threatening). Males for whom the mere neutral presence of a rival was highly disruptive had significantly higher basal cortisol concentrations than males who discriminated between the two situations. For such males, living within large and interactive baboon troops, daily life must present frequent and unpredictable social stressors. In this light, it is not surprising that they have basal cortisol concentrations more than double those of the other males.

• If a rival was actually threatening, did the male under study wait for the rival to escalate the situation to a fight, or did he initiate it himself? Males who were most likely to be initiators in such circumstances had lower basal cortisol concentrations. Moreover, in this population, initiating a fight is not usually a successful strategy (with intiators typically losing 80% of fights [Sapolsky 1982]); however, when matched by rank, these low cortisol males were mostly initiating winning fights. This implies that they were picking their fights carefully and knowledgeably, suggesting social control and savvy.

• Once the fight occurred, low basal cortisol concentrations were a marker of males who were best at differentiating between whether they had won or lost the fight. Again, this was determined by calculating transitional probabilities for behaviors. Males who did not differentiate between a positive and negative outcome (i.e., winning or losing) had high cortisol concentrations.

• If the male lost the fight, low basal cortisol concentrations were found in males who had the highest rates of displacing aggression onto third parties. This demonstrates the powers of outlets for frustrations in reducing adrenocortical secretion. This is reminiscent of the laboratory studies showing that rats getting electric shocks had lower glucocorticoid output when given wood to gnaw on or a conspecific to attack (reviewed in Levine et al. 1989).

• Lower basal cortisol concentrations were found in males who spent the most time grooming and being groomed by nonestrus females, and in interacting with females and infants (Ray and Sapolsky 1992). This is reminiscent of the finding of lower glucocorticoid concentrations in infant monkeys who, separated from their mothers, were placed with familiar rather than unfamiliar nonrelatives (Levine et al. 1989).

Collectively, low cortisol concentrations were associated with high degrees of social skillfulness and predictability (knowing that a sleeping rival is different from a threatening one, knowing which fights to pick), social control, an ability to differentiate between positive and negative reinforcers, having outlets for frustrations, and having a social support network. These are highly consonant with what is known about psychological stress and the strategies for stress management. The advantages of these styles are shown in the fact that low-cortisol dominant males remained in the upper 50% of the dominance hierarchy significantly longer than did the high-cortisol dominant males (Sapolsky and Ray 1989). Moreover, low cortisol concentrations appear to predict their successful tenure, as the trait was apparent from their first year in the dominant cohort.

In summary, what seemed to be an endocrine marker of dominance also reflects personality style. On the average, dominant individuals have lower basal cortisol concentrations than do subordinates, but within the dominant cohort, a great deal of the variability is explained by these behavioral features. What is most striking about this finding is the magnitude of the effects—the difference in basal cortisol concentrations comparing the behavioral extremes of dominant males (see figure 12.4) is greater in some cases than the difference comparing dominant and subordinate males (see figure 12.1).

These findings echo those of a classic study concerning the parents of children dying of cancer. In an important demonstration of the endocrine consequences of sustained psychological stress, such parents were shown to be hypercortisolemic (Friedman et al. 1963). The magnitude of the hypercortisolism was very sensitive to differing styles of coping of the parents. Lower cortisol concentrations occurred in parents who had a structure of religious rationalization to explain the illness, who denied the facts of the disease, or who could lose themselves in the details of managing the disease (Wolff et al. 1964).

These studies, along with those of Weiss on psychological stress discussed earlier, lead to similar conclusions. Clearly, the external reality of having a certain rank, of watching your child die of cancer, or of being subjected to mild electric shocks, can be stressful and will have a somewhat predictable effect on a physiological endpoint such as glucocorticoid concentrations. Yet these studies show that the psychological filters with which those external events are perceived alter the resultant physiology with at least as much potency as the stressor itself. This should have an even greater impact on the subtler stressors of our daily lives, in which one person's stressor—intimidating public speaking, time-wasting lines—can be challenging or calming for someone else. For us clever primates, life is filled with ambiguous events, and we differ as to whether we quench life's thirsts from glasses that are perceived as half full or half empty.

There is the tendency for many physiologists who study this system to view these ideas as valid, but bordering on the platitudinous. It might seem so, as many of these findings are eminently sensible—and the term here is pejorative. They show that even in a world full of dismal, unfair, unchangeable stressors, attitude counts to some degree; one must differentiate between what can and cannot be changed and accept the latter, and one should find footholds of control and predictability in difficult circumstances. Yet the magnitude of these effects show that they are anything but platitudes—in some of the studies cited in the last two sections, the physiological endpoint depended more on the psychological variable (changing whether there was a warning signal, an outlet for frustration, and so on) than the magnitude of the external stressor. As a physiologist, it is clear to me that physiology per se accounts for only a very small piece of these complex systems.

PERINATAL EXPERIENCE, GENETICS, AND ADULT ADRENOCORTICAL FUNCTION

When considering the findings regarding adrenocortical function and personality/rank among primates, one must wonder where these different personality styles come from. Our studies showed that these traits do not emerge as a function of dominance but are there as markers even at the beginning of their tenure. Moreover, our more recent work suggests that some of these behavioral traits are quite stable over time in these primates (Ray and Sapolsky 1992). This must move the discussion into the realm of the effects of early experience and genetics upon the adrenocortical axis.

Human and Primate Studies

A surprising amount of information is available about this subject. The strategy has been to observe very young primates—whether human or non-human—and look for differences in personality and coping styles. Most of these studies have focused on how the infant responds to novelty. One then searches for whether there are physiological correlates of these differences at these early ages. Finally, longitudinal study of these same individuals is carried out to see if these differences predict behavioral and/or physiological differences in adulthood.

The general conclusion that has emerged from these studies is that the sort of stylistic and endocrine differences that I have observed in adult baboons are remarkably stable in primates over the lifetime and are demonstrable at far earlier ages. For example, in studies of captive rhesus monkeys, some infants can be characterized as "high reactors." At their earliest stages (1 to 4 weeks of age) they show delayed sensorimotor maturation, poor muscle tone, and persistent neonatal reflexes. They are slow to explore novel stimuli. During their infancy (1 to 6 months of age) and juvenile period (6 months to 3 years), they show atypically strong responses to novelty or social isolation—they show the greater and more prolonged elevations of glucocorticoid and ACTH concentrations than do "low reactors." In addition, they have the highest rates of self-directed and passive behaviors, and the least locomotion, exploration, play, and vocalization (figure 12.5; Suomi, 1987). As adolescents, they still show the pattern of the greatest adrenocortical responsiveness to separation. Importantly, under normal social conditions (i.e., when not in a novel social setting or when not separated from an attachment object such as a mother or peer), high- and low-reactive monkeys do not differ in any of these parameters. These stylistic and endocrine differences emerge with novel and stressful social situations.

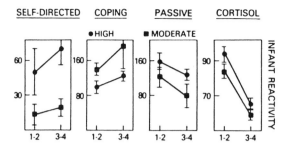

Figure 12.5. Responses of infant rhesus monkeys to a series of separation periods. Infants either came from a highly emotionally reactive pedigree (circles) or a moderately reactive pedigree (squares). During the separation period, infants of the highly reactive pedigree had far more self-directed behavior, fewer coping behaviors, were less active (i.e., more passive), and had slightly higher cortisol concentrations. (From Suomi, 1987, in Krasnegor N, et al. (eds), *Perinatal Development: A Psychobiological Perspective*. Academic Press, New York.

Similar patterns occur in humans. Most of the studies have examined behavior, but not physiology. In one such study, infants found to withdraw in the face of novelty and characterized as poor adaptors to environmental change were shown to demonstrate many of the same traits when studied as late as early adulthood (Thomas et al. 1968). Another found that infants (12 to 18 months of age) who were more "anxiously attached" to their mothers were more dependent and less exploratory in nursery school, 3 to 4 years later (Sroufe 1984). Finally, studies by Kagan and colleagues have found that infants who are the most "behaviorally inhibited" by novelty (with differences detectable at even a few months of age) show persistence of these traits for years afterward, and as young adults, are categorized as shy and anxious in social situations (Kagan and Moss 1962; Kagan et al. 1984; Garcia-Coll et al. 1984; Kagan et al. 1988). In an important recent extension, such behaviorally inhibited infants were shown to have higher urinary cortisol concentrations than their less inhibited peers (Kagan et al. 1988; Tennes 1982). As with the infant rhesus monkey, these stylistic differences in human infants were not necessarily apparent under "nonstressful" conditions, but instead emerged during periods of novelty and challenge.

Therefore, differences in behavioral styles of coping with stress and novelty are apparent in human and nonhuman primates at extremely early ages and are stable into adulthood. Moreover, the sort of physiological correlates of these differences that occur in adult baboons also occur at these younger ages. This suggests that if I examine the records of these same adult baboons when they were subordinate adolescents, there should be differing styles of subordinance that should emerge, along with endocrine correlates of these styles. Moreover, there should be stability of these differences over time, in that animals more reactive and less in control in their dominant phase of life are likely to be those showing less adaptive styles of subordinance as well. In other, more colloquial words, the glass can appear half empty or half full whether you are near the bottom or top of the dominance hierarchy, and how one views those ambiguities persists over the lifetime, independent of the absolute rank. These studies are in progress. Unfortunately, one thing I can never do with my data set is to know what the childhoods were like of these males; this is because male baboons change troops around puberty, and any of the mature individuals I have studied have grown up in troops elsewhere in the Serengeti.

These studies of infant humans and monkeys merely shift the question beginning this section to an earlier point. Rather than Where do these adult differences come from? it is now Where do these life-long differences come from? Predictably, there is evidence for genetics as well as for early environment. In a visible lead article in *Science*, Kagan and colleagues (1988) argued that the differences they had detected were genetic. Little support was given for this view, other than the idea that behavioral and physiological patterns apparent at such early ages probably reflect innate differences. This conclusion strikes me as odd, given that much of Kagan's elegant work has shown how actively infants at those very same young ages interact with their environment and are changed by it—all undermining his "If it happens early, it must be genetic" argument. On a stronger footing are studies comparing the degree of concordance of these individual traits among individuals of varying degrees of relatedness. These have shown that the closer the kinship, the more shared these behavioral traits (Plomin and Rowe 1979). However, these have the usual problems of such studies of shared kinship and shared environment covarying. As a partial control on that, some of the current studies of identical twins separated early in life suggest that the introversion/extroversion dimension is fairly strongly heritable (cf. Plomin 1990). None of these human studies have focused on issues of heritability of any physiological markers, including adrenocortical function.

More interventionist studies have been done with nonhuman primates, and these suggest that both genetics and early environment can contribute to these behavioral and physiological differences. Closer rhesus relatives share patterns of adrenocortical reactivity more than do nonrelatives (Suomi 1987). In another study, the behavioral and endocrine traits of the fathers of infants were categorized (i.e., whether they were adult versions of high or low reactors). After mating, the males are not present when the infants are raised; thus, the male contribution is solely genetic. Using such a paradigm, some evidence for heritability of these reactivity traits was found (Scanlan et al. 1985). In a subsequent study, the classic fostering approach of behavior genetics was used, in which infants were raised by other than their biological mother. The biological and foster mothers were categorized for their reactivity personalities. In addition, the foster mothers were judged for some qualities of their mothering. Rhesus mothers can differ as to how "punitive" and rejecting they are of infants, especially during weaning, or how "nurturant" they are (frequency of grooming). Infants were then studied under normal social conditions and during novel, stressful circumstances. To summarize a complex study, the biological pedigree of the infants was the best predictor of style during the stressful conditions; the offspring of biological mothers who were high reactors tended to be high reactors themselves. This finding included an apparent heritability of cortisol levels during that time; however, the effect upon cortisol was not as strong as on some of the behavioral parameters (animals at the two stylistic pedigree extremes differing perhaps 20% in their cortisol concentrations). In contrast, when in the home cage and unstressed, the style of foster mothering was the best predictor of the infant's behavior, with infants raised with more nurturant, less punitive foster mothers being more exploratory and less reactive (Suomi 1987). In studies of wild baboons, Altmann (1980) observed strong individual differences in mothering styles, and the persistent and salutary effects on the offspring of calm, nonanxious mothering.

In summary, individual differences in glucocorticoid concentrations in primates and humans can be associated with certain behavioral and personality styles. Moreover, these endocrine and behavioral differences appear fairly stable, emerging early in life, reflecting both genetic and environmental influences, with the latter reflecting styles of mothering in particular.

How do these differences in genetics and early environment produce the long-term changes in adrenocortical function? Essentially, no mechanistic information is available regarding primates or humans. For that, it is neccesary to turn to rodents.

Early Environmental Influences on Adult Adrenocortical Function in the Rodent

Probably the best-characterized example of early experience influencing the adrenocortical axis is that of neonatal *handling*, a phenomenon that has been studied for 30 years (Levine 1962). In this paradigm, handling consists of removing the mother from the litter, then placing individual pups into a new cage for 15 minutes. Afterward, pups and mothers are returned to their cage. This is done once per day for the first 3 weeks of life. Remarkably, this induces changes in adrenocortical function that persist into adulthood. Most strikingly, handled rats, as adults, have lower basal corticosterone concentrations and a faster recovery to baseline at the end of stress than do nonhandled rats (Levine et al. 1967; Ader 1970; Meaney et al. 1985b). Moreover, they are more sensitive to feedback regulation by either corticosterone or dexamethasone (Meaney et al. 1990b). The handling phenomenon could not be induced at later ages. Therefore, this represents a classic developmental example of imprinting during a critical period (in this case, of physiology rather than behavior).

The handling phenomenon quickly became a favorite of developmental psychobiology. It was not clear, however, how it worked. There was the suggestion that handling increased the numbers of hippocampal neurons. As evidence, postnatal ^{3}H-thymidine labeling in the hippocampus was increased by handling (Altman et al. 1968). However, it was later shown that handling merely accelerated normal postnatal neurogenesis, rather than enhanced it. Handled and nonhandled rats had equivalent numbers of neurons as adults, with the former reaching the plateau earlier.

In considering the endocrine changes brought about by handling, what was striking was that the variables affected were sensitive to hippocampal neuroendocrine function—basal and poststress corticosterone secretion, sensitivity to feedback regulation. The data regarding numbers of corticosteroid receptors in the hippocampus and feedback efficacy suggested to us that handling might alter numbers of such receptors. We found evidence for this (Meaney et al. 1985a,b,c). Handled rats, as adults, had an approximately 50% increase in V_{max} in the hippocampus. A smaller but significant increase occurred in frontal cortex, but not in amygdala, hypothalamus, septum, or pituitary. Subsequent study has shown that the effect is attributable to an increase in type II receptors (Sarrieau et al. 1988a). As evidence of the glucocorticoid secretory pattern being due to the increased receptor number, if adult rats (handled as infants) were exposed to enough corticosterone to down-regulate their receptors to nonhandled levels, the distinct secretory profile of handled animals disappeared (Meaney et al. 1990b).

We observed a second change in the handled rats that could also contribute to the secretory differences. Handling also decreased concentrations of CBG-like receptors in the pituitary. As reviewed, the pituitary contains a large complement of CBG-like receptors (which are either synthesized de novo in the pituitary or circulate as CBG before entering the pituitary). Such CBG-like receptors are biologically inactive (i.e., when they bind corticosterone, they do not translocate to the nucleus and interact genomically), and instead serve as a buffering system that competes with the biologically active receptors for corticosterone. If there are fewer such pituitary receptors, more corticosterone reaches the main receptors, more steroid/receptor complex reaches the nucleus, and a stronger feedback signal is triggered (Sakly and Koch 1981; Sapolsky and Meaney 1986). Therefore, handled rats should have enhanced feedback efficacy at the pituitary level as well, contributing to the low basal corticosterone concentrations and prompt shut-off of poststress secretion.

In summary, the changes in receptor patterns in handled rats probably explained why they had unique profiles of adrenocortical secretion. Why did they have changes in receptor patterns? It is probably not an autoregulatory phenomenon. That is to say, it is probably not the case that handling changes circulating corticosterone concentrations, which produces the persistent changes in receptor numbers. First, handling does not cause particularly robust changes in circulating corticosterone concentrations (Sapolsky and Meaney 1986). Second, the sort of autoregulation seen in the adult does not occur in the neonate. Therefore, exogenous administration of glucocorticoids to the neonate does not down-regulate receptors, and adrenalectomy-induced decreases in concentrations do not cause up-regulation (Meaney et al. 1985c). And even if it had, the autoregulatory changes in corticosteroid receptor profiles that are induced in the adult are nowhere near as long-lasting as the receptor changes induced by handling (Sapolsky et al. 1983d).

At this stage, a few strands have been uncovered to explain how handling increases receptor number. Administration of either triiodothyronine (T_3) or thyroxine (T_4) to nonhandled pups mimicks the handling-induced changes in

Type II receptors in the brain. Conversely, administration of propylthiouracil, a thyroid hormone synthesis inhibitor, blocks the handling effect on hippocampal receptor number (Meaney et al. 1987). A similar thyroid hormone regulation of the development of pulmonary corticosteroid receptors had been shown previously (Morishge 1982). Immediately neonatally, thyroid hormone concentrations are low (Dussault and Labrie 1975) and rise in parallel with the normal postnatal developmental increase in hippocampal corticosteroid receptors (Meaney et al. 1985c,d). Moreover, thyroid hormone secretion is stimulated by hypothermia, which could be the proximal signal during handling as pups are removed from their mother; this could be a convenient signal that has evolved to bring about the handling effect. Finally, the developing brain contains ample concentrations of receptors for thyroid hormones, and the hormones play a major role in stimulation of neuronal maturation, proliferation, and elaboration (Balazs et al. 1975; Dozin-van Roye and De Nayer 1979; Schwartz and Oppenheimer 1978); for example, postnatal hyperthyroidism enlarges a subset of mossy fiber projections within the hippocampus (Schwegler et al. 1991). Critically, neonatal handling has been shown to cause a reliable increase in thyroid hormone concentrations (Meaney et al. 1991b) (although a recent abstract failed to observe the same [Kuhn et al. 1991]).

The thyroid hormone connection does not explain the effects of handling on CBG-like receptors in the pituitary. Moreover, it is not clear how thyroid hormones trigger a lifelong increase in corticosteroid receptor number in the hippocampus. It may have something to do with serotonin. It was reported recently that serotonin increases the number of such receptors in cultured hippocampal neurons (Mitchell et al. 1990a); intriguingly, something akin to "imprinting" occurred, in that the augmentation of receptor number persisted in culture for a month after withdrawal of the serotonin (Betito et al. 1990).

Finally, it is not obvious what the handling phenomenon means; that is, why has it evolved? It seems clear that under normal circumstances, neonatal rats are never "handled," in the sense of being taken from the mother and placed temporarily in a new environment. Instead, the handling phenomenon may be what happens to the subset of rats who are more exploratory or whose mothers leave them more frequently. For the purposes of this chapter, however, what is important is that this is a powerful developmental means for producing adult variability in corticosterone secretion.

Genetics Influences on Adrenocortical Function in the Rodent

Different, yet closely related species of rodents can differ dramatically in their adrenocortical function (Treiman and Levine 1969). Within one rat species, different strains can also differ dramatically. To my knowledge, no rat strain has been bred for a feature of adrenocortical function. Rather, the differences have emerged as a by-product of breeding for related traits.

A number of strains have been defined which differ in their emotional or physiological reactivity to stress. As one example, the Roman High- and Low-Avoidance rats (RHA and RLA) were derived from the Wistar strain and originally bred for their high and low capacity, respectively, to acquire a rapid avoidance response to a two-way shuttle box (Bignami 1965). This rather specific difference was later shown to generalize to other learning tasks. Moreover, these differences also generalized to nonlearning situations, including movement in and rates of defecation in open fields, locomotor activity, and maternal behavior (reviewed in Gentsch et al. 1988). The general theme of these differences is that the RHA rats are markedly less emotional in stressful or novel situations, are more exploratory, and more capable of learning in anxiety-provoking, moderately stressful situations. The RHA rats also have somewhat higher blood pressure (Guenaire et al. 1986; Gentsch et al. 1988).

In a second example, the Maudsley Reactive (MR) and Non-reactive (MNR) rat strains have been defined for their differences in rates of defecation when placed in an open field (Broadhurst 1960, 1969). This is a very sensitive index of anxiety in a rat. As with the RHA/RLA comparison, the rather specific difference here was later found to generalize to broad MR/MNR differences in emotional reactivity during mild stress and novelty, including capacity to learn in novel situations, locomotion during novelty, and increased blood pressure (all greater in MR than in MNR rats). In a third comparison, the Spontaneously Hypertensive (SHR) rat has been bred from the normotensive Wistar-Kyoto rat (WKY). In this case, selective criteria was a purely physiological one, namely higher blood pressure in the SHR rat, which has a 100% rate of arterial hypertension (Okamoto and Aoiki 1963). Again, this narrowly defined initial breeding criteria produced strains that differ in a range of features related to emotionality. Therefore, SHR rats acquire active avoidance tasks faster than do WKY rats, defecate less, and are more active in open field settings (reviewed in Gentsch et al. 1988).

Thus, starting from very different breeding criteria—capacity to acquire a very specific learning task, emotionality in open fields, spontaneous hypertension—these different research groups have developed strains that differ in their emotional, cognitive, and physiological indices of responsivity to novel and mildly stressful situations. Importantly, they do not generally differ under basal, nonstressful situations, nor in the face of major physical stressors (Driscoll and Battig 1982; Gentsch et al. 1988). These strains differ in adrenocortical activity, with the more emotionally reactive strain showing greater adrenocortical activity under such conditions. Therefore, higher ACTH and corticosterone concentrations are observed in RLA than RHA rats (Gentsch et al. 1981a, 1982; Walker et al. 1989). Importantly, a difference does not occur basally or in response to major stressors (such as ether exposure, immobilization, or inescapable footshock). Instead, it is apparent during moderate stressors such as intraperitoneal injection, a new cage, an open field, or a shuttle box testing situation (figure 12.6; Gentsch et al. 1982). The adrenocortical axis of RHA rats is atypically hyposensitive to the mild stress, rather than the RLA system being hypersensitive (Gentsch et al. 1982).

Similar differences have been observed when comparing SHR and WKY rats, with little adrenocortical difference occurring basally, but a greater responsiveness occurring in WKY rats under conditions where they show their

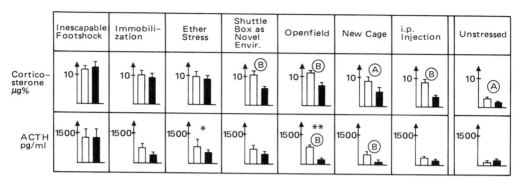

Figure 12.6. Corticosterone and ACTH responses of Roman Low-Avoidance (open bars) and Roman High-Avoidance (solid bars) rats. While the two groups did not differ in these parameters under unstressed conditions or in response to major physical stressors (inescapable footshock, immobilization, or ether exposure), corticosterone and/or ACTH concentrations tended to be higher in Low Avoidance rats in response to milder, more psychological stressors (such as injection, a novel cage, openfield exposure or a learning task). (From Gentsch et al., 1988, Experientia 44, 482.)

other indices of hyperemotionality (Yamori et al. 1973; DeVito et al. 1981; McMurtry and Wexler 1981; Sowers et al. 1981; Gentsch et al. 1981a). An identical pattern has been reported with the MR and MNR rats (Gentsch et al. 1988).

In summary, genetic strains that are more prone toward emotionality in response to mild stressors show greater adrenocortical activity at such times. What are the mechanisms to explain this? Little is known. No putative genetic markers have been found, and I would wager that it will be difficult to tie such a marker, when found, to a specific feature of adrenocortical function. Many neurochemical and morphological differences between the brains of these strains have been found (reviewed in Driscoll and Battig, 1982; Gentsch et al. 1988). Collectively, they cast only a little light on explaining the general phenomenon of differences in emotionality, let alone in adrenocortical function. Perhaps the two most interesting, in terms of making a speculative link to adrenocortical function, concern levels of binding of imipramine and of benzodiazepines. Imipramine is one of the most effective of tricyclic antidepressants. RHA rats have approximately 15% higher binding capacity for imipramine throughout a variety of brain regions, with no difference observed in affinity (Gentsch et al. 1983). As a possible link to the adrenocortical axis, hypercortisolism is seen in many cases of depression (reviewed in chapter 14) and, when tricyclics are effective in relieving depression, the hypercortisolism typically resolves as well. Therefore, RLA rats might be less sensitive to endogenous ligands for the imipramine binding site, which could produce more adrenocortical activity. This, obviously, is highly speculative, and the magnitude of the strain difference in imipramine binding is rather small.

In a slightly less speculative vein, strain differences have been found in the number of binding sites for benzodiazepines. These are the minor tranquilizers, which are extremely effective in relieving the behavioral, physiological, and cognitive indices of anxiety in rodents (Gray 1982). Moreover, benzodiazepines block adrenocortical secretion activated by mild, novel stressors. Perhaps less emotionally reactive strains have more benzodiazepine binding sites in some relevant brain region. This was observed with the MR/MNR comparison, with the former having approximately 20% greater amounts of binding of ^{3}H-diazepam than did MNR rats in a variety of brain regions examined; affinity did not differ (Robertson et al. 1978). In comparing RHA and RLA rats, one study found more binding sites in the RHA strain (Gentsch et al. 1981b), whereas two others have not (Shepard et al. 1982, 1984). Finally, no reliable differences have been observed in comparing SHR and WKY rats (Thyagarajan et al. 1983; Tunnicliff et al. 1984; Hambley et al. 1985). Therefore, while differences in benzodiazepine binding sites might explain the difference in adrenocortical reactivity between MR and MNR strains, it cannot be a general explanation. Moreover, if it were relevant to that particular pair, I do not feel that it implies that benzodiazepines directly modulate the adrenocortical axis. Rather, they modulate the perception of an external event as being anxiety-provoking or not, which, in turn, determines whether there is adrenocortical activation.

Just to make life even more complicated, the adrenocortical differences may not be so much a consequence of differences in benzodiazepine receptor number as a cause, given that glucocorticoids can modulate their numbers (cf. de Souza et al. 1986; Miller et al. 1987).

A single study has compared the dynamics of the adrenocortical axis itself between two of these strains, in this case, RHA and RHL rats. As reported previously, basal corticosterone concentrations did not differ (although RHA rats, oddly, had elevated basal ACTH concentrations, implying a basal adrenal hyporesponsiveness to the peptide). In addition, the more emotional RLA rats had greater ACTH and corticosterone responses to mild stressors. The pituitaries of RHA rats were less responsive to CRF. This was observed in vivo, measuring the ACTH response to ovine CRF, as well as in vitro, using dispersed pituitary cells from the two strains. In addition, RHA rats had more Type II corticosteroid receptors in their pituitaries, and more Type I receptors in their hippocampi (about 40% greater, in both cases) (Walker et al. 1989). This suggests some reasons why RHA rats secrete less corticosterone than do RLA rats during mild stress. The increased numbers of hippocampal Type I receptors could make the CNS locus of the axis more sensitive to glucocorticoid negative feedback. This mechanism would gain credibility if it could be shown that the adrenocortical difference between the strains was a function of differing sensitivity to negative feedback; this is not currently known.

Were this hippocampal mechanism to be important, the strains would have to differ in the amounts of one or more of the secretagogs released by the hypothalamus, with the RHA rats secreting less of the hormone(s). This has not yet been measured. These data also suggest a pituitary mechanism, in that the pituitaries of the RHA rats were less sensitive to CRF. This could be due to greater pituitary sensitivity to an inhibitory glucocorticoid feedback signal and would certainly fit with having more pituitary Type II receptors. Alternatively or additionally, it could also reflect intrinsic differences in responsiveness to CRF.

In summary, these data generate more questions than they answer. Most importantly, it is not clear whether the differences uncovered are causes or consequences of the differences in corticosterone secretion during stress. However, this is the first information available regarding neuroendocrine mechanisms that might underly these genetic differences in adrenocortical function.

ADULT EXPERIENCE AND ADRENOCORTICAL FUNCTION

As evident from the preceding section, there has been considerable interest in features of early development and genetics that will influence adult adrenocortical function. Less attention has been focused on adult manipulations. In an obvious way, stress in the adult will affect adult adrenocortical function, in that a primary effect of stress is to stimulate the axis. Of more interest, however, are a few manipulations that seem, a priori, to be rather distant from the axis but which nevertheless influence it and possibly explain sources of individual variability.

One example that I will touch on only briefly is food restriction. It has now been well more than half a century since the extraordinary, counterintuitive findings of Osborne et al. (1917) and McCay et al. (1935) that if total caloric intake in a rodent is restricted over the course of a substantial percentage of its lifespan, the animal will live approximately 20% longer. This met with considerable skepticism. However, the observation has been replicated repeatedly in different mammalian and nonmammalian species, and with a variety of different regimens of food restriction—decreasing caloric intake one seventh each daily, or fasting one day a week, restricting the numbers of calories attributable to certain nutrients, and so on. The phenomenon does not appear to be due to eliminating disease, including those of overnutrition. Were such the case, dietary restriction would make survivorship curves more rectangular, without increasing maximum lifespan. Instead, the intervention actually increases total attainable lifespan; to date, this remains one of the few demonstrated interventions capable of accomplishing this (reviewed in Holehan and Merry 1986; Weindruch and Walford 1988; Masoro 1988). The mechanisms underlying the protective effects of food restriction remain fairly obscure. Predictably, metabolic, immune, and neuroendocrine theories abound.

If food restriction retards aging of at least some organ systems, it might also retard the onset of the degenerative glucocorticoid cascade in the aging rat. The few data available are not conclusive on this point. First, it is not clear what the restriction paradigm does to adrenocortical activity in the adult rat. One study reports that after an initial period of elevated corticosterone concentrations, prolonged restriction caused decreased basal corticosterone concentrations (Holehan and Merry 1986). In contrast, another study showed a tendency toward higher basal corticosterone concentrations in adult food restricted rats; moreover, the same study showed that restriction caused a decrease in CBG concentrations, resulting in a massive increase in free corticosterone concentrations in food restricted adults, relative to ad libitum-fed controls (Sabatino et al. 1991). Two studies report that food-restricted rats in old age do not have different patterns of adrenocortical function than do aged ad libitum-fed rats; measures included basal corticosterone and ACTH concentrations, stress-responsiveness, and poststress recovery times (Dellwo and Beauchene 1990; Sabatino et al. 1991). This is surprising—the demonstration of decreased basal corticosterone concentrations in adult food-restricted rats (Holehan and Merry 1986) predicts that in old age, such rats should be spared the typical adrenocortical hyperscretion. In contrast, the demonstration of increased basal corticosterone concentrations in adult food-restricted rats (Sabatino et al. 1991) predicts that in old age, such rats should have more severe indices of adrenocortical hypersecretion. Amid the confusion of findings, the only thing not predicted was the lack of difference between aged food-restricted and aged ad libitum-fed rats. Obviously, more work is needed in this area.

CHANGES IN ADRENOCORTICAL FUNCTION AND RATE OF HIPPOCAMPAL DEGENERATION DURING AGING

Thus, rats of different genetic strains, or with different neonatal or dietary histories, differ in adrenocortical function as adults. The natural question in these cases is whether these adrenocortical differences are sufficient to alter the rate of hippocampal aging. The studies by Landfield and colleagues discussed in previous chapters showed that removal of the vast majority of circulating glucocorticoids can decelerate the rate of hippocampal aging (recall that in those studies, rats were adrenalectomized and then maintained on extremely low replacement levels of glucocorticoids). Will more subtle diminution of glucocorticoid concentrations be protective as well?

It is not known if the strains discussed differ in how their adrenocortical axes or hippocampi age. Given that these strains do not differ in their basal adrenocortical profiles or in responsiveness to major stressors, but instead differ in their responsiveness to mild, anxiety-related stressors, one might predict that differences in the rates of hippocampal aging between the more and less emotional strains might only occur in the face of frequent bouts of anxiety.

Focusing on the other model discussed, we have demonstrated that the adrenocortical changes induced by neonatal handling cause dramatic changes in the glucocorticoid cascade of aging.

The reasoning in this study was straightforward. If neonatal handling causes a reduction in basal corticosterone concentrations in the adult, and total lifetime exposure to corticosterone is a major determinant of the rate of hippocampal neuron loss during aging, then neonatally handled rats should, in their old age, have less hippocampal neuron loss. This was observed (Meaney et al. 1988). As reported previously, handled rats, as adults, had more Type II hippocampal corticosteroid receptors and lower basal corticosterone concen-

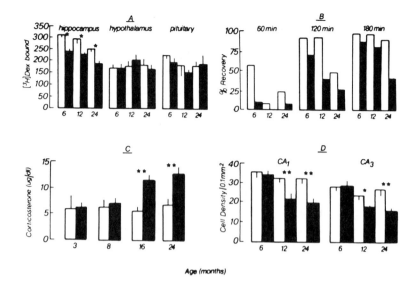

Figure 12.7. The effects of neonatal handling on various features of hippocampal and adreno-cortical senescence. Animals were either handled (open bars) or nonhandled (solid bars) during the first weeks of life and were undisturbed thereafter. A, Handled rats had an increase in corticosteroid binding sites in the hippocampus as young adults. Thus, despite sustaining a progressive loss of such receptors during aging, they still had more receptors than did nonhandled controls in old age. Handling had no effect on receptors in the hypothalamus or pituitary. B, Handling prevented the senescent phenomenon of rats being unable to terminate corticosterone secretion promptly at the end of stress. Rats were exposed to 1 hour of immobilization stress and corticosterone concentrations monitored during the 3-hour poststress recovery period. Among nonhandled control rats, aging was associated with a decreasing percentage of animals recovering to prestress corticosterone concentrations (i.e., 100% recovery) during the 3-hour period. In contrast, handled rats were relatively protected from this senescent defect. C, In nonhandled rats, aging was associated with an increase in basal corticosterone concentrations. The same was not observed in handled rats. D, In nonhandled rats, aging was associated with a loss of CA$_1$ and CA$_3$ hippocampal neurons; the same did not occur in handled rats. (From Meaney et al., 1988, Effect of neonatal handling on age-related impairments associated with the hippocampus. Science 239, 766. Copyright AAAS.)

trations (figure 12.7). The latter trend was accentuated with aging, as the normal age-related increase in basal concentrations did not occur. Moreover, handled rats did not show the typical problem in shutting off corticosterone secretion at the end of stress (figure 12.7). Therefore, given the differences in both basal and poststress adrenocortical profiles, the total lifetime exposure to corticosterone was decreased in handled rats as compared to nonhandled controls, whether there were incidences of stressors or not. This predicted that there should be less neuron loss in their aging hippocampi, and this was observed (figure 12.7). Finally, given the sensitivity of cognition to relatively small degrees of hippocampal damage, aged handled rats should have been spared some of the cognitive defects typical of aging. This was tested with the Morris swim maze, which is a sensitive measure of hippocampal-dependent spatial learning. In that task, rats must find a submerged platform in a pool of opaque water, relying entirely upon visuospatial cues from the surrounding

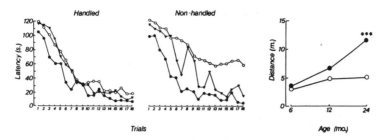

Figure 12.8. The effects of neonatal handling on hippocampal-dependent cognition during aging. *A*, Among handled rats, there was no change in the mean latency to find the platform in the Morris water maze task when comparing 6-month-olds (solid circles), 12-month-olds (triangles), and 24-month-olds (open circles). In contrast, among nonhandled rats, aging was associated with a significant increase in the latency for task completion. *B*, Mean swimming distance to the platform over the last eight trials for handled (open circle) and nonhandled (solid circle) rats of indicated ages. (From Meaney et al., 1988, Effect of neonatal handling on age-related impairments associated with the hippocampus. Science 239, 766. Copyright AAAS.)

room. Nonhandled rats had a progressive deterioration in their performance with age; in contrast, no deficits occurred in aged handled rats (figure 12.8). As an important control, when the platform was made visible above water, aged handled and nonhandled rats reached the platform at the same speed, showing that the differences when the platform was hidden represented differences in spatial skills, rather than mere motor skills.

This study seemed to show that the rate of aging of a number of parameters was retarded by neonatal handling. This was not entirely the case. In some instances, handled and nonhandled rats suffered the same rate of decline with aging; handled rats simply started with more or better and thus ended with more or better. The numbers of hippocampal corticosteroid receptors is one such case, where the slope of decline in handled and nonhandled rats were the same (see figure 12.7). Therefore, in that instance, handling did not actually retard the aging process. In some cases it did, however. For example, in young adulthood, handled and nonhandled rats did not differ in their numbers of CA_3 neurons. The age-related decline was actually prevented in handled rats.

A seeming paradox emerges in these data. Handling causes increased numbers of corticosteroid receptors in the hippocampus. Because of the role of the hippocampus in glucocorticoid negative feedback, that should cause less circulating glucocorticoids (and thus less hippocampal degeneration during aging). However, that same increase in receptor number should sensitize the hippocampus to the endangering effects of the glucocorticoids (with, thus, more hippocampal degeneration during aging). As is frequently the case with systems physiology, complex and opposing arrows wind up being predicted, and it is necessary to put the pieces together—namely, run the experiment in an intact physiological system—to see which arrow is more powerful. In this case, the end result appears to be protection of the aging hippocampus.

This strikes me as an important study for a number of reasons. First, the model presented at the end of part I of this book was meant to describe a normal and obligatory feature of aging, and these handling studies show that this degenerative cascade need not be inevitable. Instead, a physiological intervention can prevent the emergence of the degeneration. Naturally, it is striking that this protection can be caused by something so subtle, occurring so early in life. On a very pragmatic level, these results are not welcome news for gerontologists: While this may support the developmental biologists' view that early experience is enormously important and persistent, for the gerontologist, it mostly means another variable to be controlled for, and a miserably subtle one at that—entire studies of old age could be thrown off by the number of times rats were handled during cage changes 2 years earlier. That is the grim side of these results. On a more sanguine note, it shows the power of potential interventions in this system—the degeneration need not be inevitable.

CONCLUSIONS

This chapter was not meant to be exhaustive in examining all the possible sources of individual variability in the system. Instead, it was meant to touch on each of a number of different types of contributing variables—genetics, early experience, adult experience. In some of these cases, the source of variability can be explained in very mechanistic neuroendocrine terms— for example, the number of corticosteroid receptors in the hippocampus in handled rats. In some cases, the variability is best understood in the context of psychobiology—for example, the differences in the rates of psychological stressors to which animals of different ranks are exposed. Collectively, these studies seem grounds for some optimism.

What they suggest is the potential for varying degrees of intervention. At present, it is not possible to alter the genetics of the system. However, most of the other sources of variability are eminently open to manipulation, in the most positive sense of that word. Differences in early social experience, the frequency and magnitude of early stressors, adult diet, attitudinal issues concerning a sense of control—all could be relevant. What seems clear to me is that these variables are manipulated by chance anyway. Aging organisms are notorious for the variability that they present. It is only recently that investigators have begun to study this variability systematically. For example, a number of investigators have examined the cognitive capacities of aged rats and divided them into those with severe impairments and those with minimal or no impairments. Impaired rats have been found to have lower cerebral glucose utilization in many brain regions, particularly the hippocampus (Gage et al. 1984) and to be more glucose intolerant (Stone et al. 1990). Moreover, impaired rats have more deposition of the beta amyloid protein in their hippocampi, fewer receptors for NGF in their hippocampi and basal forebrains (Koh et al. 1989), more of the amyloid precursor protein containing the protease-resistant Kunitz sequnce (Higgins et al. 1990), elevated high-affinity uptake of choline in the hippocampus (Gallagher and Pelleymounter 1988), reduction of choline acetyltransferase activity (the enzyme that makes acetylcholine) in the septum (Gallagher et al. 1990), fewer synapses in the molecular layer of the dentate gyrus in the hippocampus (Geinisman et al. 1986), and fewer hippocampal neurons and higher circulating corticosterone concentrations (Issa et al. 1990). These observations make a certain amount of sense, given the roles of glucose availability, glucocorticoids, neuron number, NGF, and so on, in hippocampal-dependent cognition. But they are obviously the first of many pieces that must be collected. As this field of inquiry matures, it must take on more subtle problems, and that of individual variability is both supremely subtle and supremely important. There is considerable variability arising from many potential sources throughout the lifespan, and the variability appears to have an important impact on the aging of this system. Therefore, it must be understood in order to exploit its protective potential.

CHAPTER SUMMARY

Parts I and II of this book are grim, in that they demonstrate that glucocorticoids can accelerate brain aging and exacerbate the toxicity of a variety of insults. These findings suggest that organisms that differ in their patterns of glucocorticoid secretion may thus differ in their vulnerability to senescent brain degeneration or to neurological insults. This naturally raises the question of how much and what types of variability exist in patterns of glucocorticoid secretion in order, perhaps, to exploit their protective potential. Put most succinctly, Why might two organisms differ in the amounts of glucocorticoids that they secrete (basally, during stress or following)?

Psychological Stress

The most obvious answer to the question would be that two organisms differ in the amount of stressors to which they are exposed. That perhaps settled, one then considers very mechanistic explanations for differences in glucocorticoid secretion—two organisms may be exposed to the same frequency of stressors but may differ, for example, in ACTH half-life in the bloodstream. This analysis skips a critical intervening stage, in that the two organisms may be exposed to identical external events, but may *perceive* them differently.

The early stress physiologists utilized major stressors that tended to obliterate differences in the perception of whether an event is stressful or not; furthermore, their orientation was a very bioengineering one, seeking to define the stress-response in simple terms of the external stressful input and the endocrine output. Therefore, the perceptual, psychological component was long ignored. Any of a number of studies carried out in the 1960s showed how powerfully the physiological stress-response is modulated by the perception of the stressor. In one example, two rats might have received an identical series of shocks of the same intensity. One, however, would have a bar of wood in its cage to gnaw on after each shock. That animal, given an outlet, would have far less of a physiological response, despite experiencing the identical physical stressor. Other studies showed the highly protective effects of a warning light, a lever to press, or the presence of another rat on which to displace aggression.

Collectively, these studies show that psychological factors can modulate the response to a physical stressor, or even provoke a stress-response in the absence of a stressor. Critical factors that make for psychological stress appear to include *loss of control, loss of predictability, loss of outlets for frustration*, and *a perception of things worsening*, independent of the actual physical reality. Given the power of these variables, some psychoendocrinologists have argued that, in fact, *all* physical stressors are stressful only to the extent that they provoke these psychological states. While clearly not true (for example, anesthetized organisms have stress-responses during surgery when the first incision is made), the enormous power of psychological factors in modulating the stress-response is now accepted. Therefore, this can be a major source of individual variability.

Social Status

A body of research has shown that animals of differing rank in social dominance hierarchies differ in their adrenocortical profiles. Socially subordinate individuals generally have the highest glucocorticoid concentrations basally, smaller or sluggish stress-responses, and slow recovery. This picture is thought to reflect the fact that social subordinance carries far more psychological (and often physical) stressors—social subordinance is typically filled with lack of control, of predictability, of outlets for frustration, and so on. This has been studied in detail among wild baboons living in a national park in Africa. The elevated basal cortisol concentrations among the subordinate cohort in this population has been shown to be driven at the CNS level. This can support a "psychoendocrine" explanation for their hypercortisolism, in that they are exposed to more physical and psychological stressors than are dominant animals (and thus secrete more secretagogs). Moreover, there is a "neuroendocrine" explanation for their hypercortisolism, in that they have blunted glucocorticoid feedback sensitivity and are dexamethasone resistant. The data covered in previous chapters demonstrated how the psychoendocrine and neuroendocrine components can interact—with repeated exposure to stressors and glucocorticoid hypersecretion, feedback efficacy will be blunted.

More recent work has added some caveats to the impression that, perhaps, social subordinance is linked with hyperadrenocorticism, and obvious pathological correlates of social rank should ensue. First, in many social species, ranks change over time, so any predictions about the long-term pathological costs of rank (and their physiological correlates) must reflect this changing picture. Second, there appears to be no single picture of the physiological correlates of social rank. Rather, they appear to depend heavily on how *stable* the hierarchy is, and the relative hyposecretion of glucocorticoid by dominant animals just described is seen only when the hierarchy is stable. In contrast, dominant animals typically secrete the *most* glucocorticoids during unstable times, and this reflects the fact that a precarious hold on a dominant position in an unstable hierarchy carries none of the psychological advantages of dominance during stable times. Finally, the physiological correlates of rank are highly modulated by the individual personality of the animal. For example, among these baboons, when animals are matched by rank, there is tremendous variability in glucocorticoid profiles depending on whether the individual can differentiate between stressful and neutral social interactions with rivals, whether the animal controls when stressful interactions finally erupt into a fight, whether they can displace aggression after a frustrating event, whether they have a network of social affiliation, and so on. The relevance of these personality factors to the features of psychological stress are obvious and suggest that for the advantageous adrenocortical profiles to be seen, an organism must not only have the psychological advantages of rank available, but must have the personality that allows the perception of those advantages.

Perinatal Experience, Genetics, and Adult Adrenocortical Function

The studies of social rank lead one to conclude that while rank is important (as is the stability of the society in which it occurs), the intervening variable of personality is immensely important as well. Naturally, this raises the question of the cause of these personality differences. A body of studies suggest that some of these features exist early in development. Infant humans and primates already show strong individual differences in how aversive they find novelty to be, how exploratory they are in novel settings, how socially extroverted they are, and so on. Critically, such personality differences appear to be relatively stable into adulthood. Moreover, from the earliest of ages, these differences are correlated with physiological differences, and in general, the individuals who are more aversively reactive to and less exploratory in novel settings hypersecrete glucocorticoids. Cross-fostering studies have shown that these differences are attributable to genetics to only a small extent, but heavily reflect mothering style.

In studies of rodents, early experience has also been shown to have profound effects on life-long patterns of glucocorticoid secretion. In the well-studied case of "neonatal handling," stimulation of rats for as little as 15 minutes a day for their first few weeks of life produces animals who, as adults, secrete less glucocorticoids basally and are more sensitive to feedback regulation. Some recent studies examining the neuroendocrine mechanisms underlying this phenomenon found that they center on the hippocampus, in that neonatal handling (for complex reasons) causes a permanent increase in concentrations of hippocampal corticosteroid receptors. The route by which this can enhance feedback sensitivity has been explored in depth in earlier chapters.

Finally, a body of studies has examined the genetics of individual differences in glucocorticoid secretion in rats. A number of strains have been characterized that differ in a cluster of features of "stress-related" physiology or cognition. Critically, in these paired comparisons, the "stress-sensitive" and "stress-resistant" strains do not differ under basal, nonstressed conditions in any of these parameters, or during major physical stressors. In response to milder, more ambiguous psychological stressors, however, the more sensitive strains have higher blood pressure, less ability to learn, higher rates of defecation (a sign of anxiety in rats), less spontaneous exploration and, not surprisingly, relatively enhanced glucocorticoid secretion. Little is known about the mechanisms underlying these genetic differences.

Adult Experience and Adrenocortical Function

A number of variables will alter glucocorticoid profiles in adult animals (separate from the obvious things like differences in rates of exposure to stressors). In the mysterious but well-documented phenomenon of "dietary restriction," a substantial decrease in lifelong caloric intake will extend the total maximal lifespan of some mammals studied. The mechanisms underlying this have been debated, but in a broadly simplifying way, dietary restriction will decelerate nearly every biomarker of aging examined. At present, it is not clear what effects such restriction have on adrenocortical function in the adult or during aging.

Do These Differences Matter?

These disparate approaches have shown that adult organisms can differ tremendously in their adrenocortical profiles and thus, potentially, in their lifelong exposure to glucocorticoids. Can these differences be sufficient to alter the rate at which the degenerative glucocorticoid cascade emerges during aging? In the one explicit test of this, this was shown to be the case. These studies utilized the neonatal handling phenomenon to produce adult rats who had lower basal glucocorticoid concentrations. Followed into senescence, such handled rats were spared most of the degenerative features of the glucocorticoid cascade, including the loss of corticosteroid receptors and neurons in the hippocampus, and some of the cognitive impairments.

These studies provide some room for optimism, in that they suggest that individual differences in glucocorticoid secretion might well matter in the long run. While we rarely understand the precise mechanisms underlying these differences, some of the can be manipulated in a gross way, and might well lay the groundwork for some interventions to decrease some senescent degeneration in this system.

This orientation has been an a priori, preventive one. The next chapter examines what interventions might be made to decrease the endangering effects of glucocorticoids in the aftermath of neurological crises.

13 Interventions at the Time of Neurological Insults

SUMMARY OF THE BOOK SO FAR

Various stressors trigger the endocrine and neural adaptations that constitute the stress-response. Glucocorticoid secretion is central to this response, and it typifies the two-edged quality of the stress response: While glucocorticoids are vital for surviving acute physical stressors, prolonged glucocorticoid exposure (during exogenous glucocorticoid administration or in some instances of prolonged or repeated stressors) can cause a variety of diseases.

Part I examined how the regulation of glucocorticoid secretion is impaired during aging and how excessive exposure to glucocorticoids over the lifetime can accelerate aspects of brain aging. The data reviewed combine to form a model termed the *glucocorticoid cascade*. It attempts to link two features of aging rats—hypersecretion of glucocorticoids and degeneration of neurons in the hippocampus. The hippocampus is shown to be an important mediator of glucocorticoid feedback inhibition, such that its senescent degeneration causes glucocorticoid hypersecretion. Glucocorticoids, in turn, are shown to damage hippocampal neurons. These two regulatory features combine to form a feedforward cascade of senescent degeneration—glucocorticoids damage the hippocampus, which causes further glucocorticoid secretion (and numerous deleterious consequences for the aged rat, including further hippocampal damage).

Part II described a model by which glucocorticoids damage the hippocampus. Data were presented showing that under conditions where glucocorticoids are not themselves neurotoxic, the hormones can endanger hippocampal neurons, impairing their capacity to survive coincident insults such as hypoxiaischemia, seizure, and hypoglycemia. Therefore, glucocorticoids may not only play an important role in accelerating hippocampal damage during aging, but may also exacerbate some of the most common neurological insults to the hippocampus.

It was reviewed how these insults are toxic by activating a cascade, in which there is excessive synaptic accumulation of excitatory amino acid (EAA) neurotransmitters. This causes excessive postsynaptic mobilization of free cytosolic calcium which, in turn, causes various degenerative events in cells. Critically, these insults are energetic in nature, and a paucity of energy will impair the ability of the hippocampus to properly control the trafficking of EAAs and calcium. It was shown that glucocorticoids disrupt hippocampal neuronal energetics (most plausibly by inhibiting glucose transport in the hippocampus) and thus exacerbate this degenerative EAA/calcium cascade.

Part III considers the implications of these findings and the room for interventions. Chapter 12 focused on how altering lifelong patterns of exposure to glucocorticoids might alter the rate of hippocampal senescence. Some of the variables that give rise to individual differences in glucocorticoid secretion were reviewed, including exposure to psychological stress, social rank, early experience, and genetics. In the one model tested (neonatal handling), an intervention that decreases cumulative glucocorticoid exposure over the lifetime retards hippocampal senescence. It was concluded that there is considerable potential for modulating basal glucocorticoid secretion and thus, potentially, to modulate the rate of hippocampal aging. However, the small differences generated by these interventions are not likely to decrease the endangering effects of glucocorticoids immediately following a major neurological insult. The present chapter focuses on what might be done in those circumstances.

The previous chapter, focusing on individual differences in adrenocortical function, was most relevant to the role of glucocorticoids in the gradual accumulation of hippocampal damage *during* aging, rather than to the dramatic damage occurring *after* neurological insults. In most of the models discussed, animals with the highest and lowest basal glucocorticoid concentrations differed by perhaps two- to threefold. The question that permeated the chapter was whether these degrees of differences in glucocorticoid exposure, when extended over the lifespan, could make a difference in the rate of hippocampal aging.

What was encouraging was the suggestion in some of these studies, particularly the ones with handling of neonatal rats, that the degenerative glucocorticoid cascade need not be inevitable. This is good news, at least for the aging rodent. My bias, however, is that these differences in adrenocortical function would be swamped in the face of major stressors such as hypoxia-ischemia or status epilepticus. I would be surprised if the differences in adrenocortical function between, for example, handled and nonhandled rats, would translate into differing neuropathological outcomes following a seizure. If a theme of the previous chapter was the subtlety of interventions that can produce long-term changes in adrenocortical function, the theme of the present chapter is the unsubtle interventions needed to remove glucocorticoids from the scene immediately following a major neurological insult. I am reminded of Gandhi's statement expressing his pleasure that it was the British who were his colonial adversaries—nonviolent protest would not have worked against the Nazis, he said. In much the same way, the subtle interventions of the last chapter would probably not hold a candle against these neurological insults.

In this chapter, I review the interventions that could be carried out at the time of neurological insults to reduce the endangering impact of glucocorticoids. In most cases, it is clear what needs to be done; it is often not yet clear, however, how to do it.

The most obvious way to decrease the endangering effects of the glucocorticoids is to *block their secretion* at the time of neurological insults. This was done in the studies demonstrating the protective effects of adrenalectomy against kainic acid, hypoxia-ischemia or 3-acetylpyridine (Sapolsky 1985a,b,

1986a; Sapolsky and Pulsinelli 1985). However, in considering the clinical applicability of any of this, adrenalectomy is obviously not an option. Alternatively, there are a number of compounds available which block adrenal steroidogenesis transiently; we tried this strategy with metyrapone. The drug inhibits cortisol synthesis in primates and corticosterone synthesis in rodents by blocking 11-β-hydroxylation (Cheng et al. 1974). Importantly, in terms of potential clinical use, metyrapone is often used short-term in humans to examine the capacity of the pituitary to hypersecrete ACTH following disinhibition from cortisol-negative feedback, and long-term to control hypercortisolism secondary to ectopic ACTH-secreting tumors or adrenal neoplasms (cf. Haynes and Murad 1985; also, see Murphy 1991 for the long-term use of metyrapone in humans in a novel attempt to alleviate depressive symptoms). Therefore, the drug is both efficacious and at least reasonably safe (although not without side effects; see below).

Our first attempt at using metyrapone in a neuroprotective manner was quite encouraging. Rats were microinfused in Ammon's horn with kainic acid, and metyrapone was administered systemically at the time of the onset of seizures. This was meant to mimic the clinical picture, in which it is not possible to predict when the neurological insult will occur. As shown before in figure 7.6, the status epilepticus induced by the kainic acid caused profound corticosterone secretion in the rats; as expected, metyrapone blocked this stress-response. Hippocampal damage was decreased significantly in metyrapone-treated rats, especially in the CA_3 pyramidal layer, the cell region most vulnerable to status epilepticus seizures (figure 13.1). Importantly, the metyrapone did not alter the seizure intensity or duration, as the pattern of

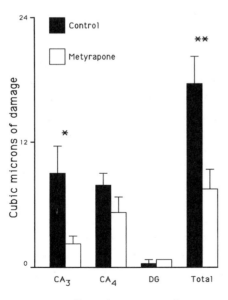

Figure 13.1. Effects of metyrapone administration on hippocampal damage produced by kainic acid microinfusion. (From Stein and Sapolsky, 1988, Brain Res 473, 175. Reprinted with permission from Elsevier Science Publishers.)

Interventions at the Time of Neurological Insults

epileptiform EEGs was not changed. A recent abstract reports that metyrapone also decreases hypoxic-ischemic injury to the hippocampus (Morse and Davis 1989). A recent report suggests an additional reason to block glucocorticoid secretion at such times—some of the drugs that might soon be used in a clinical setting to block the NMDA receptor (phencyclidine and MK-801) stimulate the adrenocortical axis (Boggan et al. 1982; Pechnick et al. 1986, 1989).

Therefore, pharmacological inhibition of glucocorticoid secretion seems a first viable intervention for protecting the hippocampus. There are obvious limitations in this strategy. First, steroidogenesis inhibitors such as metyrapone merely inhibit, rather than eliminate glucocorticoid secretion, typically stabilizing concentrations at basal values. Therefore, if even small concentrations of glucocorticoids can be endangering, this strategy is of limited use. Second, inhibitors such as metyrapone are neuroactive in a way that is poorly understood. Third, there is typically a rebound of glucocorticoid secretion once the inhibitory effects of metyrapone abates; thus, one must be certain that the rebound does not come during a period in which there is still vulnerability to glucocorticoid actions. Finally, blocking glucocorticoid synthesis/secretion as a therapy may simply come too late—an endangering amount of the steroid may be released by the time an inhibitor begins to work.

As a second and obvious strategy, if one is too late to prevent the release, *block the corticosteroid receptors*. This approach allows for a later intervention (although not by all that much time). The most likely means of doing that these days is using the specific type II antagonist RU 38486. We are currently trying this approach. As a possible limitation, while the compound is an excellent competitor with corticosterone for binding in cytosolic receptor assays, there is emerging evidence that RU 38486 has some agonist qualities in vivo (cf. Bradbury et al. 1992).

If one is too late to block the glucocorticoid secretion or its binding to its receptors, the next obvious strategy is to *block the energetic effects of glucocorticoids*. Given the dependency on protein synthesis for the sequestering of the glucose transporter, use of protein synthesis inhibitors would theoretically accomplish the task. This, however, is a very global and disruptive intervention, perhaps akin to destroying the village in order to save it. As a more selective intervention, when the specific protein responsible for sequestering the glucose transporter is identified, there might be means to inhibit its activity. The most obvious intervention, however, is to circumvent the partial inhibition of glucose transport by supplementing neurons with additional energy. As outlined, we have used this strategy in vivo and in vitro to protect hippocampal neurons from the endangering effects of glucocorticoids (Sapolsky 1986b; Sapolsky et al. 1988; Tombaugh et al. 1992). Protective compounds have included glucose itself, mannose, and the ketone β-hydroxybutyrate. Fructose, which does not penetrate the blood-brain barrier, is protective in vitro but not in vivo.

As a final intervention, if one is too late to block glucocorticoid secretion, binding to the receptors, and disruption of energetics, one can try to *protect the neuron from the consequences of the energetic disruption.* This is an intervention that has moved past the specific arena of glucocorticoid action and is instead as broad as all of neurology—block NMDA receptors, decrease the metabolic rate of neurons, block calcium channels, scavenge free radicals, and so on. A fair amount of progress has been made in recent years in using these various approaches in preclinical models. The clinical trials seem to be in progress now. Obviously, while any single one of these steps might be helpful, combinations of them are likely to be even more so, and a number of authors have speculated on the eventual development of therapeutic "cocktails." One can imagine them including NMDA receptor antagonists, calcium chelators, antioxidants, supplemental energy substrates, and perhaps corticosteroid receptor blockers.

CONCLUSIONS

Surveying this chapter, I am a bit distressed at its brevity; one would have hoped for a longer list of things to do to try to protect the hippocampus during neurological disasters. Instead, the prescriptions are brief and almost breezy. Check out the steroidogenesis inhibitors and see which works best and has the fewest side effects. Throw in some extra energy. Make an antiglucocorticoid/ anti-NMDA/antioxygen radical/anticalcium cocktail and give a bottle of it to each of your friends. What is obvious, however, is that in designing these preclinical interventions and in envisioning potential clinical studies, there will be a daunting amount of empirical work required: trying out permutations of drugs, determining proper dosages and time courses, and so on. Intellectually, this is a very different style of problem than that discussed in chapter 12. For the issues covered in that chapter, there is a lifetime of gradual glucocorticoid overexposure to be contained, and a lifetime of opportunities for subtle behavioral strategies to retard the process. In the present case, it is a tidal wave of glucocorticoids that must be contained rapidly. In the former, the interventions are pre hoc, working to prevent the disasters, and are far more psychological in flavor than biomedical. In the latter, they are post hoc, containing the disaster once it has occurred, and the interventions are outside the realm of subtle psychological manipulations. In both cases, there are some grounds for optimism, in that interventions exist to protect the aging or challenged hippocampus. The critical question, of course, is whether these threats to the hippocampus, and the means to protect it, are relevant to the human. This is the subject of the final chapter.

CHAPTER SUMMARY

Data from part II suggest that glucocorticoids exacerbate the hippocampal damage that occurs after various neurological insults. This chapter considers some interventions that might be made at such times to decrease the endangering effects of glucocorticoids.

1. As the most obvious intervention, the secretion of glucocorticoids can be blocked. This can be accomplished by adrenalectomy, but the clinical applica-

bility of this is obviously quite limited. Alternatively, one can perform a chemical adrenalectomy with drugs that transiently block adrenal steroidogenesis. In the first tests of this approach, use of the drug metyrapone decreases both seizure-induced and hypoxic-ischemic hippocampal damage in rats. The clinical applicability of this approach will obviously be limited by the side effects caused by these drugs, which are considerable in some cases.

2. Should it be too late to block glucocorticoid secretion, one might use corticosteroid receptor antagonists to block access of the steroids to their receptors. Such an approach is being tested currently.

3. Should it be too late to block glucocorticoid access to its receptors, one might attenuate the metabolic disruption caused by glucocorticoids. As outlined previously, supplementing neurons with additional energy substrates can protect them from the steroids in such circumstances.

4. Finally, should it be too late to save the hippocampus from the energetic disruption caused by glucocorticoids, it might be possible to buffer them from the most deleterious consequences of such energy crises.

While speculative, these ideas might provide a blueprint for designing rational interventions to decrease hippocampal damage following these various neurological insults.

14 Is This Relevant to the Human?

SUMMARY OF THE BOOK SO FAR

Various stressors trigger the endocrine and neural adaptations known as the stress-response. Glucocorticoid secretion is vital to such adaptations and typifies the two-edged quality of the stress-response: While glucocorticoids are needed for surviving short-term physical stressors, prolonged glucocorticoid exposure is pathogenic in a variety of ways.

Part I examined how the regulation of glucocorticoid secretion is impaired during aging, and how excessive exposure to glucocorticoids over the lifetime can accelerate aspects of brain aging. The data reviewed combine to form a model termed the *glucocorticoid cascade*. It attempts to link two features of aging rats—hypersecretion of glucocorticoids and degeneration of neurons in the hippocampus. The hippocampus is shown to be an important mediator of glucocorticoid feedback inhibition, such that its senescent degeneration causes glucocorticoid hypersecretion. Glucocorticoids, in turn, are shown to damage hippocampal neurons. These two regulatory features combine to form a feed-forward cascade of senescent degeneration—glucocorticoids damage the hippocampus, which causes further glucocorticoid secretion (and numerous deleterious consequences for the aged rat, including further hippocampal damage).

Part II presented a model by which glucocorticoids damage the hippocampus. The hormones themselves are not necessarily toxic, but rather endanger neurons by compromising the capacity of neurons to survive insults such as hypoxia-ischemia, seizure, and hypoglycemia. Therefore, glucocorticoids may not only play an important role in accelerating hippocampal damage during aging, but might also exacerbate some of the most common neurological insults to the hippocampus.

It is reviewed how these neurological insults are toxic by activating a cascade, in which there is excessive synaptic accumulation of excitatory amino acid (EAA) neurotransmitters. This causes excessive postsynaptic mobilization of free cytosolic calcium which, in turn, causes various degenerative events in the cells. Critically, these insults are energetic in nature, and a paucity of energy will impair the ability of the hippocampus to properly control the trafficking of EAAs and calcium. It is shown that glucocorticoids disrupt hippocampal neuronal energetics (most plausibly by inhibiting glucose transport in the hippocampus) and, thus, exacerbate this degenerative EAA/calcium cascade.

Part III examines what manipulations and interventions may be possible to decrease the neurodegenerative potential of glucocorticoids. Chapter 12 reviewed the sources of individual variability in basal glucocorticoid secretion—differences in psychological stress, social rank, early experience, and genetics. It is shown that manipulations of such variables which decrease lifelong glucocorticoid exposure can potentially decelerate hippocampal senescence. Chapter 13 reviewed some potential interventions that can be carried out following neurological insults to decrease the endangering effects of glucocorticoids. These include preventing glucocorticoid release, blocking access to its receptors, and reversal of its catabolic actions. Some of these strategies have been tested and shown to be protective.

Endless pages into this book, it is time to consider perhaps the most pressing questions generated by these data. Do these findings apply to the human? Is the glucocorticoid cascade a part of human aging? Can stress and glucocorticoids exacerbate neurological damage to the human hippocampus?

This chapter explores these possibilities. Of necessity, there is heavy reliance on a (sparse) nonhuman primate literature and on an even sparser human clinical literature that is mainly anecdotal. The conclusion is that while only a few pieces of the story have been tested in the human or primate, it tends to agree with the broad features outlined for the rodent in this book. Important exceptions occur, however.

In the first half of this chapter, it is neccesary to break the glucocorticoid cascade into its major regulatory arcs and to discuss whether the individual pieces occur in the human and primate. In the latter half, I will then discuss human aging and a variety of diseases in the context of these findings. For convenience, throughout the chapter, "primate" will refer to both human and nonhuman. When each is being specified alone, the latter terms will be used.

REGULATORY COMPONENTS OF THE GLUCOCORTICOID CASCADE

Is the Hippocampus a Negative Feedback Brake in the Primate?

The feedback role of the hippocampus is logical in the rodent. This is because of its sensitivity to glucocorticoids (due to the high concentrations of corticosteroid receptors) and its means of communication with the neuroendocrine regions of the hypothalamus. Therefore, one would expect the same traits were the primate hippocampus to subserve a similar feedback role. Neuroanatomically, there is considerable phylogenetic conservatism in projections among mammals, and the primate hippocampus appears to communicate with the hypothalamus as readily as does the rodent hippocampus. By the criterion of numbers of corticosteroid receptors, the nonhuman primate hippocampus appears to be as much of a glucocorticoid target tissue as is the rodent hippocampus (Gerlach et al. 1976). These studies predated the dichotomy between Types I and II receptors but were done under conditions that probably favored the labeling of the high-affinity Type I receptors. It has not been possible, of course, to conduct similar in vivo studies in humans, nor have position emission tomographic (PET) studies reached a point where quantitative data can be obtained with high resolution from individual hippocampal cell fields. However, a number of postmortem studies have demonstrated corticosteroid receptors in human brain tissue, including the hippocampus (Tsuboi et al. 1979; Yu et al. 1981; Sarrieau et al. 1988a). Moreover, these receptors show many of the same functional properties as those in the rodent (Yu et al. 1981). However, none of these studies has been sufficiently quantitative (because of technical difficulties, discussed below) to determine whether the hippocampus is as pronounced of a receptor site as in other species. Thus, while it is not yet known whether the hippocampus is a major glucocorticoid target site in the human brain, it plays this role in every other mammalian species examined, including nonhuman primates (reviewed in McEwen et al. 1986), and parsimony suggests that the same should be the case for humans.

Can the primate hippocampus inhibit adrenocortical activity? Nearly 30 years ago, it was shown that electrical stimulation of the hippocampus during neurosurgery in the human inhibited adrenocortical secretion (Mandell et al. 1963); as a control, amygdaloid stimulation did not have a similar effect. More evidence for an inhibitory hippocampal role comes from lesion data; consistently, hippocampal damage is associated with some form of hypercortisolism in the primate. This occurs in Alzheimer's disease, in which there is typically either damage to or neuroanatomical isolation of the hippocampus. Importantly, increased severity of hippocampal atrophy in the disorder is correlated with more severe hypercortisolism (De Leon et al. 1988). Moreover, among female Alzheimer's patients, more severe cognitive dysfunctions are also associated with more severe hypercortisolism (Oxenkrug et al. 1989). This will be discussed below at length.

In more controlled experimental lesions, the nonhuman primate hippocampus was also shown to be an inhibitory feedback brake (Sapolsky et al. 1991). Lesions were made in *Macaca fascicularis* monkeys. Damage to the hippocampal formation plus parahippocampal cortex, the hippocampal formation plus parahippocampal cortex plus amygdala, or fornix transection caused basal hypercortisolism in these animals. In contrast, other limbic lesions failed to do so (figure 14.1A). A number of features were observed: Such hippocampal-lesioned monkeys were also mildly, though significantly, dexamethasone resistant (figure 14.1B). It is possible that, as is seen in the human depressive literature, a stronger resistance could be detected with a smaller dose of dexamethasone. Monkeys who were most hypercortisolemic basally were also the most dexamethasone resistant. As found in the rodent, there are plasticity and recovery of function. As reviewed in chapter 5, the adrenocortical hypersecretion following hippocampal damage in the rodent tends to abate after a few weeks. This is most likely due to adaptations in the strengths of inputs of other brakes and accelerators in the system. Similarly, hypercortisolism in the primate following damage was not permanent and resolved within 15 months.

In summary, the primate hippocampus contains corticosteroid receptors and appears to be a major glucocorticoid target site within the brain. Moreover, the data from lesion and stimulation studies suggest that the hippocampus can inhibit glucocorticoid secretion.

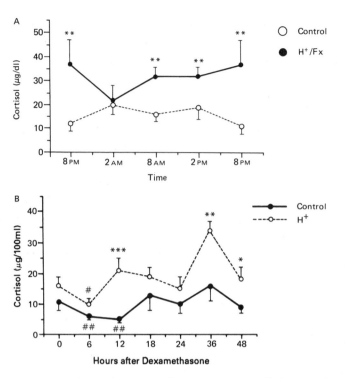

Figure 14.1. (A) Circulating cortisol concentrations (μg/dl) for control monkeys (open circles) and monkeys with hippocampal or fornix lesions (solid circles). 1991, 11, 3695 (B) Cortisol concentrations (μg/dl) following dexamethasone administration to unoperated control monkeys (solid circles) or monkeys with hippocampal lesions (open circles). (From Sapolsky et al., 1991, J Neurosci 11, 3695. Reprinted with permission of Oxford University Press.)

Regulation of Hippocampal Corticosteroid Number and Feedback Efficacy

If the primate hippocampus does indeed have the potential to inhibit gluco-corticoid concentrations, one can then ask more subtle questions about the system. Does stress and/or glucocorticoid exposure down-regulate corticos-teroid receptors in the primate hippocampus? Are hippocampal receptors *preferentially* down-regulated at those times? Does such down-regulation (inde-pendent of neuron loss) cause feedback insensitivity and/or glucocorticoid hypersecretion?

These are difficult questions, and techniques do not currently exist for answering them. Autoregulation of receptors, including steroid receptors, occurs in the primate body, and it would defy parsimony to assume that it does not occur in the brain as well. However, this has not yet been demon-strated for corticosteroid receptors. Potentially, one could study this in vivo using imaging of fluorine-substituted cortisol binding with PET scanning methods. At this stage, however, there is not sufficient anatomical sensitivity to resolve changes within hippocampal cell fields, nor the quantitative sensi-tivity to detect the subtle changes inherent in questions of stress-induced down-regulation. Moreover, some recent work with fluorine-substituted corticosteroid compounds showed either no or only poor selective accumulation and retention in the human brain (Pomper and Katzenellenbogen, personal communication).

An alternative strategy would be one utilized in many biological psychiatry studies, in which an easily obtained peripheral tissue is studied in the hopes of extrapolating from its function to that in the brain. In the version most relevant to these issues, a number of investigators have examined levels of corticosteroid receptors in circulating lymphocytes, in the hopes of inferring something about receptor function or concentrations in the brain. However, studies of rodents have shown that autoregulation of lymphoid corticosteroid receptors do not parallel such autoregulation of receptors in all brain regions (Lowy 1991; Spencer et al. 1991).

Another strategy would be to measure the receptors post mortem. For example, is there down-regulation of hippocampal corticosteroid receptors in individuals with long histories of stress or glucocorticoid exposure? As noted, corticosteroid receptors can be demonstrated post mortem in human brain. However, there are two reasons why this method will not easily answer the questions posed. First, there is considerable postmortem degradation of corticosteroid receptors in the primate brain which occurs before most autopsies are carried out. Over the course of 6 hours, ^{3}H-dexamethasone binding decays nearly 60% in macaque cortex left at room temperature (Sapolsky and Meaney 1988). When tissue is left in situ within the body, where the temperature is even warmer, decay is probably even faster. Therefore, only small amounts of receptors are demonstrable in human hippocampus by 3 to $4\frac{1}{2}$ hours post mortem, and none by 12 to 24 hours (Sapolsky and Meaney 1988). Therefore, unless autopsies are done very quickly, the data from human postmortem tissue would probably be useful only for qualitative, rather than quantitative study. Currently, few autopsies are carried out rapidly enough to study these issues.

As a second confound, there are endogenous glucocorticoids circulating at the time of death which will occupy the receptors. Given the frequent stressfulness of the agonal period, such steroid levels might be quite high. It is controversial as to whether it is possible to conduct exchange assays with corticosteroid receptors (i.e., to measure the amount of both occupied and unoccupied receptors in the cell). At present, it seems safest to say that it would not be possible to measure accurately the total number of receptors if there is even moderate degrees of endogenous occupancy at the time of death.

In summary, it is not yet possible to answer these questions in the human. It would seem natural to conduct such studies in nonhuman primates, and these are in progress. However, data are already available from the human replicating another feature of the rodent story. In the rat, some paradigms of stress and/or glucocorticoid overexposure can cause down-regulation of receptors in the hippocampus resulting in feedback resistance. While the receptor aspect of the story has not yet been studied in the human, it is clear that some stressors can cause feedback resistance in humans.

This has been seen in a number of cases. In an example that will perhaps evoke unpleasant memories among readers, medical interns were studied while scheduled with frequent nights on call coupled with first case presentations. During this very stressful situation, approximately 50% of individuals were dexamethasone resistant. After the stress had abated, resistance returned to the typical 0% to 5% rate found in healthy humans (Baumgartner et al. 1985). Similarly, humans undergoing the stressfulness of elective surgery were dexamethasone resistant at significantly higher rates the day before the surgery (Ceulemans et al. 1985). To return to the data of chapter 12, when dominant baboons undergo the stressor of dropping in rank, they become mildly hypercortisolemic and dexamethasone resistant.

In summary, sustained stress can make both the primate and the rat dexamethasone resistant. In the latter case, preferential down-regulation of hippocampal corticosteroid receptors appears to be a culprit. It can only be speculated whether the same is the case in the primate.

Can Stress Damage the Primate Hippocampus?

This is obviously the sixty-four dollar question of this whole chapter; an answer of "Yes" strikes me as nothing short of terrifying. At this stage, the answer does appear to be a tentative yes.

The human literature on this subject is extremely sparse and anecdotal. Some information comes from study of brains of Cushing's syndrome patients. Prior to current methods for managing the disorder, patients were likely to have had prolonged exposure to elevated cortisol concentrations. In one older study, the brains of such individuals were examined post mortem. A low but consistent incidence of neural atrophy and lesions in the limbic brain, frontal lobe, and hypothalamus was found (discussed in Trethowan and Cobb 1952). In a more recent but equally sparse literature, humans who have undergone sustained and profound stress—torture victims—were reported to have high incidences of cerebral atrophy, ventricular enlargement, and dementia (Jensen et al. 1982; Thygesen et al. 1970). These neurological correlates of torture appear to be transient. As more anecdotal evidence, sustained stress in humans (concentration camp victims) (Thygesen et al. 1970) and nonspecific head injuries early in life (Corkin et al. 1989) are both associated with accelerated cognitive decline during aging.

More systematic data have emerged from primate studies. In one study, dexamethasone was administered to 133-gestation day rhesus monkeys. When their fetuses were observed (either near term, or a few months post natally), total numbers of neurons were reduced dramatically in the CA_2 and CA_3 regions of the hippocampus as well as in motor and visual cortex. Less pronounced declines occurred in the CA_4 and CA_1 hippocampal cell fields and in sensory and frontal cortex. The hippocampus is cytoarchitecturally mature and differentiated in this species by the time of the dexamethasone administration; this implies that the decrement in neuron number was due to destruction of preexisting neurons rather than to arrest of subsequent neurogenesis (Uno et al. 1990).

Thus, glucocorticoids can be neurotoxic in the fetal primate hippocampus. However, it is not clear whether such stress can damage the adult hippocampus. First, the use of dexamethasone makes it impossible to decide if this is a physiological phenomenon that can be extrapolated to conditions of stress. Moreover, vulnerability of the fetal hippocampus may be different from that of the adult. A recent study of ours suggests that sustained stress can be neurotoxic to the adult hippocampus as well. The study subjects were wild-born vervet monkeys who had become agricultural pests in Kenya and were trapped and brought to a primate center in Nairobi. Some period of time into captivity, a subset of animals died spontaneously of what appeared to be a syndrome of sustained social stress. Animals had multiple gastric ulcers, hyperplastic adrenals, splenic lymphoid depletion and colitis. Although we had no behavioral data available, these appeared to have been socially subordinate animals from cages with particularly aggressive dominant individuals. The ulcerated animals came from social groups and had significantly elevated rates of canine punctures and bite scars. Other investigators have also noted high rates of gastric ulcers in vervet monkeys and, in one case where there were behavioral data available, these were socially subordinate animals (Guzman-Flores et al. 1987).

After death, brains of a dozen such animals were saved for examination and compared with brains from control animals euthanized for other experiments. Importantly, the postmortem lag times were matched between the two groups to control for artifacts of postmortem degeneration. The brains of the ulcerated animals had pronounced hippocampal degeneration. On a gross level, there was overall atrophy in the circumferential extent of Ammon's horn (figure 14.2A). At higher magnification, pyramidal neurons had reduced and irregularly shaped perikarya associated with dispersed Nissl bodies and atrophic dendritic branches (figure 14.2B). On an ultrastructural level, perikaryon size was reduced, dendritic processes were narrowed, synaptic vesicle number was reduced, and dendritic branches were swollen. These qualitative patterns of degeneration were seen in both sexes, and among males there was also a decline in overall pyramidal cell number (figure 14.3). A quarter of the animals had more than 80% of neurons with degeneration, and three quarters of the animals had more than 20% of their neurons with degeneration. In contrast, no degeneration was noted in any of the control monkeys. A similar pattern has been found in tree shrews, in which captive subordinate animals also often die from syndromes of social stress, and where the hippocampal damage can emerge as rapidly as 2 weeks after the onset of the social stress (Uno et al. 1991).

Therefore, sustained and fatal stress in the primate is associated with hippocampal damage. Importantly, it shares many features with glucocorticoid-induced neurodegeneration in the rat. The hippocampus is preferentially damaged: Some degeneration occurred in the cortex in the primate but not in thalamus, hypothalamus, caudate or pontine nucleus. Within the hippocampus,

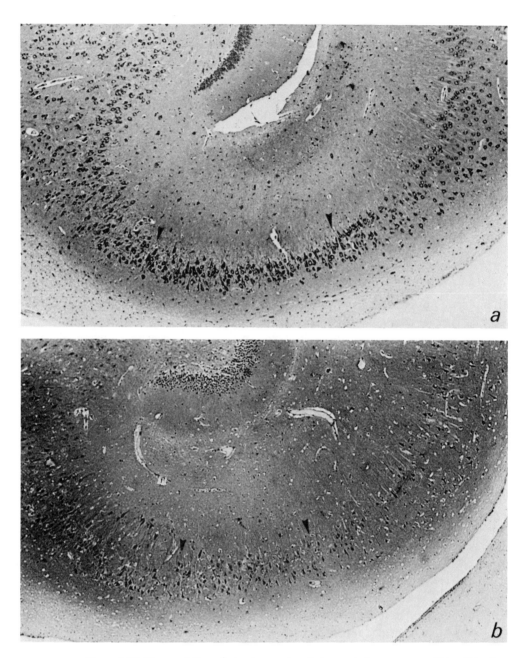

Figure 14.2. Representative photomicrographs of Ammon's horn neurons (CA_1–C_4) of a control monkey (A) compared with an ulcerated animal (B). Latter shows shrunken and sparse pyramidal neurons and reduced extent of CA_3 region (between arrowheads). ($\times$ 85) Representative photomicrographs of CA_3 neurons of a control monkey (C) and an ulcerated animal (D). Latter shows dispersed Nissl bodies and irregularly shaped perikarya with atrophic dendritic branches in the stratum lucidum. ($\times$ 500) (From Uno et al., 1989, J Neurosci 9, 1705. Reprinted with permission of Oxford University Press.)

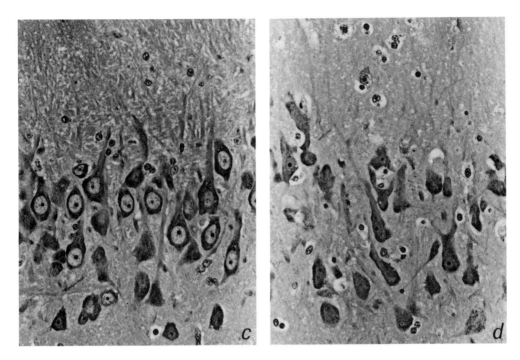

Figure 14.2 (continued)

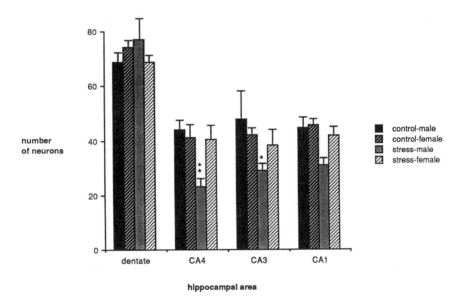

Figure 14.3. Numbers of pyramidal neurons/coronal section through Ammon's horn. Asterisks indicate significantly different from same-sex control. (From Uno et al., 1989, J Neurosci 9, 1705. Reprinted with permission of Oxford University Press.)

Is This Relevant to the Human?

pyramidal neurons of CA_3 are hardest hit, and dentate granule cells are the most resistant (Uno et al. 1989b).

Were glucocorticoids the mediators of this effect in the primate? There are several ways to test this. The most straightforward would be to expose monkeys to high cortisol concentrations in the upper stress range for a period of years and then examine the hippocampus for damage. This would produce extremely cushingoid monkeys, subject to the same opportunistic infections, myopathy, metabolic dysfunction, and probably depression as a human in a similar state. In considering the next step, this struck me as an unacceptable study. As an alternative, we studied four vervet monkeys in whom cortisol-secreting pellets were implanted into one hippocampus and cholesterol-secreting pellets into the other (as a means to control for nonspecific steroidal effects of the cortisol). After a year, the hippocampi were examined. Under these conditions, only the unilateral hippocampus, rather than the entire body, was exposed to the glucocorticoids. There were several obvious problems with this study. The sample size was quite small. Moreover, it was unclear what levels of cortisol the hippocampus would be exposed to from the pellet; thus, it is impossible to determine whether this is a physiological or pharmacological study. Finally, a year of glucocorticoid exposure is quite short if this study was meant to mimic the chronic glucocorticoid studies in the rat—one year is roughly equivalent to one month of steroid exposure for a rat, a time insufficient for inducing hippocampal damage (Nichols and Finch, personal communication).

Despite these caveats, we observed preferential damage in the cortisol-treated hippocampi. In the cholesterol side, mild cell layer irregularity was noted in two of four cases. In contrast, in all the cortisol-treated hippocampi there were at least two of the following neuropathologic markers: cell layer irregularity, dendritic atrophy, soma shrinkage and condensation, or nuclear pyknosis. Damage was severe in one case (i.e., more than 20% of neurons with some neuropathology), and was restricted to the CA_3/CA_2 cell field in all animals (Sapolsky et al. 1990b). There were no differences in neuron number; the cortisol-induced damage was qualitative.

Collectively, these rather grim studies show that sustained and severe stress can damage the primate hippocampus. Moreover, glucocorticoids alone can damage both the fetal and adult hippocampus. It is still not clear if physiologically high concentrations of glucocorticoids are neurotoxic. Such a study is necessary to verify whether glucocorticoids are the mediators of damage in the circumstances of chronic stress. If the answer is shown to be yes, it may have implications for humans exposed to sustained stress. However, the pharmacological data in hand already may have serious implications for humans exposed to pharmacological concentrations of glucocorticoids for sustained periods. This is an enormous number of people, as vast quantities of such steroids are perscribed each year to approximately 16 million people in this country (Eufermiond, 1990). Most of these cases are fairly benign, with short-term administration of rather low steroid doses. However, a substantial subset of individuals receive sustained high-dose steroid regimens to control autoimmune disorders, asthma, tumor-induced edema, and a host of other disorders. These high-dose corticosteroid regimens are known to cause transient ventricular enlargement, cerebral atrophy, and neuropsychological impairments (Bentson et al. 1978; Momose and Richardson 1968; Walkowitz et al. 1990; even moderate glucocorticoid exposure can disrupt cognition in rodents and humans [Levy and Dachir 1991; Fehm-Wolfsdorf et al. 1991]). The permanence of these deficits is unknown. Along with a number of colleagues, we are currently in the midst of the formidable task of collecting a library of brains from humans with long-term corticosteroid exposure to determine if there is hippocampal damage.

In summary, the first half of this chapter shows that the major regulatory components of the glucocorticoid cascade seem to occur, at least to some extent, in the primate. The primate hippocampus is an inhibitor of adrenocortical function, much as in the rodent. While it is not clear if glucocorticoids or stress preferentially down-regulate corticosteroid receptors in the hippocampus, the consequences of chronic stress are the same as in the rat—feedback resistance and hyperadrenocorticism. Finally, in a pair of studies, severe stress and sustained exposure to glucocorticoids were shown to damage the primate hippocampus in ways similar to that seen in the phenomenon of glucocorticoid neurotoxicity in the rodent hippocampus. The remainder of this chapter examines how these different components are relevant to human aging and to a number of human diseases.

RELEVANCE TO HUMAN AGING AND TO HUMAN DISEASE

Normal Human Aging

At first glance, the most striking feature of adrenocortical function in aged humans is its normalcy. Basal concentrations of cortisol and of the 17-hydroxycorticoids do not increase with age (West et al. 1961; Blichert-Toft and Blichert-Toft 1970; Cartlidge et al. 1970; Jensen and Blichert-Toft 1971; Kley et al. 1975; Touitou et al. 1983). Moreover, the circadian rhythm of cortisol remains intact (Serio et al. 1969; Grad et al. 1971; Tourigny-Rivard et al. 1981; Touitou et al. 1983), and CBG levels are not changed with age (Colucci et al. 1975). In addition to normal basal function, the stress-response remains intact with age. While this has been tested only rarely (for obvious ethical reasons), normal responses are seen following surgical stress, or experimental hypoglycemia (Blichert-Toft and Blichert-Toft 1970; Cartlidge et al. 1970; Blichert-Toft 1975; Muggeo et al. 1975). Whether aged humans can terminate cortisol secretion at the end of stress has not been addressed. Finally, feedback sensitivity of the axis is intact, in that there is normal responsiveness to dexamethasone (more than 50 studies reviewed in Zimmerman and Coryell 1987), as well as after disinhibition due to metyrapone administration (Blichert-Toft and Hummer 1977).

Therefore, the overall features of basal function, of the stress-response and feedback sensitivity are normal in aged humans. Most individual components of the adrenocortical axis are also intact. Adrenal sensitivity to ACTH is normal (West et al. 1961; Blichert-Toft and Blichert-Toft 1970; Kley et al. 1975; Blichert-Toft 1975; Ohashi et al. 1986; Roberts et al. 1990) as is the pituitary's responsiveness to CRF (May et al. 1987; Pavlov et al. 1986). One exception concerns basal cortisol concentrations. Ideally, if this endpoint does not change with age, it should be because the components that regulate it do not change. Instead, the stable basal concentrations result from two different and opposing changes that cancel each other out. With age, there is decreased glucocorticoid production (Serio et al. 1969) coupled with decreased clearance of glucocorticoids from the circulation. The latter manifests itself as both a longer half-life of steroids in the bloodstream (West et al. 1961), as well as lower urinary corticosteroid concentrations (West et al. 1961; Romanoff and Baxter 1975).

Overall, the adrenocortical axis of the aged human works quite adequately and is free of the dysfunctions of the aged rat. However, some subtle defects are reminiscent of the pattern in the rat. They are demonstrable in at least three ways:

1. Extremely aged humans tend to be hypercortisolemic and dexamethasone resistant. The extensive literature concerning dexamethasone sensitivity in aged humans (reviewed in Zimmerman and Coryell 1987) is based on the now-dated notion of what constitutes "aged." Therefore, while the 53 studies covered in that review showed no age-related trends, the oldest category considered was classified only as "greater than 50 years," and of the individual studies, a mean age of 68 was the oldest reported. Gerontologists would currently categorize these as only moderately aged populations. More recent studies have demonstrated significantly increased rates of dexamethasone resistance and/or basal hypercortisolism among humans 80 years or older (Nelson et al. 1984b; Davis et al. 1984; Halbreich et al. 1984; Greden et al. 1986; Weiner et al. 1987; Ferrier et al. 1988; one exception: Olsson et al. 1989), and near significant levels of hypercortisolism among individuals in their 70s (Pavlov et al. 1986). As further support for this trend, we have observed recently that the incidence of basal hypercortisolism and of dexamethasone resistance rises with age in wild baboons (Sapolsky and Altmann 1991). As discussed earlier, individual differences in dexamethasone kinetics in the bloodstream might be a major confound in cases of dexamethasone resistance, and this is a particular possibility when comparing different age groups (Weiner 1989). Thus, the reports of increased rates of dexamethasone resistance with age from the studies above should be interpreted with caution. However, the demonstration of increased rates of basal hypercortisolism with age is impressive, in that it avoids that confound.

2. The threshold for feedback resistance may be lower in aged humans. In the standard dexamethasone suppression test, 1 mg of the steroid is given, and individuals with circulating cortisol concentrations greater than 5 $\mu g/dl$ are considered to be dexamethasone resistant. However, numerous studies in biological psychiatry have used 0.5 mg doses of dexamethasone in order to unmask "borderline" cases of resistance. When tested with the lower dose,

healthy aged populations are dexamethasone resistant at a higher rate than healthy younger populations (Dilman et al. 1979; Oxenkrug et al. 1983; Branconnier et al. 1984).

3. Aged humans may have normal feedback sensitivity, but might still be close to the threshold at which they become resistant. In such a case, if aging coincides with disorders of borderline feedback resistance, the incidence of resistance should increase with age. That is to say, either having such a disorder or being aged might be insufficient to cause resistance, but the threshold is passed when both occur together. This is seen with two disorders to be discussed shortly—Alzheimer's disease and depression. Dexamethasone resistance, a common feature of both of these diseases, occurs more frequently in aged persons (see below). (A number of possible confounds should be discussed as to why aged depressives are more likely to be dexamethasone resistant than young depressives, separate from the model presented in this book. For example, aged depressives may be more resistant than young depressives because of a factor of chronicity, with more cumulative depressive episodes in an aged than a younger depressive. Moreover, aged depressives may have a higher incidence of a subtype of depression that is not yet recognized as being highly associated with resistance. In that case, the association would be between the hypersecretion and that subtype, rather than with aging. Finally, the half-life of dexamethasone might be shorter in aged humans, leading to less steroid available to exert a feedback signal. None of these possibilities has, as yet, been adequately eliminated from possibility.)

These more recent data suggest that the aged adrenocortical axis in the human has some of the same defects as in the rat, in that there is basal hypersecretion and feedback resistance. The hippocampus, as discussed, appears to inhibit glucocorticoid secretion in the primate, and the human hippocampus loses neurons with age (of a similar magnitude and pattern as in the rat [reviewed in Coleman and Flood 1987]). Yet, it is not the identical syndrome. The hypersecretion in the rat emerges relatively early in the process of senescence (by approximately 15 to 18 months of age; see chapter 3), whereas in the human, there is an emergence only in extreme old age. At earlier ages (60s and 70s), hypersecretion does not become apparent until coupled with an additional insult (such as depression) or tested more sensitively (i.e., the 0.5-mg version of the dexamethasone suppression test). Therefore, while the human and rat adrenocortical axes decline in similar ways, the former seems more robust—for the same degree of hippocampal damage, there is only the proclivity toward dysfunction until extreme old age. To use a convenient phrase that masks complete ignorance as to an explanation, the human adrenocortical axis appears to have more redundancy built into it than that of the rodent.

Depression and Hypercortisolism

It has been 30 years since the first report that humans with major depressions secreted excessive quantities of cortisol and were insensitive to glucocorticoid feedback inhibition (Gibbons and McHugh 1962). The development of the dexamethasone suppression test and the demonstration of dexamethasone resistance sent waves of excitement through the biological psychiatry community. The existence of an endocrine abnormality in affective disorders such as depression verified the biological reality of the disorder; moreover, there is at least the suggestion that the hypercortisolism might be sufficient to actually be immunosuppressive (cf. Stein et al. 1991). The fact that not all patients were hypercortisolemic suggested that the appearance of the trait could be used as a diagnostic tool and prognostic predictor. In addition, it seems that some of the excitement from that period resulted from the promise that modern psychiatrists would soon be able to rely on laboratory reports and hormone values—the sort of hard figures that often seem to evoke their envy of internal medicine. For the purposes of this book, the most interesting questions to be asked are, What are the neuroendocrine causes and neuropathologic consequences of the hypercortisolism?

In approaching the first question, it is critical to first note that the hypercortisolism is not a unitary phenomenon; depressives hypersecrete cortisol in different circumstances, and they need not all go together. There can be basal hypersecretion throughout the circadian cycle or, more typically, only during the circadian trough; moreover, the circadian rhythm can be phase-shifted (Winokur et al. 1985). Dexamethasone resistance can take the form of not suppressing endogenous cortisol secretion in response to exogenous dexamethasone, or suppression that is delayed or truncated ("early escape") (Extein et al. 1985). A recent study shows that depressives are relatively insensitive to glucocorticoid fast feedback (Young et al. 1991). Moreover, there may be abnormally large secretory responses to hypoglycemic challenges in depressives (Meller et al. 1988). Most importantly, all of these abnormalities do not necessarily appear in the same individual (APA Task Force, 1987). Therefore, there must be multiple and dissociable mechanisms of control that can go awry in the disease. Until the end of this section, *hypercortisolism* will refer to hypersecretion of cortisol under basal conditions, and/or in response to dexamethasone. The distinctions between the two will be considered later.

Of those different possible manifestations of hypercortisolism, the one most studied is the resistance to dexamethasone feedback. The dexamethasone suppression test (DST) in its standardized form consists of administering 1 mg dexamethasone at 11 PM and taking blood at 8 AM, 4, and 11 PM the next day; circulating cortisol concentrations of greater than 5 μg/dl at any of those times qualifies the person as dexamethasone resistant (Carroll et al. 1981). By those criteria, the test has a sensitivity of approximately 50% (i.e., 50% of depressives show the trait) (Carroll et al. 1981). There are a number of possible sources of error in this test. The number can be elevated spuriously by failing to exclude patients who are stressed by conducting the test in a novel setting, who are receiving or withdrawing from various drugs, who have sustained major weight loss, or who have any of a number of diseases including, obviously, most endocrine disorders. Likewise, the specificity of the test is not perfect (i.e., dexamethasone resistance can occur in other disorders, especially acute psychoses, mania, eating disorders, and various dementias). Once that is sorted out, the question becomes What is distinctive about the subset of depressives who are hypercortisolemic?

This has generally been a disappointing line of research, at least for those who hoped that the feature would immediately identify the subtype of depression being suffered, the prognosis, or the treatment outcome. Hypercortisolism does not correlate with sex, duration of symptoms, the severity of depression, or the length of hospitalization (Carroll et al. 1981). Its one major correlate is that rates of resistance become far higher in aged depressive populations. This has been shown in a veritable explosion of recent reports (Spar and La Rue 1983; Davis et al. 1984; Stokes et al. 1984; Georgotas et al. 1984; Jacobs et al. 1984; Rubinow et al. 1984; Nelson et al. 1984a; Lewis et al. 1984; Halbreich et al. 1984; Fogel et al. 1985; Hunt et al. 1989; Maes et al. 1990). Moreover, dexamethasone resistance has only limited usefulness in differentiating among different depressive subtypes. In general, there are somewhat higher rates of hypercortisolism for acute psychotic affective disorders or mixed manic-depressive states, as opposed to major depression in general (Sachar et al. 1973; Coryell et al. 1982; Asnis et al. 1982; Mendlewicz et al. 1982; Rothschild et al. 1982; Rudorfer et al. 1982; Arana et al. 1983; Krishnan et al. 1983; Evans and Nemeroff 1983; Evans et al. 1983; Stokes et al. 1984; Schatzberg et al. 1985). It has been suggested that the common theme of emotional arousal among these different depressive subtypes leads to the hypercortisolism (Lamberts 1986). Regardless of the cause, the correlation between the endocrine marker and the depressive subtype is still not very good—one certainly cannot differentiate between two of these forms of depression based merely on whether dexamethasone resistance is present. Things are not much better prognostically, with a slight suggestion that resistant patients have less favorable prognoses. With respect to treatment outcome, in general, dexamethasone status is not a strong predictor of response to electroconvulsive therapy or tricyclic antidepressants (Gitlin and Gerner 1986); there is some suggestion that dexamethasone resistant patients are less likely to respond to placebo treatment or cognitive therapy (Rush 1984; Brown et al. 1987).

In summary, some of the initial, almost fevered enthusiasm for the dexamethasone suppression test has waned. For our purposes, however, the most interesting question is, What neuroendocrine dysfunction causes such resistance? As should be obvious, I will argue that hippocampal dysfunction may contribute to the defect. What is known about the mechanisms underlying the hypercortisolism?

The first possibility is that the phenomenon could arise from a subtle but very real artifact. Perhaps dexamethasone-resistant individuals merely have a shorter half-life of dexamethasone in their bloodstream. In this scenario, less dexamethasone is available to exert a feedback signal. Suddenly the interesting possibility that dexamethasone resistance implies something distinct about neural function in some depressives is undermined—dexamethasone resistance would be due to nothing more than the liver taking out its proverbial garbage faster than usual. Research has examined this possibility, and a subset of resistant patients do have different dexamethasone pharmacokinetics that would account for the pattern; these differences are independent of age, sex, weight, body surface area, body mass index, severity of illness, hospitalization status, or gastrointestinal absorption rate, and probably mostly reflects the catabolic rate of the liver (Lowry and Meltzer 1987). This suggests that when the DST is conducted, circulating dexamethasone concentrations should be monitored, and the suppressive response should be expressed not per unit dexamethasone administered, but per unit dexamethasone that winds up in the bloodstream (APA Task Force 1987).

When this important factor is accounted for, there is still a substantial subset of depressive patients who are abnormally resistant to a dexamethasone feedback signal in the bloodstream. Moreover, there is the subset of depressives who, independent of any complexities in interpreting the DST, hypersecrete cortisol basally. Why does this happen?

The phenomenon could arise from a number of points in the adrenocortical axis. Potentially, there could be (1) adrenal hypersensitivity to ACTH; (2) pituitary resistance to GC feedback; (3) pituitary hypersensitivity to secretagogs; (4) hypothalamic secretagog hypersecretion; or (5) neural feedback resistance. A number of these occur. Of principal importance, the driving point of dysfunction appears to be at the level of the brain.

To begin with, there is considerable evidence of adrenal hypersensitivity to ACTH. First, hypercortisolism can occur in patients despite normal ACTH concentrations, implying enhanced adrenal sensitivity (Nasr et al. 1982; Gerkin and Holsboer 1986; Risch et al. 1988). This is shown more explicitly by challenging individuals with ACTH and measuring their cortisol secretory response. Adrenal hypersensitivity occurs in some hypercortisolemic depressives (Amsterdam et al. 1989). This has also been shown indirectly after CRF challenges, in which cortisol output per unit ACTH in the bloodstream can be quantified. Again, hypercortisolemic depressives secrete more cortisol per unit ACTH stimulation (Gold et al. 1986; Holsboer et al. 1984a, 1987a; Risch et al. 1988) (It should be noted that this literature has been critized [Krishnan et al. 1989], for the supraphysiologic concentrations of ACTH generated). Some evidence, free of those confounds, comes from anatomical data. Adrenals can become hyperresponsive to ACTH by enlarging, thus having more steroid synthetic capacity. Evidence for such adrenal hyperplasia in hypercortisolemic depressives has been found by measuring the adrenal in living patients by CT scanning (Amsterdam et al. 1987), or by postmortem examination of the adrenal (Dorovini-Zis and Zis 1987).

These numerous studies suggest that at least part of depressive hypercortisolism can be explained at the level of the adrenal. However, in many hypercortisolemic depressives, there is hypersecretion of ACTH (Kalin et al. 1982; Reus et al. 1982; Herevanian et al. 1983; Pfohl et al. 1985). Therefore, there must also be a problem at the level of the pituitary. Part of this is due to blunted pituitary sensitivity to glucocorticoid feedback. As evidence, more dexamethasone is required to block pituitary responsiveness to CRF in depressives than in healthy controls (Holsboer et al. 1987a; von Bardeleben and

Holsboer 1989, 1991—however, the authors interpret this as secondary to a neural defect, to be discussed below. Moreover, some of this difference could be explained by difference in dexamethasone half-life, rather than in pituitary function). Therefore, there might be a pituitary contribution as well. However, hypersecretion of a hypothalamic secretagog also contributes.

The best evidence for this came with the characterization of CRF; in the aftermath, a number of groups quickly examined pituitary sensitivity to CRF in depressives (or, more specifically, in hypercortisolemic depressives), and a pleasing consensus has emerged. Consistently, ACTH secretion in response to a CRF challenge is blunted (Holsboer et al. 1984a,b, 1986; Gold et al. 1984, 1986; Risch et al. 1987). This could be due to either of two reasons. First, in these hypercortisolemic patients, the elevated plasma glucocorticoid concentrations may cause a feedback signal strong enough to block pituitary responsiveness to CRF. This mechanism occurs in rats (Miyanaga et al. 1991); one recent report suggests the same in human depressives, in that following metyrapone administration (which blocks glucocorticoid synthesis and thus removes the steroid feedback signal), depressives have responses to CRF that are at least as large as those of normal controls (von Bardeleben et al. 1988; Lisansky et al. 1989; Ur 1991). Arguing aginst this mechanism is the report that pituitaries of depressives are less sensitive to a glucocorticoid feedback signal (Holsboer et al. 1987a). As an alternative mechanism, the pituitary may have lost its intrinsic responsiveness to CRF itself. This could be due to sustained overexposure to CRF (which down-regulates CRF receptor number [Wynn et al. 1985]). Regardless of which mechanism(s) explains the blunted pituitary sensitivity, the conclusion is similar and important: If there are elevated circulating ACTH concentrations *despite* diminished pituitary sensitivity to CRF, there must be enhanced secretagog drive from the level of the brain. (The reader will note how similar this sequence of experiments and of interpretations is to the data reviewed in chapter 12 showing that hypercortisolism of socially subordinate baboons originates at the CNS level.) This conclusion is supported further with the report that depressives also have a blunted pituitary response to vasopressin (Carroll 1972; Krahn et al. 1985).

A neural defect is also implied by the reports of elevated CSF concentrations of CRF in depressives (Nemeroff et al. 1984; Banki et al. 1987). This should be interpreted cautiously, however. Cerebrospinal fluid CRF represents an integrated measure of both "neuroendocrine" CRF (i.e., median eminance CRF destined to release ACTH from the pituitary) and "neural" CRF (CRF elsewhere in the brain serving a neurotransmitter or neuromodulatory role). As evidence that CSF CRF is a poor index of neuroendocrine CRF and adrenocortical function, its circadian rhythm is desynchronized from that of adrenocortical hormones (Garrick et al. 1987; Kalin et al. 1987).

Finally, a neural defect is suggested by the results of a very subtle experiment. Healthy humans were administered 4 mg of dexamethasone. Twelve hours later, their pituitaries still responded to CRF, implying that the dexamethasone was not working directly at the pituitary. If, at such times, dexamethasone normally suppresses ACTH concentrations (which it does), it must be due to lack of CRF secretion, since there is still responsiveness to CRF. Therefore, if dexamethasone-induced feedback at such times occurs at the brain level, dexamethasone resistance must be a failure at the brain level (Hermus et al. 1987). The only problem with this reasoning is that CRF is not the only hypothalamic secretagog, and the defect in hypercortisolism could be failure of dexamethasone to block pituitary responsiveness to one of the other hormones, such as vasopressin. As a counter to that critique, however, is the report that depressives do indeed have blunted sensitivity to vasopressin (Carroll 1972; Krahn et al. 1985).

In summary, the hypercortisolism of depression seems to involve secretagog hypersecretion by the brain, a compensatory decrease in sensitivity by the pituitary, and a hypersensitivity to ACTH at the adrenal. Gold and colleagues (1986) have synthesized these findings into a hypothesis about the temporal emergence of hypercortisolism. They believe that the hypercortisolism in acute and chronic depressions have different underpinnings. In acute depression, there are elevated concentrations of secretagogs, of ACTH, and of cortisol. With time, two changes occur that are of opposite directions—the pituitary becomes less sensitive to CRF as a compensation, and the adrenal becomes more sensitive to ACTH (i.e., it becomes hyperplastic). The net result with chronic depression is still hypercortisolism, but from different building blocks: A typical hypercortisolemic at that point would have elevated secretagog and cortisol concentrations, but near-normal ACTH concentrations. Moreover, it is only in chronic depression that there would be a blunted ACTH response to CRF, an enhanced cortisol response to ACTH, and adrenal hyperplasia.

Given the implied role of the CNS in the hypercortisolism of depression, I naturally would point a finger at the hippocampus as a possible cause. There is no evidence of hippocampal atrophy in the acute depressions that so typically give rise to hypercortisolism. Therefore, the hypercortisolism could not arise from overt hippocampal damage. My sense is that the rat model of stress-induced down-regulation of hippocampal corticosteroid receptors, discussed in chapter 5, might be relevant. Those data showed that at least some paradigms of repeated or sustained stress produce such receptor loss; feedback efficacy declines and hypersecretion ensues. Moreover, with the cessation of stress, receptor number and feedback efficacy normalize. These observations fit the depression picture quite well, it seems. Stress is frequently a predisposing factor in depression (Anisman and Zacharko 1982; Gold et al. 1988). Moreover, humans who have undergone sustained stress become dexamethasone resistant (Baumgartner et al. 1985; Ceulemans et al. 1985). In addition, the hypercortisolism of depressives typically resolves when the depression abates (Carroll 1982). Finally, such a model also explains why dexamethasone resistance becomes more common in older depressives, as that would represent the intersection of two trends—increased rates of resistance with aging, and with depression.

Given the proposed role of the hippocampus, and down-regulation of its corticosteroid receptors in the hypercortisolism of depression, which secretagog(s) is hypersecreted? The clinical literature is muddy on this question. The reports of blunted pituitary sensitivity to CRF and vasopressin in depressives do not prove that it is those secretagogs which are hypersecreted; they merely imply that at least one secretagog is hypersecreted. For example, there may be oversecretion of oxytocin, and the pituitary simply attempts to compensate by reducing sensitivity to CRF and vasopressin. The elevated CSF CRF concentrations of depressives suggests that CRF is hypersecreted. However, as discussed, CSF CRF does not automatically equal portal CRF, limiting the usefulness of that observation.

It might be that both CRF and another secretagog are oversecreted. Lamberts and colleagues (1986) suggest that it is CRF and catecholamines. As evidence, they have shown that CRF alone cannot override a dexamethasone blockade of responsiveness in rat anterior pituitary cells in culture, while a combination of CRF and catecholamines cause "dexamethasone resistance." Given how important dosages and pharmacokinetics are in this field, I feel that one cannot rely too heavily on in vitro studies such as these. In a study with human volunteers, von Bardeleben and colleagues (1985) showed that CRF and vasopressin, but not CRF alone, could override a dexamethasone blockade. The authors suggest that it is a combination of both that is hypersecreted in hypercortisolism. This study has been criticized, however (Hermus et al. 1987); these authors note that von Bardeleben et al. used human CRF, which is not as effective as ovine CRF (used in most clinical studies). Therefore, they theorized that this is why CRF alone did not override dexamethasone in this case and does not imply that CRF hypersecretion alone cannot explain hypercortisolism. In another study, von Bardeleben and Holsboer (1989) demonstrated that CRF could override an inhibitory dexamethasone signal at the pituitary of depressives, but not in healthy controls; they speculated that hypersecretion of vasopressin in depressives synergizes with the CRF to override the feedback signal.

Clearly, it is not known which secretagog(s) is hypersecreted. This reflects the difficulties of inferring physiology from pharmacological studies and trying to study one of the least accessible parts of the body in the human.

If the rat model of corticosteroid receptor down-regulation in the hippocampus does explain the hypercortisolism of the depressive, it also allows some predictions as to which secretagog mediates the hypersecretion. As will be recalled from many chapters ago, the hippocampus appears to regulate the secretion of a number of secretagogs, but under differing conditions and with different sensitivities. During either basal or moderate stress conditions, fornix-transected rats hypersecreted both vasopressin and oxytocin. During conditions of a heavy corticosterone feedback signal, fornix-transected rats hypersecreted both CRF and oxytocin. Moreover, the receptor occupancy studies showed that the relationship between occupancy and inhibition of CRF was linear. In contrast, the relationship between occupancy and inhibition of oxytocin and vasopressin were nonlinear; very small and moderate amounts of occupancy were needed to substantially inhibit vasopressin and oxytocin, respectively. These observations allow some very speculative predictions (tempered, of course, by the rodent data being derived from the unphysiologic preparation of cannulating the hypophysial portal circulation). In the rat, hippocampal corticosteroid receptors are never down-regulated more than approximately 50%. Therefore, the system cannot be down-regulated to the point of massive disinhibition of vasopressin secretion (see chapter 5). If things work similarly in the human, this predicts that hypercortisolism due to down-regulation can never be driven by vasopressin and can be driven by oxytocin only in extreme cases. CRF would be the most likely secretagog hypersecreted in such circumstances.

In summary, the model of stress-induced hippocampal receptor depletion might explain the hypercortisolism of depressives. However, two obvious problems with this model must be discussed:

It has never been shown that depressives who become dexamethasone resistant had a major stressor prior to the depression. This is certainly a problem for this model. As a possible explanation, people may differ not only in how much stress they are exposed to, but also in their intrinsic vulnerability to stress-induced down-regulation. This could arise from at least three different neuroendocrine variables (figure 14.4; Sapolsky and Plotsky 1990). First, two individuals could differ in the amount of corticosteroid receptors they have in their hippocampus prior to stress (A versus B). Under those circumstances, while both individual's receptor populations might down-regulate at the same rate in response to stress, B reaches the threshold for feedback resistance more readily. Second, two individuals might differ in the sensitivity of their receptor system to stress-induced down-regulation, such that one loses receptors faster (A versus C). Third, individuals may differ as to how much receptor loss is required to cause feedback dysfunction. The number of such hippocampal receptors is tremendously variable among rats, depending on age, sex, behavioral history, strain, and early experience. There should be at least that much among the

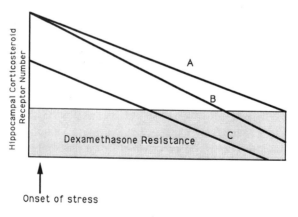

Figure 14.4. Schematic representation of possible sources of individual variability in sensitivity to stress-induced down-regulation of hippocampal corticosteroid receptors. (Reprinted by permission of Elsevier Science Publishing Company, Inc. from Hypercortisolism and its possible neural basis by R. Sapolsky and P. Plotsky, Biological Psychiatry 27, 937. Copyright 1990 by the Society of Biological Psychiatry.)

more heterogeneous humans. Given large amounts of variability, some individuals should require very little external stress to down-regulate them past the threshold; the stressor required may be so subtle that it is not discernable to the outside observer.

How can these ideas be tested? As noted, it will be difficult to quantify receptors in postmortem tissue. Two possible studies would be informative:

1. Once PET-scanning methods allow quantification of small changes within the hippocampus in binding of tagged cortisol, the following study should be conducted: Humans undergoing a period of major stress (for example, the medical interns discussed earlier) should have cortisol binding in the hippocampus quantified before and during the stressor. Binding should be assessed after metyrapone administration, to minimize endogenous competing cortisol. Previous studies predict that approximately 50% of the interns should become dexamethasone resistant during the stressor. Are these the individuals who started off with the least binding prior to the stressor, wound up with the least, lost the most binding sites during the stressor? This might piece out which variable is most critical in predicting vulnerability.

2. A pattern might exist in reviewing case histories of depressives that would allow a test of these ideas. As shown in figure 14.4, individual B requires less stress to become dexamethasone resistant than individual A. Given the progressive loss of hippocampal neurons with aging, senescent humans are more likely to resemble individual B than A, and thus require less of a stressor to be down-regulated to the point of dysfunction. This predicts that hypercortisolism as a predisposing stressor should be more tightly linked and more easily demonstrated in young depressives than in old ones—in aged subjects, the amount of stress needed to push the individual past the threshold of dysfunction may be so mild as to be undetectable to the outsider.

If hippocampal dysfunction supposedly causes depressive hypercortisolism, how can the hypersecretion come in different and dissociable forms? This is the problem discussed earlier—basal hypersecretion and dexamethasone resistance can occur independently. This initially seemed to be a problem for the "It's the hippocampus" scenario, as there is only one hippocampus and at least two different mechanisms of dysfunction implied (Sapolsky and McEwen 1988). However, a subsequent study (Sapolsky et al. 1989) provides a possible explanation. That study showed that when the hippocampus is removed from the feedback scene (by fornix transection), there is hypersecretion of secretagogs under conditions of both low and heavy feedback—but the two conditions involved different secretagogs being hypersecreted. Therefore, the hippocampus contributes to feedback by at least two different mechanisms. Following hippocampal damage, hypersecretion under low feedback conditions seems to be driven by vasopressin and oxytocin, whereas hypersecretion under heavy feedback conditions seems to be driven by CRF and oxytocin. This does not even consider heterogeneity of feedback regulation of basal adrenocortical activity (which, obviously, can never be studied with stressful portal surgery). As discussed many chapters ago, the high-affinity Type I receptors are involved in inhibiting glucocorticoid secretion during the circadian trough, whereas both Types I and II receptors are involved during the circadian peak.

In summary, so long as the dysfunction in depression impairs only a subset of hippocampal neurons, only subsets of feedback mechanisms might be impaired. One can readily imagine that there are neurons distributed throughout the hippocampus with differing feedback roles. One, for example, might inhibit CRF secretion only during the circadian trough and in the absence of stress, and only when 40% to 60% of its Type I receptors are occupied. Another might inhibit vasopressin independent of time, but only following stress and whenever its Type II are more than 70% occupied. The different profiles of hypercortisolism in different depressed individuals probably reflects only subpopulations of hippocampal neurons being impaired in their feedback roles. For example, the difference between depressives who hypersecrete cortisol only during the circadian trough versus those who hypersecrete throughout the cycle could be that only the latter have down-regulated Type II receptors, whereas both have losses of Type I receptors.

These speculative ideas focus on why the hypercortisolism of depression occurs. Another question comes to mind. In more severe cases of depressive hypercortisolism, steroid concentrations can approach the range seen in cushingoid patients. Since there is no change in levels of CBG in depressives (Leake et al. 1989), there is a vast increase in the amount of free, biologically active cortisol reaching target tissues. Numerous investigators are now exploring whether this is sufficient to, for example, suppress immune function. From the perspective of this book, an obvious question is whether the hypercortisolism of sustained depression is enough to cause hippocampal damage.

While this idea initially seems quite improbable, some evidence has been accumulating that supports this idea. One early report examined brains from depressives post mortem and found elevated rates of moderate and severe cerebral atrophy (Corsellis 1962). More recent studies, however, have taken advantage of CT and MRI scanning techniques to study structural features of the brain in living patients. A number of studies have found ventricular enlargement in depressives (reviewed in Nasrallah et al. 1989). The correlates of enlarged ventricles include being aged, having a psychotic or delusional depression, being dexamethasone resistant, and being hypercortisolemic (Schlegel and Kretzschmar 1987; Kellner et al. 1983) (It should be remembered that psychotic depression is associated with high rates of dexamethasone resistance.) In addition, scanning studies have shown some (although less consistent) evidence for cortical or cerebellar atrophy in depressives (Nasrallah et al. 1989).

While this begins to support the notion that the sustained hypercortisolism of some forms of prolonged depression could be neurodegenerative, there are obviously tremendous holes to be filled. (1) Ventricular enlargement may reflect an increase in the fluid volume of the brain, rather than a decrease in the tissue volume. Therefore, this may not reflect a loss of neurons. Furthermore, even if it did, there is no reason to suppose that such a loss is exclusive to, or even preferential in the hippocampus, as my ideas would predict. (2) It is not clear if the ventricular enlargement is permanent or resolves with recovery. If the latter, it could not be due to neuron loss (much as is the case for the transient ventricular enlargement seen in torture victims [Jensen et al. 1982]). (3) Whether reflecting a change in fluid or tissue volume, the phenomenon could be due to the drug treatment, rather than the depression itself. This is particularly the case for the possibility of a change in the fluid volume, since both lithium and tricylic antidepressants affect fluid shifts (Preskorn et al. 1982).

To control for the first two issues, postmortem neuron counts must be performed. To control for the third issue, patients must be studied who have not yet been treated pharmacologically. But controls will be difficult to perform. At this stage, the conclusion must be that there is at best only a hint that the prolonged hypercortisolism of depression may exert a neuropathologic toll.

Alzheimer's Disease, Hippocampal Damage, and Hypercortisolism

Senile dementia of the Alzheimer's type (SDAT) is among the most common of dementias. Its neurocytological hallmarks are neuritic plaques of amyloid and neurofibrillary tangles in the hippocampus and neocortex (Terry and Katzman 1983). In some cases, damage to the hippocampus itself is only moderate, but there is considerable damage to the afferent and efferent projections of the structure, isolating it neuroanatomically (Hyman et al. 1984). The disease preferentially targets neurons with certain neurochemical profiles. While a number of such vulnerabilities have been noted, the one to receive the most attention is the profound sensitivity of cholinergic neurons to SDAT damage. Considerable percentages of cholinergic neurons are lost in the nucleus basalis of Meynert; these neurons normally project into hippocampus and cortex (Bowen et al. 1982; Coyle et al. 1983). Molecular biological and genetic studies of the disorder are generating vast excitement and no small amount of confusion; these studies, which are mostly concerning with the amyloid gene and its various protein products, are beyond the scope of this chapter.

As with depression, Alzheimer's disease is associated with basal hypercortisolism and dexamethasone resistance, with an incidence of 50% and with the different manifestations of hypercortisolism being dissociable (Spar and Gerner 1982; Raskind et al. 1982; Carnes et al. 1983a,b; Balldin et al. 1983). Moreover, as with depression, the incidence of hypercortisolism increases with age among Alzheimer's patients (Greenwald et al. 1986). The assumption by most in the field is that the hypercortisolism in SDAT is driven by the brain. This has not been demonstrated very solidly, however. To my knowledge, there have been no studies giving CRF challenges to SDAT patients in order to confirm that. In addition, CSF measurements in SDAT patients have shown decreased concentrations of CRF and vasopressin (Nemeroff et al. 1984; May et al. 1987; Whitehouse et al. 1987; Mazurek et al. 1986; one study showing no change in vasopressin: Jolkkonen et al. 1989). Initially, this appears not to support the notion of hypersecretion by the brain. However, there are two explanations for this discrepancy. First, in these studies, all SDAT patients were examined, rather than limiting the study to hypercortisolemic SDAT patients. Therefore, on the average, half of the patients were not hypercortisolemic, diluting any effect. Second, as noted, CSF secretagog concentrations reflect both neuroendocrine concentrations of peptides as well as neurotransmitter concentrations. In SDAT, there is substantial loss of neurotransmitter CRF in the brain (Bissette et al. 1985), and any putative increase in the (small) pool of neuroendocrine CRF would be undiscernable in the face of this large neurotransmitter decline.

Asssuming that the hypercortisolism is indeed neurally based, it seems quite readily explained by the hippocampal damage and/or isolation typical of SDAT. To make this correlation even tighter, more severe hypercortisolism is associated with more severe hippocampal atrophy (figure 14.5; De Leon et al. 1988) and with more severe cognitive deficits (in women; Oxenkrug et al. 1989). A role for the hippocampus would also explain why hypercortisolism becomes more prevalent with aged SDAT patients, much as with aged depressives. Again, the data imply a threshold model where the tendencies toward resistance during aging and with SDAT combine.

Which secretagog is hypersecreted in SDAT? At present, there is scant clinical indications of an answer. Our rodent studies suggest a different picture than for depression. Here, the problem is not mere down-regulation of the corticosteroid receptors where one must account for there being only a 50% limit as to how far down-regulation can occur. In SDAT, there is overt damage, and it can be severe. The data discussed in chapter 5 showed that hippocampal regulation of vasopressin secretion is tighter than that for CRF, with regulation of oxytocin in between. Therefore, it takes more hippocampal damage to disinhibit vasopressin than CRF. This generates the prediction that when SDAT damage is moderate, hypercortisolism should mostly be driven by CRF. With increasing damage, however, a hyperphysiologic oxytocin signal should be added and, with more damage, an extremely augmented vasopressin signal. As with the ideas about depression, this is extremely speculative thinking.

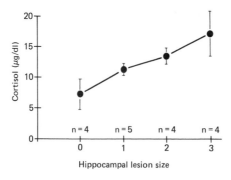

Figure 14.5. Average cortisol levels 120 minutes after intravenous glucose as a function of severity of hippocampal atrophy. (From de Leon, et al., 1988. Abnormal cortisol response in Alzheimer's disease linked to hippocampal atrophy. Lancet 2, 391–392.)

As with depression, one must explain why only some SDAT patients are hypercortisolemic and why different features of hypercortisolism can occur independently. In both cases, the answers are much as for depression. The individual variability must reflect differences in how severe the degeneration is, which hippocampal neurons are damage and/or isolated, and what that individual's threshold of damage is before hypercortisolism is triggered. The plasticity of the system adds another explanation. As discussed, the hypercortisolism and dexamethasone resistance in primates after damage to the hippocampal system is not permanent. Much as in the rat, it resolves after a time (over the course of weeks in the rats, and months to years in the primate) (Sapolsky et al. 1991a). This suggests that in SDAT patients in whom the degeneration has stabilized, there is likely to be normalization of cortisol secretion. It is not clear whether SDAT damage ever does reach a plateau.

As to why different features of resistance can occur independently, one must again invoke the data showing that the hippocampus helps regulate secretagog release under both basal and heavy feedback conditions, but in different ways and with differing roles of the two types of receptors during the circadian cycle. Therefore, there are multiple components of feedback control within the hippocampus; so long as the disease damages only a subset of the hippocampal neurons, individuals will be likely to differ as to which domains of feedback inhibition are compromised.

In considering SDAT, one must also focus on the other half of the relationship between glucocorticoids and the hippocampus—can glucocorticoid overexposure play a role in bringing about the hippocampal degeneration of SDAT? This is really two questions. Can a history of stress *cause* SDAT by damaging the hippocampus? Once the disease is established, can its degenerative features be exacerbated by glucocorticoid overexposure (either due to stress, to the hypercortisolism of the disease itself, or due to exogenous glucocorticoids taken for some other reasons)?

No answers are known for either of these questions. Six years ago, when writing about glucocorticoids as causing or exacerbating SDAT neurodegeneration, I characterized both possibilities as extremely unlikely (Sapolsky and McEwen 1986). A few very striking threads have emerged in the last few years, suggesting that glucocorticoids just might exacerbate such degeneration. Specifically, it has been shown that EAAs, calcium, and energy deprivation can cause some of the degenerative features seen in SDAT:

• Antigenic changes similar to those that occur in neurofibrillary tangles can be caused by EAAs and calcium in cultured hippocampal neurons (Mattson 1990). Such tangles contain large quantities of the protein ubiquitin, and of the phosphorylated version of a cytoskeletal protein called tau. Exposure of cultures to toxic or subtoxic doses of EAAs increase tau and ubiquitin immunoactivity; this increase is dependent on the presence of calcium in the culture medium. One should not get too excited about the implied EAA/Alzheimer's link in the ubiquitin; while the protein is a marker for tangles in Alzheimer's disease, it is a rather nonspecific marker of filamentous inclusion bodies found in a number of neurodegenerative diseases (Lowe and Mayer 1990).

• Exposure of fibroblasts from healthy human subjects to an antimetabolite (an uncoupler of oxidative phosphorylation) also causes a massive increase in tau-like immunoactivity (Blass et al. 1990).

• The β-amyloid protein that makes up amyloid plaques appears to be derived from inappropriate processing of the amyloid precursor protein (APP) (Selkoe 1990). EAAs and calcium will induce APP production (Shigematsu et al. 1991) and promote its proteolysis. Such proteolysis is calpain-dependent (Siman et al. 1990).

• The toxicity of the amyloid fragments appear to involve mechanisms similar to those for the EAA/calcium cascade. As evidence, amyloid fragments will synergize with toxicity induced by EAAs (Koh et al., 1990), hypoglycemia (Copani et al. 1991), and oxygen radicals (Saunders et al. 1991) in vitro.

As recently as a year ago, a paper linking Alzheimer's-like neurodegeneration with the EAA story was viewed as fairly speculative (see Greenamyre and Young 1989, and the peer commentary following this paper). These very recent findings suggest that the link might actually be quite meaningful. They also suggest an obvious syllogism concerning glucocorticoids: If glucocorticoids exacerbate the EAA/calcium cascade, and if the EAA/calcium cascade might cause SDAT-like degeneration, then do glucocorticoids exacerbate the induction of these degenerative features? In support of this idea, we find that glucocorticoids exacerbate EAA-induced tau immunoreactivity (Elliott et al., submitted). SDAT researchers have debated for years whether markers such as the amyloid plaques are causes or consequences of the degeneration and dementia. In the last few years, the tide has begun to shift toward the markers being damaging. For example, a pair of recent papers show that APP fragments are preferentially neurotoxic to cultured hippocampal neurons (Yankner et al. 1989, 1990), and to the hippocampus in vivo (Kowall et al. 1991).

There are also a few suggestions that glucocorticoids might modulate the pathologies of SDAT independent of the EAA cascade. For example, it was noted that SDAT involves pronounced cholinergic neuron loss, and glucocorticoids can exacerbate the toxicity of a cholinergic neurotoxin (Hortnagl et al. 1991). As another hint, in the brain, glucocorticoids also induce the expression of α-1-antichymotrypsin, which is a primary component of senile plaques in SDAT (Das et al. 1991).

At present, these are all very thin threads indeed linking glucocorticoids and SDAT. However, if glucocorticoids do exacerbate these degenerative features, it raises the very real, although still speculative, possibility that these hormones might worsen the neuropathological and/or cognitive features of this tragic disease. The test of this idea is currently underway.

Alcoholic Neurotoxicity

Alcohol is well known for its capacity to disrupt learning, memory recall, and other aspects of cognition. With prolonged periods of alcohol abuse, profound dementias (e.g., Wernicke-Korsakoff dementia) emerge. In concordance with this latter observation, chronic alcoholism can be neurotoxic. This is frequently observed at postmortem examination of such demented alcoholics. The interpretation that the neurodegeneration was due to the alcohol was confounded by the poor, vitamin-deficient diet typical of chronic alcoholics, which could be neurotoxic itself (Irle and Markowitsch 1983). With the development of animal models for chronic alcoholism (in which diets are matched with those of controls), chronic ethanol exposure was showed to be neurotoxic, particularly in the hippocampus (Walker et al. 1980; Irle and Markowitsch 1983; Lescaudron and Verna 1985; Cadete-Leite et al. 1988).

It was also observed that alcohol exposure could activate the adrenocortical axis and increase glucocorticoid secretion (Ellis 1966; Mendelson and Stein 1966; Jenkins and Connolly 1968; Stokes 1973; Kakihana and Moore 1976; Kakihana 1979; Majumdar et al. 1981; Guaza et al. 1983; Zgombick and Erwin 1988; Wand 1989). The mechanisms underlying this activation are not fully understood, but there is evidence that ethanol directly releases various secretagogs from hypothalamic neurons in vitro (Redei et al. 1988). This suggests that ethanol is not a stressor, in that it provokes some physical or psychological perturbation, as much as a nonspecific releaser.

Regardless of the mechanism for ethanol-induced glucocorticoid secretion, the two sets of data immediately suggests a hypothesis: Is the preferential hippocampal neurotoxicity of chronic alcoholism due to the glucocorticoid hypersecretion?

This possibility has been tested in a single study, and the authors concluded that such toxicity was not glucocorticoid mediated (Rachamin et al. 1989). However, I find a number of difficulties with this study which cause me to conclude that the issue has not yet been settled. First, it seems to me that the most direct way to determine whether alcoholic neurotoxicity is glucocorticoid mediated is to see if such toxicity still occurs in the absence of glucocorticoids. Thus, adrenalectomized rats would be exposed to ethanol in a manner known to cause neuronal damage in intact rats. Instead of this approach, the authors took a rather circuitous route. They reasoned that if alcoholic neurotoxicity is glucocorticoid-mediated, the neurons killed should have had large numbers of corticosteroid receptors (ie, that they were most vulnerable to glucocorticoid action). Therefore, they measured whether there was a marked loss of such receptors after chronic alcohol exposure. As an obvious drawback of this indirect approach, remaining neurons are quite capable of up-regulating their receptor concentrations to compensate for any receptor loss, obscuring the indirect endpoint that was being measured.

Most importantly, the authors measured glucocorticoid concentrations and found that alcohol-treated and control rats did not differ. Therefore, it appears that this particular paradigm of ethanol exposure did not even cause the hyperadrenocorticism which could cause neuron damage. (A recent study supports the view that the adrenocortical axis of the rat will at least partially habituate to the stressor of ethanol exposure over the course of weeks [Spencer and McEwen 1990]).

In summary, I feel that this question has not yet been fully explored. Again, the most direct test of the hypothesis would be whether alcoholic neurotoxicity still occurred in adrenalectomized animals. Should glucocorticoids be shown to mediate the neurotoxicity, I would predict that it would be via a very different mechanism than the exacerbation of the glutamate/NMDA/calcium cascade outlined in chapter 11. This is because of the recent observation that ethanol inhibits the conductance of the NMDA receptor-gated channel (Lovinger et al. 1989; Dildy and Leslie 1989; Dildy-Mayfield and Leslie 1991) and inhibits NMDA-dependent instances of long-term potentiation (Blitzer et al. 1990).

Neurological Insults in Humans and the Clinical Use of Glucocorticoids

Hypoxia-Ischemia   The number of humans who sustain hypoxic-ischemic brain damage each year numbers in the hundreds of thousands, by conservative estimates. Can glucocorticoids increase such damage? This seems a plausible possibility to me. A vast number of studies have examined whether the ability of glucocorticoids to inhibit brain tumor edema can be extended to inhibiting postischemic edema. As reviewed in chapter 11, this strategy has not proven to be protective, mostly because glucocorticoids have little impact on the cytotoxic form of edema that occurs following hypoxia or ischemia. The two most authoritative reviews on the subject (Fishman 1982; Goldstein et al. 1989) both conclude that there are no benefits to using glucocorticoids at such times. Despite this, a number of neurological texts still suggest the use of glucocorticoids following cerebral hypoxia or ischemia (Gunderson 1990; Mumenthaler 1990; Adams and Victor 1985, although this recommendation has been dropped by the next edition of Adams and Victor 1989). Thus, it appears worthwhile to add a voice to the chorus suggesting that nonglucocorticoid alternatives be used in such situations (most notably, mannitol). Parsimony suggests to me that the demonstrated ability of glucocorticoids to exacerbate hypoxic-ischemic damage in the rodent justifies examining this possibility in the primate.

Does the endogenous secretion of glucocorticoids during a hypoxic or ischemic crisis add to the damage, as it does in the rodent? There is massive glucocorticoid secretion during global ischemia in humans, and more severe damage is associated with higher circulating concentrations of the steroids (Feibel et al. 1977). Potentially, this could be because the higher glucocorticoid concentrations cause more damage. Alternatively, it could imply that more severe ischemia (which causes more damage) could be a more severe stressor. Once again, parsimony suggests that findings from the rodent might well apply to the primate brain.

Spinal Cord Injury   It is now a highly consistent finding that glucocorticoids can be protective against traumatic injury to the spine. This has been shown with numerous experimental animal models, in which functional and neuropathological endpoints have been assessed (Ducker and Hamit 1969; Black and Markowitz 1971; Richardson and Nakamura 1971; Tator 1972; Campbell et al. 1973; Hall and Braughler 1982; Hall et al. 1984; Braughler and Hall 1985, Braughler et al. 1987). These findings motivated a number of clinical trials in which protective effects against incomplete (but not complete) spinal cord injury were reported (Lucas and Ducker 1979a,b); as a problem, in these studies, steroid treatment was neither blind nor randomized. These findings led to a large, multicenter study that used megadoses of glucocorticoids and which also had the strengths of a placebo group and blind administration of drug or placebo. In a highly publicized report of these findings in the *New England Journal of Medicine* (Bracken et al. 1990), the authors concluded that glucocorticoids caused a significant and persistent improvement of outcome in cases of both complete and incomplete injury.

Glucocorticoids are most probably protective in this instance by non-specifically intercalating in cell membranes, thus stabilizing them against per-oxidative free radical attack. As discussed in chapter 11, the strongest pieces of evidence for this are the facts that the steroids are protective only at megadose concentrations that vastly saturate receptors, that nonglucocorticoid steroids such as the lazaroid compounds are protective as well, and that the degree of protection by a particular steroid is best predicted by how lipid soluble it is and how readily it inhibits lipid peroxidation. Thus, this represents a very different mechanism of action than the route by which glucocorticoids probably damage the hippocampus or by which they decrease brain tumor edema.

Regardless of precise mechanism, at present, the evidence in support of the use of glucocorticoids to decrease spinal cord injury is essentially unanimous. Despite this, there may well be a clinical shift toward the use of the synthetic 21-aminosteroid lazaroids instead, given that they are even more protective and have none of the side effects of glucocorticoids.

Brain Trauma   The very encouraging findings regarding glucocorticoids and spinal cord injury suggest that the hormones might protect against traumatic brain injury as well. However, clinical studies of this issue are very contradictory. Some investigators report protective effects (as measured by reductions in mortality and morbidity) (Ransohoff 1972; Gobiet et al. 1976; Faupel et al. 1976; Jane et al. 1984). In some cases, while there was no overall effect of the glucocorticoids, subsets of patients responded positively to the steroid (for example, the subset showing the most rapid recovery of function following injury [Saul et al. 1981], or the younger cohort [Giannotta et al. 1984]). In contrast, numerous studies have shown no protective effect of glucocorticoids (Sparacio et al. 1965; Alexander 1972; Gutterman and Shenkin 1972; Hoyt et al. 1973; Cooper et al. 1979; Gudeman et al. 1979; Braakman et al. 1983), even when considering separately the subset of patients previously identified as being responsive to the steroids (Braakman et al. 1983). Furthermore, in at least one study, glucocorticoid treatment was even associated with a worse neurological outcome (Saul et al. 1981). Finally, some investigators have criticized reports of protective effects, identifying flaws in experimental design that would have artifactually generated that observation. For example, in a critique of the work of Gobiet and colleagues (1976), it was noted that the investigators did not study the experimental and control groups concurrently, but rather drew the control data from normative populations studied previously; thus, the reported improvement might have been due to advances in management techniques, rather than to the corticosteroid administration (Cooper et al. 1979). Another study (Gianotta et al. 1984) has been studied for nonrandom distribution of patients in steroid-treated or untreated groups in a way that would bias toward a positive outcome (Cooper 1984).

Collectively, it does not appear that glucocorticoids are particularly protective against brain trauma, even when administered in the megadose range (Giannotta et al. 1984) that has been so helpful in spinal cord injury. A priori, this is surprising. Traumatic injury to the brain should be just as potent a route of oxygen radical generation as in the spinal cord, and subsequent lipid peroxidation should be just as pathogenic (Hall and Braughler, 1989). Moreover, the lipid solubility of corticosteroids should not differ substantially in the brain and spinal cord, nor should the potential for the steroids to stabilize the membrane against peroxidative attack. Why should this approach work in the brain but not in the spinal cord? Naturally, I would suggest that because in the brain, any protective antiperoxidative effects might potentially be counterbalanced by the catabolic and endangering effects of glucocorticoids on hippocampal (and to a lesser extent, cortical) neurons.

In summary, I would predict that the nonglucocorticoid lazaroids should be protective against brain trauma and that the advantages of using them over glucocorticoids will be even more apparent in cases of brain trauma than of spinal trauma.

I would also suggest that there may be an additional way to decrease damage following traumatic brain injury. Not surprisingly, such injury provokes massive elevations of endogenous glucocorticoid secretion (Bouzarth et al. 1968; King et al. 1970; Steinbok and Thompson, 1979; Robertson et al. 1985), and this is of a sufficient magnitude to cause catabolic effects outside the nervous system (Clifton et al. 1984; Robertson et al. 1985). It seems quite plausible that this endogenous hypercorticoid state is also sufficient to endanger hippocampal (and perhaps cortical) neurons, much as is the case in the rat. This suggests the following novel clinical intervention: In the aftermath of a traumatic injury to the brain, simultaneous administration of lazaroids *and* an inhibitor of glucocorticoid secretion such as metyrapone should prove even more protective than the lazaroids alone, and far more than megadoses of glucocorticoids alone. The rationale is obvious, in that by blocking endogenous glucocorticoid release, the central nervous system would be spared any of the catabolic and endangering effects of these steroids, while a megadose of the lazaroids would more than match the antiperoxidative potential of the corticosteroids. As a nonclinician, I offer these speculative interventions cheerfully; naturally, any such interventions would have to accommodate the considerable side effects that arise from metyrapone administration.

Prolonged Use of Glucocorticoids to Control Nonneurological Disorders   As noted, vast numbers of individuals take high-dose glucocorticoids each year to inhibit rejection of transplanted tissue, or to control asthma, arthritis, or an autoimmune disorder. At present, it is not clear whether such treatment damages the brain. I consider this possibility to be among the most frightening raised by this book, and the lack of any knowledge whatsoever to be among the most frustrating. Testing this possibility will be enormously difficult. First, a large collection of brains will be needed from individuals with a history of prolonged high-dose glucocorticoid exposure, with well-documented histories of the disease and of steroid use. The large sample size will be necessary in order to have brains from individuals with a broad array of diseases which, in all cases, were treated with high-dose corticosteroids. Next, a control group from healthy age-matched controls will be needed. Furthermore, a control group will be needed of individuals with similar histories of long, debilitating disease, but without the steroid treatment. This will control for the stressfulness of the chronic disease itself. Finally, the endpoint will have to be the extremely tedious measure of neuron number. Obviously, this is not a trivial undertaking, but I believe it is a necessary one. If these studies demonstrate that prolonged high-dose corticosteroid treatment accelerates hippocampal senescence, we are faced with a difficult clinical decision, indeed. It is not obvious, a priori, if this would always argue against the use of corticosteroids in such cases. Given the numerous deleterious side-effects of corticosteroids that are already recognized, they are rarely being administered capriciously. However, such knowledge will allow us to make these difficult decisions more wisely.

SUMMARY

This final chapter focuses on the relevance of the findings presented throughout the book to the primate (including human) brain. One must begin by examining the regulatory components that make up the glucocorticoid cascade model of part I and determining which occur in the primate.

Does the Primate Hippocampus Inhibit the Adrenocortical Axis?

Parsimony suggests that the hippocampus should be as sensitive a glucocorticoid target tissue in the primate as in the rodent, given the high density of corticosteroid receptors in both cases. In a recent study, monkeys that had lesions of the hippocampal system (or fornix cuts) were shown to hypersecrete glucocorticoids and to be dexamethasone resistant. Other limbic lesions did not cause such hypersecretion.

Will Stress Down-regulate Corticosteroid Receptors in the Primate Hippocampus and Thus Cause Feedback Resistance?

This is not known, given the current constraints of receptor technology as applied to humans or primates. However, in important support of this possibility, when human or primates are chronically stressed, they become feedback resistant.

Can Stress Damage the Primate Hippocampus?

In support of this, a very early literature reports "limbic atrophy" in untreated Cushing's patients, and chronically stressed humans (in this case, concentration camp survivors) have high rates of the cognitive deficits that would be expected from hippocampal damage. Until recently, little more than this anecdotal literature was available. A few recent studies, however, show that glucocorticoids and severe chronic stress can both preferentially damage the primate hippocampus, with the degeneration sharing many neuroanatomical and cellular features with that observed in the rodent.

In summary, some of the major pieces of the glucocorticoid cascade demonstrated in the rodent appear to apply to the primate as well. With this knowledge, one can then examine the implications of this for normal human aging and a variety of human diseases.

Normal Human Aging

A vast literature suggests that adrenocortical function is relatively normal in the aged human; in particular, there is little evidence for there being basal hypercortisolism or dexamethasone resistance. However, recent findings suggest some similarities between the aging rodent and human adrenocortical axis. First, the conclusion that aged humans have normal basal glucocorticoid concentrations and normal dexamethasone responsiveness is based on the now-dated notion of what constitutes "aged" humans, and is typically derived from studies of 60-year-olds. More recent studies with very aged humans show marked basal hypercortisolism and dexamethasone resistance. Second, when dexamethasone responsiveness is tested under more sensitive conditions (i.e., with 0.5 mg of dexamethasone, rather than the usual 1.0 mg), there is marked resistance in aged humans. Finally, the hypercortisolism and dexamethasone resistance that is seen in a subset of individuals with major depression or Alzheimer's disease becomes more prevalent in older populations of patients. This suggests that an adrenocortical defect may be near-penetrant in aged humans and is pushed past the threshold of expression when combined with one of these insults.

Depression

Approximately 50% of individuals with major depression show some feature of glucocorticoid hypersecretion (basal hypersecretion at all or some times of the day and/or some feature of dexamethasone resistance). In general, hypercortisolism is associated with psychotic depression, more vegetative depressions, and with depressions in aged subjects.

A considerable amount of work has examined the neuroendocrine bases of such hypersecretion, and while there are changes in peripheral components of the adrenocortical axis that contribute to it, the consensus in the field is that there is a central, neurally driven component of hypersecretion and feedback resistance; it remains unclear which secretagog(s) mediates such hypersecretion. Given the predisposing role of stress in many depressions, this suggests that such stressors may down-regulate corticosteroid receptor number in the hippocampus and thus cause the hypersecretion. Rodent studies on the relationship between hippocampal receptor occupancy and regulation of secretagogs suggest that it is CRF and, in only severe cases, oxytocin, which are hypersecreted at such times. Neither of these ideas have been tested. In addition, the clinical literature contains two seeming challenges to these ideas. First, it is not always possible to demonstrate a stressor that preceded a major depression, and a stress/depression link is not necessarily tighter in those depressives who are hypercortisolemic. As a possible explanation for this variability, humans may differ markedly in their concentrations of hippocampal corticosteroid receptors prior to the stressor, in their sensitivity to stress-induced down-regulation, and in the threshold of down-regulation at which hypersecretion ensues. As a second challenge, the heterogeneity of syndromes of depressive hypercortisolism (i.e., some individuals hypersecrete basally but are responsive to dexamethasone, others the opposite, and so on) initially seems to argue against the hippocampus as a sole cause of hypersecretion. However, the data reviewed in chapter 5 shows that the hippocampus has a variety of domains of feedback inhibition of the adrenocortical axis, and these can be dissociated.

To examine the other half of the glucocorticoid cascade model, one might posit that prolonged hypercortisolism during chronic depression can cause hippocampal damage. There is some very scant evidence to support this idea.

Alzheimer's Disease

Much as with depression, approximately 50% of Alzheimer's sufferers show some hypercortisolemic features; again, the phenomenon is more common in older sufferers. As with depression, the hypersecretion appears to originate at the brain. Given that the hippocampus is a primary site of degeneration in the disease, the data in chapter 5 suggest that this damage might underlie the hypercortisolism. Moreover, should the rodent data apply in this case, as damage becomes more severe, hypersecretion should be driven by CRF, then by CRF plus oxytocin, and finally by both plus vasopressin. As with depression, one can invoke ideas about individual differences in thresholds at which hippocampal damage induces feedback resistance in order to explain variability in the clinical pattern of hypercortisolism in the disease.

To examine the other half of the cascade model, can glucocorticoids exacerbate Alzheimer's-like damage? This seemed most unlikely and highly speculative up until the past few years. The recent demonstrations that glucocorticoids exacerbate the EAA/calcium cascade and that this cascade can cause some of the neurodegenerative features of Alzheimer's disease (inappropriate proteolysis of the amyloid precursor protein, and accumulation of tau and ubiquitin immunoreactivity) make this idea slightly more plausible. In support of that, one recent report shows that glucocorticoids can exacerbate EAA-induced tau immunoreactivity.

Alcoholic Neurotoxicity

Both acute and chronic exposure to alcohol will stimulate glucocorticoid secretion, and chronic alcoholism will preferentially damage the hippocampus. This suggests the possibility that the alcohol-induced hypersecretion of glucocorticoids may be the cause, or at least an exacerbator of the hippocampal damage. This possibility has not yet been tested very explicitly.

Neurological Insults and the Clinical Use of Corticosteroids

It is not yet known whether glucocorticoids exacerbate neurological insults in the primate or human hippocampus but, given that demonstration in a number of rodent species, parsimony suggests that this should at least be examined in the human. Should that prove to be the case, the interventions suggested in the preceding chapter might conceivably be useful in clinical settings to decrease hippocampal damage. At the least, it would caution against the use of exogenous corticosteroids in such circumstances. As discussed, many of the clinical benefits of corticosteroid use (most notably, in controlling edema) have been overemphasized in the neurological literature, and when such treatments are indeed efficacious, nonglucocorticoid substitutes (mannitol, progesterone, 21-aminosteroids) are useful as well.

At the end of the many pages of this book, we are left with a grim message. As emphasized in the very first chapter, glucocorticoids are essential to life, and few of us would survive the rigors of daily life, let alone a major stressor, without these hormones. Furthermore, they are vastly effective and helpful in the control of a variety of diseases. Nevertheless, we have known for many decades that excessive exposure to these steroids carries many deleterious consequences, and the findings presented in this book suggest that hippocampal damage can be included in this list of pathologies. Moreover, this message is made grimmer by the growing possibility that these damaging effects might occur in our own brains. We are haunted by scenarios in which we sustain some sort of grievous injury, and our lives would obviously be transformed by the loss of our eyes, a limb, or by the severing of our spine. But, as I think most readers would concur, such tremendous loss becomes almost trivial compared to what happens when we sustain major brain damage, for then we lose ourselves. It is my hope that the message from this book is not entirely disheartening; perhaps these findings will allow us to design some rational interventions to decrease the endangering effects of glucocorticoids and even to decrease the primary toxicity of these neurological insults themselves.

References

Abdul-Rahman A, Siesjo B (1980) Local cerebral glucose consumption during insulin-induced hypoglycemia, and in the recovery period following glucose administration. Acta Physiol Scand 110, 149.

Abe K, Kroning J, Greer M, Critchlow V (1979) Effects of destruction of the suprachiasmatic nuclei on the circadian rhythms in plasma corticosterone, body temperature, feeding and plasma thyrotropin. Neuroendocrinology 29, 119.

Abou-Samra A, Catt K, Aguilera G (1986a) Involvement of protein kinase C in the regulation of adrenocorticotropin release from rat anterior pituitary cells. Endocrinology 118, 212.

Abou-Samra A, Catt K, Aguilera G (1986b) Biphasic inhibition of adrenocorticotropin release by corticosterone in cultured anterior pituitary cells. Endocrinology 119, 972.

Abou-Samra A, Harwood J, Manganiello V, Catt K, Aguilera G (1987) Phorbol 12-myristate 13-acetate and vasopressin potentiate the effect of corticotropin-releasing factor on cyclic AMP production in rat anterior pituitary cells. J Biol Chem 262, 1129.

Acosta D, Kass I, Cottrell J (1987) Effect of alpha-tocopherol and free radicals on anoxic damage in the rat hippocampal slice. Exp Neurol 97, 607.

Adamo M, Wener W, Farnsworth C, Roberts T, Raizada M, LeRoith D (1988) Dexamethasone reduces steady state insulin-like growth factor I messenger RNA levels in rat neuronal and glial cells in primary culture. Endocrinology 123, 2565.

Adams R, Victor M (1985) *Principles of Neurology* (3rd ed). McGraw-Hill, New York.

Adams R, Victor M (1989) *Principles of Neurology* (4th ed). McGraw-Hill, New York.

Ader R (1970) The effect of early experience on the adrenocortical response to different magnitudes of stimulation. Physiol Behav 5, 837.

Agardh C, Siesjo B (1981) Hypoglycemic brain injury: phospholipids, free fatty acids, and cyclic nucleotides in the cerebellum of the rat after 30 and 60 minutes of severe insulin-induce hypoglycemia. J Cereb Blood Flow Metab 1, 267.

Agardh C, Kalimo H, Olsson Y, Siesjo B (1981) Hypoglycemic brain injury: Metabolic and structural findings in rat cerebeller cortex during profound insulin-induced hypoglycemia and in the recovery period following glucose administration. J Cereb Blood Flow Metab 1, 71.

Aguilera G, Harwood J, Wilson J, Morell J, Brown J, Catt K (1983) Mechanisms of action of corticotropin-releasing factor and other regulators of corticotropin release in rat pituitary cells. J Biol Chem 258, 8039.

Ahmed Z, Conner J (1980) Intracellular pH changes induced by calcium influx during elecrical activity in molluscan neurons. J Gen Physiol 75, 403.

Aitken P, Balestrin M, Somjen G (1988) NMDA antagonists: lack of protective effect against hypoxic damage in CA_1 region of hippocampal slices. Neurosci Lett 89 187.

Aizenman E, Lipton S, Loring R (1989) Selective modulation of NMDA responses by reduction and oxidation. Neuron 2, 1257.

Aizenman E, Hartnett K, Reynolds I (1990) Oxygen free radicals regulate NMDA receptor function via a redox modulatory site. Neuron 5, 841.

Akana S, Dallman M (1987) Low levels of corticosterone reverse adrenalectomy-induced immunohistochemical staining of CRF and vasopressin in the paraventricular nucleus of adrenalectomized rat. Soc Neurosci Abstr 13, 450.6.

Akana S, Shinsako J, Dallman M (1985a) Closed-loop feedback control of the nyctohemeral rise in adrenocortical system function. Fed Proc 44, 177.

Akana S, Cascio C Shinsako J, Dallman M (1985b) Corticosterone: narrow range required for normal body and thymus weight and ACTH. Am J Physiol 249, R527.

Akana S, Cascio C, Du J, Levin N, Dallman M (1986) Reset of feedback in the adrenocortical system: an apparent shift in sensitivity of adrenocorticotropin to inhibition by corticosterone between morning and evening. Endocrinology 119, 2325.

Akana S, Jacobson L, Cascio C, Shinsako J, Dallman M (1988) Constant corticosterone replacement normalizes basal ACTH but permits sustained ACTH hypersecretion after stress in adrenalectomized rats. Endocrinology 122, 1337.

Albin R, Young A, Penney J, Handelin B, Balfour R, Anderson K, Markel D, Tourtellote W, Reiner A (1990) Abnormalities of striatal projection neurons and NMDA receptors in presymptomatic Huntington's Disease. N Engl J Med 322, 1293.

Alexander E (1972) Medical management of closed head injuries. Clin Neurosurg 19, 240.

Alford S, Schofield J, Collingridge G (1991) Dendritic calcium transients associated with NMDA receptor-mediated synaptic currents in rat hippocampal slices. J Physiol 438, 255P.

Altman J, Das G, Anderson W (1968) Effects of infantile handling on morphological development of the rat brain: an exploratory study. Dev Psychobiol 1, 10.

Altman D, Young R, Yagel S (1984) Effects of dexamethasone in hypoxic-ischemic brain injury in the neonatal rat. Biol Neonate 46, 149.

Altmann J (1980) *Baboon Mothers and Infants*. Harvard University Press, Cambridge.

Amagasa M, Mizoi K, Ogawa A, Yoshimoto T (1989) Actions of brain-protecting substances against both oxygen and glucose deprivation in the guinea pig hippocampal neurons studied in vitro. Brain Res 504, 87.

Ames B (1983) Dietary carcinogens and anticarcinogens (oxygen radicals and degenerative diseases). Science 221, 1256.

Amsterdam J, Marinelli D, Arger P, Winokur A (1987) Assessment of adrenal gland volume by computed tomography in depressed patients and healthy volunteers: a pilot study. Psychiatr Res 21, 189.

Amsterdam J, Maislin G, Berwish N, Phillips J, Winokur A (1989) Enhanced adrenocortical sensitivity to submaximal doses of cosyntropin in depressed patients. Arch Gen Psychiatry 46, 550.

Anderson D, Cranford R (1979) Corticosteroids in ischemic stroke. Stroke 10, 68.

Andine P, Jacobson I, Hagberg H (1988a) Calcium uptake evoked by electrical stimulation is enhanced postischemically and precedes delayed neuronal death in CA_1 of rat hippocampus: involvement of NMDA receptors. J Cereb Blood Flow Metab 8, 799.

Andine P, Lehmann A, Ellren K, Wennberg E, Kjellmer I, Nielsen T, Hagberg H (1988b) The excitatory amino acid antagonist kyneurenic acid administered after hypoxic-ischemia in neonatal rats offers neuroprotection. Neurosci Lett 90, 208.

Ando Y, Inoue M, Hirota M, Morino Y, Araki S (1989) Effect of a superoxide dismutase derivative on cold-induced brain edema. Brain Res 477, 286.

Andreeva N, Khodorv B, Stelmashook E, Cragoe E, Victorov I (1991) Inhibition of sodium/ calcium exchange enhances delayed neuronal death elicited by glutamate in cerebellar granule cell cultures. Brain Res 548, 322.

Andreis P, Neri G, Belloni A, Mazzocchi G, Kasprzak A, Nussdorfer G (1991) Interleukin-1beta enhances corticosterone secretion by acting directly on the rat adrenal gland. Endocrinology 129, 53.

Angelucci L, Valeri P, Grossi E, Veldhuis H, Bohus B, de Kloet E (1980) Involvement of hippocampal corticosterone receptors in behavioral phenomena. In Brambilla F, Racagni G, de Wied E (eds), *Progress in Psychoneuroendocrinology*. Elsevier, Amsterdam.

Anisman H, Zacharko R (1982) Depression: the predisposing influence of stress. Behav Brain Sci 5, 89.

Antoni F (1986) Hypothalamic control of adrenocorticotropin secretion: advances since the discovery of 41-residue CRF. Endocrine Rev 7, 351.

Antoni F, Holmes M, Jones M (1983a) Oxytocin as well as vasopressin potentiates ovine CRF in vitro. Peptides 4, 411.

Antoni F, Palkovits M, Makara G, Linton E, Lowry P, Kiss J (1983b) Immunoreactive cortico- tropin-releasing hormone in the hypothalamoinfundibular tract. Neuroendocrinology 36, 415.

Antoni F, Holmes M, Kiss J (1985) Pituitary binding of vasopressin is altered by experimental manipulations of the hypothalamo-pituitary-adrenocortical axis in normal as well as homo- zygous (di/di) Brattleboro rats. Endocrinology 117, 1293.

Antoni F, Fink G, Sheward W (1990) Corticotropin-releasing peptides in rat hypophysial portal blood after paraventricular lesions: a marked reduction in the concentration of CRF, but no change in vasopressin. J Endocrinol 125, 175.

APA Taskforce on Laboratory Tests in Psychiatry (1987) The dexamethasone suppression test. An overview of its current status in psychiatry. Am J Psychiatry 144, 1253.

Arai H, Passonneau J, Lust W (1986) Energy metabolism in delayed neuron death of CA_1 neurons of the hippocampus following transient ischemia in the gerbil. Metab Brain Dis 1, 263.

Arai A, Vanderklish P, Kessler M, Lee K, Lynch G (1991) A brief period of hypoxia causes proteolysis of cytoskeletal proteins in hippocampal slices. Brain Res 555, 276.

Arako T, Kato H, Kogure K, Inoue T (1991) Regional neuroprotective effects of pentobarbital on ischemia-induced brain damage. Brain Res Bull 25, 861.

Arana G, Barreira P, Cohen B, et al (1983) The dexamethasone suppression test in psychotic disorders. Am J Psychiatry 140, 1521.

Archer J (1970) Effects of aggressive behavior on the adrenal cortex in laboratory mice. J Mammol 51, 327.

Ardeleanu A, Sterescu N (1978) RNA and DNA synthesis in developing rat brain: hormonal influences. Psychoneuroendocrinology 3, 93.

Arimura A, Bowers C, Schally A, Saito M, Miller M (1969) Effect of corticotropin-releasing factor, dexamethasone and actinomycin D on the release of ACTH from rat pituitaries in vivo and in vitro. Endocrinology 85, 300.

Armanini M, Hutchins C, Stein B, Sapolsky R (1990) Glucocorticoid endangerment of hippo-campal neurons is NMDA-receptor mediated. Brain Res 532, 7.

Armstrong D (1989) Calcium channel regulation by calcineurin, a Ca^{++}-activated phosphatase in mammalian brain. Trends Neurosci 12, 117.

Armstrong D, Neill K, Crain B, Nadler J (1989) Absence of electrographic seizures after transient forebrain ischemia in the Mongolian gerbil. Brain Res 476, 174.

Aronsson M, Fuxe K, Dong Y, Agnati L, Okret S, Gustafsson J (1988) Localization of gluco-corticoid receptor mRNA in the male rat brain by in situ hybridization. Proc Natl Acad Sci USA 85, 9331.

Arriza J, Weinberger C, Cerelli, G, Glaser T, Handelin B, Housman d, Evans R (1987) Cloning of human mineralocorticoid receptor complementary DNA: structural and functional kinship with the glucocorticoid receptor. Science 237, 268.

Arriza J, Simerly R, Swanson L, Evans R (1988) The neuronal mineralocorticoid receptor as a mediator of glucocorticoid response. Neuron 1, 887.

Ashton D, Reid K, Willems R, Wauquier A (1986) NMDA and hypoxia induced calciumchanges in the CA_1 region of the hippocampal slice. Brain Res 385, 185.

Asnis G, Halbreich U, Nathan R, et al (1982) The dexamethasone suppression test in depressive illness: clinical correlates. Psychoneuroendocrinology 7, 295.

Auer R, Siesjo B (1988) Biological differences between ischemia, hypoglycemia, and epilepsy. Ann Neurol 24, 699.

Auer R, Olsson Y, Siesjo B (1984a) Hypoglycemic brain damage: correlation with EEG iso-electric time. A quantitative study. Diabetes 33, 1090.

Auer R, Wieloch T, Olsson Y, Siesjo B (1984b) Distribution of hypoglycemic brain damage: Relationship to white matter and cerebrospinal fluid pathways. Acta Neuropathol 64, 177.

Aus der Muhlen K, Ockenfels H (1969) Morphologische Veränderungen im Diencephalon und Telencephalon nach Storngen des regelkreises Adenohypophyse-Nebennierenrinde III. Ergebnisse beim Meerschweinchen nach Verabreichung von Cortison und Hydrocortison. Z Zellforsch 93, 126.

Azrin N, Hutchinson R, Hake D (1966) Extinction induced aggression. J Exp Anal Behav 9, 191.

Babij P, Hundal H, Rennie M, Watt P (1986) Effects of corticosteroid on glutamine transport in rat skeletal muscle. J Physiol 374, 35P.

Bading H, Greenberg M (1991) Stimulation of protein tyrosine phosphorylation by NMDA receptor activation. Science 253, 912.

Bahler M, Benfenati F, Valtorta F, Greengard P (1990) The synapsins and the regulation of synaptic function. Bioessays 12, 259.

Baimbridge K, Kao J (1988) Calbinding D-28K protects against glutamate induced neurotoxicity in rat CA_1 pyramidal neuron culres. Soc Neurosci Abstr 14, 507.1.

Bakay R, Harris A (1981) Neurotransmitter, receptor and biochemical changes in monkey cortical epileptic foci. Brain Res 206, 387.

Balazs R, Cotterrell M (1972) Effect of hormonal state on cell number and functional maturation of the brain. Nature 236, 348.

Balazs R, Patel A, Hajos F (1975) Factors affecting the biochemical maturation of the brain: effects of hormones during early life. Psychoneuroendocrinology 1, 25.

Balcar V, Pumain R, Mark J, Borg J, Mandel J (1978) GABA-mediated inhibition in the epileptogenic focus, a process which may be involved in the mechanism of the cobalt-induced epilepsy. Brain Res 154, 182.

Balding F, Wolfson B, Heinemann U, Gutnick M (1986) An NMDA receptor antagonist reduces bicuculline-induced depolarization shifts in neocortical explant cultures. Neurosci Lett 70, 101.

Balldin J, Gottfries C, Karlsson I, Lindstedt G, Langstrom G, Walinder J (1983) Dexamethasone suppression test and serum prolactin in dementia disorders. Br J Psychiatry 143, 277.

Baly D, Horuk R (1988) The biology and biochemistry of the glucose transporter. Biochem Biophys Acta 947, 571.

Banki C, Bissette G, Arato M, O'Conner L, Nemeroff C (1987) CSF corticotropin-releasing factor-like immunoreactivity in depression and schizophrenia. Am J Psychiatry 144, 7.

Baran H, Lassmann H, Sperk G, Seitelberger F, Hornykiewicz O (1987) Effect of mannitol treatment on brain neurotransmitter markers in kainic acid-induced epilepsy. Neuroscience 21, 679.

Barbour B, Brew H, Attwell D (1988) Electrogenic glutamate uptake in glial cells is activated by intracellular potassium. Nature 335, 433

Barbour B, Szatkowski M, Ingledew N, Attwell D (1989) Arachidonic acid induces a prolonged inhibition of glutamate uptake into glial cells. Nature 342, 918.

Barbrosa-Coutinho L, Hartman A, Hossmann K, Ronnel T (1985) Effect of dexamethasone on serum protein extravasation in experimental brain infarcts of monkey: an immunohistochemical study. Acta Neuropathol 65, 255.

Barks J (1991) Glucocorticoid does not exacerb ate excitotoxic damage in the immature rat brain. Soc Neurosci Abstr 17, 316.8.

Barks J, Post M, Tuor U (1991). Dexamethasone prevents hypoxic-ischemic brain damage in the neonatal rat. Pediatr Res 29, 558.

Barnett S (1955) Competition among wild rats. Nature 175, 126.

Bartus R, Dean R, Eveleth D, Lutz D, Harris M, Powers J (1991) Calpain inhibitors as unique therapeutics for ischemic brain damage. Soc Neurosci Abstr 17, 500.15.

Bateman A, Singh A, Kral T, Solomon S (1984) The immune-hypothalamic-pituitary-adrenal axis. Endocr Rev 10, 92.

Baumgartner A, Graf K, Kurten I (1985) The dexamethasone suppression test in depression, in schizophrenia and during experimental stress. Biol Psychiatry 20, 675.

Bazan N (1970) Effect of ischemia and electroconvulsive shock on free fatty acid pool in the brain. Biochim Biophys Acta 218, 1.

Beal M, Marshall P, Burd G, Landis D, Martin J (1985) Excitotoxin lesions do not mimic the alteration of somatostatin in Huntington's disease. Brain Res 361, 135.

Beal M, Kowall N, Ellison D, Mazurek M, Swartz K, Martin J (1986) Replication of the neurochemical characteristics of Huntington's disease by quinolinic acid. Nature 321, 168.

Beal M, Swartz K, Finn S, Mazurek M, Kowall N (1991a) Neurochemical characterization of excitotoxin lesions in the cerebral cortex. J Neurosci 11, 147.

Beal M, Ferrante R, Swartz K, Kowall N (1991b) Chronic quinolinic acid lesions in rats closely resemble Huntington's disease. J Neurosci 11, 1649.

Beato M (1989) Gene regulation by steroid hormones. Cell 56, 335.

Beck T, Bielenberg G (1990) Failure of the lipid peroxidation inhibitor U74006F to improve neurological outcome after transient forebrain ischemia in the rat. Brain Res 532, 336.

Ben-Ari Y (1985) Limbic seizure and brain damage produced by kainic acid: mechanisms and relevance to human temporal lobe epilepsy. Neuroscience 14, 375.

Ben-Ari Y, Cherubini E (1988) Brief anoxic episodes induced long-lasting changes in synaptic properties of rat CA_3 hippocampal neurons. Neurosci Lett 90, 273.

Ben-Ari Y, Tremblay E, Ottersen O, Meldrum B (1980) The role of epileptic activity in hippocampal and "remote" cerebral lesions induced by kainic acid. Brain Res 191, 79.

Ben-Ari Y, Tremblay E, Riche E, Ghilini G, Naquet R (1981) Electrographical, clinical and pathological alterations following systemic administration of kainic acid, bicuculline, or pentelenetetrazole: metabolic mapping using the deoxyglucose method with special reference to the pathology of epilepsy. Neuroscience 6, 1361.

Ben-Yoseph O, Bachelard H, Badar-Goffer R, Dolin S, Morris P (1990) Effects of NMDA on $[Ca^{++}]i$ and the energy state in the brain by 19F- and 31P-nuclear magnetic resonance spectroscopy. J Neurochem 55, 1446.

Benson W, McLaurin R, Foulkes E (1970) Traumatic cerebral edema. An experimental model with evaluation of dexamethasone. Arch Neurol 23, 179.

Bentson J, Reza M, Winter J, Wilson G (1978) Steroids and apparent cerebral atrophy on computed tomography scans. J Comput Assist Tomogr 2, 16.

Benveniste H, Diemer N (1988) Early postischemic ^{45}Ca accumulation in rat dentate hilus. J Cereb Blood Flow Metab 8, 713.

Benveniste H, Drejer J, Schousboe A, Diemer N (1984) Elevation of extracellular concentrations of glutamate and aspartate in the rat hippocampus during transient cerebral ischemia monitored by intracerebral microdialysis. J Neurochem 43, 1369.

Benzi G, Pastoris O, Vercesi L, Gorini A, Viganotti C, Villa R (1987) Energetic state of aged brain during hypoxia. Gerontology 33, 207.

Berdichevsky E, Riveros N, Sanchez-Armass S, Orrego F (1983) Kainate, NMDA and other excitatory amino acids increase calcium influx into rat brain cortex cells in vitro. Neurosci Lett 36, 75.

Berdichevsky E, Munoz C, Riveros N, Cartier L, Orrego F (1987) Neuropathologic changes in the rat brain cortex in vitro: effects of kainic acid and of ion substitutions. Brain Res 423, 213.

Bereiter D, Plotsky P, Gann D (1982) Tooth pulp stimulation potentiates the adrenocortical response to hemorrhage in cats. Endocrinology 111, 1127.

Bering E (1974) Effect of profound hypothermia and circulatory arrest on cerebral oxygen metabolism and cerebrospinal fluid electrolyte composition in dogs. J Neurosurg 39, 199.

Berk M, Finkelstein J (1981) Afferent projections to the preoptic and hypothalamic regions in the rat brain. Neuroscience 6, 1601.

Berkenbosch F, van Oers J, del Rey A, Tilders F, Besedovsky H (1987) Corticotropin-releasing factor-producing neurons in the rat activated by Interleukin-1. Sciences 238, 524.

Bernstein J, Fisher R, Zaczek R, Coyle J (1985) Dipeptides of glutamate and aspartate may be endogenous neuroexcitants in the rat hippocampal slice. J Neurosci 5, 1429.

Berntman L, Welsh F, Harp J (1981) Cerebral protective effect of low-grade of hypothermia. Anesthesiology 55, 495.

Bertoni J, Sprenkle P (1988) Inhibitors of cation pump enzyme activity present in normal and ischemic gerbil brain. Life Sci 42, 1955.

Betito K, Mitchell J, Rowe W, Boksa P, Meaney M (1990) Serotonin regulation of corticosteroid receptor binding in cultured hippocampal cells: the role of ^5HT-induced increases in cAMP levels. Soc Neurosci Abstr 16, 439.3.

Betz A (1985) Identification of hypoxanthine transport and xanthine oxidase activity in brain capillaries. J Neurochem 44, 574.

Betz A, Coester H (1990) Effect of steroids on edema and sodium uptake of the brain during focal ischemia in rats. Stroke 21, 1199.

Betz A, Gilboe D, Drewes L (1974) Effects of anoxia on net uptake and unidirectional transport of glucose into the isolated dog brain. Brain Res 67, 307.

Betz A, Randall J, Martz D (1991) Xanthine oxidase is not a major source of free radicals in focal cerebral ischemia. Am J Physiol 260, H563.

Beyer H, Matta S, Sharp B 1988 Regulation of the messenger ribonucleic acid for corticotropin-releasing factor in the paraventricular nucleus and other brain sites of the rat. Endocrinology 123, 2117.

Bhatnagar S, Viau V, Meaney M (1991) HPA respones to acute restraint stress following chronic exposure to cold in handled and nonhandled rats. Soc Neurosci Abstr 17, 621.3.

Bignami G (1965) Selection for high rates and low rates of avoidance conditioning in the rat. Anim Behav 13, 221.

Bilezikjian L, Vale W (1983) Glucocorticoids inhibit corticotrophin-releasing factor-induced production of adenosine 3',5'-monophosphate in cultured anterior pituitary cells. Endocrinology 113, 657.

Bilezikjian L, Vale W (1987) Regulation of ACTH secretion from corticotrophs: The interaction of vasopressin and CRF. Ann NY Acad Sci 512, 85.

Bilezikjian L, Blount A, Vale W (1987) The cellular actions of vasopressin on corticotrophs of the anterior pituitary: resistance to glucocorticoid action. Mol Endocrinol 1, 451.

Bing G, Vielkind U, Bohn M (1989) Glucocorticoid receptor expression in primary hippocampal neuronal cultures. Soc Neurosci Abstr 15, 290.12.

Birren J, Schaie K (1985) *Handbook of the Psychology of Aging.* Van Nostrand, New York.

Bissette G, Reynolds G, Kilts C, Widerlov E, Nemeroff C (1985) Corticotropin-releasing factor-like immunoreactivity in senile dementia of the Alzheimer type. JAMA 254, 3067.

Bittner S, Wielckens K (1988) Glucocorticoid-induced lymphoma cell growth inhibition: the role of leukotriene B4. Endocrinology 123, 991.

Black P, Markowitz R (1971) Experimental spinal cord injury in monkeys; comparison of steroids and local hypothermia. Surg Forum 22, 409.

Blackwell G, Carnuccio R, DiRosa M, Flower R, Parente L, Persico P (1980) Macrocortin: a polypeptide causing the anti-phospholipoase effect of glucocorticoids. Nature 287, 147.

Blakely R, Robinson M, Thompson R, Coyle J 1988 Hydrolysis of the brain dipeptide N-acetyl-L-aspartyl-L-glutamate: subcellular and regional distribution, ontogeny, and the effect of lesions on N-acetylated-alpha-linked acidic dipeptidase activity. J Neurochem 50, 1200.

Blass J, Baker A, Ko L, Black R (1990) Induction of Alzheimer antigens by an uncoupler of oxidative phosphorylation. Arch Neurol 47, 864.

Blaustein M (1988) Calcium transport and buffering in neurons. Trends Neurosci 11, 438.

Blennow G, Nilsson B, Siesjo B (1985) Influence of reduced oxygen availability on cerebral metabolic changes during bicuculline-induced seizures in rats. J Cereb Blood FLow Metab 5, 439.

Blichert-Toft M (1975) Secretion of corticotrophin and somatotrophin by the senescent adenohypophysis in man. Acta Endocrinol 78 (Suppl 195) 1.

Blichert-Toft B, Blichert-Toft M (1970) Adrenocortical function in the aged assessed by the rapid corticotropin test. Acta Endocrinol (Copenh) 64, 410.

Blichert-Toft M, Hummer L (1977) Serum immunoreactive corticotropin and response to metyrapone in old age in man. Gerontology 23, 236.

Blitzer R, Gil O, Landau E (1990) Long-term potentiation in rat hippocampus is inhibited by low concentrations of ethanol. Brain Res 537, 203.

Block G, Pulsinelli W (1987) Excitatory amino acid receptor antagonists: failure to prevent ischemic neuronal damage. J Cereb Blood Flow Metab 7 (Suppl 1) S149.

Boakye P, White E, Clark J (1991) Protection of ischaemic synaptosomes from calcium overlod by addition of exogenous lactate. J Neurochem 57, 88.

Boast C, Hoffman C (1991) Neuroprotection by MK801 in temperature maintained gerbils. Soc Neurosci Abstr 17, 235.14.

Boast C, Gerhardt S, Janak P (1987) Systemic AP7 reduces ischemic brain damage in gerbils. In Hicks T, Lodge D, McLennan H (eds), Excitatory Amino Acid Transmission Liss, New York.

Boast C, Gerhardt S, Pastor G (1988) The NMDA antagonists CGS 19755 and CPP reduce ischemic brain damage in gerbils. Brain Res 442, 345.

Bodsch W, Barbier A, Oehmichen M, Gosse-Ophoff B, Hossman K (1986) Recovery of monkey brain after prolonged ischemia. II. Protein synthesis and morphological alterations. J Cereb Blood Flow Metab 6, 22.

Boegman R, Smith Y, Parent A (1987) Quinolinic acid does not spare striatal neuropeptide Y-immunoreactive neurons. Brain Res 415, 178.

Boggan W, Wallis C, Owens M (1982) Effect of phencyclidine on plasma corticosterone in mice. Life Sci 30, 1581.

Bohn M (1980) Granule cell genesis in the hippocampus of rats treated neonatally with hydrocortisone. Neuroscience 5, 2003.

Bohn M, Lauder J (1978) The effects of hydrocortisone on rat cerebellar development. Dev Neurosci 1, 250.

Bohus B, de Kloet E (1981) Adrenal steroids and extinction behavior: antagonism by progesterone, deoxycorticosterone and dexamethasone of a specific effect of corticosterone. Life Sci 28, 433.

Bohus B, de Kloet E, Veldhuis H (1982) Adrenal steroids and behavioural adaptation: Relationship to brain corticoid receptors. In Ganten D, Pfaff D (eds), Current Topics in Neuroendocrinology, Adrenal Action on Brain. Springer-Verlag, New York.

Booker R, Truman J (1987) Postembryonic neurogenesis in the CNS of the tobacco hornworm, Manduca sexta. II. Hormonal control of imaginal nest cell degeneration and differentiation during metamorphosis. J Neurosci 7, 4107.

Bosley T, Woodhams P, Gordon R, Balazs R (1983) Effects of anoxia on the stimulated release of amino acid neurotransmitters in the cerebellum in vitro. J Neurochem 40, 189.

Bouchelouche P, Belhage B, Frandsen A, Drejer J, Schousboe A (1989) Glutamate receptor activation in cultured cerebellar granule cells increases cytosolic free calcium by mobilization of cellular calcium and activation of calcium influx. Exp Brain Res 76, 281.

Bouzarth W, Shenkin H, Feldman W (1968) Adrenocortical response to craniocerebral trauma. Surg Gynecol Obstet 126, 995.

Bowen D, Benton J, Spillane J, Smith C, Allen S (1982) Choline acetyltransferase activity and histopathology of frontal neocortex from biopsies of demented patients. J Neurol Sci 57, 191.

Braakman R, Schouten H, Blaauw-van Dischoeck M, Minderhoud J (1983) Megadose steroids in severe head injury: results of a prospective double-blind clinical trial. J Neurosurg 58, 326.

Bracken M, Collins W, Freeman D, et al (1984) Efficacy of methylprednisolone in acute spinal cord injury. JAMA 251, 45.

Bracken M, Shepard M, Hellenbrand K, et al (1985) Methylprednisolone and neurological function one year after spinal cord injury. J Neurosurg 63, 704.

Bracken M, Shepard M, Collins W, Holford T, Young W, Baskin D, Eisenberg H, Flamm E, Leo-Summers L, Maroon J, Marshall L, Perot P, Piepmeier J, Sonntag VB, Wagner F, Wilberger J, Winn H (1990) A randomized controlled trial of methylprednisolone or naloxone in the treatment of acute spinal cord injury. N Engl J Med 322, 1405.

Bradbury M, Dallman M (1989) Effects of hippocampal Type I and Type II glucocorticoid receptor antagonists on ACTH levels in the PM. Soc Neurosci Abstr 15, 290.4.

Bradbury M, Cascio C, Scribner K, Dallman M (1991) Stress-induced ACTH secretion: diurnal responses and decreases during stress in the evening are not dependent on corticosterone. Endocrinology 128, 680.

Bradbury M, Akana S, Cascio C, Levin N, Jacobson L, Dallman M (1992) Regulation of basal ACTH secretion by corticosterone is mediated by both Type I and Type II receptors in rat brain. J Steroid Biochem Suppl, in press.

Bradford H, Young A, Crowder J (1987) Continuous glutamate leakage from brain cells is balanced by compensatory high-affinity reuptake transport. Neurosci Lett 81, 296.

Bradshaw H, Vedeckis W (1983) Glucocorticoid effects on thymidine incorporation into the DNA of S49 lymphoma cells. J Steroid Biochem 18, 691.

Branconnier R, Oxenkrug G, McIntyre I, et al (1984) Prediction of serum cortisol response to dexamethasone in normal volunteers: a multivariate approach. Psychopharmacology 84, 274.

Braughler J, Hall E (1984) Effects of multi-dose methylprednisolone sodium succinate administration on injured cat spinal cord neurofilmanet degradation and energy metabolism. J Neurosurg 61, 290.

Braughler J, Hall E (1985a) Current application of high dose steroid therapy for CNS trauma. J Neurosurg 62, 806.

Braughler J, Hall E (1985b) Current application of "high-dose" steroid therapy for CNS injury: A pharmacological perspective. J Neurosurg 63, 714.

Braughler J, Hall E, Means E, Waters T, Anderson D (1987) Evaluation of an intensive methylprednisolone sodium succinate dosing regimen in experimental spinal cord injury. J Neurosurg 67, 102.

Bredt D, Hwang P, Glatt C, Lowenstein C, Reed R, Snyder S (1991) Cloned and expressed nitric oxide synthase structurally resembles cytochrome P-450 reductase. Nature 351, 714.

Bremer A, Yamada K, West C (1980) Ischemic cerebral edema in primates: effects of acetazolamide, phenytoin, sorbitol, dexamethasone, and methylprednisolone on brain water and electrolytes. Neurosurgery 6, 149.

Brett L, Chong G, Coyle S (1983) The pituitary-adrenal response to novel stimulation and ether stress in young adult and aged rats. Neurobiol Aging 4, 133.

Brett L, Levine R, Levine S (1986) Bidirectional response of the pituitary-adrenal system in old and young male and female rats. Neurobiol Aging 7, 153.

Bridges R, Koh J, Hatalski C, Cotman C (1991) Increased excitotoxic vulnerability of cortical cultures with reduced levels of glutathione. Eur J Pharmacol 192, 199.

Brier A, Albus M, Pickar D, Zahn T, Wolkowitz O, Paul S 1987 Controllable and uncontrollable stress in humans: alterations in mood and neuroendocrine and psychophysiological function. Am J Psychiatry 144, 11.

Brierley J (1976) Cerebral hypoxia. In Blackwood W, Corsellis J (eds) *Greenfield's Neuropathology*. Year Book Medical Publishers, Chicago, p 43.

Brierley J, Graham D (1984) Hypoxia and vascular disorders of the central nervous system. In Adams J, Coprsellis J, Duchen L (eds), *Greenfield's Neuropathology* (4th ed). Wiley, New York.

Brinton R, McEwen B (1988) Regional distinctions in the regulation of Type I and Type II adrenal steroid receptors in the central nervous system. Neurosci Res Commun 2, 37.

Britton G, Rotenberg S, Freeman C (1975) Regulation of corticosterone levels and liver enzyme activity in aging rats. Adv Exp Med Biol 61, 209.

Brizzee K, Ordy J (1979) Age pigments, cell loss and hippocampal function. Mech Ageing Dev 9, 143.

Broadhurst P (1960) Experiments in psychogenetics: application of biometrical genetics to behavior. In Eysenck H (ed), *Experiments in Personality, vol 1. Psychogenetics and Psychopharmacology*. Routledge and Kegan Paul, London.

Broadhurst P (1969) Psychogenetics of emotionality in the rat. Ann NY Acad Sci 159, 806.

Brodish A, Odio M (1989) Age-dependent effects of chronic stress on ACTH and corticosterone responses to an acute novel stress. Neuroendocrinology 49, 496.

Bronson F, Eleftheriou B (1964) Chronic physiologic effects of fighting on mice. Gen Comp Endocrinol 4, 9.

Brown W, Shrivastava R, Arato M (1987) Pretreatment pituitary-adrenocortical status and placebo response in depression. Psychopharmacol Bull 23, 155.

Brush F, Nagase Shain C (1989) Endogenous opioids and behavior. In Levine S, Brush F (eds), *Psychoendocrinology*. Academic Press, New York.

Bryan R, King J (1988) Glucocorticoids modulate the effect of plasma epinephrine on regional glucose utilization. Soc Neurosci Abstr 14, 399.11.

Bucala R, Fishman J, Cerami A (1982) Formation of covalent adducts between cortisol and 16-alpha-hydroxyestrone and protein: possible role in the pathogenesis of cortisol toxicity and systemic lupus erythematosus. Proc Natl Acad Sci USA 79, 3320.

Buchan A (1990) Do NMDA antagonists protect against cerebral ischemia: are clinical trials warranted? Cerebrovasc Brain Metab Rev 2, 1.

Buchan A, Pulsinelli W (1990a) Hypothermia but not the NMDA antagonist, MK-801, attenuates neuronal damage in gerbils subjected to transient global ischemia. J Neurosci 10, 311.

Buchan A, Pulsinelli W 1990b Septo-hippocampal deafferentation protects CA_1 neurons against ischemic injury. Brain Res 512, 7.

Buckingham J (1979b) The influence of corticosteroids on the secretion of corticotrophin and its hypothalamic releasing hormone. J Physiol 286, 331.

Buckingham J, Hodges J (1977) Production of corticotropin releasing hormone by the isolated hypothalamus of the rat. J Physiol 272, 469.

Buckley D, Ramachandran J 1981 Characterization of corticotropin receptors on adrenocortical cells. Proc Natl Acad Sci USA 78, 7431.

Bugnon C, Fellmann D, Gouget A (1983) Changes in corticoliberin and vasopressin-like immunoreactivity in the zona externa of the median eminence in adrenalectomized rats. Neurosci Lett 37, 43.

Burgoyne R, Pearce I, Cambray-Deakin M (1988) NMDA raises cytosolic calcium concentration in rat cerebellar granule cells in culture. Neurosci Lett 91, 47.

Burke S, Nadler J (1989) Effects of glucose deficiency on glutamate/aspartate release and excitatory synaptic responses in the hippocampal CA_1 area in vitro. Brain Res 500, 333.

Burnstein K, Cidlowski J (1989) Regulation of gene expression by glucocorticoids. Annu Rev Physiol 51, 683.

Burnstein K, Bellingham D, Jewell C, Powell-Liver F, Cidlowski J (1991) Autoregulation of glucocorticoid receptor gene expression. Steroids 56, 52.

Burton A, Storr J, Dunn W (1967) Cytolytic action of corticosteroids on thymus and lymphoma cells in vitro. Can J Biochem 45, 289.

Butcher S, Hagberg H, Sandberg M, Hamberger A (1987a) Extracellular purine catabolite and amino acid levels in the rat striatum during severe hypoglycemia: effect of 2-amino-5-phosphonovalerate. Neurochem Int 11, 95.

Butcher S, Lazarewicz J, Hamberger A (1987b) In vivo microdialysis studies on the effects of decortication and excitotoxic lesions on kainic acid-induced calcium fluxes, and endogenous amino acid release, in the rat striatum. J Neurochem 49, 1355.

Buzsaki G, Freund T, Bayardo F, Somogyi P (1989) Ischemia-induced changes in the electrical activity of the hippocampus. Exp Brain Res 78, 268.

Cadete-Leite A, Tavares M, Paula-Barbosa M (1988) Alcohol withdrawal does not impede hippocampal granule cell progressive loss in chronic alcohol-fed rats. Neurosci Lett 86, 45.

Cambronero J, Borrell J, Guaza C (1989) Glucocorticoids modulate rat hypothalamic CRF release induced by interleukin-1. J Neurosci Res 24, 470.

Campbell J, DeCrescito V, Tomasula J, Demopoulos H, Flamm E, Ransohoff J (1973) Experimental treatment of spinal cord contusion in the cat. Surg Neurol 1, 102.

Cao W, Carney J, Duchon A, Floyd R, Chefvion M (1988) Oxygen free radical involvement in ischemia and reperfusion injury to the brain. Neurosci Lett 88, 233.

Carlsson C, Hagerdal M, Siesjo B (1976) Protective effect of hypothermia in cerebral oxygen deficiency caused by arterial hypoxia. Anesthesiology 44, 27.

Carnes M, Smith J, Kalin N (1983a) Effects of chronic medical illness and dementia on the dexamethasone suppression test. J Am Geriatr Soc 31, 267.

Carnes M, Smith J, Kalin N (1983b) The dexamethasone suppression test in demented outpatients with and without depression. Psychiatr Res 9, 337.

Carpenter C, Marks S, Watson D, Greenberg D (1988) Dextromethorphan and dextrorphan as calcium channel antagonists. Brain Res 439, 372.

Carroll B 1972 Stimulation tests in depression. In Davies B, et al. (eds), *Depressive Illness: Some Research Studies*. C C Thomas, Springfield.

Carroll B (1982) The dexamethasone suppression test for melancholia. Br J Psychiatry 140, 292.

Carroll B, Feinberg M, Greden J, Tarika J, Albala A, Haskett R, James N, Kronfol Z, Lohr N, Steiner M, de Vigne J, Young E (1981) A specific laboratory test for the diagnosis of melancholia. Arch Gen Psychiatry 38, 15.

Carter-Su C, Okamoto K (1985) Effects of glucocorticoids on hexose transport in rat adipocytes: evidence for decreased transporters in the plasma membrane. J Biol Chem 260, 11091.

Cartlidge N, Black M, Hall M (1970) Pituitary function in the elderly. Gerontol Clin 12, 65.

Casady R, Taylor A (1976) Effect of electrical stimulation of the hippocampus upon corticosteroid levels in the freely-behaving, non-stressed rat. Neuroendocrinology 35, 205.

Cascio C, Shinsako J, Dallman M (1987) The suprachiasmatic nuclei stimulate evening ACTH secretion in the rat. Brain Res 423, 173.

Cascio C, Jacobson L, Akana S, Sapolsky R, Dallman M (1989) Occupancy of hippocampal Type I, corticosterone-preferring receptors correlates with the inhibition of plasma ACTH in adrenalectomized rats. Endocr Abstr 71, 1745.

Ceulemans D, Westenberg H, van Praag H (1985) The effect of stress on the dexamethasone suppression test. Psychiatry Res 14, 189.

Chamove A, Bowman R (1976) Rank, rhesus social behavior, and stress. Folia Primatol 26, 57.

Chan P, Fishman R (1978) Brain edema: induction in cortical slices by polyunsaturated fatty acids. Science 201, 358.

Chan P, Fishman R, Caronna J, Schmidley J, Prioleau G, Lee J (1983) Induction of brain edema following intracerebral injection of arachidonic acid. Ann Neurol 13, 625.

Chan P, Chu L, Fishman R (1988) Reduction of activities of superoxide dismutase but not of glutathione peroxidase in rat brain regions following decapitation ischemia. Brain Res 439, 388.

Chan P, Yang G, Chen S, Carlson E, Epstein C (1991) Cold-induced brain edema and infarction are reduced in transgenic mice overexpressing CuZn-superoxide dismutase. Ann Neurol 29, 482.

Chance B (1965) The energy-linked reaction of calcium with mitochondria. J Biol Chem 240, 2729.

Chang J, Martin D, Johnson E (1990) Interferon suppresses sympathetic neuronal cell death caused by nerve growth factor deprivation. J Neurochem 55, 436.

Chang M, Baldwin R, Bruce C, Wisnieski B (1989) Second cytotoxic pathway of diphtheria toxin suggested by nuclease activity. Science 246, 1165.

Chao H, Choo P, McEwen B (1989) Glucocorticoid and mineralocorticoid receptor mRNA expression in rat brain. Neuroendocrinology 50, 365.

Chaplin E, Free R, Goldstein G (1981) Inhibition by steroids of the uptake of potassium by capillaries isolated from rat brain. Biochem Pharm 30, 241.

Chapman A, Meldrum B, Siesjo B (1977) Cerebral metabolic changes during porolonged epileptic seizures in rats. J Neurochem 28, 1025.

Chapman A, Cheetham S, Hart G, Meldrum B, Westerberg E (1985) Effects of two convulsant beta-carboline derivatives, DMCM and beta-CCCM, on regional neurotransmitter amino acid levels and on in vitro d-^{3}H-aspartate release in rodents. J Neurochem 45, 370.

Charlton B (1990) Adrenal cortical innervation and glucocorticoid secretion. J Endocrinol 126, 5.

Cheng B, Horst I, Mader S, Kowal J (1990) Diminished adrenal steroidogenic activity in aging rats: new evidence from adrenal cells cultured from young and aged normal and hypoxic animals. Mol Cell Endocrinol 73, R7.

Cheng S, Harding B, Carballeira A (1974) Effects of metyrapone on pregnenolone biosynthesis and on cholesterol-cytochrome P-450 interaction in the adrenal. Endocrinology 94, 1451.

Chesler M (1990) The regulation and modulation of pH in the nervous system. Prog Neurobiol 34, 401.

Cheung J, Bonventre J, Malis C, Leaf A (1986) Calcium and ischemic injury. N Engl J Med 26, 1670.

Childs G, Morell J, Niendorf A, Aguilera G (1986) Cytochemical studies of CRF receptors in anterior lobe corticotropes: binding, glucocorticoid regulation, and endocytosis of [Biotinyl-Ser1]CRF. Endocrinology 119, 2129.

Childs G, Unabia G, Burke J, Marchetti C (1987) Secretion from corticotropes after avidin-fluorescein stains for biotinylated ligans (CRF and AVO). Am J Physiol 252, E349.

Chiueh C, Nespor S, Rapoport S (1980) Cardiovascular, sympathetic and adrenal corticoal responsiveness of aged Fischer-344 rats to stress. Neurobiol Aging 1, 157.

Choi D (1985) Glutamate neurotoxicity in cortical cell culture is calcium dependent. Neurosci Lett 58, 293.

Choi D (1987a) Glutamate neurotoxicity in cortical cell culture. J Neurosci 7, 357.

Choi D (1987b) Ionic dependence of glutamate neurotoxicity. J Neurosci 7, 369.

Choi D (1987c) Dextrorphan and dextromethorphan attenuate glutamate neurotoxicity. Brain Res 403, 333.

Choi D (1988) Calcium-mediated neurotoxicity: relationship to specific channel types and role in ischemic damage. Trends Neurosci 11, 465.

Choi D (1990) Cerebral hypoxia: some new approaches and unanswered questions. J Neurosci 10, 2493.

Choi D, Koh J, Peters S (1988) Pharmacology of glutamate neurotoxicity in cortical cell culture: attenuation by NMDA antagonists. J Neurosci 8, 185.

Chopp M, Welch K, Tidwell C, Knight R, Helpern J (1988) Effect of mild hyperthermia on recovery of metabolic function after global cerebral ischemia in cats. Stroke 19, 1521.

Chopp M, Knight R, Tidwell C, Helpern J, Brown E, Welch K (1989) The metabolic effects of mild hypothermia on global cerebral ischemia and recirculation in the cat: comparison to normothermia and hyperthermia. J Cereb Blood Flow Metab 9, 141.

Chopp M, Chen H, Dereski M, Garcia J (1991) Mild hypothermic intervention after graded ischemic stress in rats. Stroke 22, 37.

Chou Y, Luttge W (1988) Activated type II receptors in brain cannot rebind glucocorticoids: relationship to progesterone's antiglucocorticoid action. Brain Res 440, 67.

Christie-Pope B, Palmer G (1986) Modulation of ischemic-induced damage to cerebral adenylate cyclase in gerbils by calcium channel blockers. Metab Brain Dis 1, 249.

Christine C, Choi D (1990) Effect of zinc on NMDA receptor-mediated channel currents in cortical neurons. J Neurosci 10, 108.

Chun J, Nakamura M, Shatz C (1987) Transient cells of the developing mammalian telencephalon are peptide-immunoreactive neurons. Nature 325, 617.

Church J, Zeman S (1991) Ketamine promotes hippocampal CA_1 pyramidal neuron loss after a short-duration ischemic insult in rats. Neurosci Lett 123, 65.

Church J, Zeemans S, Lodge D (1988) Ketamine and MK-801 as neuroprotective agents in cerebral ischemia/hypoxia. In Domino E, Kamenka J (eds), *Sigma and Phencyclidine-like Compounds as Molecular Probes in Biology*. NPP Books, Ann Arbor.

Cidlowski J (1982) Glucocorticoids stimulate ribonucleic acid degradation in isolated rat thymic lymphocytes in vitro. Endocrinology 11, 184.

Clark A, Cotman C (1990) Adrenal hormone effects on hippocampal excitatory amino acid receptor binding. Soc Neurosci Abstr 16, 351.3.

Clark G, Rothman S (1987) Blockade of excitatory amino acid receptors protects anoxic hippocampal slices. Neuroscience 21, 665.

Clifford D, Olney J, Benz A, Fuller T, Zorumsky C (1990) Ketamine, phencyclidine, and MK-801 protect against kainic acid-induced seizure-related brain damage. Epilepsia 31, 382.

Clifton G, Robertson C, Grossman R (1984) The metabolic response to severe head injury. J Neurosurg 60, 687.

Coe C, Mendoza S, Levine S (1979) Social status constrains the stress response in the squirrel monkey. Physiol Behav 23, 633.

Coe C, Stanton M, Levine S (1983) Adrenal responses to reinforcement and extinction: role of expectancy vs. instrumental responding. Behav Neurosci 97, 654.

Cohen J, Duke R (1984) Glucocorticoid activation of a calcium-dependent endonuclease in thymocyte nuclei leads to cell death. J Immunol 132, 38.

Cohen M, Sridhara N, Ramchand C (1988) Glutamine synthetase inhibition by methionine-sulfoximine fails to modify kainic acid induced striatal damage. Res Commun Psychol Psychiatry Behav 13, 309.

Coleman G, Barthold S, Osbaldiston G, Foster S, Jonas A (1977) Pathological changes during aging in barrier-reared Fischer 344 male rats. J Gerontol 32, 258.

Coleman P, Flood D (1987) Neuron numbers and dendritic extent in normal aging and Alzheimer's disease. Neurobiol Aging 8, 521.

Collingridge G, Bliss T, (1987) NMDA receptors—their role in long-term potentiation. Trends Neurosci 10, 288.

Collins G, Anson J, Surtees L (1983) Presynpatic kainate and NMDA receptors regulate excitatory amino acid release in the olfactory cortex. Brain Res 265, 157.

Colucci C, D'Alessandro B, Bellastella A, Montalbetti N (1975) Circadian rhythm of plasma cortisol in the aged (Cosinor method). Gerontol Clin 17, 89.

Combs D, Dempsey R, Maley M, Donaldson D, Smith C (1990) Relationship between plasma glucose, brain lactate, and intracellular pH during cerebral ischemia in gerbils. Stroke 21, 936.

Compton M, Cidlowski J (1986) Rapid in vivo effects of glucocorticoids on the integrity of rat lymphocyte genomic deoxyribonucleic acid. Endocrinology 118, 38.

Compton M, Cidlowski J (1987) Identification of a glucocorticoid-induced nuclease in thymocytes: a potential "lysis gene" product. J Biol Chem 262, 8288.

Compton M, Haskill J, Cidlowski J (1988) Analysis of glucocorticoid actions on rat thymocyte deoxyribonucleic acid by fluorescence-activated flow cytometry. Endocrinology 122, 2158.

Conforti N, Feldman S (1976) Effects of dorsal fornix section and hippocampectomy on adrenocortical responses to sensory stimulation in the rat. Neuroendocrinology 22, 1.

Conner J, Wadman W, Hockberger P, Wong R (1988) Sustained dendritic gradients of calcium induced by excitatory amino acids in CA_1 hippocampal neurons. Science 240, 649.

Cooper H, Zalewska T, Kawakami S, Hossmann K, Kleihues P (1977) The effect of ischemia and recirculation on protein synthesis in the rat brain. J Neurochem 28, 929.

Cooper P (1984) Commentary following the paper by Gianotta et al. Neurosurgery 15, 501.

Cooper P, Moody S, Clark W (1979) Dexamethasone and severe head injury: a prospective double-blind study. J Neurosurg 51, 307.

Coover G (1983) The rat's reward environment and pituitary-adrenal activity. In Ursin H, Murison R (eds), Biological and Psychological Basis of Psychosomatic Disease. Permanon Press, Oxford.

Coover G, Goldman L, Levine S (1971) Plasma corticosterone levels during extinction of a lever-press response in hippocampectomized rats. Physiol Behav 7, 727.

Coover G, Ursin H, Levine S (1973) Plasma corticosterone levels during active avoidance learning in rats. J Comp Physiol Psychol 82, 170.

Copani A, Koh J, Cotman C (1991) Beta-amyloid protein potentiates injury by glucose deprivation in neuronal cultures. Soc Neurosci Abstr 17, 572.13.

Corbett R, Laptook A, Nunnally R, Hassan A, Jackson J (1988) Intracellular pH, lactate, and energy metabolism in neonatal brain during partial ischemia measured in vivo by ^{31}P and ^{1}H nuclear magnetic resonance spectroscopy. J Neurochem 51, 1501.

Corkin S, Rosen T, Sullivan E, Clegg R (1989) Penetrating head injury in young adulthood exacerbates cognitive decline in later years. J Neurosci 9, 3876.

Corsellis J (1962) *Mental Illness and the Ageing Brain*. Oxford University Press, Oxford.

Corsellis J, Meldrum B (1976) The pathology of epilepsy. In Blackwood W, Corsellis J (eds), *Greenfield's Neuropathology* Arnold, London, p 771.

Coryell W, Gaffney G, Burkhardt P (1982) DSM-III melancholia and the primary-secondary distinction: a comparison of concurrent validity by means of the dexamethasone suppression test. Am J Psychiatry 130, 120.

Cos D, Bachelard H (1988) On the relationship between the excitability of dentate granule cell field potentials and their sensitivity to low glucose. Brain Res 440, 195.

Cotman C, Monaghan D, Otterson O, Storm-Mathisen J (1987) Anatomical organization of excitatory amino acid receptors and their pathways. Trends Neurosci 10, 273.

Cotman C, Bridges R, Taube J, Clark A, Geddes J, Monaghan D (1989) The role of the NMDA receptor in central nervous system plasticity and pathology. J NIH Res 1, 65.

Cotterrell M, Balazs R, Johnson A (1972) Effects of corticosteroids on the biochemical maturation of rat brain: postnatal cell formation. J Neurochem 19, 2151.

Cowan W, Fawcett J, O'Leary D, Stanfield B (1984) Regressive events in neurogenesis. Science 225, 1258.

Cox J, Lysko P, Henneberry R (1989) Excitatory amino acid neurotoxicity at the NMDA receptor in cultured neurons: role of the voltage-dependent magnesium block. Brain Res 499, 267.

Coyle J (1983) Neurotoxic action of kainic acid. J Neurochem 41, 1.

Coyle J, Schwarcz R (1976) Lesion of striatal neurones with kainic acid provides a model for Huntington's chorea. Nature 263, 244.

Coyle J, Price D, DeLong M (1983) Alzheimer's disease: disorder of cortical cholinergic innervation. Science 219, 1184.

Crowder J, Croucher M, Bradford H, Collins F (1987) Excitatory amino acid receptors and depolarization-induced calcium influx into hippocampal slices. J Neurochem 48, 1917.

Cull-Candy S, Usowicz M (1987) Multiple-conductance channels activated by excitatory amino acids in cerebellar neurons. Nature 325, 525.

Cullinan W, Herman J, Watson S (1991) Morphological evidence for hippocampal interaction with the hypothalamic paraventricular nucleus. Soc Neurosci Abstr 17, 395.2.

Cupps T, Fauci A (1982) Corticosteroid-mediated immunoregulation in man. Immunol Rev 65, 133.

Curtis D, Watkins J (1960) The excitation and depression of spinal neurons by structurally related amino acids. J Neurochem 6, 117.

Cushman S, Wardzala L (1980) Potential mechanisms of insulin action on glucose transport in the isolated rat adipose cell: apparent translocation of intracellular transport systems to the plasma membrane. J Biol Chem 255, 4758.

Dagani F, Erecinska M (1987) Relationship among ATP synthesis, potassium gradients, and neurotransmitter amino acid levels in isolated rat brain synaptosomes. J Neurochem 49, 1229.

Dallman M (1985) Control of adrenocortical growth in vitro. Endocr Res 10, 213.

Dallman M, Jones M (1973a) Corticosteroid feedback control of stress-induced ACTH secretion. In Brodish A, Redgate E (eds), *Brain-Pituitary-Adrenal Interrelationships*. S Karger, Basal, p 176.

Dallman M, Jones M (1973b) Corticoteroid feedback control of ACTH secretion: effects of stress-induced corticosterone secretion on subsequent stress responses in the rat. Endocrinology 92, 1367.

Dallman M, Yates F (1968) Anatomical and functional mapping of central neural input and feedback pathways of the adrenocortical system. Mem Soc Endocrinol 17, 39.

Dallman M, Yates F (1969) Dynamic asymmetries in the corticoid feedback path and distribution-metabolism-binding elements of the adrenocortical system. Ann NY Acad Sci 156, 696.

Dallman M, Engeland W, Rose J, Wilkinson C, Shinsako J, Siedenburg F (1978) Nycthemeral rhythm in adrenal responsiveness to ACTH. Am J Physiol 235, R210.

Dallman M, Engeland W, Holzwarth M, Scholz P (1981) Adrenocorticotropin inhibits compensatory adrenal growth after unilateral adrenalectomy. Endocrinology 107, 1397.

Dallman M, Makara G, Roberts J, Levin N, Blum M (1985) Corticotrope response to removal of releasing factors and corticosteroids in vivo. Endocrinology 117, 2190.

Dallman M, Akana S, Cascio C, Darlington D, Jacobson L, Levin N 1987 Regulation of ACTH secretion: variations on a theme of B. Recent Prog Horm Res 43, 113.

Dallman M, Levin N, Cascio C, Akana S, Jacobson L, Kuhn R (1989) Pharmacological evidence that the inhibition of diurnal adrenocorticotropin secretion by corticosteroids is mediated via Type I corticosterone-preferring receptors. Endocrinology 124, 2844.

Daniels W, Jaffer A, Engelbrecht A, Rusell V, Taljaard J (1990) The effect of intrahippocampal injection of kainic acid on corticosterone release in rats. Neurochem Res 15, 495.

Dantzer R, Mormede P (1981) Pituitary-adrenal consequences of adjunctive activities in pigs. Horm Behav 15, 386.

Darlington D, Shinsako J, Dallman M (1986) Responses of ACTH, epinephrine, norepinephrine, and cardiovascular system to hemorrhage. Am J Physiol 251, H612.

Darlington D, Neves R, Ha T, Chew G, Dallman M (1990a) Fed, but not fasted, adrenalectomized rats survive the stress of hemorrhage and hypovolemia. Endocrinology 127, 759.

Darlington D, Chew G, Ha T, Keil L, Dallman M (1990b) Corticosterone, but not glucose, treatment enables fasted adrenalectomized rats to survive moderate hemorrhage. Endocrinology 127, 766.

Das S, Nelson R, Potter H (1991) Dexamethasone and dibutyryl cyclic AMP induce the expression of alpha-1-antichymotrypsin in rat astrocytes: implications for Alzheimer's disease. Soc Neurosci Abstr 17, 423.16.

Dave J, Eiden L, Lozovsky D, Waschek J, Eskay R (1987) Calcium-independent and calcium-dependent mechanisms regulate corticotropin-releasing factor–stimulated propiomelanocortin peptide secretion and messenger ribonucleic acid production. Endocrinology 120, 305.

Davies S, Roberts P (1988) Sparing of cholinergic neurons following quinolinic acid lesions of the rat striatum. Neuroscience 26, 387.

Davis D, Christian J (1957) Relation of adrenal weight to social rank of mice. Proc Soc Exp Biol Med 94, 728.

Davis H, Porter J, Livingstone J (1977) Pituitary-adrenal activity and lever press shock escape behavior. Physiol Psychol 5, 280.

Davis K, Davis B, Mathe A, et al. (1984) Age and the dexamethasone suppression test. Am J Psychiatry 141, 872.

Davis L, Arentzen R, Reid J, Manning R, Wolfson B, Lawrence K, Baldino F (1986) Glucocorticoid sensitivity of vasopressin mRNA levels in the paraventricular nucleus of the rat. Proc Natl Acad Sci USA 83, 1145.

Dawson T, Bredt D, Fotuhi M, Hwang P, Snyder S (1991) Nitric oxide synthase and neuronal NADPH diaphorase are identical in brain and peripheral tissues. Proc Natl Acad Sci USA 88, 7797.

Dawson V, Dawson T, London E, Bredt D, Snyder S (1991) Nitric oxide mediates glutamate neurotoxicity in primary cortical culres. Proc Natl Acad Sci USA 88, 6368.

Deardeu N, Gibson J, McDowall D, Gibson R, Cameron M (1986) Effect of high-dose dexamethasone on outcome from severe head injury. J Neurosurg 64, 81.

de Goeij D, Kvetnansky R, Whitnall M, Jezova D, Berkenbosch F, Tilders F (1991) Repeated stress-induced activation of CRF neurons enhances vasopressin stores and colocalization with CRF in the median eminence of rats. Neuroendocrinology 53, 150.

de Kloet E, Reul J (1987) Feedback action and tonic influence of corticosteroids on brain functions: a concept arising from the heterogeneity of brain receptor systems. Psychoneuroendocrinology 12, 83.

de Kloet E, Kovacs G, Szabo G, Telegdy G, Bohus B, Versteeg D (1982) Decreased serotonin turnover in the dorsal hippocampus of rat brain shortly after adrenalectomy: selective normalization after corticosterone substitution. Brain Res 239, 659.

de Kloet E, Sybesma H, Reul J (1986) Selective control of serotonin receptor capacity in raphe-hippocampal system. Neuroendocrinology 42, 513.

de Kloet E, Ratka A, Reul J, Sutanto W, van Eekelen J (1987) Corticosteroid receptor types in brain: regulation and putative function. Ann NY Acad Sci 512, 351.

de Kloet E, de Kock s, Schild V, Veldhuis H (1988a) Antiglucocorticoid RU 38486 attenuates retention of a behaviour and disinhibits the hypothalamic-pituitary-adrenal axis at different brain sites. Neuroendocrinology 47, 109.

de Kloet E, Rosenfeld P, van Eekelen J, Sutanto W, Levine S (1988b) Stress, glucocorticoids and development. Prog Brain Res 73, p 101.

de Kloet E, Reul J, Sutanto W (1990) Corticosteroids and the brain. J Steroid Biochem Molec Biol 37, 387.

DeKosky S, Scheff S, Cotman C (1984) Elevated corticosterone levels: a mechanism for impaired sprouting in the aged hippocampus. Neuroendocrinology 38, 33.

DeLaTorre J, Surgeon J (1976) Dexamethasone and DMSO in experimental transorbital cerebral infarction. Stroke 7, 577.

DeLeo J, Toth L, Schubert P, Rudolphi K, Kreutzberg G (1987) Ischemia-induced neuronal cell death, calcium accumulation and glia response in the hippocampus of the mongolian gerbil and protection by propentofylline (HWA 285). J Cereb Blood Flow Metab 7, 745.

De Leon M, McRae T, Tsai J, George A, Marcus D, Freedman M, Wolf A, McEwen B (1988) Abnormal cortisol response in Alzheimer's disease linked to hippocampal atrophy. Lancet 2, 391.

Dellwo M, Beauchene R (1990) The effect of exercise, diet restriction, and aging on the pituitary-adrenal axis in the rat. Exp Gerontol 25, 553.

Deshpande J, Siesjo B, Wieloch T (1987) Calcium accumulation and neuronal damage in the rat hippocampus following cerebral ischemia. J Cereb Blood Flow Metab 7, 89.

de Souza E, van Loon G (1982) Stress-induced inhibition of the plasma corticosterone response to a subsequent stress in rats: a nonadrenocorticotropin-mediated mechanism. Endocrinology 110, 23.

de Souza E, van Loon G (1989) Rate-sensitive glucocorticoid feedback inhibition of ACTH and beta-endorphin/beta-lipotropin secretion in rats. Endocrinology 125, 2927.

de Souza E, Goeders N, Kuhar M (1986) Benzodiazepine receptors in rat brain are altered by adrenalectomy. Brain Res 381, 176.

Dess-Beech N, Linwick D, Patterson J, Overmier J (1983) Immediate and proactive effects of controllability and predictability on plasma cortisol resposnes to shocks in dogs. Behav Neurosci 97, 1005.

Devenport L, Knehans A, Sundstrom A, Thomas T (1989) Corticosterone's dual metabolic actions. Life Sci 45, 1389.

DeVito W, Sutterer J, Brush F (1981) The pituitary-adrenal response to ether stress in the spontaneously hypertensive and normotensive rat. Life Sci 28, 1489.

de Waal F (1982) *Chimpanzee Politics*. Harper Colophon, New York.

de Wied D (1964) The site of the blocking action of dexamethasone on stress-induced pituitary ACTH release. J Endocrinol 29, 29.

Diamond M, Miner J, Yoshinaga S, Yamamoto K (1990) Transcription factor interactions: selectors of positive or negative regulation from a single DNA element. Science 249, 1266.

Dienel G (1984) Regional accumulation of calcium in post-ischemic rat brain. J Neurochem 43, 913.

Dienel G, Pulsinelli W, Duffy T (1980) Regional protein synthesis in rat brain following acute hemispheric ischemia. J Neurochem 35, 1216.

Dienel G, Kiessling M, Jacewicz M, Pulsinelli W (1986) Synthesis of heat shock proteins in rat brain cortex after transient ischemia. J Cereb Blood Flow Metab 6, 505.

Dietrich W, Busto R, Yoshida S, Ginsberg M (1987) Histopathological and hemodynamic consequences of complete versus incomplete ischemia in the rat. J Cereb Blood Flow Metab 7, 300.

Dildy J, Leslie S (1989) Ethanol inhibits NMDA-induced increases in free intracellular calcium in dissociated brain cells. Brain Res 499, 383.

Dildy-Mayfield J, Leslie S (1991) Mechanism of inhibition of NMDA-stimulated increases in free intracellular calcium concentration by ethanol. J Neurochem 56, 1536.

Dilman V, Lapin I, Oxenkrug G (1979) Serotonin and aging. In Essman W (ed), *Serotonin in Health and Disease*. Spectrum Press, New York.

Di Stasi A, Gallo V, Ceccarini M, Petrucci T (1991) Neuronal fodrin proteolysis occurs independently of excitatory amino acid—induced neurotoxicity. Neuron 6, 445.

Dodd P, Bradford H (1976) Release of amino acids from the maturing cobalt-induced epileptic focus. Brain Res 111, 377.

Dodd P, Bradford H, Abdul-Ghani A, Cox D, Continho-Netto J (1980) Release of amino acids from chronic epileptic and subepileptic foci in vivo. Brain Res 193, 505.

Dolphin A, Archer E (1983) An adenosine agonist inhibits and a cyclic AMP analogue enhances the release of glutamate but not GABA from slices of rat dentate gyrus. Neurosci Lett 43, 49.

Domer F, Mori K, Dinarello C, Sokoloff L (1988) Effects of leukocyte pyrogen (Interleukin-1) on local cerebral utilization in rats with and without premedication with indomethacin or dexamethasone. J Cereb Blood Flow Metab 8, 173.

Dong Y, Poellinger L, Gustafsson J, Okret S (1988) Regulation of glucocorticoid receptor expression: evidence for transcriptional and posttranslational mechanisms. Mol Endocrinol 2, 1256.

Donley R, Sundt T (1973) The effect of dexamethasone on the edema of focal cerebral ischemia. Stroke 4, 148.

Dorovini-Zis K, Zis A (1987) Increased adrenal weight in victims of violent suicide. Am J Psychiatry 144, 1214.

Dourmashkin R (1980) Electron microscopic demonstration of lesions in target cell membranes associated with antibody-dependent cellular cytotoxicity. Clin Exp Immunol 42, 554.

Dozin-van Roye B, De Nayer P (1979) Nuclear triiodothyronine receptors in rat brain during maturation. Brain Res 177, 551.

Drejer J, Benveniste H, Diemer N, Schousboe A (1985) Cellular origin of ischemia-induced glutamate release from brain tissue in vivo and in vitro. J Neurochem 34, 145.

Drian M, Kamenka J, Pirat J, Privat A (1991) Non-competitive antagonists of NMDA prevent spontaneous neuronal death in primary cultures of embryonic rat cortex. J Neurosci Res 29, 133.

Driscoll P, Battig K (1982) Behavioral, emotional and neurochemical profiles of rats selected for extreme differences in active, two-way avoidance performance. In Lieblich I (ed), *Genetics of the Brain*. Elsevier, Amsterdam.

Dubinsky J, Rothman S (1991) Intracellular calcium concentrations during "chemical hypoxia" and excitotoxic neuronal injury. J Neurosci 11, 2545.

Duchen M, Valdeolmillos M, O'Neill S, Eisner D (1990) Effects of metabolic blockade on the regulation of intracellular calcium in dissociated mouse sensory neurones. J Physiol 424, 411.

Ducker T, Hamit H (1979) Experimental treatments of acute spinal cord injury. J Neurosurg 30, 693.

Dumuis A, Sebben M, Haynes L, Pin J, Bockaert J (1988) NMDA receptors activate the arachidonic acid cascade system in striatal neurons. Nature 336, 68.

Dunn A (1989) Psychoimmunology for the psychoneuroendocrinologist: a review of animal studies of nervous system-immune system interactions. Psychoneuroendocrinology 14, 251.

Dunn J, Critchlow V (1973) Pituitary-adrenal function following ablation of medial basal hypothalamus. Proc Soc Exp Biol Med 142, 749.

Dunn J, Orr S (1984) Differential plasma corticosterone responses to hippocampal stimulation. Exp Brain Res 54, 1.

Dunwiddie T, Lynch G (1979) The relationship between extracellular calcium concentration and the induction of hippocampal long-term potentiation. Brain Res 169, 103.

Dupont A, Bastarache E, Endroczi E (1972) Hippocampal stimulation on plasma thyrotropin and corticosterone responses to acute cold-exposure in rat. Can J Physiol Pharm 50, 364.

Dussault J, Labrie F (1975) Development of the hypothalamic-pituitary-thyroid axis in the neonatal rat. Endocrinology 97, 1321.

Duverger D, Benavides J, Cudennec A, MacKenzie E, Scatton B, Seylax J, Verecchia C (1987) A glutamate antagonist reduces infarction size following focal cerebral ischemia independently of vascular and metabolic changes. J Cereb Blood Flow Metab 7 (Suppl 1), S144.

Dykens J, Stern A, Trenkner J (1987) Mechanism of kainate toxicity to cerebeller neurons in vitro is analogous to reperfusion tissue injury. J Neurochem 49, 1222.

Eaton G, Resko J (1974) Plasma testosterone and male dominance in a Japanese macaque (*Macaca fuscata*) troop compared with repeated measures of testosterone in laboratory males. Horm Behav 5, 251.

Eberhart J, Keverne E (1979) Influences of the dominance hierarchy on LH, testosterone and prolactin in male talapoin monkeys. J Endocrinol 83, 42.

Eberwine J, Roberts J (1984) Glucocorticoid regulation of pro-opiomelanocortin gene transcription in the rat pituitary. J Biol Chem 259, 2166.

Eberwine J, Jonassen J, Evinger M, Roberts J (1987) Complex transcriptional regulation by glucocorticoids and CRH of POMC gene expression in rat pituitary cultures. DNA 6, 483.

Eisenberg H, Barlow C, Lorenzo A (1970) Effect of dexamethasone on altered brain vascular permeability. Arch Neurol 23, 18.

Ejike C, Schreck C (1980) Stress and social heirarchy rank in coho salmon. Trans Am Fisheries Soc 109, 423.

Eldridge J, Landfield P (1990) Cannabinoid interactions with the glucocorticoid receptors in rat hippocampus. Brain Res 534, 135.

Eldridge J, Fleenor D, Kerr D, Landfield P (1989a) Impaired up-regulation of type II corticosteroid receptors in hippocampus of aged rats. Brain Res 478, 248.

Eldridge J, Brodish A, Kute T, Landfield P (1989b) Apparent age-related resistance of Type II hippocampal corticosteroid receptors to down-regulation during chronic escape training. J Neurosci 9, 3237.

Elliott E, Sapolsky R (1992) Corticosterone enhances kainic acid-induced calcium mobilization in cultured hippocampal neurons. J Neurochem, in press.

Elliott E, Mattson M, Vanderklish P, Lynch G, Chang I, Sapolsky R (1992) Corticosterone exacerbates kainate-induced alterations in hippocampal tau immunoreactivity and spectrin proteolysis in vivo. Submitted.

Ellis F (1966) Effect of ethanol on plasma corticosterone levels. J Pharmacol Exp Ther 153, 121.

Endroczi E, Lissak K (1962) Interrelations between paleocortical activity and pituitary-adrenocortical function. Acta Physiol Acad Sci Hung 21, 257.

Endroczi E, Lissak K, Bohus B (1959) The inhibitory influence of archicortical structures on pituitary adrenal function. Acta Physiol Acad Sci Hung 16, 17.

Engeland W, Shinsako J, Winget C, Vernikos-Danellis J, Dallman M (1977) Circadian patterns of stress-induced ACTH secretion are modified by corticosterone responses. Endocrinology 100, 138.

Engeland W, Byrnes G, Presnell K Gann D (1981) Adrenocortical sensitivity to ACTH in awake dogs changes as a function of the time of observation and after hemorrhage independently of changes in ACTH. Endocrinology 108, 2149.

English H, Kyprianou N, Isaacs J (1989) Relationship between DNA fragmentation and apoptosis in the rat prostate following castration. Prostate 15, 233.

Erecinska M, Silver I (1989) ATP and brain function. J Cereb Blood Flow Metab 9, 2.

Erisman S, Carnes M, Takahashi L, Lent S (1990) The effects of stress on plasma ACTH and corticosterone in young and aging pregnant rats and their fetuses. Life Sci 47, 1527.

Eufermiond M (1990) Advances in the therapy of steroid-induced osteoporosis. Geriatric Med Today, February.

Evans D, Nemeroff C (1983) Use of the dexamethsone suppression test using DSM-III criteria on an inpatient psychiatric unit. Biol Psychiatry 18, 505.

Evans D, Burnett G, Nemeroff C (1983) The dexamethasone suppression test in the clinical setting. Am J Psychiatry 140, 586.

Evans M, Meldrum B (1984) Regional brain glucose metabolism in chemically-induced seizures in the rat. Brain Res 297, 235.

Evans M, Swan J, Meldrum B (1988) An adenosine analogue, 2-chloroadenosine, protects against long term development of ischemic cell loss in the rat hippocampus. Neurosci Lett 83, 287.

Evans R (1988) The steroid and thyroid hormone receptor superfamily. Science 240, 889.

Evans R, Arriza J (1989) A molecular framework for the actions of glucocorticoid hormones in the nervous system. Neuron 2, 1105.

Extein I, Pottash A, Gold M (1985) Number of cortisol time-points and dexamethasone suppression test sensitivity for major depression. Psychoneuroendocrinology 10, 281.

Faden A, Siman R (1988) A potential role for excitotoxins in the pathophysiology of spinal cord injury. Ann Neurol 23, 623.

Faden A, Demediuk P, Panter S, Vink R (1989) The role of excitatory amino acids and NMDA receptors in traumatic brain injury. Science 244, 798.

Fahrbach S, Truman J (1987) Autoradiographic studies of ecdysteroid binding in the nervous system of Manduca sexta. Soc Neurosci Abstr 13, 1518.

Fan P, O'Regan P, Szerb J (1988) Effect of low glucose concentration on synaptic transmission in the rat hippocampal slice. Brain Res Bull 21, 741.

Farah J, Rao T, Mick S, Coyne IK, Iyengar S (1991) NMDA treatment increases circulating ACTH and LH in the rat. Endocrinology 128, 1875.

Farias L, Smith E, Markov A (1990) Prevention of ischemic-hypoxic brain injury and death in rabbits with fructose-1,6-diphosphate. Stroke 21, 606.

Faupel G, Reulen H, Muller D, Schurmann K (1976) Double-blind study on the effects of steroids on severe closed head injury. In Pappiu H, Feindel W (eds), Dynamics of Brain Edema. Springer-Verlag, Berlin, p 337.

Favaron M, Manev H, Alho H, Bertolino M, Ferret B, Guidotti A, Costa A (1988) Gangliosides prevent glutamate and kainate neurotoxicity in primary neuronal cultures of neonatal rat cerebellum and cortex. Proc Natl Acad Sci USA 85, 7351.

Federoff H, Grabczyk E, Fishman M (1988) Corticosteroids suppress expression of GAP-43. Soc Neurosci Abstr 14, 112.7.

Fehm H, Voigt K, Kummer G, Lang R, Pfeiffer E (1979) Differential and integral corticosteroid feedback effect on ACTH secretion in hypoadrenocorticism. J Clin Invest 63, 247.

Fehm-Wolfsdorf G, Nagel D, Fehm H (1991) Stress induced cortisol secretion influences information processing in man. Soc Neurosci Abstr 17, 561.6.

Feibel J, Hardi P, Campbell M, Goldstein N, Joynt R (1977) Prognostic value of the stress response following stroke. JAMA 238, 1374.

Feldman S, Conforti N (1976) Feedback effects of dexamethasone on adrenocortical responses of rats with fornix section. Horm Res 7, 56.

Feldman S, Conforti N (1979) Effect of dorsal hippocampectomy or fimbria section on adrenocortical responses in rats. Isr J Med Sci 15, 539.

Feldman S, Conforti N (1980) Participation of the dorsal hippocampus in the glucocorticoid feedback effect on adrenocortical activity. Neuroendocrinology 30, 52.

Feldman S, Chowers I, Conforti N (1973) Effect of dexamethasone on adrenocortical response in intact and hypothalamic deafferented rats. Acta Endocrinol (Copenh) 73, 660.

Feldman S, Conforti N, Siegel R (1982) Adrenocortical responses following limbic stimulation in rats with hypothalamic deafferentations. Neuroendocrinology 35, 205.

Feldman S, Saphier D, Conforti N (1987) Hypothalamic afferent connections mediating adreno-cortical respones that follow hippocampal stimulation. Exp Neurol 98, 103.

Felt B, Sapolsky R, McEwen B (1984) Regulation of hippocampal corticosterone receptors by a vasopressin analogue. Peptides 5, 1225.

Fendler K, Karmos G, Telegdy M (1961) The effect of hippocampal lesions on pituitary-adrenal function. Acta Endocrinol (Copenh) 73, 660.

Fenske A, Fisher M, Regli F, Hase U (1979) The response of focal ischemic cerebral edema to dexamethasone. J Neurol 220, 199.

Ferkany J, Coyle J (1983) Kainic acid selectively stimulates the release of endogenous excitatory acidic amino acids. J Pharmacol Exp Ther 225, 399.

Ferrante R, Kowall N, Beal M, Richardson E, Bird E, Martin J (1985) Selective sparing of a class of striatal neurons in Huntington's disease. Science 230, 561.

Ferrara C, Cocchi D, Muller E (1991) Somatostatin in the hippocampus mediates dexamethasone-induced suppression of corticosterone secretion in the rat. Neuroendocrinology 53, 428.

Ferrier I, Pascual J, Charlton B, Wright C, Leake A (1988) Cortisol, ACTH and dexamethasone concentrations in a psychogeriatric population. Biol Psychiatry 23, 252.

Finch C (1990) Longevity, Senescence, and the Genome. University of Chicago Press, Chicago.

Finch C, Felicio L, Mobbs C, Nelson J (1984) Ovarian and steroidal influences on neuroendocrine aging processes in female rodents. Endocr Rev 5, 467.

Fink G, Robinson I, Tannahill L (1988) Effects of adrenalectomy and glucocorticoids on the peptides CRF-41, AVP and oxytocin in rat hypophysial portal blood. J Physiol 401, 329.

Fischette C, Komisurak B, Edinger H, Feder H, Siegel A (1980) Differential fornix ablations and the circadian rhythmicity of adrenal corticosterone secretion. Brain Res 195, 373.

Fishman R (1982) Steroid in the treatment of brain edema. N Engl J Med 306, 359.

Fishman R, Chan P (1981) Hypothesis: membrane phospholipids degradation and polyunsaturated fatty acids play a key role in the pathogenesis of brain edema. Ann Neurol 10, 75.

Flower R (1974) Drugs which inhibit prostaglandin biosynthesis. Pharmacol Rev 26, 33.

Flower R (1986) The mediators of steroid action. Nature 320, 20.

Floyd R (1991) Oxidative damage to behavior during aging. Science 254, 1597.

Fogel B, Satel S, Levy S (1985) Occurrence of high concentrations of postdexamethasone cortisol in elderly psychiatric inpatients. Psychiatry Res 15, 85.

Foley J, Jeffries M, Munck A (1980) Glucocorticoid effects on incorporation of lipid and protein precursors into rat thymus cell fractions. J Steroid Biochem 12, 231.

Fortier C, Dalgado A, Ducummon P, Ducummon S, DuPont A, Jobin M, Kraicer J, MacIntosh-Hardt B, Marceau H, Maihle P, Miahle-Voiloss C, Rerup C, Van Rees G (1970) Functional interrelationship between the adrenohypophysis, thyroid, adrenal cortex, and gonads. Can Med Assoc J 103, 864.

Fowler J (1989) Adenosine antagonists delay hypoxia-induced depression of neuronal activity in hippocampal brain slice. Brain Res 490, 378.

Fox M, Andrews R (1973) Physiologic and biochemical correlates of individual differences in behavior of wolf cubs. Behavior 46, 129.

Frairia R, Agrimonti F, Fortunati N, Fazzari A, Gennari P, Berta L (1988) Influence of naturally occurring and synthetic glucocorticoids on CBG-steroid interaction in human peripheral plasma. Ann NY Acad Sci 538, 287.

Francis A, Pulsinelli W (1982) The response of GABAergic and cholinergic neurons to transient cerebral ischemia. Brain Res 243, 271.

Franck J, Kunkel D, Baskin D, Schwartzkroin P (1988) Inhibition in kainate-lesioned hyperexcitable hippocampi: physiologic, autoradiographic, and immunocytochemical observations. J Neurosci 8, 1991.

Frandsen A, Schousboe A (1991) Dantrolene prevents glutamate cytotoxicity and calcium release from intracellular stores in cultured cerebral cortical neurons. J Neurochem 56, 1075.

Frankenhaeuser M (1980) Psychoneuroendocrine approaches to the study of stressful person-environment transactions. In Selye H (ed), Selye's Guide to Stress Research. Van Nostrand, New York.

Fredholm B, Dunwiddie T (1988) How does adenosine inhibit transmitter release? Trends Pharmacol Sci 8, 130.

Freeman E, Damron D, Terrian D, Dorman R (1991) 12-Lipoxygenase products attenuate the glutamate release and caclium accumulation evoked by depolarization of hippocampal mossy fiber nerve endings. J Neurochem 56, 1079.

Freund T, Buzsaki G, Leon A, Somogyi P (1990a) Hippocampal cell death following ischemia: effects of brain temperature and anesthesia. Exp Neurol 108, 251.

Freund T, Buzsaki G, Leon A, Baimbridge K, Somogyi P (1990b) Relationship of neuronal vulnerability and calcium binding protein immunoreactivity in ischemia. Exp Brain Res 83, 55.

Friedman H, Booth-Kewley S (1987) The "disease-prone personality": a meta-analytic view of the construct. Am Psychol 42, 539.

Friedman S, Mason J, Hamburg D (1963) Urinary 17-hydroxycorticosteroid levels in parents of children with neoplastic disease: a study of chronic psychological stress. Psychosom Med 25, 364.

Frotscher M, Zimmer J (1987) GABAergic non-pyramidal neurons in intracerebral transplants of the rat hippocampus: a combined light and electron microscopic immunocytochemical study. J Comp Neurol 259, 266.

Fujimori H, Pan-Hou H (1991) Effect of nitric oxide on L-[^{3}H]glutamate binding in rat brain synaptic membranes. Brain Res 554, 355.

Fujisawa A, Matsumoto M, Matsuyamat I (1986) The effect of the calcium antagonist nimodipine on the gerbil model of experimental cerebral ischemia. Stroke 17, 748.

Funder J (1991) Corticosteroid receptors in the brain. In Motta M (ed), Brain Endocrinology (2nd ed). Raven Press, New York, p 133.

Funder J, Sheppard K (1987) Adrenocortical steroids and the brain. Annu Rev Physiol 49, 397.

Funder J, Pearce P, Smith R, Smith A (1988) Mineralocorticoid action: target tissue specificity is enzyme, not receptor, mediated. Science 242, 583.

Furukawa K, Yamana K, Kogure K (1990) Postischemic alterations of spontaneous activities in rat hippocampal CA_1 neurons. Brain Res 530, 257.

Fuxe K, Wikstronm A, Okret S, Agnati L, Harfstrand A, Yu Z, Granholm L, Zoli M, Vale W, Gustafsson J (1985) Mapping of glucocorticoid receptor immunoreactive neurons in the rat tel- and diencephalon using a monoclonal antibody against a rat liver glucocorticoid receptor. Endocrinology 117, 1803.

Gage F, Kelly P, Bjorklund A (1984) Regional changes in brain glucose metabolism reflect cognitive impairments in aged rats. J Neurosci 4, 2856.

Gagner J, Drouin J (1987) Tissue-specific regulation of pituitary POMC gene transcription by CRH, 3',5'-cyclic adenosine monophosphate, and glucocorticoids. Mol Endocrinol 1, 677.

Gaillard R, Riondel A, Muller A, Herrmann W, Baulieu E (1984) RU 486: a steroid with anti-glucocorticosteroid activity that only disinhibits the human pituitary-adrenal system at a specific time of day. Proc Natl Acad Sci USA 81, 3879.

Gaillard S, Dupont J (1990) Ionic control of intracellular pH in rat cerebellar Purkinje cells maintained in culture. J Physiol 425, 71.

Galicich J, French L (1961) Use of dexamethasone in treatment of cerebral edema resulting from brain tumor and brain surgery. Am Prac Dig Treat 12, 169.

Galicich J, French L, Melly J (1961) Use of dexamethasone in treatment of cerebral edema associated with brain tumor. J Lancet 81, 46.

Gallagher M, Pelleymounter M (1988) An age-related spatial learning deficit: choline uptake distinguishes impaired and unimpaired rats. Neurobiol Aging 9, 363.

Gallagher M, Burwell R, Kidsi M, McKinney M, Southerland S, Vella-Rountree L, Lewis M (1990) Markers for biogenic amines in aged rat brain: relationship to decline in spatial learning ability. Neurobiol Aging 11, 507.

Gametchu B (1987) Glucocorticoid receptor-like antigen in lymphoma cell membranes: correlation to cell lysis. Science 236, 456.

Gann D (1969) Parameters of the stimulus initiating the adrenocortical response to hemorrhage. Ann NY Acad Sci 156, 740.

Gann D, Cryer G (1973) Feedback control of ACTH secretion by cortisol. In Brodish A, Redgate E (eds), *Brain-Pituitary-Adrenal Interrelationships*. S Karger, Basel, p 197.

Gann D, Cryer G, Pirkle J (1977) Physiological inhibition and facilitation of the adrenocortical response to hemorrhage. Am J Physiol 232, R5.

Gannon R, Terrian D (1991) Presynpatic modulation of glutamate and dynorphin release by excitatory amino acids in the guinea-pig hippocampus. Neuroscience 41, 401.

Ganong W, Hume D (1955) Effect of hypothalamic lesions on steroid-induced atrophy of the adrenal cortex in the dog. Proc Soc Exp Biol Med 88, 528.

Garcia-Coll C, Kagan J, Resnick J (1984) Behavioral inhibition in young children. Child Dev 55, 1005.

Garrick N, Hill J, Szele F, Tomai T, Gold P, Murphy D (1987) Corticotropin-releasing factor: a marked circadian rhythm in primate cerebrospinal fluid peaks in the evening and is inversely related to the cortisol circadian rhythm. Endocrinology 121, 1329.

Garthwaite G, Garthwaite J (1986) Neurotoxicity of excitatory amino acid receptor agonists in rat cerebeller slices: dependence on calcium concentration. Neurosci Lett 66, 193.

Garthwaite G, Garthwaite J (1988) Cyclid GMP and cell death in rat cerebellar slices. Neuroscience 26, 321.

Garthwaite G, Hajos F, Garthwaite J (1986) Ionic requirements for neurotoxic effects of excitatory amino acid analogues in rat cerebeller slices. Neuroscience 18, 437.

Garthwaite J (1991) Glutamate, nitric oxide and cell-cell signalling in the nervous system. Trends Neurosci 14, 60.

Garvey W, Huecksteadt T, Lima F, Birnbaum M (1989a) Expression of a glucose transporter gene cloned from brain in cellular models of insulin resistance: dexamethasone decreases transporter mRNA in primary cultured adipocytes. Mol Endocrinol 3, 1132.

Garvey W, Huecksteadt T, Monzon R, Marshall S (1989b) Dexamethasone regulates the glucose transport system in primary cultured adipocytes: different mechanisms of insulin resistance after acute and chronic exposure. Endocrinology 124, 2063.

Gaudet R, Levine L (1979) Transient cerebral ischemia and brain prostaglandins. Biochem Biophys Res Comm 86, 893.

Gbadebo D, Hamm R, Lyeth B, Jenkins L, Stewart J, Porter J (1991) Corticosterone's mediation of traumatic brain injury. Soc Neurosci Abstr 17, 65.7.

Gehring U (1986) Genetics of glucocorticoid receptors. Mol Cell Endocrinol 48, 89.

Geinisman Y, deToledo-Morrell L, Morrell F (1986) Loss of perforated synapses in the dentate gyrus: morphological substrate of memory deficit in aged rats. Proc Natl Acad Sci USA 83, 3027.

Gentsch C, Lichtsteiner M, Feer H (1981a) Locomotor activity, defecation score and corticosterone levels during an openfield exposure: a comparison among individually and group-housed rats, and genetically selected rat lines. Physiol Behav 27, 183.

Gentsch C, Lichtsteiner M, Feer H (1981b) ³H-diazepam binding sites in Roman high- and Roman low-avoidance rats. Experientia 37, 1315.

Gentsch C, Lichtsteiner M, Driscoll P, Feer H (1982) Differential hormonal and physiological responses to stress in Roman high- and low-avoidance rats. Physiol Behav 28, 259.

Gentsch C, Lichsteiner M, Feer H (1983) Regional distribution of ³H-imipramine binding sites in the CNS of Roman high and low avoidance rats. Eur J Pharmacol 88, 259.

Gentsch C, Lichtsteiner M, Feer H (1988) Genetic and environmental influences on behavioral and neurochemical aspects of emotionality in rats. Experientia 44, 482.

George C, Goldberg M, Choi D, Steinberg G (1988) Dextromethorphan reduces neocortical ischemic neuronal damage in vivo. Brain Res 440, 375.

Georgotas A, Stokes P, Krakowski M, Fanelli C, Cooper T (1984) Hypothalamic-pituitary-adrenocortica function in geriatric depression: diagnostic and treatment implications. Biol Psychiatry 19, 685.

Gerkin A, Holsboer F (1986) Cortisol and corticosterone response after syn-corticotropin in relationship to the suppressibility of cortisol. Psychoneuroendocrinology 11, 185.

Gerlach J, McEwen B, Pfaff D, Moskowitz S, Ferin M, Carmel P, Zimmerman E (1976) Cells in regions of rhesus monkey brain and pituitary retain radioactive estradiol, corticosterone and cortisol differentially. Brain Res 103, 603.

Germano I, Pitts L, Meldrum B, Bartkowski H, Simon R (1987) Kynurenate inhibition of cell excitation decreases stroke size and deficits. Ann Neurol 22, 730.

Gertz B, Contreras L, McComb D, Kovacs, K Tyrrell J, Dallman M (1987) Chronic administration of CRF increases pituitary corticotroph number. Endocrinology 120, 381.

Giannotta S, Weiss M, Apuzzo M, Martin E (1984) High dose glucocorticoids in the management of severe head injury. Neurosurgery 15, 497.

Gibbons J, McHugh P (1962) Plasma cortisol in depressive illness. Psychiatry Res 1, 162.

Gibbs D (1986) Vasopressin and oxytocin: hypothalamic modulators of the stress response: a review. Psychoneuroendocrinology 11, 131.

Gibbs D, Vale W, Rivier J, Yen S (1984) Oxytocin potentiates the ACTH-releasing activity of CRF but not vasopressin. Life Sci 34, 2245.

Gibbs F (1970) Circadian variation of ether-induced corticosterone secretion in the rat. Am J Physiol 219, 288.

Giffard R, Monyer H, Christine C, Choi D (1990a) Acidosis reduces NMDA receptor activation, glutamate neurotoxicity, and oxygen-glucose deprivation neuronal injury in cortical cultures. Brain Res 506, 339.

Giffard R, Monyer H, Choi D (1990b) Selective vulnerability of cultured cortical glia to injury by extracellular acidosis. Brain Res 530, 138.

Giguere V, Labrie F (1982) Vasopressin potentiates cytosolic AMP accumulation and ACTH release induced by corticotropin-releasing factor in rat anterior pituitary cells in culture. Endocrinology 111, 1752.

Giguere V, Labrie F (1983) Additive effects of epinephrine and CRF on adrenocorticotropin release in rat anterior pituitary cells. Biochem Biophys Res Commun 110, 456.

Giguere V, Labrie F, Cote J, Coy D, Sueiras-Diaz J, Schally A (1982) Stimulation of cyclic AMP accumulation and corticotropin release by synthetic ovine CRF in rat anterior pituitary cells: site of glucocorticoid action. Proc Natl Acad Sci USA 79, 3466.

Gilbert J, Sawas A (1983) ATPase activities and lipid peroxidation in rat cerebral cortex synaptosomes. Arch Int Pharmacodyn 263, 189.

Gill R, Foster A, Woodruff G (1987) Systemic administration of MK-801 protects against ischemia-induced hippocampal neurodegeneration in the gerbil. J Neurosci 7, 3343.

Gill R, Foster A Woodruff G (1988) MK-801 is neuroprotective in gerbils when administered during the post-ischemic period. Neuroscience 25, 847.

Gillies G, Linton E, Lowry P (1982) Corticotropin releasing activity of the new CRF is potentiated several times by vasopressin. Nature 299, 355.

Ginsberg M, Welsh F, Budd W (1980) Deleterious effect of glucose pretreatment on recovery from diffuse cerebral ischemia in the cat. I. Local cerebral blood flow and glucose utilization. Stroke 11, 347.

Gitlin M, Gerner R (1986) The dexamethasone suppression test and response to somatic treatment: a review. J Clin Psychiatry 47, 16.

Globus M, Busto R, Martinez E, Valdes I, Dietrich W, Ginsberg M (1991) Comparative effect of transient global ischemia on extracellular levels of glutamate, glycine, and GABA in vulnerable and nonvulnerable brain regions in the rat. J Neurochem 57, 470.

Gobiet W (1976) Influence of various doses of dexamethasone on intracranial pressure in patients with severe head injury. In Pappiu H, Feindel W (eds), *Dynamics of Brain Edema*. Springer-Verlag, Berlin.

Gobiet W, Bock W, Liesgang J, Grote W (1976) Treatment of acute cerebral edema with high dose of dexamethasone. In Beks J, Bosch D, Brock M (eds), *Intracranial Pressure III*. Springer-Verlag, New York.

Gold P, Chrousos G, Kellner C, Post R, Roy A, Avgerinos P, Schulte H, Oldfield E, Loriaux D (1984) Psychiatric implications of basic and clinical studies with CRF. Am J Psychiatry 141, 619.

Gold P, Loriaux L, Roy A, et al. (1986) Responses to corticotropin-releasing hormone in the hypercortisolism of depression and Cushing's disease. N Engl J Med 314, 1329.

Gold P, Goodwin F, Chrousos G (1988) Clinical and biochemical manifestations of depression: relation to the neurobiology of stress. N Engl J Med 319, 348.

Goldberg M, Weiss J, Pham P, Choi D (1987) NMDA receptors mediate hypoxic neuronal injury in cortical culture. J Pharm Exp Ther 243, 784.

Goldberg M, Monyer H, Weiss J, Choi D (1988) Adenosine reduces cortical neuronal injury induced by oxygen or glucose deprivation in vitro. Neurosci Lett 89, 323.

Goldberg W, Watson B, Busto R, Kurchner H, Santiso M, Ginsberg M (1984) Concurrent measurement of (Na$^+$, K$^+$)-ATPase activity and lipid peroxides in rat brain following reversible global ischemia. Neurochem Res 9, 1737.

Goldberg W, Kadingo R, Barrett J (1986) Effects of ischemia-like conditions on cultured neurons: protection by low sodium, low calcium solutions. J Neurosci 6, 3144.

Goldman S, Pulsinelli W, Clarke W, Kraig R, Plum F (1989) The effects of extracellular acidosis on neurons and glia in vitro. J Cereb Blood Flow Metab 9, 471.

Goldstein A, Wells B, Keats A (1966) Increased tolerance to cerebral anoxia by pentobarbital. Arch Int Pharmcodyn Ther 161, 138.

Goldstein M, Barnett H, Orgogozo J, Sartorious N, Symon L, Verschagin N (1989) Recommendations on stroke prevention, diagnosis and therapy: report of the WHO task force on stroke and other cerebrovascular disorders. Stroke 20, 1407.

Goodall J (1986) *The Chimpanzees of Gombe*. Belknap Press, Cambridge.

Goodman H (1980) The pancreas and regulation of metabolism. In Mountcastle V (ed), *Medical Physiology* (14th ed). Mosby, St. Louis.

Gordon T, Rose R, Bernstein I (1976) Seasonal rhythm in plasma testosterone levels in the rhesus monkey (*Macaca mulatta*): a three year study. Horm Behav 7, 229.

Gould E, Woolley C, McEwen B (1990) Short-term glucocorticoid manipulations affect neuronal morphology and survival in the adult dentate gyrus. Neuroscience 37, 367.

Grad B, Rosenberg G, Liberman H (1971) Diurnal variation of serum cortisol level of geriatric subjects. J Gerontol 26, 351.

Graf M, Kastin A, Coy D, Fischman A (1985) Delta-sleep-inducing peptide reduces CRF-induced corticosterone release. Neuroendocrinology 41, 353.

Graf M, Fischman A, Kastin A, Moldow R (1988) Circadian variation in response to CRF-41 and AVP. Am J Physiol 255, E265.

Grafton S, Longstretch W (1988) Steroids after cardiac arrest: a retrospective study with concurrent nonrandomized controls. Neurology 38, 1315.

Grantyn R, Lux H (1988) Similarity and mutual exclusion of NMDA- and proton-activated transient sodium currents in rat tectal neurons. Neurosci Lett 89, 198.

Gray G, Bergfors A, Levine R, Levine S (1978) Comparison of the effects of restricted morning or evening water intake on adrenocortical activity in female rats. Neuroendocrinology 25, 236.

Gray J (1982) *The Neuropsychology of Anxiety: An Enquiry into the Function of the Septo-Hippocampal System*. Oxford University Press, Oxford.

Greden J, Flegel P, Haskett R, Dilsaver S, Carroll B, Grunhaus L (1986) Age effects in serial hypothalamic-pituitary-adrenal monitoring. Psychoneuroendocrinology 11, 195.

Greenamyre J, Young A (1989) Excitatory amino acids and Alzheimer's disease. Neurobiol Aging 10, 593.

Greene R, Haas H (1991) The electrophysiology of adenosine in the mammalian central nervous system. Prog Neurobiol 36, 329.

Greenwald B, Mathe A, Mohs R, Levy M, Johns C, Davis K (1986) Cortisol in Alzheimer's disease. II. Dexamethasone suppression, dementia severity and affective symptoms. Am J Psychiatry 143, 442.

Grossman A, Tsagarakis S (1989) Hunt for the CIA factors which demonstrate corticotropin inhibitory activity. J Endocrinol 123, 169.

Grossman A, Delitala G, Mannelli M, Al-Damluji S, Coy D, Besser G (1986) An analogue of met-enkephalin attenuates the pituitary adrenal response to oCRF. Clin Endocrinol 25, 421.

Grover A, Samson S (1988) Effect of superoxide radical on calcium pumps of coronary artery. Am J Physiol 255, C297.

Guaza C, Torrellas A, Borell S (1983) Adrenocortical response to acute and chronic ethanol administration in rats. Psychopharmacology 79, 173.

Gudeman S, Miller J, Becker D (1979) Failure of high-dose steroid therapy to influence intracranial pressure in patients with severe head injury. J Neurosurg 51, 301.

Guenaire C, Feghall G, Senault B, Delacour J (1986) Psychophysiological profiles of the Roman strains of rats. Physiol Behav 37, 423.

Gumbinas M, Oda M, Huttenlocher P (1973) The effects of corticosteroids on myelination of the developing rat brain. Biol Neonate 22, 355.

Gunderson C (1990) *Essentials of Clinical Neurology*. Raven Press, New York.

Gustafsson J, Carlstedt-Duke J, Poellinger L, Okret S, Wikstrom A, Bronnegard M, Gillner M, Dong Y, Fuxe K, Cintra A, Harfstrand A, Agnati L (1987) Biochemistry, molecular biology and physiology of the glucocorticoid receptor. Endocr Rev 8, 185.

Gutierrez P, Meyer J (1988) Inhibition of hippocampal cell proliferation by stress in developing rats. Soc Neurosci Abstr 14, 112.4.

Gutterman P, Shenkin H (1972) Prognostic features in recovery from traumatic decerebration. J Neurosurg 32, 330.

Guzman-Flores C, Alcaraz M, Garcia-Castells E, Ervin F, Juarez J (1987) Estudio experimental de la depresión por estres social. Bol Estud Med Biol 35, 11.

Hagberg H, Lehman A, Sandberg M, Nystrom B, Jacobson I, Hamberger A (1985) Ischemia-induced shift of inhibitory and excitatory amino acids from intra- to extracellular compartments. J Cereb Blood Flow Metab 5, 413.

Hahn J, Aizenman E, Lipton S (1988) Central mammalian neurons normally resistant to glutamate toxicity are made sensitive by elevated extracellular calcium: toxicity is blocked by the NMDA antagonist MK-801. Proc Natl Acad Sci USA 85, 6556.

Hajos F, Garthwaite G, Garthwaite J (1986) Reversible and irreversible neuronal damage caused by excitatory amino acid analogues in rat cerebellar slices. Neuroscience 18, 417.

Hakim A (1987) The cerebral ischemic penumbra. Can J Neurol Sci 14, 557.

Hakim G, Itano T, Verma A, Penniston J (1982) Purification of the calcium and magnesium-requiring ATPase from rat brain synaptic plasma membrane. Biochem J 207, 225.

Halasz B, Slusher M, Gorski R (1967) Adrenocorticotrophic hormone secretion in rats alters partial or total deafferentation of the medial basal hypothalamus. Neuroendocrinology 2, 43.

Halbreich U, Asnis G, Zumoff B, Nathan R, Shindledecker R (1984) Effect of age and sex on cortisol secretion in depressives and normals. Psychiatry Res 13, 221.

Hall E (1985) High-dose glucocorticoid treatment improves neurological recovery in head-injured mice. J Neurosurg 62, 883.

Hall E (1990) Steroids and neuronal destruction or stabilization. Steroids and neuronal activity. Wiley, Chicester (Ciba Foundation Symposium 153), p 206.

Hall E, Braughler J (1982) Glucocorticoid mechanisms in acute spinal cord injury: a review and therapeutic rationale. Surg Neurol 18, 320.

Hall E, Braughler J (1989) Central nervous system trauma and stroke II. Physiological and pharmacological evidence for involvement of oxygen radicals and lipid peroxidation. Free Radical Biol Med 6, 303.

Hall E, Wolf D, Braughler J (1984) Effects of a single large dose of methylprednisolone sodium succinate on posttraumatic spinal cord ischemia; dose response and time-action analysis. J Neurosurg 61, 124.

Hall E, McCall J, Chase R, Yonkers P, Braughler J (1987) A nonglucocorticoid steroid analog of methylprednisolone duplicates its high-dose pharmacology in models of central nervous system trauma and neruonal membrane damage. J Pharm Exp Ther 242, 137.

Hall E, Pazara K, Braughler J (1988) 21-Aminosteroid lipid peroxidation inhibitor U74006F protects against cerebral ischemia in gerbils. Stroke 19, 997.

Halliwell B, Gutteridge J (1985) Oxygen radicals and the nervous systems. Trends Neurosci, January, 22.

Halpain S, McEwen B (1989) Corticosteroid decreases ^{3}H-glutamate binding in rat hippocampal formation. Neuroendocrinology 48, 235.

Hambley J, Johnston G, Shaw J (1985) The central GABA system in the spontaneously hypertensive rat: effects of pretreatments with hydralazine. Aust NZ J Med 15, Suppl 2, 529.

Hamburger V, Oppenheim R (1982) Naturally occurring neuronal death in vertebrates. Neurosci Comm 1, 39.

Hamilton WD (1964) The genetical evolution of social behaviour: I and II. J Theroretical Biol 7, 1.

Hammond G (1990) Molecular properties of CBG and the sex-steroid binding proteins. Endocr Rev 11, 65.

Hamon B, Heinemann U (1986) Effects of GABA and bicuculline on NMDA and quisqualate-induced reductions in extracellular free calcium in area CA_1 of the hippocampal slice. Exp Brain Res 64, 27.

Hansen A (1985) Effect of anoxia on ion distribution in the brain. Physiol Rev 65, 101.

Hansen A, Zuethen T (1981) Extracellular ion concentrations during spreading depression and ischemia in the rat brain cortex. Acta Physiol Scand 113, 437.

Hanson J, Larson M, Snowdon C (1976) The effects of control over high intensity noise on plasma cortisol levels in rhesus monkeys. Behav Biol 16, 333.

Hara H, Kato H, Kogure K (1990) Protective effect of alpha-tocopherol on ischemic neuronal damage in the gerbil hippocampus. Brain Res 510, 335.

Harmon D (1984) Free radical theory of aging: the "free radical" diseases. Age 7, 111.

Harmon J, Horman M, Fowles B, Thompson E (1979) Dexamethasone induces irreversible G1 arrest and death of a human lymphoid cell line. J Cell Physiol 98, 267.

Harris K, Rulf D, Rosenberg P (1990) A role for glutamate uptake in modulating glutamate neurotoxicity in cultures of rat cerebral cortex. Soc Neurosci Abstr 16, 192.

Harris R, Wieloch T, Symon L, Siesjo B (1984) Cerebral extracellular calcium activity in severe hypoglycemia: relation to extracellular potassium and energy charge. J Cereb Blood Flow Metab 4, 187.

Harrison M, Brownbill D, Lewis P, Russell R (1973) Cerebral edema following carotid artery ligation in the gerbil. Arch Neurol 28, 389.

Hashimoto H, Marystone J, Greenough W, Bohn M (1989) Neonatal adrenalectomy alters dendritic branching of hippocampal granule cells. Exp Neurol 104, 62.

Hattori H, Wasterlain C (1989) Posthypoxic glucose supplement reduces hypoxic-ischemic brain damage in the neonatal rat. Soc Neurosci Abstr 15, 529.8.

Hauger R, Millan M, Catt K, Aguilera G (1987) Differential regulation of brain and pituitary CRF receptors by corticosterone. Endocrinology 120, 1527.

Hauger R, Millan M, Lorang M, Harwood J, Aguilera G (1988) Corticotropin-releasing factor receptors and pituitary adrenal responses during immobilization stress. Endocrinology 123, 396.

Hauger R, Lorang M, Irwin M, Aguilera G (1990) CRF receptor regulation and sensitization of ACTH responses to acute ether stress during chronic intermittent immobilization stress. Brain Res 532, 34.

Hauser W, Kurland L (1975) The epidemiology of epilepsy in Rochester, Minnesota. Epilepsia 16, 1.

Haynes R, Murad F (1985) Adrenocorticotropic hormone; adrenocortical steroids and their synthetic analogs, inhibitors of adrenocortical steroid biosynthesis. In Gilman A, Goodman L, Rall T, Murad F (eds). *The Pharmacological Basis of Therapeutics* (7th ed). Macmillan, New York.

Hedley-Whyte E, Hsu D (1986) Effect of dexamethasone on blood-brain barrier in the normal mouse. Ann Neurol 19, 373.

Heinemann U, Pumain R (1980) Extracellular calcium activity changes in cat sensorimotor cortex induced by iontophoretic application of amino acids. Exp Brain Res 40, 247.

Hennessy J, Levine S (1979) Stress, arousal and the pituitary-adrenal system: a psychoendocrine model. In Sprague J, Epstein A (eds), *Progress in Psychobiology and Physiological Psychology*. Academic Press, New York.

Hennessy J, King M, McClure T, Levine S (1977) Uncertainty, as defined by the contingency between environmental events, and the adrenocortical response of the rat to electric shock. J Comp Physiol Psychol 91, 1447.

Hennessy M, Heybach J, Vernikos J, Levine S (1979) Plasma corticosterone concentrations sensitively reflect levels of stimulus intensity in the rat. Physiol Behav 22, 821.

Herbert J, Keverne E, Yodyingyuad U (1986) Modulation by social status of the relationship between cerebrospinal fluid and serum cortisol levels in male talapoin monkeys. Neuroendocrinology 42, 436.

Herevanian B, Woolf P, Iker H (1983) Plasma ACTH levels in depression before and after recovery: relationship to the dexamethasone suppression test. Psychiatry Res 10, 175.

Herman J, Patel P, Akil H, Watson S (1989a) Localization and regulation of glucocorticoid and mineralocorticoid receptor messenger RNAs in the hippocampal formation of the rat. Mol Endocrinol 3, 1886.

Herman J, Schafer M, Young E, Thompson R, Douglass J, Akil H, Watson S (1989b) Evidence for hippocampal regulation of neuroendocrine neurons of the hypothalamo-pituitary-adrenocortical axis. J Neurosci 9, 3072.

Herman J, Watson S, Spencer R (1990) Treatment with the type I glucocorticoid antagonist RU 28318 alters circadian patterns of CRH mRNA expression in the hypothalamic paraventricular nucleus. Endocrine Abstr 72, 289.

Hermus A, Pieters G, Pesman G, Hofman J, Smals G, Benraad T, Kloppenborg P (1987) Escape from dexamethasone-induced ACTH and cortisol suppression by corticotropin-releasing hormone: modulatory effect of basal dexamethasone levels. Clin Endocrinol 26, 67.

Hernandez-Cruz A, Sala F, Adams P (1990) Subcellular calcium transients visualized by confocal microscopy in a voltage-clamped vertebrate neuron. Science 247, 858.

Heroux J, Grigoriadis D, de Souza E (1991) Age-related decreases in corticotropin-releasing factor (CRF) receptors in rat brain and anterior pituitary gland. Brain Res 542, 155.

Herrero I, Miras-Portugal M, Sanchez-Prieto J (1991) Inhibition of glutamate release by arachidonic acid in rat cerebrocortical synaptosomes. J Neurochem 57, 718.

Hertz L, Kvamme E, McGreer E, Schousboe E (eds) (1983a) *Glutamine, Glutamate and GABA in the Central Nervous System.* Liss, New York.

Hertz L, Yu A, Potter R, Fisher T, Schousboe A (1983b) Metabolic fluxes from glutamate and towards glutamate in neurons and astrocytes in primary cultures. In Hertz L, Kvamme E, McGeer E, Schousboe A (eds), *Glutamine, Glutamate and GABA in the Central Nervous System.* Liss, New York, p 327.

Hertz L, Drejer J, Schousboe A (1988) Energy metabolism in glutamatergic neurons, GABAergic neurons and astrocytes in primary cultures. Neurochem Res 13, 605.

Hess G, Riegle G (1970) Adrenocortical responsiveness to stress and ACTH in aging rats. J Gerontol 25, 354.

Hess G, Riegle G (1972) Effects of chronic ACTH stimulation on adrenocortical function in young and aged rats. Am J Physiol 222, 1458.

Hexum T, Fried R (1979) Effects of superoxide radicals on transport of Na-K-adenosine triphosphatase and protection by superoxide dismutase. Neurochem Res 4, 73.

Heybach J, Vernikos-Danellis J (1979) Inhibition of adrenocorticotrophin secretion during deprivation-induced eating and drinking in rats. Neuroendocrinology 28, 329.

Hicks S (1955) Pathologic effects of antimetabolites. I. Acute lesions in hypothalamus, peripheral ganglia and adrenal medulla caused by 3-acetylpyridine and prevented by nicotinamide. Am J Pathol 31, 189.

Higgins G, Oyler G, Neve R, Chen K, Gage F (1990) Altered levels of amyloid protein precursor transcripts in the basal forebrain of behaviorally impaired aged rats. Proc Natl Acad Sci USA 87, 3032.

Hirata F (1981) The regulation of lipomodulin, a phospholipase inhibitory protein, in rabbit neutropils by phosphorylation. J Biol Chem 256, 7730.

Hirata F, Schiffmann E, Venkatasubamanian K, Salomon D, Axelrod J (1980) A phospholipase A2 inhibitory protein in rabbit neutrophils induced by glucocorticoids. Proc Natl Acad Sci USA 77, 2533.

Hiroshige T, Sato T (1970) Postnatal development of circadian rhythm of corticotropin-releasing activity in the rat hypothalamus. Endocrinol Jpn 17, 1.

Hodges J, Vernikos J (1960) The effect of hydrocortisone on the level of corticotrophin in the blood and pituitary glands of adrenalectomized and of stressed adrenalectomized rats. J Physiol 150, 683.

Hoehn K, White T (1990a) Role of excitatory amino acid receptors in K^+ and glutamate-evoked release of endogenous adenosine from rat cortical slices. J Neurochem 54, 256.

Hoehn K, White T (1990b) Glutamate-evoked release of endogenous adenosine from rat cortical synaptosomes is mediated by glutamate uptake and not by receptors. J Neurochem 54, 1716.

Hoffman W, Pelligrino D, Miletich D, Albrecht R (1985) Berain metabolic changes in young versus aged rats during hypoxia. Stroke 16, 860.

Holehan A, Merry B (1986) The experimental manipulation of ageing by diet. Biol Rev 61, 329.

Hollenberg S, Weinberger C, Ong E, Cerelli G, Oro A, Lebo R, Thompson E, Rosenfeld M, Evans R (1985) Primary structure and expression of a functional human glucocorticoid receptor cDNA. Nature 318, 635.

Holler M, Dierking H, Dengler K, Tegtmeier F, Peters T (1986) Effect of flunarizine on extracellular ion concentration in the rat brain under hypoxia and ischemia. In Battistina N, Fiorani P, Courbier R, Plum F, Fieschi C (eds), *Acute Brain Ischemia, Medical and Surgical Therapy*. Raven Press, New York.

Holmes M, Antoni F, Szentendrei T (1984) Pituitary receptors for CRF: no effect of vasopressin on binding or activation of adenylate cyclase. Neuroendocrinology 39, 162.

Holmes M, Antoni F, Catt K, Aguilera G (1986) Predominant release of vaspressin versus CRF from the isolated median eminence after adrenalectomy. Neuroendocrinology 43, 245.

Holsboer F, von Bardeleben U, Gerken A, Stalla G, Muller O (1984a) Blunted corticotropin and normal cortisol response to human corticotropin-releasing factor in depression. N Engl J Med 311, 1127.

Holsboer F, Muller O, Doerr H, Sippell W, Stalla G, Gerken A, Steiger A, Boll E, Benkert O (1984b) ACTH and multisteroid responses to CRF in depressive illness: relationship to multisteroid responses after ACTH stimulation and dexamethasone suppression. Psychoneuroendocrinology 9, 147.

Holsboer F, Gerken A, von Bardeleben U, Grimm W, Stalla G, Muller O (1986) Human CRH in depression. Biol Psychiatry 21, 601.

Holsboer F, Gerken A, Stalla G, Muller O (1987a) Blunted aldosterone and ACTH release after human CRH administration in depressed patients. Am J Psychiatry 144, 229.

Holsboer F, von Bardeleben U, Wiedemann K, Muller O, Stalla G (1987b) Serial assessment of corticotropin-releasing hormone response after dexamethasone in depression: implications for pathophysiology of DST nonsuppression. Biol Psychiatry 22, 228.

Hori N, French-Mullen J, Carpenter D (1985) Kainic acid responses and toxicity show pronounced calcium dependence. Brain Res 358, 380.

Hori N, Doi N, Miyahara S, Shinoda Y, Carpenter D (1991) Appearance of NMDA receptors triggered by anoxia independent of voltage in vivo and in vitro. Exp Neurol 112, 304.

Horner H, Munck A, Lienhard G (1987) Dexamethasone causes translocation of glucose transporters from the plasma membrane to an intracellular site in human fibroblasts. J Biol Chem 262, 17696.

Horner H, Packan D, Sapolsky R (1990) Glucocorticoids inhibit glucose transport in cultured hippocampal neurons and glia. Neuroendocrinology 52, 57.

Hortnagl H, Berger M, Hornykiewicz O (1991) Glucocorticoids aggravate the cholinergic deficit induced by ethylcholine aziridinium (AF64A) in rat hippocampus. Soc Neurosci Abstr 17, 285.1.

Hossmann K, Paschen W, Csiba L (1983) Relationship between calcium accumulation and recovery of cat brain after prolonged cerebral ischemia. J Cereb Blood Flow Metab 3, 346.

Hassmann K, Grosse Ophoff B, Schmidt-Kastner R, Oschlies (1985) Mitochondrial calcium sequestration in cortical and hippocampal neurons after prolonged ischemia of the brain. Acta Neuropathol (Berl) 68, 230.

Houser C, Harris A, Vaughn J (1986) Time course of the reduction of GABA terminals in a model of focal epilepsy: a glutamic acid decarboxylase immunocytochemical study. Brain Res 383, 129.

Howard E (1965) Effects of corticosterone and food restriction on growth and on DNA, RNA and cholesterol contents of the brain and liver in infant mice. J Neurochem 12, 181.

Howard E (1968) Reductions in size and total DNA of cerebrum and cerebellum in adult mice after corticosterone treatment in infancy. Exp Neurol 22, 191.

Howard E, Benjamin J (1975) DNA, ganglioside and sulfatide in brains of rats given corticosterond in infancy, with an estimate of cell loss during development. Brain Res 92, 73.

Howell G, Gustafsson J, Lefebvre Y (1990) Glucocorticoid receptor identified on nuclear envelopes of male rat livers by affinity labelling and immunochemistry. Endocrinology 127, 1087.

Hoyt H, Goldstein F, Reigel D, Holst R (1973) Clinical evaluation of highly water-soluble steroids in the treatment of cerebral edema of traumatic origin (double-blind study). Clin Pharmacol Ther 13, 141.

Hua S, Chen Y (1989) Membrane receptor-mediated electrophysiological effects of glucocorticoids on mammalian neurons. Endocrinology 124, 687.

Huang S, Sun G (1986) Cerebral ischemia induced quantitative changes in rat brain membrane lipids involved in phosphoinositide metabolism. Neurochem Int 9, 185.

Huettner J (1989) Indole-2-carboxylic acid: a competitive antagonist of potentiation by glycine at the NMDA receptor. Science 243 1611.

Humphrey J, Dourmashkin R (1969) The lesions in cell membranes caused by complement. Adv Immunol 11, 75.

Hunt G, Johnson G, Caterson I (1989) The effect of age on cortisol and plasma dexamethasone concentrations in depressed patients and controls. J Affect Disorders 17, 21.

Hylka V, Sonntag W, Meites J (1984) Reduced ability of old male rats to release ACTH and corticosterone in response to CRF administration. Proc Soc Exp Biol Med 175, 1.

Hyman B, Van Hoesen G, Damasio A, Barnes C (1984) Alzheimer's disease: cell-specific pathology isolates the hippocampal formation. Science 225, 1168.

Iacopino A, Christakos S (1991) Corticosterone regulates Calbindin-D28K mRNA and protein levels in rat hippocampus. J Biol Chem 265, 10177.

Iannotti F, Crockard A, ladds G, Symon L (1981) Are prostaglandins involved in experimental ischemic edema in gerbils? Stroke 12, 301.

Ida Y, Tanaka M, Tsuda A (1984) Recovery of stress-induced increases in noradrenaline turnover is delayed in specific brain regions of old rats. Life Sci 34, 2357.

Ikeda M, Yoshida S, Busto R, Santiso M, Ginsberg M (1986) Polyphosphoinositides as a probable source of brain free fatty acids accumulated at the onset of ischemia. J Neurochem 47, 123.

Ikeda M, Nakazawa T, Abe K, Kaneko T, Yamatsu K (1989) Extracellular accumulation of glutamate in the hippocampus induced by ischemia is not calcium dependent—in vitro and in vivo evidence. Neurosci Lett 96 202.

Ikonomidoua C, Mosinger J, Salles K, Labruyere J, Olney J (1989) Sensitivity of the developing rat brain to hypobaric-ischemic damage parallels sensitivity to N-methyl-aspartate neurotoxicity. J Neurosci 9, 2809.

Imdahl A, Hossmann K (1986) Morphometric evaluation of post-ischemic capillary perfusion in selectively vulnerable areas of the gerbil brain. Acta Neuropathol 69, 267.

Imon H, Mitani A, Andou Y, Arai T, Kataoka K (1991) Delayed neuronal death is induced without postischemic hyperexcitability: continuous multiple-unit recording from ischemic CA_1 neurons. J Cereb Blood Flow Metab 11, 819.

Ingraham F, MAtson D, McLaurin R (1952) Cortisone and ACTH as an adjunct to the surgery of craniopharyngiomas. N Engl J Med 246, 1422.

Ingvar M, Folbegrova J, Siesjo B (1987) Metabolic alterations underlying the development of hypermetabolic necrosis in the substantia nigra in status epilepticus. J Cereb Blood Flow Metab 7, 103.

Irle E, Markowitsch H (1983) Widespread neuroanatomical damage and learning deficits following chronic alcohol consumption or vitamin-B$_1$ deficiency in rats. Behav Brain Res 9, 277.

Issa A, Rowe W, Gauthier S, Meaney M (1990) Hypothalamic-pituitary-adrenaactivity in aged, cognitively impaired and cognitively unimpaired rats. J Neurosci 10, 3247.

Jacewicz M, Kiessling M, Pulsinelli W (1986) Selective gene expression in focal cerebral ischemia. J Cereb Blood Flow Metab 6, 263.

Jacobs S, Mason J, Kosten T, Brown S, Ostfeld A (1984) Urinary-free cortisol excretion in relation to age in acutely stressed persons with depressive symptoms. Psychosom Med 46, 213.

Jacobson L, Sapolsky R (1991a) Stress-induced hypersecretion of ACTH in adrenalectomized rats replaced with constant corticosterone is normalized by an acute increase in corticosterone. Soc Neurosci Abstr 17, 542.6.

Jacobson L, Sapolsky R (1991b) The role of the hippocampus in feedback regulation of the hypothalamic-pituitary-adrenocortial axis. Endocr Rev 12, 118.

Jacobson L, Akana S, Cascio C, Shinsako J, Dallman M (1988) Circadian variations in plasma corticosterone permit normal termination of adrenocorticotropin responses to stress. Endocrinology 122, 1343.

Jacobson L, Akana S, Cascio C, Scribner K, Shinsako J, Dallman M (1989) The adrenocortical system responds slowly to removal of corticosterone in the absence of concurrent stress. Endocrinology 124, 2144.

Jacquin T, Fortin G, Pasquier C, Gillet B, Beloeil J, Champagnat J (1988) Metabolic acidosis induced by NMDA in brain slices of the neonatal rat: ^{31}P- and ^{1}H-magnetic resonance spectroscopy.

Jakubovicz D, Klip A (1989) Lactic acid-induced swelling in C6 glial cells via Na^+/H^+ exchange. Brain Res 485, 215.

Jane J, Rimel R, Pobereskin L (1984) Outcome and pathology of head injury. In Grossman R, Gildenberg P (eds), *Head Injury: Basic and Clinical Aspects*. Raven Press, New York.

Jarrott D, Domer F (1980) A gerbil model of cerebral ischemia suitable for drug evaluation. Stroke 11, 203.

Jastremski M, Sutton-Tyrrell P, Vaagenes N, Abramson D, Heiselman J, Safer P (1989) Glucocorticoid treatment does not improve neurological recovery following cardiac arrest. JAMA 262, 3427.

Jenkins J, Connolly J (1968) Adrenocortical response to ethanol in man. Br Med J 11, 804.

Jensen H, Blichert-Toft M (1971) Serum corticotrophin, plasma cortisol, and urinary excretion of 17-ketogenic steroids in the elderly (age group 66–94 years). Acta Endocrinol 66, 25.

Jensen M, Auer R (1988) Ketamine fails to protect against ischaemic neuronal necrosis in the rat. Br J Anaesth 61, 206.

Jensen M, Auer R (1989) Intraventricular infusion of APH mitigates ischemic brain damage. Neurol Res 11, 37.

Jensen M, Lambert J, Johansen F (1991) Electrophysiological recordsing from rat hippocampal slices following in vivo brain ischemia. Brain Res 554, 166.

Jensen T, Genefke I, Hyldebrandt N (1982) Cerebral atrophy in young torture victims. N Engl J Med 307, 1341.

Jia L, Canny B, Orth D, Leong D (1991) Distinct classes of corticotropes mediate corticotropin-releasing hormone- and arginine vasopressin-stimulated adrenocorticotropin release. Endocrinology 128, 197.

Jia L, Canny B, Leong D (1992) Paracrine communication regulates adrenocorticotropin secretion. Endocrinology 130, 534.

Jingami H, Matsukura S, Numa S, Imura H (1985) Effects of adrenalectomy and dexamethasone administration of the level of prepro-corticotropin-releasing factor mRNA in the hypothalamus and adrenocorticotropin/beta-lipotropin precursor mRNA in the pituitary in rats. Endocrinology 117, 1314.

Joels M, de Kloet E (1989) Effects of glucocorticoids and norepinephrine on the excitability in the hippocampus. Science 245, 1502.

Joels M, de Kloet E (1989b) Mineralocorticoid receptor-mediated changes in membrane properties of rat CA_1 pyramidal neurons in vitro. Proc Natl Acad Sci USA 87, 4495.

Joels M, Hesen W, de Kloet E (1991) Mineralocorticoid hormones suppress serotonin-induced hyperpolarization of rat hippocampal CA_1 neurons. J Neurosci 11, 2288.

Johansen F, Diemer N (1986) Influence of the plasma glucose level on brain damage after systemic kainic acid injection in the rat. Acta Neuropathol 71, 46.

Johansen F, Diemer N (1990) Temporal profile of interneuron and pyramidal cell protein synthesis in rat hippocampus following cerebral ischemia. Acta Neuropathol 81, 14.

Johansen F, Jorgensen M, Diemer N (1987) Ischemia induces delayed neuronal death in the CA_1 hippocampus is dependent on intact glutamatergic innervation. In Hicks T, Lodge D, McLennan H (eds), *Excitatory Amino Acid Transmission*. Liss, New York.

Johansen F, Christensen T, Jensen M, Valente E, Jensen C, Nathan T, Lambert J, Diemer N (1991) Inhibition of postichemic rat hippocampus: GABA receptors, GABA release, and inhibitory postsynaptic potentials. Brain Res 84, 529.

Johnson J, Ascher P (1987) Glycine potentiates the NMDA response in cultured mouse brain neurons. Nature 325, 529.

Johnston G, Kennedy S, Twitchlin (1979) Action of the neurotoxin kainic acid on high affinity uptake of L-glutamic acid in rat brain slices. J Neurochem 32, 121.

Jolkkonen J, Helkala E, Kutvonen R, Lehtinen M, Riekkinen P (1989) Vasopressin levels in CSF of Alzheimer patients: correlations with monoamine metabolites and neuropsychological test performance. Psychoneuroendocrinology 14, 89.

Jolly A (1985) *The Evolution of Primate Behavior*. Macmillan, New York.

Jones C, Edwards A (1990) Adrenal responses to CRF in conscious hypophysectomized calves. J Physiol 430, 25.

Jones D, McConkey D, Nicotera P, Orrenius S (1989) Calcium-activated DNA fragmentation in rat liver nuclei. J Biol Chem 264, 6398.

Jones M, Hillhouse E (1976) Structure-activity relationship and mode of action of corticosteroid feedback on the secretion of CRF (corticoliberin). J Steroid Biochem 7, 1189.

Jones M, Stockham M (1966) The effect of previous stimulation of the adrenal cortex by ACTH on the function of the pituitary-adrenocortical axis in response to stress. J Physiol 184, 741.

Jones M, Tiptaft E (1977) Structure-activity relationship of various corticosteroids on the feedback control of corticotrophin secretion. Br J Pharmacol 59, 35.

Jones M, Brush F, Neame R (1972) Characteristics of fast feedback control of corticotrophin release by corticosteroids. J Endocrinol 55, 489.

Jones M, Tiptaft E, Brush F, Furgusson D, Neame R (1974) Evidence for dual corticosteroid-receptor mechanisms in the control of adrenocorticotrophin secretion. J Endocrinol 60, 223.

Jones M, Hillhouse E, Burden J (1977) Dynamics and mechanics of corticosteroid feedback at the hypothalamus and anterior pituitary gland. J Endocrinol 73, 405.

Jones M, Gillham B, Greenstein B, Beckford U, Holmes M (1982) Feedback actions of adrenal steroid hormones. In Ganten D, Pfaff D (eds), *Current Topics in Neuroendocrinology. Vol 2.* Springer-Verlag, New York, pp 45–48.

Jones R (1988) Epileptiform events induced by GABA-antagonists in entorhinal cortical cells in vitro are partly mediated by NMDA receptors. Brain Res 457, 113.

Jorgensen M, Johansen F, Diemer N (1987) Removal of the entorhinal cortex protects hippocampal CA_1 neurons from ischemic damage. Acta Neuropathol (Berl) 73, 189.

Jubiz W, Matsukura S, Meikle A, Harada G, West C, Tyler F (1970) Plasma metyrapone, adrenocorticotropic hormone, cortisol and deoxycortisol levels. Arch Intern Med 125, 468.

Kadekaro M, Masanori I, Gross P (1988) Local cerebral glucose utilization is increased in acutely adrenalectomized rats. Neuroendocrinology 47, 329.

Kagan J (1982) Heart rate and heart rate variability as signs of temperamental dimension in infants. In Izard C (ed), *Measuring Emotions in Infants and Young Children.* Cambridge University Press, New York.

Kagan J, Moss H (1962) *Birth to Maturity.* Wiley, New York.

Kagan J, Reznick J, Clarke C, Snidman N, Garcia-Coll C (1984) Behavioral inhibition to the unfamiliar. Child Develop 55, 2212.

Kagan J, Reznick J, Snidman N (1988) Biological bases of childhood shyness. Science 240, 167

Kaiser P, Lei S, Aggarwal S, Lipton S (1991) The antihypertensive drugs nitroprusside and nitroglycerin inhibit excitatory amino acid responses. Soc Neurosci Abstr 17, 163.18.

Kakihana R (1979) Alcohol intoxication and withdrawal in inbred strains of mice: behavioral and endocrine studies. Behav Neural Biol 26, 97.

Kakihana R, Moore J (1976) Circadian rhythm of corticosterone in mice: the effect of chronic consumption of alcohol. Psychopharmacology 46, 301.

Kaku D, Goldberg M, Choi D (1991) Antagonism of non-NMDA receptors augments the neuroprotective effect of NMDA receptor blockade in cortical cultures subjected to prolonged deprivation of oxygen and glucose. Brain Res 554, 344.

Kalimo H, Rehncrona B, Soderfeldt B, Olsson Y, Siesjo B (1981) Brain lactic acidosis and ischemic cell damage: II. Histopathology. J Cereb Blood Flow Metab 1, 313.

Kalin N, Weiler S, Shelton S (1982) Plasma ACTH and cortisol concentrations before and after dexamethasone. Psychiatr Res 7, 87.

Kalin N, Shelton S, Barksdale C, Brownfield M (1987) A diurnal rhythm in cerebrospinal fluid corticotropin-releasing hormone different from the rhythm of pituitary-adrenal activity. Brain Res 426, 385.

Kalinyak J, Dorin R, Hoffman A, Perlman A (1987) Tissue-specific regulation of glucocorticoid receptor mRNA by dexamethasone. J Biol Chem 262, 10441.

Kaneko M, Hiroshige T, Shinsako J, Dallman M (1980) Diurnal changes in amplification of hormone rhythms in the adrenocortical system. Am J Physiol 234, R309.

Kaneko M, Kaneko K, Shinsako J, Dallman M (1981) Adrenal sensitivity to adrenocorticotropin varies diurnally. Endocrinology 109, 70.

Kant G, Meyerhoff J, Jarrad L (1984) Biochemical indices of reactivity and habituation in rats with hippocampal lesions. Pharmacol Biochem Behav 20, 793.

Kant G, Mougey E, Meyerhoff J (1986) Diurnal variation in neuroendocrine responses to stress in rats: plasma ACTH, beta-endorphin, beta-LPH, corticosterone, prolactin, and pituitary cyclic AMP responses. Neuroendocrinology 43, 383.

Kaplan J, Manuck S, Clarkson T, Lusso F, Taub D (1982) Social status, environment, and atherosclerosis in cynomolgus monkeys. Arteriosclerosis 2, 359.

Kaplan T, Lasner T, Nadler V, Crain B (1989) Lesions of excitatory pathways reduce hippocampal cell death after transient forebrain ischemia in the gerbil. Acta Neuropathol (Berl) 78, 283.

Karteszi M, Dallman M, Makara G, Stark E (1982) Regulation of the adrenocortical response to insulin-induced hypoglycemia. Endocrinology 111, 535.

Kasambalides E, Lanks K (1983) Dexamethasone can modulate glucose-regulated and heat shock protein synthesis. J Cell Physiol 114, 93.

Kass I, Lipton P (1982) Mechanisms involved in irreversible anoxic damage to the in vitro rat hippocampal slice. J Physiol 332, 459.

Kass I, Lipton P (1986) Calcium and long-term transmission damage following anoxia in dentate gyrus and CA_1 regions of the rat hippocampal slice. J Physiol 378 313.

Kato H, Araki T, Kogure K (1990) Role of the excitotoxic mechanism in the development of neuronal damage following repeated brief cerebral ischemia in the gerbil: protective effects of MK-801 and pentobarbital. Brain Res 516, 175.

Kato H, Araki T, Kogure K (1991) Postischemic spontaneous hyperthermia is not a major aggravating factor for neuronal damage following repeated brief cerebral ischemia in the gerbil. Neurosci Lett 126, 21.

Kauppinen R, Enkvist K, Holopainen I, Akerman K (1988a) Glucose deprivation depolarizes plasma membrane of cultured astrocytes and collapses transmembrane potassium and glutamate gradiants. Neuroscience 26, 283.

Kauppinen R, McMahon H, Nicholls D (1988b) Calcium-dependent and calcium-independent glutamaterelease, energy status and cytosolic free calcium concentration in isolated nerve terminals following metabolic inhibition: possible relevance to hypoglycaemia and anoxia. Neuroscience 27, 175.

Kawakami M, Seto K, Terasawa E, Yoshida K, Miyamoto T, Sekiguchi M, Hattori Y (1968) Influence of electrical stimulation and lesion in limbic structure upon biosynthesis of adreno-corticoid in the rabbit. Neuroendocrinology 3, 377.

Kearley R, van Hartesveldt C, Woodruff M (1974) Behavioral and hormonal effects of hippo-campal lesions on male and female rats. Physiol Psychol 2, 187.

Keith L, Tam B, Greer M (1986) Stimulation of corticosterone secretion in vitro by brief ACTH exposure. Am J Physiol 250, E629.

Keller-Wood M, Dallman M 1984 Corticosteroid inhibition of ACTH secretion. Endocr Rev 5, 1.

Keller-Wood M, Shinsako J, Dallman M (1983a) Integral as well as proportional adrenal responses to ACTH. Am J Physiol 245, R53.

Keller-Wood M, Shinsako J, Dallman M (1983b) Inhibition of ACTH and corticosteroid responses to hypoglycemia after prior stress. Endocrinology 113, 491.

Keller-Wood M, Shinsako J, Dallman M (1983c) Feedback inhibition of adrenocorticotropic hormone by physiological increases in plasma corticosteroids in conscious dogs. J Clin Invest 71, 859.

Keller-Wood M, Shinsako J, Dallman M (1984) Interaction between stimulus intensity and corticosteroid feedback control of ACTH. Am J Physiol 247, E489.

Keller-Wood M, Kimura B, Shinsako J, Phillips M (1986) Interaction between CRF and angiotensin II in control of ACTH and adrenal steroids. Am J PHysiol 250, R396.

Kellner H, Rubinow D, Gold P (1983) Relationship of cortisol hypersecretion to brain CT scan alters in depressed patients. Psychiatry Res 8, 191.

Kemp J, Foster A, Wong E (1987) Non-competitive antagonists of excitatory amino acid receptors. Trends Neurosci 10, 2994.

Kennedy M (1989) Regulation of synaptic transmission in the central nervous system: long-term potentiation. Cell 59, 777.

Kent L, Zobre C, Miller M (1991) Calpain inhibition and neuroprotection. Soc Neurosci Abstr 17, 500.14.

Kerr D, Campbell L, Hao S, Landfield P (1989) Corticosteroid modulation of hippocampal potentials: increased effect with aging. Science 245, 1505.

Kerr D, Campbell L, Applegate M, Brodish A, Landfield P (1991) Chronic stress-induced acceleration of electrophysiologic and morphometric biomarkers of hippocampal aging. J Neurosci 11, 1316.

Keverne E, Meller R, Eberhart J (1982) Dominance and subordination: concepts or physiological states? In Chiarelli V, Corruccini J (eds), *Advanced Views in Primate Biology*. Springer-Verlag, New York.

Kieslling M, Dienel G, Jacewicz M, Pulsinelli W (1986) Protein synthesis in postischemic rat brain: a two-dimensional electrophoretic analysis. J Cereb Blood Flow Metab 6, 642.

Kim C, Kim C (1961) Effect of partial hippocampal resection on stress mechanisms in rats. Am J Physiol 201, 337.

Kimelberg H, Norenberg M (1989) Astrocytes. Sci Am April, 66.

Kimelberg H, Goderie S, Higman S, Pang S, Waniewski R (1990) Swelling-induced release of glutamate, aspartate, and taurine from astrocyte cultures. J Neurosci 10, 1583.

King L, McLaurin R, Lewis H, Knowles H (1970) Plasma cortisol levels after head injury. Ann Surg 172, 975.

Kinuta Y, Kimura M, Ktokawa Y, Ishikawa M, Kikuchi H (1989) Changes in xanthine oxidase in ischemic rat brain. J Neurosurg 71, 417.

Kirino T (1982) Delayed neuronal death in the gerbil hippocampus following ischemia. Brain Res 239, 57.

Kirino T, Sano K (1984) Selective vulnerability in the gerbil hippocampus following transient ischemia. Acta Neuropathol (Berl) 61, 201.

Kirino T, Tamura A, Sano K (1984) delayed neuronal death in the rat hippocampus following transient ischemia. Acta Neuropathol (Berl) 64, 139.

Kiss J, Mezey E, Skirboll L (1984) Corticotropin-releasing factor-immunoreactive neurons of the paraventricular nucleus become vasopressin positive after adrenalectomy. Proc Natl Acad Sci USA 81, 1854.

Kitagawa k, Matsumoto M, Oda T, Niinobe M (1990) Free radical generation during brief period of cerebral ischemia may trigger delayed neuronal death. Neuroscience 35, 551.

Kitagawa K, Matsumoto M, Tagaya M, Kuwabara K, et al. (1991) Hyperthermia-induced neuronal protection against ischemic injury in gerbils. J Cereb Blood Flow Metab 11, 449.

Kleihues P, Hossmann K (1971) Protein synthesis in the cat brain after prolonged cerebral ischemia. Brain Res 35, 409.

Kleihues P, Kobayashi K, Hossmann K (1974) Purine nucleotide metabolism in the cat brain after one hour of complete ischemia. J Neurochem 23, 417.

Kley H, Nieschlag E, Kruskemper H (1975) Age dependence of plasma oestrogen response to HCG and ACTH in men. Acta Endocrinol (Copenh) 79, 95.

Knigge K (1961) Adrenocortical response to stress in rats with lesions in hippocampus and amygdala. Proc Soc Exp Biol Med 108, 18.

Knigge K, Hays M (1963) Evidence of inhibitive role of hippocampus in neural regulation of ACTH release. Proc Soc Exp Biol Med 114, 67.

Knigge K, Penrod C, Schindler W (1959) In vitro and in vivo adrenal corticosteroid secretion following stress. Am J Physiol 196, 579.

Knopfel T, Spuler A, Grafe P, Gahwiler B (1990) Cytosolic calcium during glucose deprivation in hippocampal pyramidal cells of rats. Neurosci Lett 117, 295.

Koch B, Lutz-Bucher B (1985) Specific receptors for vasopressin in the pituitary gland: evidence for down-regulation and desensitization to adrenocorticotropin-releasing factors. Endocrinology 116, 671.

Kochbar A, Zivin J, Lyden P, Mazzarella V (1988) Glutamate antagonist therapy reduces neurologic deficits produced by focal CNS ischemia. Arch Neurol 45, 148.

Kogure K (1990) Trans-NMDA receptor signalling in ischemia-induced brain cell damage. Trans Am Soc Neurochem 21, 185.

Koh J, Choi D (1987) Quantitative determination of glutamate mediated cortical neuronal injury in cell culture by lactate dehydrogenase efflux assay. J Neurosci Methods 20, 83.

Koh J, Choi D (1988) Vulnerability of cultured cortical neurons to damage by excitotoxins: Differential susceptibility of neurons containing NADPH-diaphorase. J Neurosci 8, 2153.

Koh J, Peters S, Choi D (1986) Neurons containing NADPH-diaphorase are selectively resistant to quinolinate toxicity. Science 234, 73.

Koh J, Goldberg M, Hartley D, Choi D (1990a) Non-NMDA receptor-mediated neurotoxicity in cortical culture. J Neurosci 10, 693.

Koh J, Yang L, Cotman C (1990b) Beta-amyloid protein increases the vulnerability of cultured cortical neurons to excitotoxic damage. Brain Res 533, 315.

Koh S, Chang P, Collier T, Loy R (1989) Loss of NGF receptor immunoreactivity in basal forebrain neurons of aged rats: correlation with spatial memory impairment. Brain Res 498, 397.

Kohler C, Schwarcz R (1981) Monosodium glutamate: increased neurotoxicity after removal of neuronal re-uptake sites. Brain Res 211, 485.

Kohler C, Schwarcz R, Fuxe K (1978) Perforant path transections protect hippocampal granule cells from kainate lesion. Neurosci Lett 10, 241.

Koide T, Wieloch T, Siesjo B (1986) Chornic dexamethasone pretreatment aggravates ischemic neuronal necrosis. J Cereb Blood Flow Metab 6, 395.

Koike T, Martin D, Johnson E (1989) Depolarization prevents trophic factor deprivation induced neuronal death: the role of non-inactivating calcium channels. Abstract 45, Molecular and Cellular Mechanisms of Neuronal Plasticity in Aging and Alzheimer's Disease. NIA Meeting, May, 1989.

Komatsumoto S, Greenberg J, Hickey W, Reivich M (1988) Effect of the ganglioside GM1 on neurologic function, electroencephalogram amplitude, and histology in chronic middle crerebral artery occlussion in cats. Stroke 19, 1027.

Korf J, Klein H, Venema K, Postema F (1988) Increases in striatal and hippocampal impedance and extracellular levels of amino acids by cardiac arrest in freely moving rats. J Neurochem 50, 1087.

Kovachich G, Mishra O (1981) Partial inactivation of Na,K-ATPase in cortical brain slices incubated in normal Krebs-Ringer phosphate medium at 1 and at 10 atm oxygen pressures. J Neurochem 36, 333.

Kovacs K, Antoni F (1990) Atriopeptin inhibits stimulated secretion of adrenocorticotropin in rats: evidence for a pituitary site of action. Endocrinology 127, 3003.

Kovacs K, Mezey E (1987) Dexamethasone inhibits CRF gene expression in the rat paraventricular nucleus. Neuroendocrinology 46, 365.

Kovacs K, Kiss J, Makara G (1986) Glucocorticoid implants around the hypothalamic paraventricular nucleus prevent the increase of corticotropin-releasing factor and arginine vasopressin immunostaining induced by adrenalectomy. Neuroendocrinology 44, 229.

Kowall N, Ferrante R, Martin J (1987) Patterns of cell loss in Huntington's disease. Trends Neurosci 10, 24.

Kowall N, Beal M, Busciglio J, Duffy L, Yankner B (1991) An in vivo model for the neurodegenerative effects of beta amyloid and protection by substance P. Proc Natl Acad Sci USA 88, 7247.

Kracier J, Gosbee J, Bencosme S (1973) Pars intermedia and pars distalis: two sites of ACTH production in the rat hypophysis. Neuroendocrinology 11, 156.

Krahn D, Meller W, Shafter R, Morley J (1985) Cortisol response to vasopressin in depression. Biol Psychiatry 20, 918.

Kraig R, Pulsinelli W, Plum F (1985a) Hydrogen ion buffering during complete brain ischemia. Brain Res 342, 281.

Kraig R, Pulsinelli W, Plum F (1985b) Heterogeneous distribution of hydrogen and bicarbonate ions during complete brain ischemia. In Kogure K, Hossman K, Siesjo B, Welsh F (eds), *Molecular Mechanisms of Ischemic Brain Damage: Progress Brain Research* Vol 63, Elsevier, New York, p 155.

Kraig R, Petito C, Plum F, Pulsinelli W (1987) Hydrogen ions kill brain at concentrations reached in ischemia. J Cereb Blood Flow Metab 7, 379.

Krebs J, Woods J, Alberto L (1975) Hyperlactatemia and lactic acidosis. Essay Med Biochem 1, 81.

Krespan B, Berl S, Nicklas W (1982) Alterations in neuronal glial metabolism of glutamate by the neurotoxin kainic acid. J Neurochem 38, 509.

Krieger D (1982) *Cushing's Syndrome. Monographs in Endocrinology*, Vol 22. Springer-Verlag, Berlin.

Krieger D, Hauser H, Krey L (1977) Suprachiasmatic nuclear lesions do not abolish food-shifted circadian adrenal and temperature rhythmicity. Science 197, 398.

Krishnan K, Ritchie J, Manepalli A, Nemeroff C, Carroll B (1989) Adrenocortical sensitivity to ACTH in man. Biol Psychiatry 27, 930.

Krishnan R, Maltbie A, Davidson J (1983) Abnormal cortisol suppression in bipolar patients with simultaneous manic and depressive symptoms. Am J Psychiatry 140, 203.

Kudo YH, Ogura A (1986) Glutamate-induced increase in intracellular calcium concentration in isolated hippocampal neurons. Br J Pharmacol 89, 191.

Kuhn C, Eck J, Francis R (1991) Endocrine response of infant rats to handling. Soc Neurosci Abstr 17, 621.4.

Kuhr W, van den Berg C, Korf J (1988) In vivo identification and quantitative evaluation of carrier-mediated transport of lactate at the cellular level in the striatum of conscious, freely moving rats. J Cereb Blood Flow Metab 8, 848.

Kuo C, Ichida S, Matsuda T, Kakiuchi S, Yoshida H (1979) Regulation of ATP-dependent Ca-uptake of synaptic plasma membranes by Ca-dependent modulation protein. Life Sci 25, 235.

Kurland L (1988) Amyotrophic lateral sclerosis and Parkinson's disease complex on Guam linked to an environmental neurotoxin. Trends Neurosci 11, 51.

Kuroiwa T, Bonnekoh P, Hossmann K (1990) Prevention of postischemic hyperthermia prevents ischemic injury of CA_1 neurons in gerbils. J Cereb Blood Flow Metab 10, 550.

Labrie F, Veilleux R, Lefevre G, Coy D, Sueiras-Diaz J, Schally A (1982) Corticotropin-releasing factor stimulates accumulation of adenosine 3',5'-monophosphate in rat pituitary corticotrophs. Science 216, 1007.

Labrie F, Giguiere V, Meunier H, Simard J, Gossard F, Raymond V (1987) Multiple factors controlling ACTH secretion at the anterior pituitary level. Ann NY Acad Sci 512, 97.

Lai J, DiLorenzo J, Sheu K (1988) Pyruvate dehydrogenase complex is inhibited in calcium-loaded cerebrocortical mitochondria. Neurochem Res 11, 1043.

Lakshamanan J, Padmanaban G (1974) Effect of some strong excitants of central neurons on the uptake of glutamate and aspartate by synaptosomes. Biochem Biophys Res Comm 58, 690.

Lakshmi V, Sakai R, McEwen B, Monder C (1991) Regional distribution of 11β-hydroxysteroid dehydrogenase in rat brain. Endocrinology 128, 1741.

Lambert J, Peters J, Cottrell G (1987) Actions of synthetic and endogenous steroids on the $GABA_A$ receptor. Trends Pharmacol Sci 8, 224.

Lamberts S (1986) Neuroendocrine aspects of the DST in psychiatry. Life Sci 39, 91.

Lamberts S, Bons E, Zuiderwijk J (1986) High concentrations of catecholamines selectively diminish the sensitivity of CRF-stimulated ACTH release by cultured rat pituitary cells to the suppressive effects of dexamethasone. Life Sci 39, 97.

Landfield P, Pitler T (1984) Prolonged calcium-dependent afterhyperpolarizations in hippocampal neurons of aged rats. Science 226, 1089.

Landfield P, Rose G, Sandles L, Wohlstadter T, Lynch G (1977) Patterns of astroglial hypertrophy and neuronal degeneration in the hippocampus of aged, memory-deficient rats. J Gerontol 32, 3.

Landfield P, Waymire J, Lynch G (1978) Hippocampal aging and adrenocorticoids: a quantitative correlation. Science 202, 1098.

Landfield P, Baskin R, Pitler T (1981a) Brain-aging correlates: retardation by hormonal-pharmacological treatments. Science 214, 581.

Landfield P, Braun T, Pitler T, Lindsay J, Lynch G (1981b) Hippocampal aging in rats: a morphometric study of mulitple variables in semithin sections. Neurobiol Aging 2, 265.

Landfield P, Pitler T, Applegate M (1986) The effects of high magnesium/calcium ratios on in vitro hippocampal frequency potentiation in young and aged rats. J Neurophysiol 56, 797.

Lanier L, van Hartesveldt C, Weis B, Isaacson R (1975) Effects of differential hippocampal damage upon rhythmic and stress-induced corticosterone secretion in the rat. Neuroendocrinology 18, 154.

Lanier W, Perkins W, Karlsson B, Milde J, Scheithauer B, Shearman G, Michenfelder J (1990) The effects of dizolcilpine maleste (MK-801), an antagonist of the NMDA receptor, on neurologic recovery and histopathology following complete cerebral ischemia in primates. J Cereb Blood Flow Metab 10, 252.

Lassmann H, Petsche Y, Kitz K, Baran H, Sperk G, Seitelberger F, Hornykiewicz O (1984) The role of the brain edema in epileptic brain damage induced by systemic kainic acid injection. Neuroscience 13, 691.

Lazarewicz J, Lehmann A, Hagberg H, Hamberger A (1986) Effects of kainic acid on brain calcium fluxes studied in vivo and in vitro. J Neurochem 46, 494.

Lazarewicz J, Lehmann A, Hamberger A (1987) Effects of calcium entry blockers on kainate-induced changes in extracellular amino acids and calcium in vivo. J Neurosci Res 18, 341.

Lazarewicz J, Wroblewski J, Costa E (1990) NMDA-sensitive glutamate receptors induce calcium-mediated arachidonic acid release in primary cultures of cerebellar granule cells. J Neurochem 55, 1875.

Leake A, Griffiths HK, Pascual J, Ferrier I (1989) Corticosteroid-binding globulin in depression. Clin Endocrinol 30, 39.

Lee K, Frank S, Vanderklish P, Arai A, Lynch G (1991) Inhibition of proteolysis protects hippocampal neurons from ischemia. Proc Natl Acad Sci USA 88, 7233.

Lee M, Mastri A, Waltz A, Loewenson R (1974) Ineffectiveness of dexamethasone for treatment of experimental cerebral infarction. Stroke 5, 216.

Lee P, Grimes L, Hong J (1989) Glucocorticoids potentiate kainic acid-induced seizures and wet dog shakes. Brain Res 480, 322.

Lees G, Lehmann A, Sandberg M, Hamberger A (1990) The neurotoxicity of ouabain, a sodium-potassium ATPase inhibitor, in the rat hippocampus. Neurosci Lett 120, 159.

Lehmann A, Hansson E (1988) Kainate-induced stimulation of amino acid release from primary astroglial cultures of the rat hippocampus. Neurochem Int 13, 557.

Lehmann A, Sandberg M, Huxtable R (1986) In vivo release of neuroactive amins and amino acids from the hippocampus of seizure-resistant and seizure-susceptible rats. Neurochem Int 8, 513.

Lengvari I, Halasz B (1973) Evidence for a diurnal fluctuation in plasma corticosterone levels after fornix transection in the rat. Neuroendocrinology 11, 191.

Leprince P, Lefebvre P, Rigo J, Delree P, Rogister B, Moonen G (1989) Cultured astroglia release a neuronotoxic activity that is not related to the excitotoxins. Brain Res 502, 21.

Lescaudron L, Verna A (1985) Effects of chronic ethanol consumption on pyramidal neurons of the mouse dorsal and ventral hippocampus: a quantitative histological analysis. Exp Brain Res 58, 362.

Levi-Montalcini R (1987) The nerve growth factor 35 years later. Science 237, 1154.

Levin N, Akana S, Jacobson L, Kuhn R, Siiteri P, Dallman M (1987) Plasma adrenocorticotropin is more sensitive than transcortin production or thymus weight to inhibition by corticosterone in rats. Endocrinology 121, 1104.

Levin N, Shinsako J, Dallman M (1988) Corticosterone acts on the brain to inhibit adrenalectomy-induced adrenocorticotropin secretion. Endocrinology 122, 694.

Levine S (1962) Plasma-free corticosteroid response to electric shock in rats stimulated in infancy. Science 135, 795.

Levine S (1978) Cortisol changes following repeated experiences with parachute training. In Ursin H, Baade E, Levine S (eds), *Psychobiology of Stress: A Study of Coping Men*. Academic Press, New York.

Levine S, Haltmeyer G, Karas G, Denenberg V (1967) Physiological and behavioral effects of infantile stimulation. Physiol Behav 2, 55.

Levine S, Goldman L, Coover G (1972) Expectancy and the pituitary-adrenal system. In Porter R, Knight J (eds), *Physiology, Emotion and Psychosomatic Illness*. CIBA Foundation Symposium 8. Elsevier, Amsterdam.

Levine S, Weinberg J, Brett L (1979) Inhibition of pituitary-adrenal activity as a consequence of consummatory behavior. Psychoneuroendocrinology, 4, 275.

Levine S, Coe C, Wiener S (1989) The psychoneuroendocrinology of stres—a psychobiological perspective. In Levine S, Brush R (eds), *Psychoendocrinology*. Academic Press, New York.

Levitsky D, Collier G (1968) Schedule-induced wheel running. Physiol Behav 3, 571.

Levy A, Dachir S (1991) Subchronic corticosterond treatment leads to minor learning impairments in the radial arm maze in young rats. Soc Neurosci Abstr 17, 58.9.

Levy D, Caronna J, Singer B (1985) Predicting outcome from hypoxic-ischemic coma. JAMA 253, 1420.

Levy D, Sucher N, Lipton S (1990) Redox modulation of NMDA receptor-mediated toxicity in mammalian central neurons. Neurosci Lett 110, 291.

Lewis B, Wexler B (1974) Serum insulin changes in male rats associated with age and reproductive activity. J Gerontol 20, 204.

Lewis D, Pfohl B, Schlechte J, Coryell W (1984) Influence of age on the cortisol response to dexamethasone. Psychiatry Res 13, 213.

Lewis L, Ljunggren B, Norberg K, Siesjo B (1974) Changes in carbohydrate substrates, amino acids and ammonia in the brain during insulin induced hypoglycemia. J Neurochem 23, 659.

Lin Y, Phillis J (1991) Oxypurinol reduces focal ischemic brain injury in the rat. Neurosci Lett 126, 187.

Ling E, Leblond C (1973) Investigation of glial cells in semithin sections. I. Variations with age in the numbers of the various glial cell types in rat cortex and corpus callosum. J Comp Neurol 149, 73.

Liotta A, Krieger D (1983) Pro-opiomelanocortin-related and other pituitary hormones in the central nervous system. In Krieger D, Brownstein M, Martin J (eds), *Brain Peptides*. Wiley, New York, p 613.

Lipton P, Whittingham T (1979) The effect of hypoxia on evoked potentials in the in vitro hippocampus. J Physiol 287, 427.

Lipton P, Whittinghamn T (1982) Reduced ATP concentrations as a basis for synaptic transmission failure during hypoxia in the in vitro guinea-pig hippocampus. J Physiol 325 51.

Lisansky J, Peake G, Strassman R, Qualls C, Meikle A, Risch S, Fava G, Zownir-Brazis M, Hochla P, Britton D (1989) Augmented pituitary corticotropin response to a threshold dosage of human corticotropin-releasing hormone in depressives pretreated with metyrapone. Arch Gen Psychiatry 46, 641.

Ljunggren B, Norberg K, Siesjo B (1974) Influence of tissue acidosis upon restitution of brain energy metabolism following total ischemia. Brain Res 77, 173.

Lobner D, Lipton P (1990) Sigma-ligands and non-competitive NMDA antagonists inhibit glutamate release during cerebral ischemia. Neursoci Lett 117, 169.

Lockshin R, Zakeri Z (1990) Programmed cell death: new thoughts and relevance to aging. J Gerontol 45, B135.

Lodge D, O'Shaughnessy C, Zeman S (1986) Reduction of ischemia-induced brain damage and of glutamate-induced calcium uptake by subanesthetic concentrations of ketamine. Neurosci Lett Suppl 24, 535.

Loeffler J, Kley N, Pittius C, Hollt V (1986) Calcium ion and cyclic adenosine 3',5'-monophosphatre regulate POMC mRNA levels in rat intermediate and anterior pituitary lobes. Endocrinology 110, 2840.

Longstreth W, Diehr P, Inui T (1983) Prediction of awakening after out-of-hospital cardiac arrest. N Engl J Med 308, 1378.

Lorens S, Hata N, Handa R, Van de kar L, Guschwan M, Goral J, Lee J, Hamilton M, Bethea C, Clancy J (1990) Neurochemical, endocrine and immunological responses to stress in young and old Fischer 344 male rats. Neurobiol Aging 11, 139.

Lothman E, Collins R (1981) Kainic acid induced limbic seizures: metabolic, behavioural, electro-encephalographic, and neuropathological correlates. Brain Res 218, 299.

Louch C, Higginbotham M (1967) The relation between social rank and plasma corticosterone levels in mice. Gen Comp Endocrinol 8, 441.

Lovinger D, White G, Weight F (1989) Ethanol inhibits NMDA-activated ion currents in hippocampal neurons. Science 243, 1721.

Low P, Waugh S, Zinke K, Drenckhahn D (1985) The role of hemoglobin denaturation and band 3 clustering in red blood cell aging. Science 227, 531.

Lowe J, Mayer R (1990) Ubiquitin, cell stress and diseases of the nervous system. Neuropathol Appl Neurobiol 16, 281.

Lowy M (1990) Reserpine-induced decrease in Type I and II corticosteroid receptors in neuronal and lymphoid tissues of adrenalectomized rats. Neuroendocrinology 51, 190.

Lowy M (1991) Corticosterone regulation of brain and lymhpoid corticosteroid receptors. J Steroid Biochem Mol Biol 39, 147.

Lowry M, Meltzer H (1987) Dexamethasone bioavailability: implications for DST research. Biol Psychiatry 22, 373.

Lucas d, Newhouse J (1957). The toxic effect of sodium L-glutamate on the inner layers of the retina. Arch Ophthalmol 58, 193.

Lucas J, Ducker T (1979a) Recovery in spinal cord injuries. Adv Neurosurg 7, 281.

Lucas J, Ducker T (1979b) Motor classification of spinal cord injuries with mobility, morbidity and recovery indices. Am Surg 45, 151.

Luisi B, Xu W, Otwinowski Z, Freedman L, Yamamoto K, Sigler P (1991) Crystallographic analysis of the interaction of the glucocorticoid receptor with DNA. Nature 352, 497.

Lundgren J, Smith M, Siesjo B (1991a) Influence of moderate hypothermia on ischemic brain damage incurred under hyperglycemic conditions. Exp Brain Res 84, 91.

Lundgren J, Zhang H, Agardh C, Smith M, Evans P, Halliwell B, Siesjo B (1991b) Acidosis-induced ischemic brain damage: are free radicals involved? J Cereb Blood Flow Metab 11, 587.

Luttge W, Rupp M (1990) Differential up- and down-regulation of type I and type II adreno-corticosteroid receptors in mouse brain. Steroids, in press.

Luttge W, Davda M, Rupp M, Kang C (1989a) High affinity binding and regulatory actions of dexamethasone-Type I receptor complexes in mouse brain. Endocrinology 125, 1194.

Luttge W, Rupp M, Davda M (1989b) Aldosterone-stimulated down-regulation of both Type I and Type II adrenocorticosteroid receptors in mouse brain is mediated via Type I receptors. Endocrinology 125, 817.

Lynch G, Larson J, Kelso S, Barrioneuvo G, Schottler F (1983) Intracellular injections of EGTA block the induction of hippocampal long-term potentiation. Nature 305, 719.

Lynch M, Voss K (1990) Arachidonic acid increases inositol phospholipid metabolism and glutamate release in synaptosomes prepared from hippocampal tissue. J Neurochem 55, 215.

Lyons M, Anderson R, Meyer F (1991) Corticotropin releasing factor antagonist reduces ischemic hippocampal neuronal injury. Brain Res 545, 339.

Lyons W, Puttfarcken P, Coyle J (1991) Protection against kainic acid toxicity with lipophilic antioxidants in cerebellar granule cell cultures. Soc Neurosci Abstr 17, 314.17.

Lysko P, Cox J, Alessandra Givano M, Henneberry R (1989) Excitatory amino acid neurotoxicity at the NMDA receptor in cultured neurons: pharmacological characterization. Brain Res 499, 258.

Mabe H, Nagai H, Takagi T (1986) Effect of nimodipine on cerebral functional and metabolic recovery following ischemia in the rat brain. Stroke 17, 501.

Maccari S, Piazza P, Deminiere J, Lemaire V, Mormeded P, Simon H, Angelucci L, Le Moal M (1991a) Life events-induced decrease of corticosteroid Type I receptors is associated with reduced corticosterone feedback and enhanced vulnerability to amphetamine self-administration. Brain Res 547, 7.

Maccari S, Piazza P, Deminiere J, Angelucci L, Simon H, Le Moal M (1991b) Hippocampal Type I and Type II corticosteroid receptor affinities are reduced in rats predisposed to develop amphetmaine self-administration. Brain Res 548, 305.

MacDermott A, Dale N (1987) Receptors ion channels and synaptic potentials underlying the integrative actions of excitatory amino acids. Trends Neurosci 10, 280.

MacDermott A, Mayer M, Westbrook M, Smith G Barker J (1986) NMDA-receptor activation increases cytoplasmic calcium concentration in cultured spinal cord neurones. Nature 321, 519.

MacDonald R, Martin T, Cidlowski J (1980) Glucocorticoids stimulate protein degradation in lymphocytes: a possible mechanism for steroid-induced cell death. Endocrinology 107, 1512.

Maclusky N (1987) Relationship between nuclear steroid binding and steroid-induced responses. In Clark C (ed), *Steroid Hormone Receptors*. Horwood, Chicester.

MacMillan V (1982) Cerebral Na^+, K^+-ATPase activity during exposure to and recovery from acute ischemia. J Cereb Blood Flow Metab 2, 457.

MacVicar B, Baker K, Crichton S (1988) Kainic acid evokes a potassium efflux from astrocytes. Neuroscience 25, 721.

Maderdrut J, Oppenheim R, Prevette D (1988) Enhancement of naturally occurring cell death in the sympathetic and parasympathetic ganglia of the chicken embryo following blockade of ganglionic transmission. Brain Res 444, 189.

Madison D, Niedermeyer E (1970) Epileptic seizures resulting from acute cerebral anoxia. J Neurol Neurosurg Psychiatry 33, 381.

Maehlen J, Torvik A (1990) Necrosis of granule cells of hippocampus in adrenocortical failure. Acta Neuropathol 80, 85.

Maes M, Jacobs M, Suy E, Minner B, Raus J (1990) Prediction of the DST results in depressives by means of urinary-free cortisol excretion, dexamethasone levels, and age. Biol Psychiatry 28, 349.

Margarinos A, Somoza G, DeNicola A (1987) Glucocorticoid negative feedback and glucocorticoid receptors after hippocampectomy in rats. Horm Metab Res 19, 105.

Mahmoud S, Scaccianoce S, Scraggs P, Nicholson S, Gillham B, Jones M (1984) Characteristics of corticosteroid inhibition of adrenocorticotropin release from the anterior pituitary gland of the rat. J Endocrinol 102, 33.

Majewska M, Harrison N, Schwartz R, Barker T, Paul S (1986) Steroid hormone metabolites are barbiturate-like modulators of the GABA receptor. Science 232, 1004.

Majewska M, Bell J, London E (1990) Regulation of the NMDA receptor by redox phenomena: inhibitory role of ascorbate. Brain Res 537, 328.

Majumdar S, Shaw G, Thomson A, Bridges P (1981) Serum cortisol concentrations and the effect of chlormethiazole on them in chronic alcoholics. Neuropharmacology 20, 1357.

Makara G, Stark E, Martezi M, Palkovits M, Rappay G (1981) Effects of paraventricular lesions of stimulated ACTH release and CRF in stalk-median eminence of the rat. Am J Physiol 240, E441.

Makara G, Stark E, Kapocs G, Antoni F (1986) Long-term effects of hypothalamic paraventricular lesion on CRF content and stimulated ACTH secretion. Am J Physiol 250, E319.

Makman M, Dvorkin B, White A (1966) Alterations in protein and nucleic acid metabolism of thymocytes produced by adrenal steroids. J Biol Chem 241, 1646.

Makman M, Dvorkin B, White A (1968) Influence of cortisol on the utilization of precursors of nucleic acids and protein by lymphoid cells in vitro. J Biol Chem 243, 1485.

Malamed S, Carsia R (1983) Aging of the rat adrenocortical cell response to ACTH and cyclic AMP in vitro. J Gerontol 38, 130.

Mandell A, Chapman L, Rand R, Walter R (1963) Plasma corticosteroids: changes in concentration after stimulation of hippocampus and amygdala. Science 139, 1212.

Manogue K, Leshner A, Candland D (1975) Dominance status and adrenocortical reactivity to stress in squirrel monkeys (Saimiri sciureus). Primates 16, 457.

Manzoni O, Fagni L, Marin P, Prezeau L, Sahuquet A, Sladeczeck FR, Bockaert J (1991) Nitric oxide selectively inhibits NMDA receptor activation via a cGMP-independent pathway. Soc Neurosci Abstr 17, 32.14.

Marcoux F, Goodrich J, Dominick M (1988) Ketamine prevents ischemic neuronal injury. Brain Res 452, 329.

Martin D, Schmidt R, DiStefano P, Lowry O, Carter J, Johnson E (1988) Inhibitors of protein synthesis and RNA synthesis prevent neuronal death caused by nerve growth factor deprivation. J Cell Biol 106, 829.

Martin D, Wallace T, Johnson E (1990) Cytosine arabinoside kills postmitotic neurons in a fashion resembling trophic factor deprivation: evidence that a deoxycytidine-dependent process may be required for nerve growth factor signal transduction. J Neurosci 10, 184.

Martinez A, Vitorica J, Bogonez E, Satrustegui J (1987) Differential effects of age on the pathways of calcium influx into nerve terminals. Brain Res 435, 249.

Martins E, Inamura K, Themner K, Malmqvuist K, Siesjo B (1988) Accumulation of calcium and loss of potassium in the hippocampus following transient cerebral ischemia: a proton microprobe study. J Cereb Blood Flow Metab 8, 531.

Mason J (1958) The central nervous system regulation of ACTH secretion. In Jasper H, Proctor L, Knighton R, Noshay W, Costello R (eds), The Reticular Formation of the Brain. Little, Brown, Boston, p 645.

Mason J (1968) A review of psychoendocrine research on the pituitary-adrenal cortical system. Psychosom Med 30, 576.

Mason J (1975a) A historical view of the stress field I. J Human Stress 1, 6.

Mason J (1975b) A historical view of the stress field II. J Human Stress 1, 22.

Masoro E (1988) Food restriction in rodents: an evaluation of its role in the study of aging. J Gerontol 43, B59.

Masson D, Tschopp J (1985) Isolation of a lytic, pore-forming protein (perforin) from cytolytic T-lymphocytes. J Biol Chem 260, 9069.

Masters J, Finch C, Sapolsky R (1989) Glucocorticoid endangerment of hippocampal neurons does not involve DNA cleavage. Endocrinology 124, 3083.

Mattson M (1990) Antigenic changes similar to those seen in neurofibrillary tangles are elicited by glutamate and calcium influx in cultured hippocampal neurons. Neuron 2, 105.

Mattson M, Kater S (1989) Development and selective neurodegeneration in cell cultures from different hippocampal regions. Brain Res 490, 110.

Mattson M, Rychlik B (1990) Glia protect hippocampal neurons against excitatory amino acid-induced degeneration: involvement of fibroblast growth factor. Int J Dev Neurosci 8, 399.

Mattson M, Guthrie P, Hayes B, Kater S (1989) Roles for mitotic history in the generation and degeneration of hippocampal neuroarchitecture. J Neurosci 9 1223.

Mattson M, Engle M, Rychlik B (1991a) Effects of elevated intracellular calcium levels on the cytoskeleton and tau in cultured human cortical neurons. Mol Chem Neuropathol, in press.

Mattson M, Rychlik B, Christakos S (1991b) Evidence for calcium-reducing and excitoprotective roles for the calcium binding protein calbindin-D28K in cultured hippocampal neurons. Neuron 6, 41.

Max S, Mill J, Mearow K, Konagaya M, Konagaya Y, Thomas J, Banner C, Vitkovic L (1988) Dexamethasone regulates glutamine synthetase expression in rat skeletal muscles. Am J Physiol 255, E397.

May C, Rapoport S, Tomai T, Chrousos G, Gold P (1987) CSF concentrations of corticotropin releasing hormone (CRF) and corticotropin are reduced in patients with Alzheimer's disease. Neurology 37, 535.

Mayer M, Wesbrook G, Guthrie P (1984) Voltage-dependent block by Mg of NMDA respones in spinal cord neurones. Nature 309, 261.

Mazurek M, Growdon J, Beal M, Martin J (1986) CSF vasopressin concentration is reduced in Alzheimer's disease. Neurology 36, 1133.

McBain C, Traynelis S, Dingledine R (1990) Regional variation of extracellular space in the hippocampus. Science 249, 675.

McBeen G, Roberts P (1985) Neurotoxicity of L-glutamate and DL-threo-3-hydroxyaspartate in the rat striatum. J Neurochem 44, 247.

McBurney R, Neering I (1987) Neuronal calcium homeostasis. Trends Neurosci 10, 164.

McCarty R (1986) Age-related alterations in sympathetic-adrenal medullary responses to stress. Gerontology 32, 172.

McCay C, Crowell M, Maynard L (1935) The effect of retarded growth upon the length of the life span and upon the ultimate body size. J Nutrit 10, 63.

McConkey D, Hartzell P, Duddy S, Hakansson H, Orrenius S (1988) 2,3,7,8-tetrachlorodibenzo-p-dioxin kills immature thymocytes by calcium-mediated endonuclease activation. Science 242, 256.

McCord J (1985) Oxygen-derived free radicals in post-ischemic tissue injury. N Engl J Med 312, 159.

McDonald J, Silverstein F, Johnston M (1987) MK-801 protects the neonatal brain from hypoxic-ischemic damage. Eur J Pharmacol 140, 359.

McEwen B, Weiss J, Schwartz L (1968) Selective retention of corticosterone by limbic structures in rat brain. Nature 220, 911.

McEwen B, Wallach G, Magnus C (1974) Corticosterond binding to hippocampus: immediate and delayed influences in the absence of adrenal secretion. Brain Res 70, 321.

McEwen B, Stephenson B, Krey L (1980) Radioimmunoassay of brain tissue and cell nuclear corticosteroid. J Neurosci Methods 3, 57.

McEwen B, de Kloet E, Rostene W (1986) Adrenal steroid receptors and actions in the nervous system. Physiol Rev 66, 1121.

McGeer E, McGeer P (1976) Duplication of biochemical changes in Huntington's chorea by intrastriatal injections of glutamic and kainic acids. Nature 263, 517.

McGeer E, McGeer P, Singh K (1978) Kainate induced degeneration of neostriatal neurons: dependency upon the corticostriatal tract. Brain Res 132, 381.

McIntosh T, Faden A, Bendall M, Vink R (1987) Traumatic brain injury in the rat: alterations in brain lactate and pH as characterized by ^{1}H and ^{31}P nuclear magnetic resonance. J Neurochem 49, 1530.

McIntosh T, Vink R, Yamakami I, Faden A (1989) Magnesium protects against neurological deficit after brain injury. Brain Res 482, 252.

McMahon H, Nicholls D (1990) Glutamine and aspartate loading of synaptosomes: a re-evaluation of effects on calcium-dependent excitatory amino acid release. J Neurochem 54, 373.

McMurtry J, Wexler B (1981) Hypersensitivity of spontaneously hypertensive rats (SHR) to heat, ether, and immobilization. Endocrinology 108, 1730.

McNeill T, Masters J, Finch C (1990) Effect of chronic adrenalectomy on neuron loss and distribution of sulfated glycoprotein-2 in the dentate gyrus of the prepubertal rats. Exp Neurol 111, 140.

Meaney M, Aitken D (1985) The effects of early, postnatal handling on the development of hippocampal glucocorticoid receptors: temporal parameters. Dev Brain Res 22, 301.

Meaney M, Aitken D, Bodniff S, Iny L, Tatarewicz J, Sapolsky R (1985a) Early, postnatal handling alters glucocorticoid receptor concentrations in selected brain regions. Behav Neurosci 99, 760.

Meaney M, Aitken D, Bodnoff S, Iny L, Sapolsky R (1985b) The effects of postnatal handling on the development of the glucocorticoid receptor systems and stress recovery in the rat. Prog Neuropsychopharmacol Biol Psychiatry 9, 731.

Meaney M, Sapolsky R, McEwen B (1985c) The development of the glucocorticoid receptor system in the rat limbic brain. I. Ontogeny and autoregulation. Dev Brain Res 18, 159.

Meaney M, Sapolsky R, McEwen B (1985d) The development of the glucocorticoid receptor system in the rat limbic brain. II. An autoradiographic study. Dev Brain Res 18, 165.

Meaney M, Aitken D, Sapolsky R (1987) Thyroid hormones influence the development of hippocampal glucocorticoid receptors in the rat: a mechanism for the effects of postnatal handling on the development of the adrenocortical stress response. Neuroendocrinology 45, 278.

Meaney M, Aitken D, Bhatnager S, van Berkel C, Sapolsky R (1988b) Effect of neonatal handling on age-related impairments associated with the hippocampus. Science 239, 766.

Meaney M, Aitken D, Sharma S, Viau V (1990a) Basal ACTH, corticosterone and corticosterone-binding globulin levels over the diurnal cycle, and hippocampal type I and type II corticosteroid receptors in young and old, handled and nonhandled rats. Neuroendocrinology, in press.

Meaney M, Aitken D, Sharma V, Viau V, Sarrieau A (1990b) Postnatal handling of rats alters adrenocortical negative feedback: a model for individual differences in the neuroendocrine response to stress. Neuroendocrinology 50, 597.

Meaney M, Aitken D, Sapolsky R 1991a Postnatal handling attenuates neuroendocrine, anatomical and cognitive dysfunctions associated with aging in female rats. Neurobiol Aging, 12, 31.

Meaney M, Viau V, Bhatnager S, Betito K, Iny L, O'Donnell D, Mitchell J (1991b) Cellular mechanisms underlying the development and expression of individual differences in the hypothalamic-pituitary-adrenal stress response. J Steroid Biochem Molec Biol 39, 265.

Meech R (1974) The sensitivity of *Helix aspersa* neurons to injected calcium ions. J Physiol 237, 259.

Mela L, Miller L, Nicholas G (1972) Influence of cellular acidosis and altered cation concentration on shock-induced mitochondrial damage. Surgery 72, 102.

Meldelosi J, Volpe P, Pozzan T (1988) The intracellular distribution of calcium. Trends Neurosci 11, 449.

Meldrum B (1983) Metabolic factors during prolonged seizures and their relation to nerve cell death. In Delgado-Escueta A, Wasterlain C, Treiman D, Porter R (eds), *Advances in Neurology, vol 34*. Raven Press, New York.

Meldrum B, Vigoroux R, Brierley J (1973) Systemic factors and epileptic brain damage. Prolonged seizures in paralysed, artifically ventilated baboons. Arch Neurol 29, 82.

Meller W, Kathol R, Jaeckle R, Grambsch P, Lopez J (1988) HPA axis abnormalities in depressed patients with normal response to the DST. Am J Psychiatry 145, 3.

Mendelson J, Stein S (1966) Serum cortisol levels in alcoholic and non-alcoholic subjects during experimentally induced intoxication. Psychosom Med 28, 616.

Mendlewicz J, Charles G, Franckson J (1982) The dexamethasone suppression test in affective disorder: relationship to clinical and genetic subgroups. Br J Psychiatry 141, 464.

Mendoza S, Coe C, Lowe E, Levine S (1979) The physiological response to group formation in adult male squirrel monkeys. Psychoneuroendocrinology 3, 221.

Merchenthaler I, Vigh S, Petrusz P, Schally A (1983) The paraventriculo-infundibular corticotropin-releasing factor (CRF) pathway as revealed by immunocytochemistry in long term hypophysectomized or adrenalectomized rats. Regul Pept 5, 295.

Meyer J (1985) Biochemical effects of corticosteroids on neural tissues. Physiol Rev 65, 946.

Meyer J, Luine V, Khylchevskaya R, McEwen B (1979) Glucocorticoids and hippocampal enzyme activity. Brain Res 166, 172.

Mezey E, Reisine T, Palkovits M, Brownstein M, Axelrod J (1983) Direct stimulation fo β2-adrenergic receptors in rat anterior pituitary induces the release of adrenocorticotropin in vivo. Proc Natl Acad Sci USA 80, 6728.

Micco D, McEwen B (1980) Glucocorticoids, the hippocampus and behaviour: interactive relation between task activation and steroid hormone binding specificity. J Comp Physiol Psychol 94, 624.

Michaels R, Rothman S (1990) Glutamate neurotoxicity in vitro: antagonist pharmacology and intracellular calcium concentrations. J Neurosci 10, 283.

Micheau J, Destrada C, Soumireu-Mourat B (1985) Time-dependent effects of post-training intrahippocampal injections of corticosterone on retention of repetitive learning tasks in mice. Eur J Pharmacol 106, 39.

Michenfelder J, Richard A, Theye A (1970) The effect of anesthesia and hypothermia on canine cerebral ATP and lactate during anoxia produced by decapitation. Anesthesiology 33, 430.

Michenfelder J, Milde J, Sundt T (1976) Cerebral protection by barbiturate anesthesia. Arch Neurol 33, 345.

Milani D, Guidolin D, Facci L, Pozzan T, Buso M, Leon A, Skaper S (1991) Excitatory amino acid-induced alterations of cytoplasmic free calcium in individual cerebellar granule neurons: role in neurotoxicity. J Neurosci Res 28, 434.

Miller G, Davis J (1991) Post-ischemic surge in corticosteroids aggravates ischemic damage to gerbil CA_1 pyramidal cells. Soc Neurosci Abtr 17, 302.4.

Miller L, Thompson M, Greenblatt D, Deutsch S, Shader R, Paul S (1987) Rapid increase in brain benzodiazepine receptor binding following defeat stress in mice. Brain Res 414, 395.

Miller R (1987) Multiple calcium channels and neuronal function. Science 235, 46.

Mink R, Dutka A, Kumaroo K, Hallenbeck J (1990) No conversion of xanthine dehydrogenase to oxidase in canine cerebral ischemia. Am J Physiol 259, H1655.

Mitchell J, Iny L, Meaney M (1990a) The role of serotonin in the development and environmental regulation of Type II corticosteroid receptor binding in rat hippocampus. Dev Brain Res 55, 231.

Mitchell J, Rowe W, Boksa P, Meaney M (1990b) Seotonin regulates Type II corticosteroid receptor binding in hippocampal cell cultures. J Neurosci 10, 1745.

Miyamoto M, Murphy T, Schnaar R, Coyle J (1988) Antioxidants protect against glutamate cytotoxicity in a neuronal cell line. Soc Neurosci Abstr 14, 169.19.

Miyanaga K, Miyabo S, Ooya E (1991) negative feedback by corticosterone is the major mechanism responsible for CRF-induced desensitization. J Neuroendocrinol 2, 36.

Moberg G, Scapagnini U, de Groot J, Ganong W (1971) Effect of sectioning the fornix on diurnal fluctuations in plasma corticosterone levels in the rat. Neuroendocrinology 7, 11.

Mody I, Heinemann U (1986) Laminar profiles of the changes in extracellular calcium concentration induced by repetitive stimulation and excitatory amino acids in the rat dentate gyrus. Neurosci Lett 69, 137.

Mody I, Heinemann U (1987) NMDA receptors of dentate gyrus granule cells participate in synaptic transmission following kindling. Nature 326, 701.

Mody I, MacDonald J, Baimbridge K (1988) Release of intracellular calcium following activation of excitatory amino acid receptors in cultured hippocampal neurons. Soc Neurosci Abstr 14, 40.4

Moisan M, Seckl J, Edwards C (1990) 11β-Hydroxysteroid dehydrogenase bioactivity and messenger RNA expression in rat forebrain: localization in hypothalamus, hippocampus, and cortex. Endocrinology 127, 1450.

Momose R, Richardson E (1968) The neurological manifestations of systemic lupus erythematosus. A clinical-pathological study of 24 cases and review of the literature. Medicine 47, 337.

Moncada S, Palmer R (1991) Inhibition of the induction of nitric oxide synthase by glucocorticoids: yet another explanation for their anti-inflammatory effects? Trends Pharmacol Sci 12, 130.

Monyer H, Choi D (1988) Morphinans attenuate cortical neuronal injury induced by glucose deprivation in vitro. Brain Res 446, 144.

Monyer H, Goldberg M, Choi D (1989) Glucose deprivation neuronal injury in cortical culture. Brain Res 483, 347.

Monyer H, Hartley D, Choi D (1990) 21-Aminosteroids attenuate excitotoxic neuronal injury in cortical cell cultures. Neuron 5, 121.

Moody W (1984) Effects of intracellular H^+ on the electrical properties of excitable cells. Annu Rev Neurosci 7, 257.

Moore D (1989) Promiscuous behaviour in the steroid hormone receptor superfamily. Trends Neurosci 12, 165.

Moore R, Eichler V (1972) Loss of a circadian adrenal corticosterone rhythm following suprachiasmatic lesions in the rat. Brain Res 42, 201.

Morad M, Dichter M, Tang C (1988) The NMDA activated current in hippocampal neurons is highly sensitive to $[H^+]_0$. Soc Neurosci Abstr 14, 318.18.

Morano M, Akil H (1990) Effects of aging on the hippocampal glucocorticoid and mineralocorticoid receptors. Soc Neurosci Abstr 16, 439.8.

Morishige W (1982) Thyroid hormone influences glucocorticoid recptor levels in the neonatal rat lung. Endocrinology 111, 1017.

Morse J, Davis J (1989) Chemical adrenalectomy protects hippocampal cells following ischemia. Soc Neurosci Abstr 15, 149.4.

Morse J, Davis J (1990a) Hippocampal damage following ischemia: temperature maintenence blocks protective effects of the antiglucocorticoid metapyrone. Soc Neurosci Abstr 16, 118.16.

Morse J, Davis J (1990b) Regulation of ischemic hippocampal damage in the gerbil: adrenalectomy alters the rate of CA_1 cell disappearance. Exp Neurol 110, 86.

Moskowitz M, Kiwak K, Hekimian K, Levine L (1984) Synthesis of compounds with properties of leukotrienes C4 and D4 in gerbil brains after ischemia and reperfusion. Science 224, 886.

Muggeo M, Fedele D, Tiengo A, Milinari M, Crepaldi G (1975) Human growth hormone and cortisol resposne to insulin stimulation in aging. J Gerontol 30, 546.

Mulder G, Smelik P (1977) A superfusion system technique for the study of the sites of action of glucocorticoids in the rat hypothalamus-pituitary-adrenal system in vitro. I. Pituitary cell superfusion. Endocrinology 100, 1143.

Mumenthaler M (1990) *Neurology* (3rd ed). Thieme, Stuttgart.

Munck A (1971) Glucocorticoid inhibition of glucose uptake by peripheral tissues: old and new evidence, molecular mechanisms and physiological significance. Perspect Biol Med 14, 265.

Munck A, Crabtree G (1981) Glucocorticoid-induced cell death. In Bowen I, Lockshin R (eds), *Cell Death in Biology and Pathology.* Chapman and Hall, London, p 329.

Munck A, Guyre P, Holbrook N (1984) Physiological actions of glucocorticoids in stress and their relation to pharmacological actions. Endocr Rev 5, 25.

Murphy B (1991) Treatment of major depression with steroid suppressive drugs. J Steroid Biochem Molec Biol 39, 239.

Murphy T, Miuyamoto M, Sastre A, Schnaar R, Coyle J (1989) Glutamate toxicity in a neuronal cell line involves inhibition of cystine transport leading to oxidative stress. Neuron 2, 1547.

Myers R (1979) Lactic acid accumulation as a cause of brain edema and cerebral necrosis resulting from oxygen deprivation. In Korobkin R, Guillemineault G (eds), *Advances in Perinatal Neurology.* Spectrum, New York.

Myers R, Yamaguchi S (1977) Nervous system effects of cardiac arrest in monkeys: Preservation of vision. Arch Neurol 34, 65.

Nadler J, Cuthbertson G (1980) Kainic acid neurotoxicity towards hippocampal formation: dependence on specific excitatory pathways. Brain Res 195, 47.

Nahorski S (1988) Inositol polyphosphates and neuronal calcium homeostasis. Trends Neurosci 11, 444.

Nakadate G, DeGroot J (1963) Fornix transection and adrenocortical function in rats. Anat Rec 145, 338.

Nakano S, Kogure K, Fujikura H (1990) Ischemia-induced slowly progressive neuronal damage in the rat brain. Neuroscience 38, 115.

Nasr s, Rodgers G, Pandey E (1982) ACTH, cortisol and the DST in depressed outpatients. Proc Soc Biol Psychiatry 37, 68.

Nasrallah H, Coffman J, Olson S (1989) Structural brain-imaging findings in affective disorders: an overview. J Neuropsychiatry 1, 21.

Nedergaard M, Goldman S, Desai S, Pulsinelli W (1991) Acid-induced death in neurons and glia. J Neurosci 11, 2489.

Nelson W, Orr W, Shane S, et al, (1984a) Occurrence of high concentrations of postdexamethasone cortisol in elderly psychiatric inpatients. J Clin Psychiatry 45, 120.

Nelson W, Orr W, Shane S, Stevenson J (1984b) Hypothalamic-pituitary-adrenal axis activity and age in major depression. J Clin Psychiatry 45, 120.

Nemeroff C, Widerlov E, Bisette G, Walleus H, Karlsson I, Eklund K, Kilts C, Loosen P, Vale W (1984) Elevated concentrations of CSF corticotropin-releasing factor-like immunoreactivity in depressed patients. Science 226, 1342.

Nemoto E, Frinak S (1988) Brain tissue pH after global brain ischemia and barbiturate loading in rats. Stroke 12, 77.

Nestler E, Rainbow T, McEwen B, Greengard P (1981) Corticosterone increases the amount of protein 1, a neuron-specific phosphoprotein, in rat hippocampus. Science 212, 1162.

Nevander G, Ingvar M, Auer R, Siesjo B (1985) Status epilepticus in well-oxygenated rats causes neuronal necrosis. Ann Neurol 18, 281.

Nicholls D (1989) Release of glutamate, aspartate and GABA from isolated nerve terminals. J Neurochem 52, 331.

Nicholls D, Sihra T (1986) Synaptosomes possess an exocytotic pool of glutamate. Nature 321, 772.

Nicholson C, Bruggencate G, Steinberg R, Stockle H (1977) Calcium modulation in brain extracellular microenvironment demonstrated with ion-selective micropipette. Proc Natl Acad Sci USA 74, 1287.

Nicholson S, Mahmoud S, Sutanto W, Gillham B, Jones M (1986) The combination of 17α-hydroxyprogesterone and 11-epicortisol prevents the delayed feedback effect of natural and synthetic glucocorticoids. Neuroendocrinology 43, 491.

Nitsch C (1991) relationship of presence of the calcim-binding protein parvalbumin in GABAergic interneurons and their survival after transient global ischemia. Soc Neurosci Abstr 17, 77.6.

Nordstrom C, Rehncrona S, Siesjo B (1976) Restitution of cerebral energy state after complete and incomplete ischemia of 30 minute duration. Acta Physiol Scand 97, 270.

Norenberg M, Martinez-Hernandez A (1979) Fine structural localization of glutamine synthetase in astrocytes of rat brain. Brain Res 161, 303.

Norris J, Hacinski J (1986) High dose steroid treatment in cerebral infarction. Br Med J 292, 21.

Novelli A, Reilly J, Lysko P, Henneberry R (1988) Glutamate becomes neurotoxic via the NMDA receptor when intracellular energy levels are reduced. Brain Res 451, 205.

Nowak L, Bregestowski P, Ascher P (1984) Magnesium gates glutamate-activated channels in mouse central neurons. Nature 307, 462.

Nowak T (1985) Synthesis of a stress protein following transient ischemia in the gerbil. J Neurochem 45, 1635.

Nowak T (1991) Localzation of 70 kDa stress protein mRNA induction in gerbil brain after ischemia. J Cereb Blood Flow Metab 11, 432.

Nussmeier N, Ralund C, Slogoff S (1986) Neuropsychiatric complications after cardiopulmonary bypass: cerebral protection by a barbiturate. Anesthesiology 64, 165.

Odio M, Brodish A (1988) Effects of age on metabolic responses to acute and chronic stress. Am J Physiol 254, E617.

Odio M, Brodish A (1989) Age-related adaptation of pituitary-adrenocortical responses to stress. Neuroendocrinology 49, 382.

Oda M, Huttenlocher (1974) The effect of corticosteroids on dendritic development in the rat brain. Yale J Biol Med 3, 155.

Ogura A, Miyamoto M, Kudo Y (1988) Neuronal death in vitro: parallelism between survivability of hippocampal neurones and sustained elevation of cytosolic calcium after exposure to glutamate receptor agonist. Exp Brain Res 73, 447.

Ogura A, Akita K, Kudo Y (1990) Non-NMDA receptor mediates cytoplasmic calcium elevation in cultured hippocampal neurones. Neurosci Res 9, 103.

Ohashi M, Kato K, Nawata H, et al. (1986) Adrenocortical responsiveness to graded ACTH infusions in normal young and elderly human subjects. Gerontology 32, 43.

Okada Y, Tanimoto M, Yoneda K (1988) The protective efect of hypothermia on reversibility in the neuronal function of the hippocampal slice during long lasting anoxia. Neurosci Lett 84, 277.

Okajima T, Hertting G (1986) Delta-sleep-inducing peptide inhibited CRF-induced ACTH secretion from rat anterior pituitary gland in vitro. Horm Metab Res 18, 497.

Okamoto K, Aoiki K (1963) Development of a strain of spontaneously hypertensive rats. Jpn Circ J 27, 282.

Okazaki M, Nadler J (1988) Protective effects of mossy fiber lesions against kainic acid-induced seizures and neuronal degeneration. Neuroscience 26, 763.

Okret S, Poellinger L, Fong Y, Gustafsson J (1986) Down-regulation of glucocorticoid receptor mRNA by glucocorticoid hormones and recognition of a specific binding sequence within a receptor cDNA clone. Proc Natl Acad Sci USA 83, 5899.

Olgemoller B, Schon J, Wieland O (1985) Endothelial plasma membrane is a glucocortiocid-regulated barrier for the uptake of glucose into the cell. Mol Cell Endocrinol 43, 165.

Olney J (1978) Neurotoxicity of excitatory amino acids. In McGeer E, Olney J, McGeer P (eds), *Kainic Acid as a Tool in Neurobiology.* Raven Press, New York.

Olney J (1990) Excitotoxin-mediated neuron death in young and old age. Prog Brain Res 86, 37.

Olney J, Ho O, Rhee V (1971) Cytotoxic effects of acidic and sulphur-containing amino acids on the infant mouse central nervous system. Exp Brain Res 14, 61.

Olpe H, McEwen B (1976) Glucocorticoid binding to receptor-like proteins in rat brain and pituitary: ontogenetic and experimentally induced changes. Brain Res 105, 121.

Olsson T, Viitanen M, Hagg E, Asplund K, Grankvist K, Eriksson S, Gustafson Y (1989) Hormones in "young" and "old" elderly: pituitary-thyroid and pituitary-adrenal axes. Gerontology 35, 144.

Onadera H, Sato G, Kogure K (1986) Lesions to Schaffer collaterals prevent ischemic death of pyramidal cells. Neurosci Lett 68, 169.

Oppenheim R (1985) Cyclic GMP and neurone death. Nature 313, 248.

Oppenheim R, Prevette D (1988) Reduction of naturally occurring neuronal death in vivo by the inhibition of protein and RNA synthesis. Soc Neurosci Abstr 14, 150.14.

Orchinik M, Murray T, Moore F (1991a) A corticosteroid receptor in neuronal membranes. Science 252, 1848.

Orchinik M, Murray T, Moore F (1991b) Membrane-bound corticosteroid receptor is coupled to a G-protein. Soc Neurosci Abstr 17, 561.2.

Osborne T, Mendel L, Ferry E (1917) The effect of retardation of growth upon the breeding period and duration of life in rats. Science 45, 294.

O'Steen W, Brodish A (1985) Neuronal damage in the rat retina after chronic stress. Brain Res 344, 231.

O'Steen W, Donnelly J (1982) Antagonistic effects of adrenalectomy and ether—surgical stress on light-induced photoreceptor damage. Invest Ophthalmol Vis Sci 22, 1.

Ostergaard H, Kane K, Mescher M, Clark W (1987) Cytotoxic T lymphocyte mediated lysis without release of serine esterase. Nature 330, 71.

Oxenkrug G, Pmara N, McIntyre I, et al. (1983) Aging and cortisol resistance to suppression by dexamethasone: a positive correlation. Psychiatry Res 10, 125.

Oxenkrug G, Mcintyre I, Stanley M, Gershon S (1984a) Dexamethasone suppression test: experimental model in rats, and effect of age. Biol Psychiatry 19, 413.

Oxenkrug G, McIntyre I, Gershon M (1984b) Effects of pinealectomy and aging on the serum corticosterone circadian rhythm in rats. J Pineal Res 1, 181.

Oxenkrug G, Gurevich D, Siegel B, Dumlao M, Gershon S (1989) Correlation between brain-adrenal axis activation and cognitive impairment in Alzheimer's disease: Is there a gender effect? Psychiatry Res 29, 169.

Oxyurt E, Graham D, Woodruff G, McCulloch J (1988) Protective effect of the glutamate antagonist, MK-801 in focal cerebral ischemia in the cat. J Cereb Blood Flow Metab 8, 138.

Ozawa S, Nakamura T, Yuzaki M (1988) Cation permeability change caused by L-glutamate in cultured rat hippocampal neurons. Brain Res 443, 85.

Packan D, Sapolsky R (1990) Glucocorticoid endangerment of the hippocmapus: tissue, steroid and receptor specificity. Neuroendocrinology 51, 613.

Pai K, Ravindranath V (1991) Toxicity of N-acetylaspartylglutamate and its protection by NMDA and non-NMDA receptor antagonists. Neurosci Lett 126, 49.

Palacios J, Neihoff D, Kuhar M (1981) Receptor-autoradiography with tritium-sensitive film: potential for computerized densitometry. Neurosci Lett 25, 102.

Palmer G, Palmer S, Christie-Pope C, Callahan A, Taylor M, Eddy L (1985) Classification of ischemic-induced damage to Na^+, K^+-ATPase in gerbil forebrain. Neuropharmacology 24, 509.

Palmer G, Palmer S, Christie-Pope B (1988) Protective action of calcium channel blockers on Na,K-ATPase in gerbil cerebral cortex following ischemia. J Neurosci Res 19, 252.

Parce J, Owicki J, Kercso K, Sigal G, Wada H, Muir V, Bousse L, Ross K, Sikic B, McConnell H (1989) Detection of cell-affecting agents with a silicon biosensor. Science 246, 243.

Park C, Nehls D, Graham D, Teasdale G, McCulloch J (1988) Focal cerebral ischaemia in the cat: treatment with the glutamate antagonist MK-801 after induction of ischaemia. J Cereb Blood Flow Metab 8, 757.

Parks T, Artman L, Alasti N, Nemeth E (1991) Modulation of NMDA receptor-mediated increases in cytosolic calcium in cultured rat cerebellar granule cells. Brain Res 552, 13.

Pastuszko A, Wilson D, Erecinska F (1984) Effects of kainic acid in rat brain synaptosomes: the involvement of calcium. J Neurochem 43, 747.

Patacchioli F, Amenta F, Tamacci M, Taglialatela G, Maccari S, Angelucci L (1989) Acetyl-L-carnitine reduces the age-dependent loss of glucocorticoid receptors in the rat hippocampus: an autoradiographic study. J Neurosci Res 23, 462.

Patel A, Hunt A, Tahourdin C (1983) Regulation of in vivo glutamine synthetase activity by glucocorticoids in the developing rat brain. Dev Brain Res 10, 83.

Patel M, Peoples R, Yim G, Isom G (1991) Enhancement of NMDA-mediated responses by cyanide. Soc Neurosci Abstr 17, 464.13.

Paull W, Gibbs F (1983) The corticotropin-releasing factor neurosecretory system in intact, adrenalectomized, and adrenalectized-dexamethasone treated rats. Histochemistry 78, 303.

Pauwels P, van Assouw H, Leysen J (1989) Attenuation of neurotoxicity following anoxia or glutamate receptor activation in EGF- and hippocampal extract−treated neuronal cultures. Cell Signal 1, 45.

Pavlov E, Harman S, Chrousos G, Loriaux D, Blacman M (1986) Responses of plasma adreno-corticotropin, cortisol, and dehydroepiandrosterone to ovine CRH in healthy aging men. J Clin Endocrinol Metab 62, 767.

Pearl R (1929) *The Rate of Living*. Alfred Knopf, New York.

Pechnick R, George R, Lee R, Poland R (1986) The effects of the acute administration of phencyclidine hydrochloride (PCP) on the release of corticosterone, growth hormone and prolactin in the rat. Life Sci 38, 291.

Pechnick R, George R, Poland R (1989) Characterization of the effects of the acute and repeated administration of MK-801 on the release of adrenocorticotropin, corticosterone and prolactin in the rat. Eur J Pharmacol 164, 257.

Pechnick R, Wong C, George R, Thurkauf A, Jacobson A, Rice K (1989) Comparison of the effects of the acute administration of dexoxadrol, levoxadrol, MK-801 and phencyclidine on body temperature in the rat. Neuropharmacology 28, 829.

Peiffer A, Barden N, Meaney M (1989) Age-related changes in Type II glucocorticoid receptor mRNA levels in pituitary and selected brain regions in the rat. Soc Neurosi Abstr 15, 290.6.

Peiffer A, Barden N, Meaney M (1991) Age-related changes in glucocorticoid receptor binding and mRNA levels in the rat brain and pituitary. Neurobiol Aging 12, 475.

Pellegrini-Giampietro D, Cherici G, Alesiani M, Carla V, Moroni F (1988) Excitatory amino acid release from rat hippocampal slices as a consequence of free-radical formation. J Neurochem 51, 1960.

Pellegrini-Giampietro D, Cherici G, Alesiani M, Carla V, Moroni F (1990) Excitatory amino acid release and free radical formation may cooperate in the genesis of ischemia-induced neuronal damage. J Neurosci 10, 1035.

Pelligrino D, Almquist L, Siesjo B (1981) Effects of insulin-induced hypoglycemia on intracellular pH and impedance in the cerebral cortex of the rat. Brain Res 221, 129.

Pepin M, Barden N (1991) Increased levels of glucocorticoid receptor mRNA, glucocorticoid binding and sensitivity to glucocorticoids in cell cultures and in mouse brain following antidepressant treatment. Soc Neurosci Abstr 17, 42.3.

Pesce G, Guillaume V, Jezova D, Faudon M, Grino M, Oliver C (1990) Epinephrine in rat hypophysial portal blood is derived mainly from the adrenal medulla. Neuroendocrinology 52, 322.

Peters T (1986) Calcium in physiological and pathological cell function. Eur Neurol 25 (suppl) 27.

Petito C, Feldman E, Pulsinelli W, Plum F (1987) Delayed hippocampal damage in humans following cardiorespiratory arrest. Neurology 37, 1281.

Pfohl B, Sherman B, Schlechte J, Stone R (1985) Pituitary-adrenal axis rhythm disturbances in psychiatric depression. Arch Gen Psychiatry 42, 897.

Phillips M, Tashjian A (1982) Characterization of an early inhibitory effect of glucocorticoids on stimulated ACTH and endorphin release from a clonal strain of mouse pituitary cells. Endocrinology 110, 892.

Phillis J, Simpson R, Walter G (1990) The effect of hyperglycemia on extracellular levels of adenosine in the hypoxic rat cerebral cortex. Brain Res 524, 336.

Piatt J, Schiff S (1984) High dose barbiturate therapy in neurosurgery and intensive care. Neurosurgery 15, 427.

Picard D, Khursheed B, Garabedian M, Fortin M, Lindquist S, Yamamoto K (1990) Reduced levels of hsp90 compromise steroid receptor action in vivo. Nature 348, 166.

Pitler T, Landfield P (1990) Aging-related prolongation of calcium spike duration in rat hippocampal slice neurons. Brain Res 508, 1.

Plaitakis A, Caroscio J (1987) Abnormal glutamate metabolism in amyotrophic lateral sclerosis. Ann Neurol 22, 575.

Plaitakis A, Berl S, Yahr M (1982) Abnormal glutamate metabolism in an adult-onset degenerative neurological disorder. Science 216, 193.

Plomin R (1990) *Nature and Nurture: An Introduction to Human Behavioral Genetics.* Brooks/Cole, Pacific Grove, Ca.

Plomin R, Rowe C (1979) Genetic and environmental etiology of social behavior in infancy. Devel Psychobiol 15, 62.

Plotsky P (1988) Hypophysiotropic regulation of stress-induced ACTH secretion. In Chrousos G, Loriaux D, Gold P (eds), *Mechanisms of Physical and Emotional Stress.* Plenum Press, New York.

Plotsky P, Sawchenko P (1987) Hypophysial-portal plasma levels, median eminence content, and immunohistochemical staining of corticotropin-releasing factor, arginine vasopresin, and oxytocin after pharmacological adrenalectomy. Endocrinology 120, 1361.

Plotsky P, Vale W (1984) Hemorrhage-induced secretion of corticotropin-releasing factor-like immunoactivity into the rat hypophysial portal circulation and its inhibition by glucocorticoids. Endocrinology 114, 164.

Plotsky P, Bruhn T, Vale W (1985a) Evidence for multifactor regulation of the adrenocorticotropin secretory response to hemodynamic stimuli. Endocrinology 116, 633.

Plotsky P, Bruhn T, Vale W (1985b) Hypophysiotropic regulation of ACTH secretion in response to insulin-induced hypoglycemia. Endocrinology 117, 323.

Plotsky P, Otto S, Sapolsky R (1986) Inhibition of immunoreactive corticotropin-releasing factor secretion into the hypophysial-portal circulation by delayed glucocorticoid feedback. Endocrinology 119, 1126.

Plotsky P, Cunningham E, Widmaier E (1989) Catecholaminergic modulation of CRF and adrenocorticotropin secretion. Endocr Rev 10, 437.

Plum F, Alvord E, Posner J (1963) Effect of steroids on experimental cerebral infarction. Arch Neurol 9, 571.

Pocock J, Murphie H, Nicholls D (1988) Kainic acid inhibits the synaptosomal plasma membrane glutamate carrier and allows glutamate leakage from the cytoplasm but does not affect glutamate exocytosis. J Neurochem 50, 745.

Podack E, Dennert G (1983) Assembly of two types of tubules with putative cytolytic funciton by cloned natural killer cells. Nature 302, 442.

Podack E, Young J, Cohn Z (1985) Isolation and biochemical and functional characterization of perforin 1 from cytolytic T-cell granules. Proc Natl Acad Sci USA 82, 8629.

Poolos N, Kocsis J (1990) Elevated extracellular potassium concentration enhances synaptic activation of NMDA receptors in hippocampus. Brain Res 508, 7.

Popova N, Naumenko E (1972) Dominance relation and the pituitary-adrenal system in rats. Anim Behav 20, 108.

Popplewell P, Azhar S (1987) Effects of aging on cholesterol content and cholesterol-metabolizing enzymes in the rat adrenal gland. Endocrinology 121, 64.

Popplewell P, Tsubokawa M, Ramachandran J, Azhar S (1986) Differential effects of aging on ACTH receptors, adenosine 3',5' cyclic monophosphate response and corticosterone secretion in adrenocortical cells from Sprague-Dawley rats. Endocrinology 119, 2206.

Popplewell P, Butte J, Azhar S (1987) The influence of age on steroidogenic enzyme activitieis of the rat adrenal gland: enhanced expression of cholesterol side-chain cleavage activity. Endocrinology 120, 2521.

Porter R (1954) The central nervous system and stress-induced eosinopenia. Rec Prog Horm Res 10, 1.

Prados M, Strawger R, Feindel W (1945) Studies on cerebral edema. II Reaction of the brain to exposure to air; physiologic changes. Arch Neurol Psych 54, 290.

Pratt W (1990) Interaction of hsp90 with steroid receptors: organizing some diverse observations and presenting the newest concepts. Mol Cell Endocrinol 74, C69.

Preskorn S, Hartman B, Irwin C (1982) Roles of the central adrenergic system in mediating amytriptyline-induced alteration in the mammalian blood-brain barrier in vivo. J Pharmacol Exp Ther 233, 388.

Price M, Olney J, Samson L, Labruyere J (1985) Calcium influx accompanies but does not cause excitotoxin-induced neuronal necrosis in retina. Brain Res Bull 14, 369.

Prince D, Feeser H (1988) Dextromethorphan protects against cerebral infarction in a rat model of hypoxia-ischemia. Neurosci Lett 85, 291.

Pritchett J, Sartin J, Marple D (1979) Interaction of aging with in vitro adrenocortical responsiveness to ACTH and cyclic AMP. Horm Res 10, 96.

Pulsinelli W (1985a) Deafferentation of the hippocampus protects CA_1 pyramidal neurons against ischemic injury. Stroke 16, 144.

Pulsinelli W (1985b) Selective neuronal vulnerability: morphological and molecular characteristics. Prog Brain Res 63, 29.

Pulsinelli W, Duffy T (1983) Regional energy balance in rat brain after transient forebrain ischemia. J Neurochem 40, 1500.

Pulsinelli W, Waldman S, Rawlinson D, Plum F (1982a) Moderate hyperglycemia augments ischemic brain damage: a neuropathologic study in the rat. Neurology 32, 1239.

Pulsinelli W, Brierley J, Plum F (1982b) Temporal profile of neuronal damage in a model of transient forebrain ischemia. Ann Neurol 11, 491.

Pulsinelli W, Levy D, Sigsbee B (1983) Increased damage after ischemic stroke in patients with hyperglycemia with or without diabetes meliitus. Am J Med 74, 540.

Pumain R, Heinemann U (1985) Stimulus- and amino acid–induced calcium and potassium changes in rat neocortex. J Neurophysiol 53, 1.

Puttfarcken P, Lyons W, Coyle J (1991) Dissociation of nitric oxide generation and kainate-mediated neuronal degeneration in cerebellar granule cells. Soc Neurosci Abstr 17, 314.18.

Quelle F, Smith R, Hrycyna C, Kaliban T, Crooks J, O'Brien J (1988) ^{3}H-Dexamethasone binding to plasma membrane-enriched fractions from liver of nonadrenalectomized rats. Endocrinology 123, 1642.

Rachamin G, Luttge W, Hunter B, Walker D (1989) Neither chronic exposure to ethanol nor aging affects Type I or Type II corticosteroid receptors in rat hippocampus. Exp Neurol 106, 164.

Raff H, Shinsako J, Dallman M (1982) Surgery potentiates the adrenocortical responses to hypoxia in dogs. Proc Soc Exp Biol Med 172, 400.

Raff H, Sandri R, Segerson T (1986) Renin, ACTH and adrenocortical function during hypoxia and hemorrhage in conscious rats. Am J Physiol 250, R240.

Raff H, Flemma R, Findling J (1988) Fast cortisol-induced inhibition of the adrenocorticotropin response to surgery in humans. J Clin Endocrinol Metab 67, 1146.

Raffin C, Sick T, Rosenthal M (1988) Inhibition of glycolysis alters potassium ion transport and mitochondrial redox activity in rat brain. J Cereb Blood Flow Metab 8, 857.

Rakic P, Bourgeois J, Eckenhoff M, Zecevic N, Goldman-Rakic P (1986) Concurrent over-production of synapses in diverse regions of the primate cerebral cortex. Science 232, 232.

Raley K, Lipton P (1988) Protein synthesis and ATP in different cell populations in the rat hippocampal slice: role of calcium and NMDA receptor activation. Soc Neurosci Abstr 14.

Raley K, Lipton P (1990) NMDA receptor activation accelerates ischemic energy depletion in the hippocampal slice and the demonstration of a threshold for ischemic damage to protein synthesis. Neurosci Lett 110, 118.

Raley-Susman K, Lipton P (1990) In vitro ischemia and protein synthesis in the rat hippocampal slice: the role of calcium and NMDA receptor activation. Brain Res 515, 27.

Raley-Susman K, Cragoe E, Sapolsky R, Kopito R (1991) Regulation of intracellular pH in cultured hippocampal neurons by an amiloride-insensitive Na^+/H^+ exchanger. J Biol Chem 266, 2739.

Raley-Susman K, Kercso K, Owicki J, Sapolsky R (1992) Effects of excitotoxin exposure on metabolic rate of primary hippocampal cultures: application of silicon microphysiometry to neurobiology. J Neurosci, in press.

Randall A, Schofield J, Collingridge G (1990) Whole-cell patch-clamp recordings of an NMDA receptor-mediated synaptic current in rat hippocampal slices. Neurosci Lett 114, 191.

Ransohoff J (1972) The effects of steroids on brain edema in man. In Reulen H, Schurmann K (eds), *Steroids and Brain Edema*. Springer-Verlag, Berlin.

Rao M, Stefan H, Bauser J (1989) Epileptic but not psychogenic seizures are accompanied by simultaneous elevation of serum pituitary hormones and cortisol levels. Neuroendocrinology 49, 33.

Rapaport P, Allaire Y, Bourliere F (1964) Réactivité au "stress" et capicité d'adaptation à une situation inhabituelle chez le rat jeune, adulte et âgé. Gerontology 10, 20.

Raskind M, Peskind E, Rivard M (1982) Dexamethasone suppression test and cortisol and circadian rhythm in primary degenerative dementia. Am J Psychiatry 139, 1468.

Rasmussen T, Gulati D (1962) Cortisone in the treatment of postoperative cerebral oedema. J Neurosurg 19, 535.

Ratka A, Sutanto W, Bloemers M, de Kloet E (1989) On the role of the brain mineralocorticoid (Type I) and glucocorticoid (Type II) receptors in neuroendocrine regulation. Neuroendocrinology 50, 117.

Ray J, Sapolsky R (1992) Styles of male social behavior and their endocrine correlates among high-ranking wild baboons. Am J Primatol, in press.

Raymond V, Leung P, Veilleux R, Labrie F (1985) Vasopressin rapidly stimulates phosphatidic acid-phosphatidylinositol turnover in rat anterior pituitary cells. FEBS Lett 182, 196.

Redei E, Branch B, Gholami S, Lin E, Taylor A (1988) Effects of ethanol on CRF release in vitro. Endocrinology 123, 2736.

Rees H, Stumpf W, Sar M (1966) Autoradiographic studies with ^{3}H-dexamethasone in the rat brain and pituitary. In Stumpf W, Grant L (eds), *Anatomical Neuroendocrinology*. Karger, Basel, p 262.

Rehncrona S, Rosen I, Siesjo B (1981) Brain lactic acidosis and ischemic cell damage: 1. Biochemistry and neurophysiology. J Cereb Blood Flow Metab 1, 297.

Reid A, Teasdale G, McCulloch J (1983a) The effect of dexamethasone administration and withdrawal on water permeability across the blood-brain barrier. Ann Neurol 13, 28.

Reid A, Teasdale G, McCulloch J (1983b) Hormonal influence on water permeability across the blood-brain barrier. Clin Exp Neurol 19, 50.

Reid I (1989) Pathogenesis and treatment of steroid osteoporosis. Clin Endocrinol 30, 83.

Reisine T, Hoffman A (1983) Desensitization of corticotropin-releasing factor receptors. Biochem Biophys Res Commun 111, 919.

Reul J, de Kloet E (1985) Two receptor systems for corticosterone in rat brain: microdistribution and differential occupation. Endocrinology 117, 2505.

Reul J, de Kloet E (1986) Anatomical resolution of two types of corticosterone receptor sites in rat brain with in vitro autoradiography and computerized image analysis. J Steroid Biochem 24, 269.

Reul J, van den Bosch F, de Kloet E (1987a) Relative occupation of Type I and Type II corticosteroid receptors in rat brain following stress and dexamethasone treatment: functional implications. J Endocrinol 115, 459.

Reul J, van den Bosch F, de Kloet E (1987b) Differential response of type I and type II corticosteroid receptors to changes in plasma steroid level and circadian rhythmicity. Neuroendocrinology 45, 407.

Reul J, Tonnaer J, de Kloet E (1988) Neurotrophic ACTH analogue promotes plasticity of Type I corticosteroid receptor in brain of senescent male rats. Neurobiol Aging 9, 253.

Reul J, Pearce P, Funder J, Krozowski Z (1989) Type I and Type II corticosteroid receptor gene expression in the rat: effect of adrenalectomy and dexamethasone administration. Mol Endocrinol 3, 1674.

Reul J, de kloet E, van Sluijs F, Rijnberk A, Rothuizen J (1990) Binding characteristics of mineralocorticoid and glucocorticoid receptors in dog brain and pituitary. Endocrinology 127, 907.

Reus V, Joseph M, Dallman M (1982) ACTH levels after the dexamethasone suppression test in depression. N Engl J Med 306, 238.

Revzin A, Maickel R (1966) Failure of fornix section to block ACTH hypersecretion elicited by reserpine or cold exposure. Life Sci 5, 253.

Reynolds J, Carlen P (1989) Diminished calcium currents in aged hippocampal dentate gyrus granule neurones. Brain Res 479, 384.

Ribak C, Harris A, Vaughn J, Roberts E (1979) Inhibitory, GABAergic nerve terminals decrease at sites of focal epilepsy. Science 205, 211.

Ribak C, Hunt C, Bakay R, Oertel W (1986) A decrease in the number of GABAergic somata is associated with the preferential loss of GABAergic terminals at epileptic foci. Brain Res 363, 78.

Rich K, Hollowell J (1990) Flunarizine protects neurons from death after axotomy or NGF deprivation. Science 248, 1419.

Richardson H, Nakamura S (1971) An electron microscopic study of spinal cord edema and the effect of treatment with steroids, mannitol and hypothermia. In *Proceedings of the Veterans Administration Spinal Cord Injury Conference*, 18, 10.

Richter C, Frei B (1988) Calcium release from mitochondria induced by prooxidants. Free Radical Biol Med 4, 365.

Riegle G (1973) Chronic stress effects on adrenocortical responsiveness in young and aged rats. Neuroendocrinology 11, 1.

Riegle G, Hess G (1972) Chronic and acute dexamethasone suppression of stress activation of the adrenal cortex in young and aged rats. Neuroendocrinology 9, 175.

Rigter H, Veldhuis H, de Kloet E (1984) Spatial orientation and the hippocampal corticoterone receptor systems of old rats: effect of ACTH4-9 analogue ORG2766. Brain Res 309, 393.

Riley V (1981) Psychoneuroendocrine influences on immunocompetence and neoplasia. Science 212, 1100.

Risch C, Golshan S, Rapaport M, Dupont R, Outenreath R, Gillin J, Janowsky D (1988) Neuroendocrine effects of intravenous ovine CRF in affective disorder patients and normal controls. Biol Psychiatry 23, 755.

Rivier C, Vale W (1983a) Interaction of corticotropin-releasing factor and arginine vasopressin on adrenocorticotropin secretion in vivo. Endocrinology 113, 939.

Rivier C, Vale W (1983b) Influence of the frequency of ovine corticotropin-releasing factor administration on adrenocorticotropin and coticosterone secretion in the rat. Endocrinology 113, 1422.

Rivier C Brownstein M, Spiess J, Rivier J, Vale W (1982) In vivo corticotropin-releasing factor-induced secretion of adrenocorticotropin, beta-endorphin, and corticosterone. Endocrinology 110, 272.

Roberts J, Johnson L, Baxter J, Budarf M, Allen R, Herbert E (1979) Effect of glucocorticoids on the synthesis and processing of the common precursor to ACTH and endorphin in mouse pituitary tumor cells. In Sato G, Ross R (eds), *Hormones and Cell Cultures, Book B*. Cold Spring Harbor Laboratories, Cold Spring Harbor, p 827.

Roberts N, Barton R, Horan M (1990) Ageing and the sensitivity of the adrenal gland to physiological doses of ACTH in man. J Endocrinol 126, 507.

Robertson C, Clifton G, Goodman J (1985) Steroid administration and nitrogen excretion in the head-injured patient. J Neurosurg 63, 714.

Robertson H, Martin I, Candy J (1978) Differences in benzodiazepine receptor binding in Maudsley reactive and Maudsley non-reactive rats. Eur J Pharmacol 50, 455.

Robinson A, Seif S, Verbalis J, Brownstein M (1983) Quantification of changes in the content of neurohypophyseal peptides in hypothalamic nuclei after ADX. Neuroendocrinology 36, 347.

Romanoff L, Baxter M (1975) The secretion rates of deoxycorticosterone and corticosterone in young and elderly men. J Clin Endocrinol Metab 41, 630.

Romijn H, Ruijter J, Wolters P (1988) Hypoxia preferentially destroys GABAergic neurons in developing rat neocortex explants in culture. Exp Neurol 100, 332.

Roos A, Boron W (1981) Intracellular pH. Physiol Rev 61, 296.

Rordorf G, Koroshetz W, Nemenoff R, Vonventre J (1991) Glutamate modulates phospholipase A2 activity in cultured cortical neurons. Soc Neurosci Abstr 17, 6.2.

Rose R (1985) Psychoendocrinology. In Wilson J, Foster D (eds), *Textbook of Endocrinology* (7th ed). Saunders, Philadelphia.

Rose R, Holaday J, Bernstein I (1971) Plasma testosterone, rank and aggressive behavior in male rhesus monkeys. Nature 231, 366.

Rose R, Bernstein I, Gordon T (1975) Consequences of social conflict on plasma testosterone levels in rhesus monkeys. Psychosom Med 37, 50.

Rosen J, Fina J, Milholland R, Rosen F (1972) Inhibitory effect of cortisol in vitro on 2-deoxy-glucose uptake and RNA and protein metabolism in lymphosarcoma P1798. Cancer Res 32, 350.

Rosenberg P (1988) Catecholamine toxicity in cerebral cortex in dissociated cell culture. J Neurosci 8 2887.

Rosenberg P (1991) Accumulation of extracellular glutamate and neuronal death in astrocyte-poor cortical cultures exposed to glutamine. Glia 4, 91.

Rosenberg P, Aizenman E (1989) Hundred-fold increase in neuronal vulnerability to glutamate toxicity in astrocyte-poor cultures of rat cerebral cortex. Neurosci Lett 103, 162.

Rosenberg P, Amin S, Leitner M (1992) Glutamate uptake disguises neurotoxic potency of glutamate agonists in cerebral cortex in dissociated cell culture. J Neurosci 12, 56.

Rosewicz S, McDonald A, Maddux B, Goldfind I, Miesfeld R, Logsdon C (1988) Mechanism of glucocorticoid receptor down-regulation by glucocorticoids. J Biol Chem 263, 2581.

Rosner W (1990) The functions of CBG and sex hormone-binding globulin: recent advances. Endocrine Rev 11, 80.

Rotello J, Hocker M, Berschenson L (1989) Biochemical evidence for programmed cell death in rabbit uterine epithelium. Am J Pathol 134, 491.

Rothman S (1983) Synaptic activity mediates death of hypoxic neurons. Science 220, 536.

Rothman S (1984) Synaptic release of excitatory amino acid neurotransmitter mediates anoxic neuronal death. J Neurosci 4, 1884.

Rothman S (1985) The neurotoxicity of excitatory amino acids is produced by passive chloride influx. J Neurosci 5, 1483.

Rothman S, Thurston J, Hauhart R (1987) Delayed neurotoxicity of excitatory amino acids in vitro. Neuroscience 22, 471.

Rothschild A, Schatzberg A, Rosenbaum A, et a.l (1982) The dexamethasone suppression test as a discriminator among subtypes of psychotic patients. Br J Psychiatry 141, 471.

Rothstein J, Tabakoff B (1985) Alteration of striatal glutamate release after glutamine synthetase inhibition. J Neurochem 43, 1438.

Roy E, Lynn D, Bemm C (1990) Individual variations in hippocampal dentate degeneration following adrenalectomy. Behav Neurol Biol 54, 330.

Rubinow D, Post R, Savard R, Gold P (1984) Cortisol hypersecretion and cognitive impairment in depression. Arch Gen Psychiatry 41, 279.

Rubner M (1908) *Das Problem der Lebensdauer und seine Beziehungen zum Wachstum und Ernährung.* Oldenbourg, Munchen.

Rudorfer M, Hwu H, Clayton P (1982) Dexamethasone suppression test in primary depression: significance of family history and psychosis. Biol Psychiatry 7, 41.

Rush A (1984) A phase II study of cognitive therapy of depression. In Williams J, Spitzer R (eds), *Psychotherapy Research.* Guilford Press, New York.

Russell D, Haddox M, Gehring U (1981) Effects of dexamethasone and cyclic AMP on polyamine synthesizing enzymes in mouse lymphoma cells. J Cell Physiol 106, 375.

Russell S, Dhariwal A, McCann S, Yates F (1969) Inhibition by dexamethsone of the in vivo pituitary response to corticotropin-releasing factor. Endocrinology 85, 512.

Sabatino F, Masoro E, McMahan C, Kuhn R (1991) Assessment of the role of the glucocorticoid system in aging processes and in the action of food restriction. J Gerontol 46, B171.

Sachar E, Hellman L, Roffway H, Halpern F, Fukushima D, Gallagher T (1973) Disrupted 24-hour patterns of cortisol secretion in psychotic depression. Arch Gen Psychiatry 18, 19.

Saez J, Kessler J, Bennett M, Spray D (1987) Superoxide dismutase protects cultured neurons against death by starvation. Proc Natl Acad Sci USA 84, 3056.

Safar P (1980) Amelioration of post-ischemic brain damage with barbiturate. Stroke 2, 565.

Saito T (1990) Glucose-supported oxidative metabolism and evoked potentials are sensitive to fluoroacetate, an inhibitor of glial tricarboxylic acid cycle in the olfactory cortex slice. Brain Res 535, 205.

Sakai R, Lakshmi V, Monder C, McEwen B (1989) Presence of 11-beta-hydroxysteroid dehydrogenase in the hippocampus of the rat. Soc Neurosci Abstr 15, 290.9.

Sakai R, Weiss S, Blanchard C, Blanchard R, Spencer R, McEwen B (1991) Effect of social stress and housing conditions on neuroendocrine measures. Soc Neurosci Abstr 17, 621.1.

Sakamoto A, Ohnishi S, Ohnishi T, Ogawa R (1991) Relationship between free radical production and lipid peroxidation during ischemic-reperfusion injury in the rat brain. Brain Res 554, 186.

Sakellaris P, Vernikos-Danellis J (1975) Increased rate of response of the pituitary-adrenal system in the rats adapted to chronic stress. Endocrinology 97, 597.

Sakly M, Koch B (1981) Ontogenesis of glucocorticoid receptors in anterior pituitary gland: transient dissociation among cytoplasmic receptor density, nuclear uptake, and regulation of corticotropic activity. Endocrinology 108, 591.

Sanchez-Prieto J, Gonzalez P (1988) Occurrence of a large calcium-independent release of glutamate during anoxia in isolated nerve terminals (synaptosomes). J Neurochem 50, 1322.

Sandberg A, Slaunwhite J (1959) Tanscortin: a corticosteroid-binding protein of plasma. II. Levels in various conditions and the effects of estrogens. J Clin Invest 38, 1290.

Sandberg M, Butcher S, Hagberg H (1986) Extracellular overflow of neuroactive amino acids during severe insulin-induced hypoglycemia: in vivo dialysis of the rat hippocampus. J Neurochem 47, 178.

Schwegler H, Crusio W, Lipp H, Brust I, Mueller G (1991) Early postnatal hyperthyroidism alters hippocampal circuitry and improves radial-maze learning in a dult mice. J Neurosci 11, 2102.

Scribner K, Walker C, Cascio C, Dallman M (1991) Chronic streptozotocin diabetes in rats facilitates the acute stress response without altering pituitary or adrenal responsiveness to secretagogues. Endocrinology 129, 99.

Seckl J, Dow R, Low S, Edwards C, Fink G (1991) 11-beta-Hydroxysteroid dehydrogenase mRNA expression in paraventricular nucleus: enzyme inhibition reduces portal blood CRF. Soc Neurosci Abstr 17, 434.11.

Selander M, Hoyer S, Frotscher M (1988) Glutamate decarboxylase-immunoreactive neurons in the aging rat hippocampus are more resistant to ischemia than CA_1 pyramidal cells. Neurosci Lett 91, 241.

Selkoe D (1990) Deciphering Alzheimer's disease: the amyloid precursor protein yields new clues. Science 248, 1058.

Selye H (1936) A syndrome produced by diverse nocuous agents. Nature 138, 32.

Selye H (1975) Confusion and controversy in the stress field. J Human Stress 1, 37

Selye H (1976) *The Stress of Life*. McGraw-Hill, New York.

Selye H, Tuchweber B (1976) Stress in relation to aging and disease. In Everitt A, Burgess J (eds), *Hypothalamus, Pituitary and Aging*. CC Thomas, Springfield, p 557.

Sencar-Cupovic I, Milkovic S (1976) The development of sex differences in adrenal morphology and responsiveness in stress of rats from birth to end of life. Mech Ageing Devel 5, 1.

Seren M, Aldinio C, Zanoni R, Leon A, Nicoletti F (1989) Stimulation of inositol phospholipid hydrolysis by excitatory amino acids is enhanced in brain slices from vulnerable regions after transient global ischemia. J Neurochem 53, 1700.

Serio M, Piolanti P, Cappelli G (1969) The miscible pool and turnover rate of cortisol with aging and variations in relation to time of day. Exp Gerontol 4, 95.

Seubert P, Lee K, Lynch G (1989) Ischemia triggers NMDA receptor-linked cytoskeletal proteolysis in hippocampus. Brain Res 492, 366.

Shapira Y, Davidson E, Weidenfeld Y, Cotev S, Shohami E (1988) Dexamethasone and indomethacin do not affect brain edema following head injury in rats. J Cereb Blood Flow Metab 8, 395.

Sheardown M, Nielsen E, Hansen A, Jacobsen P, Honore T (1990) 2,3-Dihydroxy-6-nitro-7-sulfamoyl-benzo(F)quinoxaline: a neuroprotectant for cerebral ischemia. Science 247, 571.

Shepard R, Nielsen E, Broadhurst P (1982) Sex and strain differences in benzodiazepine receptor binding in Roman rat strains. Eur J Pharmacol 77, 327.

Shepard R, Jackson H, Broadhurst P, Deakin J (1984) Relationship between hyponeophagia, diazepam sensitivity and benzodiazepine receptor binding in eighteen rat genotypes. Pharmacol Biochem Behav 20, 845.

Sheppard K, Roberts J, Blum M (1990) Differential regulation of Type II corticosteroid receptor mRNA expression in the anterior pituitary and hippocampus. Endocrinology 127, 431.

Sheppard K, Roberts J, Blum M (1991) Adrenocorticotropin-releasing factor down-regulates glucocorticoid receptor expression in mouse corticotrope tumor cells via an adenylate cyclase-dependent mechanism. Endocrinology 120, 663.

Sheward W, Fink G (1991) Effects of corticosteroid on the secretion of CRF, arginine vasopressin and oxytocin into hypophysial portal blood in long-term hypophysectomized rats. J Endocrinol 129, 91.

Shigematsu K, Ishii T, McGeer P (1991) Kainic acid induces production of amyloid precursor protein in rat neurons. Soc Neurosci Abstr 17, 302.13.

Shinkai Y, Takio K, Okumura K (1988) Homology of perforin to the ninth component of complement (C9). Nature 334, 525.

Shipston M, Antoni F (1991) Early glucocorticoid feedback in anterior pituitary corticotrophs: differential inhibition of hormone release induced by vasopressin and CRF in vitro. J Endocrinol 129, 261.

Shively C, Kaplan J (1984) Effects of social factors on adrenal weight and related physiology of *Macaca fascicularis*. Phys Behav 33, 777.

Shock N (1977) Systems integration. In Finch C, Hayflick L (eds), *Handbook of the Biology of Aging*. Van Nostrand, New York.

Shohami E, Rosenthal J, Lavy S (1982) The effect of incomplete cerebral ischemia on prostaglandin levels in rat brain. Stroke 123, 494.

Shohami E, Shapira Y, Sidi A, Cotev S (1987) Head injury induces increased protaglandin synthesis in rat brain. J Cereb Blood Flow Metab 7, 58.

Siesjo B (1978) *Brain Energy Metabolism*. Wiley, New York.

Siesjo B (1981) Cell damage in the brain: a speculative synthesis. J Cereb Blood Flow Metab 1, 155.

Siesjo B (1988) Acidosis and ischemic brain damage. Neurochem Pathol 9, 31.

Siesjo B, Agardh C (1983) Hypoglycemia. In Lajtha A (ed), *Handbook of Neurochemistry, vol 3*. Plenum, New York.

Siesjo B, Bengtsson F (1989) Calcium fluxes, calcium antagonists and calcium-related pathology in brain ischemia, hypoglycemia and spreading depression: a unifying hypothesis. J Cereb Blood Flow Metab 9, 127.

Siesjo B, Wieloch T (1986) Epileptic brain damage: pathophysiology and neurochemical pathology. Adv Neurol 44, 813.

Siesjo B, Ingvar M, Westerberg E (1982) The influence of bicuculline-induced seizures on free fatty acid concentrations in cerebral cortex, hippocampus, and cerebellum. J Neurochem 39, 796.

Silverman A, Hoffman D, Zimmerman E (1981) The descending afferent connections of the paraventricular nucleus of the hypothalamus. Brain Res Bull 6, 47.

Siman P, Noszek J (1988) Excitatory amino acids activate calpain I and induce structural protein breakdown in vivo. Neuron 1, 279.

Siman R, Gall C, Perlmutter L, Christian C, Baudry M, Lynch G (1985) Distribution of calpain I, an enzyme associated with degenerative activity, in rat brain. Brain Res 347, 399.

Siman R, Noszek J, Kegerise C (1989) Calpain I activation is specifically related to excitatory amino acid induction of hippocampal damage. J Neurosci 9, 1579.

Siman R, Card J, Davis L (1990) Proteolytic processing of beta-amyloid precursor by Calpain I. J Neurosci 10, 2400.

Simon R, Swan J, Griffiths T, Meldrum B (1984a) Blockade of N-methyl-D-aspartate receptors may protect against ischemic damage in brain. Science 226, 850.

Simon R, Griffith T, Evans M, Swan J, Meldrum B (1984b) Calcium overload in selectively vulnerable neurons of the hippocampus during and after ischemia: an electron microscopic study in the rat. J Cereb Blood Flow Metab 4, 350.

Simon R, Schmidley J, Swan J, Meldrum B (1986) Neuronal alterations in hippocampus following severe hypoglycemia: a light microscopic and ultrastructural study in the rat. Neuropathol Appl Neurobiol 12, 11.

Siperstein E, Miller K (1970) Further cytophysiologic evidence for the identify of cells that produce ACTH. Endocrinology 86, 451.

Sklar L, Anisman H (1979) Stress and coping factors influence tumor growth. Science 205, 513.

Sloviter R (1987) Decreased hippocampal inhibition and a selective loss of interneurons in experimental epilepsy. Science 235, 73.

Sloviter R, Valiquette G, Abrams G, Rink E, Sollas A, Paul L, Neubort S (1989) Selective loss of hippocampal granule cells in the mature rat brain after adrenalectomy. Science 243, 535.

Slusher M, Hyde J (1961) Effect of limbic stimulation on release of corticosteroids into the adrenal venous effluent of the cat. Endocrinology 69, 1080.

Smelik P (1963) Relation between blood levels of corticoids and their inhibiting effect on the hypophyseal stress response. Proc Soc Exp Biol Med 113, 616.

Smith J, Dwyer S, Smith L (1989) Lowering extracellular pH evokes inositol polyphosphate formation and calcium mobilization. J Biol Chem 264, 8723.

Smith M, Booze R (1991) Calcium binding proteins in the septo-hippocampal system of young and aged rats. Soc Neurosci Abstr 17, 26.3.

Smither T, Flower R, Buckingham J (1990) Effects of dexamethasone treatment on the lipocortin 1 content of specific brain nuclei in the rat. J Endocrinol 120, 49.

Smuts B (1986) Sex and Friendship in Baboons. Aldine Press, Hawthorne.

Snyder S, Bredt D (1991) Nitric oxide as a neuronal messenger. Trends Pharmacol Sci 12, 125.

Sommer B, Keinanen K, Verdoorn T, Wisden W, Burnashev N, Herb A, Kohler M, Takagi T, Sakmann B, Seeburg P (1990) Flip and flop: a cell-specific functional switch in glutamate-operate channels of the CNS. Science 249, 1580.

Sonntag W, Goliszek A, Brodish A, Eldridge J (1987) Diminished diurnal secretion of adreno-corticotropin but not corticosterone in old male rats: possible relation to increased adrenal sensitivity to ACTH in vivo. Endocrinology 120, 2308.

Sousa R, Tannery N, Lafter E (1989) In situ hybridization mapping of glucocorticoid receptor mRNA in rat brain. Mol Endocrinol 3, 481.

Southwick C, Bland V (1959) Effect of population density on adrenal glands and reproductive organs of CFW mice. Am J Physiol 197, 111.

Sowers J, Tuck M, Asp N, Sollars E (1981) Plasma aldosterone and corticosterone response to adrenocorticotropin, angiotensin, potassium and stress in sopntaneously hypertensive rats. Endocrinology 108, 1216.

Spar J, Gerner R (1982) Does the dexamethasone suppression test distinguish dementia from depression? Am J Psychiatry 139, 238.

Spar J, La Rue A (1983) Major depression in the elderly: DSM-III criteria and the dexamethasone suppression test as predictors of treatment response. Am J Psychiatry 140, 844.

Sparacio R, Lin T, Cook A (1965) Methylprednisolone sodium succinate in acute craniocerebral trauma. Surg Gynecol Obstet 121, 513.

Spencer R, McEwen B (1990) Adaptation of the hypothalamic-pituitary-adrenal axis to chronic ethanol stress. Neuroendocrinology 52, 481.

Spencer R, Young E, Choo P, McEwen B (1990) Glucocorticoid Type I and Type II receptor binding: estimates of in vivo receptor number, occupancy, and activation with varying level of steroid. Brain Res 514, 37.

Spencer R, Miller A, Stein M, McEwen B (1991) Corticosterone regulation of Type I and Type II adrenal steroid receptors in brain, pituitary, and immune tissue. Brain Res 549, 236.

Sperk G, Lassmann H, Baran H, Kish S, Seitelberger F, Hornykiewicz O (1983) Kainic acid induced seizures: neurochemical and histopathological changes. Neuroscience 10, 1301.

Spielmeyer W (1922) *Histopathologie des Nervensystem.* Springer, Berlin.

Spinedi E, Giacomini M, Jacquier M, Gaillard R (1991) Changes in the hypothalamo-corticotrope axis after bilateral adrenalectomy: evidence for a median eminence site of glucocorticoid action. Neuroendocrinology 53, 160.

Squire L (1986) Mechanisms of memory. Science 232, 1612.

Sroufe L (1984) Infant-caregiver attachment and patterns of adaptation in preschool: the roots of maladaption and competence. In Perlmutter M (ed), *Minnesota Symposium in Child Psychology, vol 16.* Erlbaum, Hillsdale, NJ.

Standish-Barry H, Bouras N, Hale A, Bridges P, Bartlett J (1986) Ventricular size and CSF transmitter metabolite concentrations in severe endogenous depression. Br J Psychiatry 148, 386.

Stanley K, Luzio P (1988) A family of killer proteins. Nature 334, 475.

Stanton M, Gutierrez Y, Levine S (1988) Maternal deprivation potentiates pituitary-adrenal stress responses in infant rats. Behav Neurosci 102, 692.

Stark E, Makara G, Marton J, Palkovits M (1973) ACTH release in rats after removal of the medial hypothalamus. Neuroendocrinology 13, 224.

Steen P, Michenfelder J (1978) Cerebral protection with barbiturates, relation to anesthetic effect. Stroke 9, 140.

Steen P, Michenfelder J, Milde J (1979) Incomplete versus complete cerebral ischemia: improved outcome with a minimal blood flow. Ann Neurol 6, 389.

Stein B, Sapolsky R (1988) Chemical adrenalectomy reduces hippocampal damage induced by kainic acid. Brain Res 473, 175.

Stein M, Miller A, Trestman R (1991) Depression, the immune system, and health and illness. Arch Gen Psychiatry 48, 171.

Stein-Behrens B, Elliott E, Miller C, Schilling J, Newcombe R, Sapolsky R (1992) Glucocorticoids exacerbate kainic acid–induced extracellular accumulation of excitatory amino acids in the rat hippocampus. J Neurochem 58, 1730.

Steinberg G, Saleh J, Kunis D (1988) Delayed treatment with dextromethorphan and dextrorphan reduces cerebral damage after transient focal ischemia. Neurosci Lett 89, 193.

Steinbok P, Thompson G (1979) Serum cortisol abnormalities after craniocerebral trauma. Neurosurgery 5, 559.

Stephen F, Zucker I (1972) Circadian rhythms in drinking behavior and locomotor activity of rats are eliminated by hypothalamic lesions. Proc Natl Acad Sci USA 69, 1583.

Stephenson G, Funder J (1987) Hippocampal and renal type I receptors are differentially regulated. Am J Physiol 252, E525.

Stillman M, Recht L, Rosario S, Seif S, Robinson A, Zimmerman E (1977) The effects of ADX and glucocorticoid replacement on vasopressin and vasopressin-neurophysin in the Zona Externa of the median eminence of the rat. Endocrinology 101, 42.

Stokes P (1973) Adrenocortical activation in alcoholics during chronic drinking. Ann NY Acad Sci 215, 77.

Stokes P, Stoll P, Koslow S, Maas J, Davis J, Swann A, Robins E (1984) Pretreatment DST and hypothalamic-pituitary-adrenocortical function in depressed patients and comparison groups. Arch Gen Psychiatry 41, 257.

Stone W, Wenk G, Olton D, Gold P (1990) Poor blood glucose regulation predicts sleep and memory deficits in normal aged rats. J Gerontol 45, B169.

Strijbos P, Tilders F, Carey F, Forder R, Rothwell N (1991) Localization of immunoreactive lipocortin-1 in the brain and pituitary gland of the rat. Effects of adrenalectomy, dexamethasone and colchicine treatment. Brain Res 553, 249.

Stumpf W (1971) Autoradiographic techniques and the localization of estrogen, androgen and glucocorticoid in the pituitary and brain. Am Zool 11, 725.

Su T, London E, Jaffe J (1988) Steroid binding at sigma receptors suggests a link between endocrine, nervous and immune systems. Science 240, 219.

Sucher N, Aizenman E, Lipton S (1991) NMDA antagonists prevent kainate neurotoxicity in rat retinal ganglion cells in vitro. J Neurosci 11, 966.

Suda T, Tozawa F, Ushiyama T, Tomori N (1980) Effects of protein kinase-C—related adreno-corticotropin secretagogues and interleukin-1 on propiomelanocortin gene expression in rat anterior pituitary cells. Endocrinology 124, 1444.

Suda T, Tomori N, Tozawa F, Mouri T, Demura H, Shizume K (1983) Effects of bilateral adrenalectomy on immunoreactive CRF in the rat median eminence and intermediate-posterior pituitary. Endocrinology 113, 1182.

Suda T, Yajima F, Tomori N, Demura H, Shizume K (1985) In vitro study of immunoreactive CRF release from the rat hypothalamus. Life Sci 37, 14599.

Sugiyama K, Brunori A, Mayer M (1989) Glial uptake of excitatory amino acids influences neuronal survival in cultures of mouse hippocampus. Neuroscience 32, 779.

Sumners C, Fregley M (1989) Modulation of angiotensin II binding sites in neuronal cultures by mineralocorticoids. Am J Physiol 256, C121.

Sun A (1972) The effect of lipoxidation on synaptosomal (Na^+K^+)-ATPase isolated from the cerebral cortex of squirrel monkey. Biochem Biophys Acta 266, 350.

Suomi S (1987) Genetic and maternal contributions to individual differences in rhesus monkey biobehavioral development. In Krasnegor N, Blass E, Hofer M, Smotherman W (eds), *Perinatal Development: A Psychobiological Perspective*. Academic Press, New York.

Sutanto W, de Kloet E (1987) Species-specificity of corticosteroid receptors in hamster and rat brains. Endocrinology 121, 1405.

Suzuki K, Kono T (1980) Evidence that insulin causes translocation of glucose transport activity to the plasma membrane from an intracellular storage site. Proc Natl Acad Sci USA 77, 2542.

Suzuki O, Takanohashi M, Yagi K (1987) Protective effect of dexamethasone on enhancement of blood-brain barrier permeability caused by electroconvulsive shock. Drug Res 26, 533.

Suzuki R, Yamaguchi T, Choh-Luh L, Klatzo I (1983) The effects of 5-minute ischemia in Mongolian gerbils. II. Changes of spontaneous neuronal activity in cerebral cortex and CA_1 sector of hippocampus. Acta Neuropathol (Berl) 60, 217.

Svec F, Rudis M (1981) Glucocorticoids regulate the glucocorticoid receptor in the AtT-20 cell. J Biol Chem 256, 5984.

Swan J, Evans M, Meldrum B (1988) Long-term development of selective neuronal loss and the mechanism of protection by 2-amino-7-phosphonoheptanoate in a rat model of incomplete forebrain ischaemia. J Cereb Blood Flow Metab 8, 64.

Swanson L, Simmons D (1989) Differential steroid hormone and neural influences on peptide mRNA levels in CRH cells of the paraventricular nucleus: a hybridization histochemical study in the rat. J Comp Neurol 285, 413.

Swanson L, Sawchenko P, Rivier J, Vale W (1983) Organization of ovine CRF immunoreactive cells and fibers in the rat brain: an immunohistochemical study. Neuroendocrinology 36, 165.

Swanson R, Choi D (1990) The vulnerability of cultured cortical neurons to glucose-deprivation-induced injury is influenced by glial glycogen stores. Soc Neurosci Abstr 16, 18.

Swanson R, Yu A, Chan P, Sharp F (1990) Glutamate increases glycogen content and reduces glucose utilization in primary astrocyte culture. J Neurochem 54, 490.

Swenson R, Vogel W (1983) Plasma catecholamine and corticosterone as well as brain catecholamine changes during coping in rats exposed to stressful foot shock. Pharmacol Biochem Behav 18, 689.

Szatkowsski M, Barbour B, Attwell D (1990) Non-vesicular release of glutamate from glial cells by reversed electrogenic glutamate uptake. Nature 348, 443.

Szerb J (1988) Changes in the relative amounts of aspartate and glutamate released and retained in hippocampal slices during stimulation. J Neurochem 50, 219.

Szerb J, O'Regan P (1988) Increase in the stimulation-induced overflow of excitatory amino acids from hippocampal slices: interaction between low glucose concentration and fluoroacetate. Neurosci Lett 86, 207.

Sztriha L, Joo F, Szerdahelyi P, Koltai M (1986) Effect of dexamethasone on brain oedema induced by kainic acid. Neuroscience 17, 107.

Taft W, Tennes-Rees K, Blair R, Clifton G, DeLorenzo R (1988) Cerebral ischemia decreases endogenous calcium-dependent protein phosphoryolation in gerbil brain. Brain Res 447, 159.

Tanaka S, Sako K, Tanaka T, Yonemasu Y (1989) Regional calcium accumulation and kainic acid (KA)–induced limbic seizure status in rats. Brain Res 478, 385.

Tang C, Dichter M, Morad M (1990) Modulation of the NMDA channel by extracellular H^+. Proc Natl Acad Sci USA 87, 6445.

Tang G, Phillips R (1978a) Some age-related changes in pituitary-adrenal function in the male laboratory rat. J Gerontol 33, 377.

Tang G, Phillips R (1978b) Some age-related changes in pituitary-adrenal function in young and aged rats. Am J Physiol 222, 1458.

Tanimoto M, Okada Y (1987) The protective effect of hypothermia on hippocampal slices from guinea pig during deprivation of oxygen and glucose. Brain Res 417, 239.

Tannahill L, Sheward W, Robinson I, Fink G (1991) CRF-41, vasopressin and oxytocin release into hypophysial portal blood in the rat: effects of electrical stimulation of the hypothalamus, amygdala and hippocampus. J Endocrinol 129, 99.

Tator C (1972) Acute spinal cord injury: a review of recent studies of treatment and pathophysiology. Can Med Assoc J 107, 143.

Taylor A, Fishman L (1988) Corticotropin-releasing hormone. N Engl J Med 319, 213.

Taylor M, Palmer G, Callahan A (1984) Protective action by methylprednisolone, allopurinol and indomethacin against stroke-induced damage to adenylate cyclase in gerbil cerebral cortex. Stroke 15, 329.

Taylor M, Mellert T, Permentier J, Eddy L (1985) Pharmacological protection of reoxygenation damage to in vitro brain slice tissue. Brain Res 347, 268.

Temesvari P, Joo F, Koltai M, Eck E, Adam G, Siklos L, Boda D (1984) Cerebroprotective effect of dexamethasone by increasing the tolerance to hypoxia and preventing brain oedema in newborn piglets with experimetnal pneumothorax. Neurosci Lett 49, 87.

Tennes K (1982) The role of hormones in mother-infant transactions. In Emde R, Harmon R (eds), *Development of Attachment and Affiliative Systems*. Plenum, New York.

Terry R, Katzman R (1983) Senile dementia of the Alzheimer type. Neurology 14, 497.

Theoret Y, Caldwell-Kenkel J, Krigman M (1985) The role of neuronal metabolic insult in organometal neurotoxicity. Toxicologist 6, abstract 491.

Thilmann R, Xie Y, Kleihues P, Kiessling M (1986) Persistent inhibition of protein synthesis precedes delayed neuronal death in postischemic gerbil hippocampus. Acta Neuropathol (Berl) 71, 88.

Thomas A, Chess S, Birch H (1968) *Temperament and Behavior Disorders in Children*. New York University Press, New York.

Thyagarajan R, Brennan T, Ticku M (1983) GABA and benzodiazepine binding sites in spontaneously hypertensive rats. Eur J Pharmacol 93, 127.

Thygesen P, Harmann K, Willanger R (1970) Concentration camp survivors in Denmark: persecution, disease, disability, compensation. Dan Med Bull 17, 65.

Todd M, Chardwick H, Shapiro H, Dunlap M, Marchall L, Dueck R (1982) The neurologic effects of thiopental therapy following experimental cardiac arrest in cats. Anesthesiology 57, 76.

Tombaugh G, Sapolsky R (1990a) Mild acidosis protects hippocampal neurons from injury induced by oxygen and glucose deprivation. Brain Res 506, 343.

Tombaugh G, Sapolsky R (1990b) Mechanistic distinctions between excitotoxic and acidotic hippocampal damage in an in vitro model of ischemia. J Cereb Blood Flow Metab 10, 527.

Tombaugh G, Sapolsky R (1990c) Hippocampal glutamine synthetase: insensitivity to glucocorticoids and stress. Am J Physiol 258, E894.

Tombaugh G, Sapolsky R (1992) Endocrine features of glucocorticoid endangerment in hippocampal astrocytes. Neuroendocrinology, in press.

Tombaugh G, Yang S, Swanson R, Sapolsky R (1992) Glucocorticoids exacerbate hypoxic and hypoglycemic hippocampal injury in vitro: biochemical correlates and a role for astrocytes. J Neurochem, in press.

Tominaga T, Katagi H, Ohnishi S (1988) Is calcium-activated potassium efflux involved in the formation of ischemic brain edema? Brain Res 460, 376.

Tominaga T, Fukata J, Naito Y, Nakai Y, Funakoshi S, Fujii N, Imura H (1990) Effects of corticostatin-I on rat adrenal cells in vitro. J Endocrinol 125, 287.

Ton H, Arai A, Eveleth D, Lynch G, Bartus R (1991) Novel calpain inhibitors offer greater hypoxic protection of synaptic transmission in hippocampal slices. Soc Neurosci Abstr 17, 500.16.

Tornello S, Orti F, De Nicola A, Rainbow T, McEwen B (1982) Regulation of glucocorticoid receptors in brain by corticosterone treatment of adrenalectomized rats. Neuroendocrinology 35, 411.

Tornheim P, McLaurin R (1978) Effect of dexamethasone on cerebral edema from cranial impact in the cat. J Neurosurg 48, 220.

Torp R, Andine P, Hagber H, Kargulle T, Blackstad T, Otterson O (1991) Cellular and sub-cellular distribution of glutamate-, glutamine- and taurine-like immunoreactivity during fore-brain ischemia: a semiquantitative electron microscopic study in rat hippocampus. Neuroscience 41, 433.

Touitou Y, Sulon J, Bogdan A (1983) The adrenocortical hormones, aging and mental condition: seasonal and circadian rhythm of plasma 18-OH-11-DOC total and free cortisol and urinary corticosteroids. J Endocrinol 96, 53.

Tourigny-Rivard M, Raskind M, Rivard D (1981) The dexamethasone suppression test in an elderly population. Biol Psychiatry 16, 1177.

Towle A, Sze P (1983) Steroid binding to synaptic plasma membrane: differential binding of glucocorticoids and gonadal steroids. J Steroid Biochem 18, 135.

Tramu G, Croix C, Pillez A (1983) Ability of the CRF immunoreactive neurons of the paraventri-cular nucleus to produce a vasopressin-like material. Neuroendocrinology 37, 467.

Traynelis S, Cull-Candy S (1990) Proton inhibition of NMDA receptors in cerebellar neurons. Nature 345, 347.

Treiman D, Levine S (1969) Plasma corticosteroid response to stress in four species of wild mice. Endocrinology 84, 676.

Trethowan W, Cobb S (1952) Neuropsychiatric aspects of Cushing's syndrome. Arch Neurol Psychiatry 67, 283.

Trivedi B, Danforth W (1966) Effect of pH on the kinetics of frog muscle phosphofructokinase. J Biol Chem 241, 4110.

Truman J (1984) Cell death in invertebrate nervous system. Annu Rev Neurosci 7, 171.

Truman J, Schwartz L (1984) Steroid regulation of neuronal death in the moth nervous system. J Neurosci 4, 274.

Truman J, Fahrbach S, Kimura K (1989) Hormones and programmed cell death: insights from invertebrate studies. Abstract 3, Molecular and Cellular Mechanisms of Neuronal Plasticity in Aging and Alzheimer's Disease. NIA Meeting, May, 1989.

Tsuboi S, Kawashima R, Tomioka O, Nakata M, Sakamoto N, Fujita T (1979) Glucocorticoid binding proteins of human brain cytosol. Brain Res 179, 181.

Tsuda T, Kogure K, Nishioka K, Watanabe T (1991) Magnesium administered up to 24 hours following reperfusion prevents ischemic damage of the CA_1 neurons in the rat hippocampus. Neuroscience 44, 335.

Tunnicliff G, Welborn K, Head R (1984) The GABA/benzodiazepine receptor complex in the nervous system of a hypertensive strain of rat. Neurochem Res 9, 1033.

Turner B (1986) Tissue differences in the up-regulation of glucocorticoid-binding proteins in the rat. Endocrinology 118, 1211.

Turner P, Westwood T, Regen C, Steinhardt R (1988) Increased protein degradation results from elevated free calcium levels found in muscle from mdx mice. Nature 335, 735.

Turski L, Bressler K, Rettig K, Loschman P, Wachtel H (1991) Protection of substantia nigra from MPP neurotoxicity by NMDA antagonists. Nature 349, 414.

Ucker D (1987) Cytotoxic T lymphocytes and glucocorticoids activate an endogenous suicide process in target cells. Nature 327, 62.

Uemura Y, Kowall N, Beal M (1991) Global ischemia induces NMDA receptor-mediated c-fos expression in neurons resistant to injury in gerbil hippocampus. Brain Res 542, 343.

Umansky S, Korol B, Nelipovich P (1981) In vivo degradation in thymocytes of irradiated or hydrocortisone-treated rats. Biochim Biophys Acta 655, 9.

Uno H, Schroeder B, Alsum P, Takahashi I, Kalin N (1989a) The effect of prenatal stress on the hippocampus in rats. Soc Neurosci Abstr 15, 110.6.

Uno H, Tarara R, Else J, Suleman M, Sapolsky R (1989b) Hippocampal damage associated with prolonged and fatal stress in primates. J Neurosci 9, 1705.

Uno H, Lohmiller L, Thieme C, Kemnitz J, Engle M, Roecker E, Farrell P (1990) Brain damage induced by prenatal exposure to dexamethasone in fetal rhesus macaques. I. Hippocampus. Dev Brain Res 53, 157.

Uno H, Flugge G, Thieme C, Johren O, Fuchs E (1991) Degeneration of the hippocampal pyramidal neurons in the socially stressed tree shrew. Soc Neurosci Abstr 17, 52.20.

Ur E (1991) Psychological aspects of hypothalamo-pituitary-adrenal activity. Bailliere's Clin Endocrinol Metab 5, 79.

Urban L, Neill K, Crain B, Nadler J, Somjen G (1989) Postischemic synaptic physiology in area CA_1 of the gerbil hippocampus studied in vitro. J Neurosci 9, 3966.

Urban L, Neill K, Crain B, Nadler J, Somjen G (1990) Postischemic synaptic excitation and NMDA receptor activation in gerbils. Stroke 21, 23 (suppl).

Vale W, Spiess J, Rivier C, Rivier J (1981) Characterization of a 4l-residue ovine hypothalamic peptide that stimulates secretion of corticotropin and beta-endorphin. Science 213, 1394.

Vale W, Vaughan J, Smith M, Yamamoto G, Rivier J, Rivier C (1983) Effects of synthetic ovine CRF, glucocorticoids, catecholamines, neurohypophysial peptides, and other substances on cultured corticotrophic cells. Endocrinology 13, 1121.

Vallette G, Vanet A, Sumida C, Nunez E (1991) Modulatory effects of unsaturated fatty acids on the binding of glucocorticoids to rat liver glucocorticoid receptors. Endocrinology 129, 1363.

Van den Berg D, de Kloet E, de Jong W (1990) Differential central effects of mineralocorticoid and glucocorticoid agonists and antagonists on blood pressure. Endocrinology 126, 118.

van der Kuil J, Korf J (1991) On-line monitoring of extracellular brain glucose using micro-dialysis and a NADPH-linked enzymatic assay. J Neurochem 57, 648.

van Eekelen A (1990) Neuroendocrine implications of brain corticosteroid receptor diversity. Doctoral dissertation, University of Utrecht.

van Eekelen J, Kiss J, Westphal H, de Kloet E (1987) Immunocytochemical study on the intracellular localization of the Type II glucocorticoid receptor in the rat brain. Brain Res 436, 120.

van Eekelen J, Jiang W, de Kloet E, Bohn M (1988) Distribution of the mineralocorticoid and the glucocorticoid receptor mRNAs in the rat hippocampus. J Neurosci Res 21, 88.

van Eekelen J, Rots N, Sutanto W, de Kloet E (1991) The effect of aging on stess responsiveness and central corticosteroid receptors in the brown Norway rat. Neurobiol Aging 13, 159.

van Oers J, Hinson J, Binnekade R, Tilders F (1992) Physiological role of CRF in the control of adrenocorticotropin-mediated corticosterone relase from the rat adrenal gland. Endocrinology 130, 282.

Vass K, Welch W, Nowak T (1988) Localation of 70 kDa stress protein induction in gerbil brain after ischemia. Acta Neuropathol (Berl) 77, 128.

Vaughan D, Peters A (1974) Neuroglial cells in the cerebral cortex of rats from young adulthood to old age. An electron microscope study. J Neurocytol 3, 405.

Veldhuis H, de Kloet E (1982a) Significance of ACTH4-10 in the control of hippocampal corticosterone receptor capacity of hypophysectomized rats. Neuroendocrinology 34, 374.

Veldhuis H, de Kloet E (1982b) Vasopressin related peptides increase the hippocampal corticosterone receptor capacity of diabetes insipidus (Brattleboro rat). Endocrinology 110, 153.

Vermes I, Mulder G, Smelik P (1977) A superfusion system technique for the study of the sites of action of glucocorticoids in the rat hypothalamus-pituitary-adrenal system in vitro. II. Hypothalamus-pituitary-adrenal cell superfusion. Endocrinology 100, 1153.

Vernikos J, Dallman M, Bonner C, Katzen A, Shinsako J (1982) Pituitary-adrenal function in rats chronically exposed to cold. Endocrinology 110, 413.

Vibulsreth S, Hefti F, Ginsberg M, Dietrich W, Busto R (1987) Astrocytes protect cultured neurons from degeneration induced by anoxia. Brain Res 422, 303.

Vielkind U, Walencewicz A, Levine J, Bohn M (1990) Type II glucocorticoid receptors are expressed in oligodendrocytes and astrocytes. J Neurosci Res 27, 360.

Vijayan V, Cotman C (1987) Hydrocortisone administration alters glial reaction to entorhinal lesion in the rat dentate gyrus. Exp Neurol 96, 307.

Vink R, McIntosh T, Demediuk P, Faden A (1987) Decrease in total and free magnesium concentration following traumatic brain injury in rats. Biochem. Biophys Res Commun 149, 594.

Vink R, McIntosh T, Faden A (1988a) Treatment with the thyrotropin-releasing hormone analog CG3703 restores magnesium homeostasis following traumatic brain injury in rats. Brain Res 460, 184.

Vink R, McIntosh T, Demediuk P, Weiner M, Faden A (1988b) Decline in intracellular free magnesium is associated with irreversible tissue injury after brain trauma. J Biol Chem 263, 757.

Virgin C, Ha T, Packan D, Tombaugh G, Yang S, Horner H, Sapolsky R (1991) Glucocorticoids inhibit glucose transport and glutamate uptake in hippocampal astrocytes: implications for glucocorticoid neurotoxicity. J Neurochem 57, 1422.

Visintainer M, Volpicelli J, Seligman M (1982) Tumor rejection in rats after inescapable or escapable shock. Science 216, 437.

Volicer L, Crino P (1990) Involvement of free radicals in dementia of the Alzheimer type: a hypothesis. Neurobiol Aging 11, 567.

Voll C, Auer R (1991) Postischemic seizures and necrotizing ischemic brain damage: neuroprotective effect of postischemic diazepam and insulin. Neurology 41, 423.

von Bardeleben U, Holsboer F (1989) Cortisol response to a combined dexamethasone-human CRH challenge in patients with depression. J Neuroendocrinol 1, 485.

von Bardeleben U, Holsboer F (1991) Effect of age on the cortisol response to human CRH in depressed patients pretreated with dexamethasone. Biol Psychiatry 29, 1042.

von Bardeleben U, Holsboer F, Stalla G, Muller O (1985) Combined administration of human corticotropin-releasing factor and lysine vasopressin induces cortisol escape from dexametahsone suppression in healthy subjects. Life Sci 37, 1613.

von Bardeleben U, Holsboer F, Stalla G, Muller O (1988) Blunting of ACTH response to h-CRH in depressed patients avoided through metyrapone induced cortisol decrease. Biol Psychiatry 24, 782.

von Lubitz D, Dambrosia J, Kempski O, Redmond D (1988) Cyclohexyl adenosine protects against neuronal death following ischemia in the CA_1 region of gerbil hippocampus. Stroke 19, 1133.

Vornov J, Coyle J (1991) Enhancement of NMDA receptor-mediated neurotoxicity in the hippocampal slice by depolarization and ischemia. Brain Res 555, 99.

Vorstrup S, Jensen K, Thomsen C, Henriksen O, Lassen N, Paulson O (1989) Neuronal pH regulation: constant normal intracellular pH is maintained in brain during low extracellular ph induced by acetazolamide—^{31}P NMR study. J Cereb Blood Flow Metab 9, 417.

Vyklicky L, Vlachova V, Krusek J (1990) The effect of external pH changes on responses to excitatory amino acids in mouse hippocampal neurones. J Physiol 430, 497.

Walker C, Rivest R, Meaney M, Aubert M (1989) Differential activation of the pituitary-adrenocortical axis after stress in the rat: use of two genetically selected lines (RLA and RHA) as a model. J Endocrinol 123, 477.

Walker D, Barnes D, Zornetzer S, Hunter B, Kubanis P (1980) Neuronal loss in hippocampus induced by prolonged ethanol consumption in rats. Science 209, 711.

Walkowitz O, Reus V, Weingartner H, Thompson K, Breier A, Doran A, Rubinow D, Pickar D (1990) Cognitive effects of corticosteroids. Am J Psychiatry 140, 1297.

Wallner B, Mattaliano R, Hession C, Cate R, Tizard R, Sinclair L, Foeller C, Pingchang C, Browning J, Ramachandran K, Pepinsky R (1986) Cloning and expression of human lipocortin, a phospholipase A2 inhibitor with potential anti-inflammatory activity. Nature 320, 77.

Walz W (1989) Role of glial cells in the regulation of the brain ion microenvironment. Prog Neurobiol 33, 309.

Wand G (1989) Ethanol differentially regulates proadrenocorticotropin/endorphin production and corticosterone secretion in LS and SS lines of mice. Endocrinology 24, 518.

Wand G, Eipper B (1987) Effect of chronic secretagogue exposure on proadrenocorticotropin/endorphin production and secretion in primary cultures of rat anterior pituitary. Endocrinology 120, 953.

Wand G, May V, Eipper B (1988) Comparison of acute and chronic secretagogue regulation of proadrenocorticotropin/endorphin synthesis, secretion and messenger ribonucleic acid production in primary cultures of rat anterior pituitary. Endocrinology 123, 1153.

Wand G, Takiyyuddin M, O'Connor D, Levine M (1991) A proposed role for chromogranin A as a glucocorticoid-responsive autocrine inhibitor of proopiomelanocortin secretion. Endocrinology 128, 1345.

Ward J, Becker D, Miller D, Choy S, Marmarou A, Wood C, Newlon P, Keenan R (1985) Failure of prophylactic barbiturate coma in the treatment of severe head trauma. J Neurosurg 62, 383.

Warembourg M (1975) Radioautographic study of the rat brain and pituitary after injection of ^{3}H-dexamethasone. Cell Tissue Res 161, 183.

Warner M, Neill K, Nadler J, Crain B (1991) Regionally selective effects of NMDA receptor antagonists against ischemic brain damage in the gerbil. J Cereb Blood Flow Metab 11, 600.

Warren M (1983) Effects of undernutrition on reproductive function in the human. Endocrine Rev 4, 363.

Wasterlain C, Massarweh W, Sollas A, Rouk E, Sloviter R (1988) Selective vulnerability of neurons to hypoxia-ischemia: role of calcium-binding protein. Soci Neurosci Abstr 14, 429.2.

Watabe T, Tanaka K, Kumagae M, Itoh S (1988) Role of endogenous AVP in potentiating CRH-stimulated corticotropin secretion in man. J Clin Endocrinol Metab 66, 1132.

Watanabe K, Hara K, Miyazaki S, Hakamada S (1980) The role of perinatal brain injury in the genesis of childhood epilepsy. Folia Psychiatr Neurol Jpn 34, 227.

Watson S, Sherman T, Schafer K, Patel P, Herman J, Akil H (1989) Regulation of mRNA in peptidergic systems: quantitative and in situ studies. In McKerns K, Chretien M (eds), *Molecular Biology of Brain and Endocrine Peptidergic Systems*. Plenum, New York.

Weeks J, Truman J (1985) Independent steroid control of the fates of motoneurons and their muscles during insect metamorphosis. J Neurosci 5 2290.

Weeks J, Truman J (1986) Hormonally-mediated reprogramming of muscles and motoneurons during the larval-pupal transformation of the tobacco hornworm, *Manduca sexta*. J Exp Biol 125, 1.

Weichsel M (1974) Glucocorticoid effect upon thymidine kinase in the developing cerebellum. Pediatr Res 8, 843.

Weidenfeld J, Siegel R, Conforti N, Chowers I, Feldman S (1984) A temporal study of post-adrenalectomy increase in ACTH secretion in the rat: effect of various hypothalamic deafferentations. Brain Res 322, 329.

Weidenfeld J, Lysy J, Shohami E (1987) The effect of dexamethasone on prostaglandin synthesis in various brain areas of the rat. J Neurochem 48, 1351.

Weill C, Greene D (1984) Prevention of natural motoneurone cell death by dibutyryl cyclic GMP. Nature 308, 452.

Weindruch R, Walford R (1988) *The Retardation of Aging and Disease by Dietary Restriction*. C C Thomas, Springfield, Ill.

Weiner M (1989) Age and corticol suppression by dexamethasone normal subjects. J Psychiat Res 23, 163.

Weiner M, Davis B, Mohs R, Davis K (1987) Influence of age and relative weight on cortisol suppression in normal subjects. Am J Psychiatry 144, 646.

Weismann A (1889) The duration of life. In Poulton B, Schonland S, Shipley A (eds), *Essays upon Heredity and Kindred Biological Problems*. Clarendon Press, Oxford.

Weiss J (1971a) Effects of coping behavior in different warning signal conditions on stress pathology in rats. J Comp Physiol Psychol 77, 1.

Weiss J (1971b) Effects of punishing the coping respose (conflict) on stress pathology in rats. J Comp Physiol Psychol 77, 14.

Weiss J (1971c) Effects of coping behavior with and without a feedback signal on stress pathology in rats. J Comp Physiol Psychol 77, 22.

Weiss J 1984 Behavioral and psychological influences on gastrointestinal pathology. In Gentry W (ed), *Handbook of Behavioral Medicine*. The Guilford Press, New York.

Weiss J, Goldberg M, Choi D (1986) Ketamine protects cultured neocortical neurons from hypoxic injury. Brain Res 390, 186.

Weiss J, Hartley D, Koh J, Choi D (1990) The calcium channel blocker nifedipine attenuates slow excitatory amino acid neurotoxicity. Science 247, 1474.

Weiss S (1989) Tissue destruction by neutrophils. N Engl J Med 320, 365.

Welsh F, Harris V (1991) Postischemic hypothermia fails to reduce ischemic injury in gerbil hippocampus. J Cereb Blood Flow Metab 11, 617.

Welsh F, Sims R, Harris V (1990) Mild hypothermia prevents ischemic injury in gerbil hippocampus. J Cereb Blood Flow Metab 10, 557.

Wertheimer E, Sasson S, Cerasi E, Ben-Neriah Y (1991) The ubiquitous glucose transporter GLUT-1 belongs to the glucose-regulated protein family of stress-inducible proteins. Proc Natl Acad Sci USA 88, 2525.

West C, Brown H, Simons E, Carter D, Kumagai L, Engelbert E (1961) Adrenocortical function and cortisol metabolism in old age. J Clin Endocrinol Metab 21, 1197.

Westbrook G, Mayer M (1987) Micromolar concentrations of Zn^{++} antagonize NMDA and GABA responses of hippocampal neurons. Nature 328, 212.

Westerberg E, Deshpande J, Wieloch T (1987) Regional differences in arachidonic acid release in rat hippocampal CA_1 and CA_3 regions during cerebral ischemia. J Cereb Blood Flow Metab 7, 189.

Westerberg E, Kehr J, Ungerstedt U, Wieloch T (1988) The NMDA-antagonist MK-801 reduces extracellular amino acid levels during hypoglycemia and prevents striatal damage. Neurosci Res Commun 3, 151.

Westlund K, Aguilera G, Childs G (1985) Quantification of morphological changes in pituitary corticotropes produced by in vivo corticotropin-releasing factor stimulation and adrenalectomy. Endocrinology 155, 439.

Westphal U (1971) *Steroid-Protein Interactions.* Springer-Verlag, New York.

Wexler B, McMurty J (1983) Cushingoid pathophysiology of old, massively obese, spontaneously hypertensive rats (SHR). J Gerontol 38, 148.

Whitehouse P, Vale W, Zweig R, Singer H, Mayeux R, Kuhar M, Price D, De Souza E (1987) Reductions in CRF-like immunoreactivity in cerebral cortex in Alzheimer's disease, Parkinson's disease, and progressive supranuclear palsy. Neurology 37, 905.

Whitnall M, (1988) Distributions of pro-vasopressin expressing and pro-vasopressin deficient CRH neurons in the paraventricular hypothalamic nucleus of colchicine-treated normal and adrenalectomized rats. J Comp Neurol 275, 13.

Whitnall M (1990) Subpopulations of CRH neurosecretory cells distinguished by presence or absence of vasopressin: confirmation with multiple CRH antisera. Neuroscience 36, 201.

Whitnall M, Smyth D, Gainer H (1987) Vasopressin coexists in half of the corticotropin-releasing factor axons present in the external zone of the median eminence in normal rats. Neuroendocrinology 45, 420.

Widmaier E, Dallman M (1984) The effects of CRF on ACTH secretion from perifused pituitaries in vitro: rapid inhibition by glucocorticoids. Endocrinology 115, 2368.

Widmaier E, Plotsky P, Sutton S, Vale W (1988) Regulation of CRF secretion in vitro by glucose. Am J Physiol 255, E287.

Widmann R, Kuroiwa T, Bonnekoh P, Hossmann K (1991) ^{14}C-Leucine incorporation into brain proteins in gerbils after transient ischemia: relationship to selective vulnerability of hippocampus. J Neurochem 56, 789.

Wielckens K, Delfs T (1986) Glucocorticoid-induced cell death and poly[adenosine diphosphate(ADP)-ribosyl]ation: increased toxicity of dexamethasone on mouse S49.1 lymphoma cells with the poly(ADP-Ribsyl)ation inhibitor benzamide. Endocrinology 119, 2383.

Wielckens K, Delfs T, Muth A, Freese V, Kleeberg H (1987) Glucocorticoid-induced lymphoma cell death: the good and the evil. J Steroid Biochem 27, 413.

Wieloch T (1985) Hypoglycemia-induced neuronal damage prevented by an N-methyl-D-aspartate antagonist. Science 230, 681.

Wieloch T, Engelsen G, Westerberg E, Auer R (1985a) Lesions of the glutamatergic corticostriatal projections in the rat ameliorate hypoglycemic brain damage in the striatum. Neurosci Lett 58, 25.

Wieloch T, Lindvall O, Blomqvuist P, Gage F (1985b) Evidence for amelioration of ischemic neuronal damage in the hippocampal formation by lesions of the perforant path. Neurol Res 7, 24.

Wieloch T, Gustafson I, Westerberg E (1989) The NMDA antagonist, MK-801, is cerebro-protective in situations where some energy production prevails but not under conditions of complete energy deprivation. J Cereb Blood Flow Metab 9 (suppl 1), S6.

Wilkinson C, Shinsako J, Dallman M (1981) Return of pituitary-adrenal function after adrenal enucleation or transplantation: diurnal rhythms and responses to ether. Endocrinology 109, 162.

Williams J, Errington M, Lynch M, Blisds T (1989) Arachidonic acid induces a long-term activity-dependent enhancement of synaptic transmission in the hippocampus. Nature 341, 739.

Williams M (1989) Adenosine: the prototypic neuromodulator. Neurochem Int 14, 249.

Wilson M (1975) Effect of hippocampectomy on dexamethasone suppression of corticosteroid-sensitive stress responses. Anat Rec 181, 511.

Wilson M, Critchlow (1973a) Effect of fornix transection or hippocampectomy on rhythmic pituitary-adrenal function in the rat. Neuroendocrinology 13, 29.

Wilson M, Critchlow V (1973b) Effect of partial hippocampal resection on stress mechanisms in rats. Am J Physiol 201, 337.

Wilson M, Critchlow V (1975) Absence of circadian rhythm in persisting corticosterone fluctuations following surgical isolation of the medial basal hypothalamus. Neuroendocrinology 19, 185.

Wilson M, Greer S, Greer M, Roberts L (1980) Hippocampal inhibition of pituitary-adreno-cortical function in female rats. Brain Res 197, 433.

Wilson M, Greer S, Greer M (1983) Nycterohemeral difference in inhibition of stress-induced ACTH in adrenalectomized rats. Am J Physiol 244, E186.

Winick M, Coscia A (1968) Cortisone induced growth failure in neonatal rats. Pediatr Res 2, 451.

Winokur G, Pfohl B, Sherman B (1985) The relationships of historically defined subtypes of depression to ACTH and cortisol levels in dpression: preliminary study. Biol Psychiatry 20, 751.

Wisniewski H, Terry T (1973) Morphology of the aging brain: human and animal. Prog Brain Res 40, 167.

Wolff B, Dickson R, Hanover J (1987) A nuclear localization signal in steroid hormone receptors? Trends Pharmacol Sci 8, 119.

Wolff C, Friedman S, Hofer M, Mason J (1964) Relationship between psychological defenses and mean urinary 17-hydroxycorticosteroid excretion rates. Psychosom Med 26, 576.

Wolfson B, Manning R, Davis L, Arntzen R, Baldino F (1985) Co-localization of corticotropin releasing factor and vasopressin mRNA in neurons after adrenalectomy. Nature 315, 59.

Wolkowitz O, Rubinow D, Doran A, Breier A, Berrettini W, Kling M, Pickar D (1990) Prednisone effects on neurochemistry and behavior. Arch Gen Psychiatry 47, 963.

Won J, Jap T, Ching K, Chiang B (1987) Modulatory effects of CRF on the delayed corti-costeroid feedback in humans: implications of feedback sites. Metabolism 36, 935.

Wong B, Coulter D, Choi D, Prince D (1988) Dextrorphan and dextromethorphan, common antitussives, are antiepileptic and antagonize NMDA in brain slices. Neurosci Lett 85, 261.

Woolley C, Gould E, McEwen B (1990) Exposure to excess glucocorticoids alters dendritic morphology of adult hippocampal pyramidal neurons. Brain Res, in press.

Woolley C, Gould E, Sakai R, Spencer R, McEwen B (1991) Effects of aldosterone or RU28362 treatment on adrenalectomy-induced cell death in the dentate gyrus in the adult rat. Brain Res 554, 312.

Wurtman R, Axelrod J (1966) Control of enzymatic synthesis of adrenaline in the adrenal medulla by adrenal cortical steroids. J Biol Chem 241, 2301.

Wyllie A (1980) Glucocorticoid-induced thymocyte apoptosis is associated with endogenous endonuclease activation. Nature 284, 555.

Wyllie A, Morris R, Smith A, Dunlop D (1984) Chromatin cleavage in apoptosis: association with condensed chromatin morphology and dependence on macromolecular synthesis. J Pathol 142, 67.

Wynn P, Harwood J, Catt K, Aguilera G (1985) Regulation of CRF receptors in the rat pituitary gland: effects of adrenalectomy on CRF receptors and corticotroph responses. Endocrinology 116, 1653.

Wynne-Edwards V (1962) Animal Dispersion in Relation to Social Behavior. Hafner, New York.

Yakovlev A, de Bernardi M, Fabrazzo M, Brooker G, Costa E, Mocchetti I (1990) Regulation of nerve growth factor receptor mRNA content by dexamethasone: in vitro and in vivo studies. Neurosci Lett 116, 216.

Yamada T, McGeer P, Baimbridge K McGeer E (1990) Relative sparing in Parkinson's disease of substantia nigra dopamine neurons containing calbindin-D28K. Brain Res 526, 303.

Yamamoto K (1985) Steroid receptor regulated transcription of specific genes and gene networks. Annu Rev Genet 19, 209.

Yamamoto M, Shima T, Uozumi T, Sogabe T, Yamada K, Kawasaki T (1983) A possible role of lipid peroxidation in cellular damages caused by cerebral ischemia and the protective effect of alpha-tocopherol administration. Stroke 14, 977.

Yamasaki Y, Kogure K, Hara H, Ban H, Akaike N (1991) The possible involvement of tetrodotoxin-sensitive ion channels in ischemic neuronal damage in the rat hippocampus. Neurosci Lett 121, 251.

Yamori Y, Ooshima A, Okamoto K (1973) Metabolism of adrenal corticosteroids in spontaneously hypertensive rats. Jpn Heart J 14, 162.

Yanagihara T (1976) Cerebral anoxia: effect on neuron-glia fractions and polysomal protein synthesis. J Neurochem 27, 539.

Yanagihara T, McCall J (1982) Ionic shifts in cerebral ischemia. Life Sci 30, 1921.

Yang G, Matocha M, Rapoport S (1988) Localization of glucocorticoid receptor mRNA in hippocampus of rat brain using in situ hybridization. Mol Endocrinol 2, 682.

Yankner B, Dawes L, Fisher S, Villa-Komaroff L, Oster-Granite M, Neve R (1989) Neurotoxicity of a fragment of the amyloid precursor associated with Alzheimer's disease. Science 245, 417.

Yankner B, Duffy L, Kirschner D (1990) Neurotrophic and neurotoxic effects of amyloid beta protein: reversal by tachykinin neuropeptides. Science 250, 279.

Yasuda N, Takabe K, Greer M (1976) Evidence of nycterohemeral periodicity in stress-induced pituitary-adrenal activation. Neuroendocrinology 21, 214.

Yates F (1981) Analysis of endocrine signals: the engineering and physics of biochemical communication systems. Biol Reprod 24, 73.

Yates F, Maran J (1974) Stimulation and inhibition of adrenocorticotropin release. In Greep R, Astwood E, Knobil E, Sawyer W, Geiger S (eds), Handbook of Physiology Section 7; Endocrinology, Vol 4: The Pituitary Gland and Its Neuroendocrine Control, part 2. Williams and Wilkins, Baltimore, p 367.

Yates F, Brennan R, Urquhart J (1969) Adrenal glucocorticoid control system. Fed Proc 28, 71.

Yates F, Russell S, Dallman M, Hedge G, McCann S, Dhariwal A (1971) Potentiation by vasopressin of corticotropin release induced by CRF. Endocrinology 88, 3.

Yatsu F (1983) Pharmacologic protection against ischemic brain damage. Neurol Clin 1, 37.

Yehuda R, Fairman K, Meyer J (1985) Early adrenalectomy promotes brain cell proliferation in rats. Soc Neurosci Abstr 11, 899.

Yi-Li Y, Jin-Xing T, Ren-Bao S (1989) Down-regulation of glucocorticoid receptor and its relationship to the induction of rat liver tyrosine aminotransferase. J Steroid Biochem 32, 99.

Yoneda K, Okada Y (1989) Effects of anoxia and recovery on the neurotransmission and level of high-energy phosphates in thin hippocampal slices from the guinea-pig. Neuroscience 28, 401.

Yoon K, Rothman S (1991) Adenosine inhibits excitatory but not inhibitory synaptic transmission in the hippocampus. J Neurosci 11, 1375.

Yoshida S, Inoh s, Asano T, Sano K, Kubota M, Shimazaki H, Ueta N (1980) Effect of transient ischemia on free fatty acids and phospholipids in the gerbil brain. Lipid peroxidation as possible cause of postischemic injury. J Neurosurg 53, 323.

Young A, Greenamyre J, Hollingsworth Z (1988) NMDA receptor losses in putamen from patients with Huntington's disease. Science 241, 981.

Young E, Akana S, Dallman M (1990a) Decreased sensitivity to glucocorticoid fast feedback in chronically stressed rats. Neuroendocrinology 51, 536.

Young E, Spencer R, McEwen B (1990b) Changes at multiple levels of the hypothalamo-pituitary-adrenal axis following repeated electrically induced seizures. Psychoneuroendocrinology 15, 165.

Young E, Haskett R, Murphy-Weinberg V, Watson S, Akil H (1991) Loss of glucocorticoid fast feedback in depression. Arch Gen Psychiatry 48, 693.

Young J (1986) Purifaction and characterization of a cytolytic pore-forming protein from granules of cloned lymphocytes with natural killer activity. Cell 44, 849.

Young J, Cohn Z (1986) Cell-mediated killing: a common mechanism? Cell 46, 641.

Young J, Peterson C, Venge P, Cohn Z (1986) Mechanism of membrane damage mediated by human eosinophil cationic protein. Nature 321, 613.

Young W, Flamm E (1982) Effect of high-dose corticosteroid therapy on blood flow, evoked potentials, and extracellular calcium in experimental spinal injury. J Neurosurg 57, 667.

Young W, Mezey E, Siegel R (1986) Quantitative in situ hybridization histochemistry reveals increased levels of corticotropin releasing factor mRNA after adrenalectomy in rats. Neurosci Lett 70, 198.

Yu A, Chan P (1988) Synergistic effects of arachidonic acid and glutamate on the injury of astrocytes in culture. Soc Neurosci Abstr 14, 205.2.

Yu Z, Wrange O, Boethius J, Gustafsson J, Granholm L (1981) A qualitative comparison of the glucocorticoid receptor in cytosol from human brain and rat brain. Brain Res 223, 325.

Zeelan F (1990) Determination of the affinity of a steroid for its receptor is not sufficient to measure its intrinsic hormonal activity. Steroids 55, 325.

Zgombick J, Erwin G (1988) Ethanol differentially enhances adrenocortical response in LS and SS mice. Alcohol 5, 287.

Zimmerman M, Coryell W (1987) The dexamethasone suppresion test in healthy controls. Psychoneuroendocrinology 12, 245.

Zimmermann E, Critchlow V (1967) Effects of diurnal variation in plasma corticosterone levels on adrenocortical resposne to stress. Proc Soc Exp Biol Med 125, 658.

Zimmermann E, Critchlow V (1969) Suppression of pituitary-adrenal function with plasma levels of corticosterone. Neuroendocrinology 5, 183.

Ziylan Y, Lefauconnier J, Bernard G, Bourre J (1989) Regional alterations in blood-to-brain transfer of alpha-aminoisobutyric acid and sucrose, after chronic administration and withdrawal of dexamethasone. J Neurochem 52, 684.

Zoli M, Ferraguti F, Gustafsson J, Toffano G, Fuxe K, Agnati L (1991a) Selective reduction of glucocorticoid receptor immunoreactivity in the hippocampal formation and central amygdaloid nucleus of the aged rat. Brain Res 545, 199.

Zoli M, Ferraguti F, Biagini G, Cintra AN, Fuxe K, Agnati L (1991b) Corticosterone treatment counteracts lesions induced by neonatal treatment with monosodium glutamate in the mediobasal hypothalamus of the male rat. Neurosci Lett 132, 225.

Index